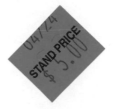

From Boys to Men

A Woman's Guide to the Health of
Husbands, Partners, Sons, Fathers, and Brothers

EMILY SENAY, M.D.,
and
ROB WATERS

SCRIBNER
NEW YORK LONDON TORONTO SYDNEY

SCRIBNER
1230 Avenue of the Americas
New York, NY 10020

SCRIBNER and design are trademarks of
Macmillan Library Reference USA, Inc., used under license
by Simon & Schuster, the publisher of this work.

For information about special discounts for bulk purchases,
please contact Simon & Schuster Special Sales:
1-800-456-6798 or business@simonandschuster.com

Designed by Kyoko Watanabe

Text set in Minion

Manufactured in the United States of America

1   3   5   7   9   10   8   6   4   2

Library of Congress Cataloging-in-Publication Data is available.

ISBN 0-7432-2594-5

Names that appear in the text with an asterisk (*) have been changed by the author.
Websites are subject to change. Websites listed in the text were the most current at the time of printing.

For our families
Emily's: Avery, Harry, Ruby, and Lucy
and Rob's: Maury and Elly, George and Judy, Lenore, and especially Josh

Contents

Foreword by Eli H. Newberger, M.D.   *ix*

Introduction   1

Overview: Being a Man May Be Dangerous to Your Health   7

PART ONE: SONS

1: It's a Boy! (But First It's a Girl)   21

2: Snips and Snails   75

3: Boys and Accidents and Injuries   108

4: Boys and Body Control   121

5: The Care and Feeding of Boys   133

6: When Things Go Wrong   140

7: *Sturm und Drang*? The Teen Years   179

8: Boys and Sex   210

9: Boys and Sports   235

PART TWO: HUSBANDS, PARTNERS, LOVERS

10: Husbands, Partners, Lovers   259

11: An Ounce—or Two—of Prevention   285

12: Bad Habits   347

13: Dealing with Emergencies   358

14: "Houston, We've Had a Problem"   368

15: The Usual Suspects — 393

16: Alcoholism: The Hidden Epidemic — 441

17: Cancer — 452

18: Male Trouble: A Gland That Doesn't Always Behave — 472

19: The Emotional Male — 494

20: Tossin', Turnin', Cuttin' Zs — 516

21: Boomeritis — 520

22: Men and Sex — 523

23: Narcissus—What a Guy! — 545

Afterword — 549

Resources for Part One: Sons — 551

Resources for Part Two: Husbands, Partners, Lovers — 573

Selected Bibliography — 593

Acknowledgments — 599

Subject Index — 601

Symptoms Index — 621

Foreword

We males are curious creatures. From infancy, we are preoccupied with locating ourselves in the pecking order. Our rough and tumble play, risk-taking, and passionate pursuit of winning the game of life set us up for injury, rejection, and isolation. The poet Anaïs Nïn asked in "The Four-Chambered Heart," "Why do men live on shoals?" As we grow up, our struggle to find and define ourselves pitches us in and out of jobs, relationships, and marriages. It's hard for us to stay the course; far more of those fathers in the elevator on the way to my sixth floor pediatric clinic seek divorce, for example, than fathers of children in good health. We men live shorter lives, not least because we don't take care of ourselves. With reason, it is said that few of us really ever grow up.

This book by Emily Senay and Rob Waters gave me new insight and reframed my doctor's worldview in a way that I've rarely experienced in my thirty-eight-year career. Dr. Senay discovered, from her unique perspective as a discerning connoisseur of medical science, as well as daughter, spouse, and mother, that not only do most men remain boys at heart, but that the keys to their health and survival are often held by women.

The publication of this book represents a remarkable and significant event, both for women and for men. Never before has there been presented in one volume a compendium of information that turns on its head all previous notions of where the real power resides, and who conducts the most important interventions to advance the health of boys and men. And it's not that we men can't take care of ourselves. We should, but we mostly don't—although I think that if every man and every physician read this book, that would change. It's that women appear to have far greater capacity and interest, not to say the commitment and courage, to care for us and attend to what's important in sustaining us from infancy to old age.

Acknowledging this, and celebrating it, should elevate our respect and esteem for what our mothers and partners do for us. One important way to do this would be to take better care of ourselves—and to better appreciate their vital role in our lives. Dr. Senay and Waters's remarkable insight requires the tools with which to guide and support their life-saving and life-enhancing work. She has provided here exactly this tool kit to all who would use it. All of us can, and should.

Perhaps because of her career as a health journalist for a leading television network, but also because of the deeply embedded sense of responsibility that flows from these pages, Dr. Senay selects the important issues unerringly. She is on target about which prevention activities are essential, those symptoms that require urgent attention, and whom we can turn to for specialized care at every age, in every organ system, and from every medical specialty vantage point. If there was truth in the proclamation on the cover of my mother's favorite cookbook that the way to a man's heart is through his stomach, now it can be said that the way to a man's health is through a woman reading this book.

This is a work of stunning breadth and depth that can and should be read from cover to cover, but will also save lives and sustain loving relationships, as specific male symptoms and illnesses inevitably rear their heads. I stand in admiration of what Emily Senay and Rob Waters have accomplished in writing it and do not doubt it will assume its deserved place among the few classics in medicine that can be appreciated and enjoyed by everyone.

Well, by at least half of us.

Eli H. Newberger, M.D.,
Department of Pediatrics, Harvard Medical School,
author of *The Men They Will Become:*
The Nature and Nurture of Male Character

Introduction

Men are the weaker sex. I don't say this to be glib; I say it because it's a fact. I know what you're probably thinking. Men are stronger. They have bigger muscles. They have more power. And they make more money, too. You're right about all that, of course. But it's not really that simple. The truth is that at every age and stage of life, the male of our species is less healthy and more vulnerable than females. They begin life as more fragile beings, then compound it with an attraction to risk, an aversion to self-care, and an arsenal of unhealthy habits. Consider:

- For every 100 females, 120 males are conceived, but the males are far less likely to survive. By the time of birth, that ratio has changed: 105 boys are born for every 100 girls.

- Boys are more likely than girls to die from nearly every cause imaginable, from sudden infant death syndrome (SIDS) to drowning, from suffocation to car accidents. They're more likely to be injured in falls, and even to be bitten by dogs!

- Teenage boys are three times as likely as girls to die of any cause. They're twice as likely to be killed in a crash, and nearly five times as likely to be murdered or to take their own lives. And although it's uncommon, teenage boys are also more likely to die from cancer, heart disease, birth defects, asthma, and flu.

- In young adulthood—through the twenties and thirties—this mortality gap grows, so that men now die at nearly four times the rate of women. As a result, women begin to outnumber men for the first time at age thirty-six. Men are almost three times as likely to die in a car crash, almost five times as likely to commit suicide, and four times as likely to be murdered. They're also more likely to die of heart disease, AIDS (acquired immune deficiency syndrome), diabetes, and liver disease (thanks to their much higher rates of alcohol consumption). They're even three times more likely to be poisoned. Young women die more often from only one cause—cancer—but men will soon catch up.

- At age forty-two, heart disease becomes the leading killer of men. Overall, men have twice as many heart attacks as women and are nearly twice as likely to die from heart disease. And from the age of fifty on, men are more likely to die of cancer as well, along with every other leading cause of death.

- Men are more likely to be killed on the job. Between 1980 and 1997, nearly 104,000 American workers were killed at work and more than 90 percent were men. That's because men do the most hazardous jobs, making up over 98 percent of firefighters, coal miners, loggers, and truck drivers.

- These problems are compounded by men's lack of attention to their own health care. Recent surveys show that one man in three has no regular doctor to go to. And one third of men say they would not go to a doctor even if they were experiencing severe chest pains or shortness of breath—two of the most common signs of a heart attack.

- The end result is a glaring longevity gap. Men die, on average, about five and a half years younger than women. Among people over eighty-five, there are only thirty-nine men to every one hundred women. By age one hundred, there is only one man for every five women.

But what does this have to do with us—women? Why should we care—and what should we do—about men's health? On a political or societal level, these are thorny questions, but on a personal level, the answers are obvious: We care about the health of males because we are married to them, we are raising them, we have brothers and fathers, and we love them. And we want them to live long, healthy lives.

We know that as women, we do a lot to make that happen. We take our boys to the pediatrician and stay up with them when they're sick. We make sure our husbands and boyfriends go to the doctor; we remind them to take their medications. We try to make sure that everyone eats right. In doing all this, we take on a role we never really asked for—medical manager for our family. We do it because we love them. Indeed, we love them, in part, for many of the same characteristics that make it hard for them to admit illness or look after themselves—their strength, their physicality, their maleness. We do it because we're observant and often see them struggling with a problem long before they admit it to themselves or anyone else. And we do it because their health affects us—our physical and mental health, our strength, the very quality of our lives.

For the most part, we're happy to do these things, yet it's hard not to be exasperated sometimes by the lack of attention our men give to their health and their bodies. We want them to be healthy, *and* we want them to change. We want them to become more aware and more responsible about their health. And most of all, we want our sons and grandsons to grow up with a different attitude toward health care.

I haven't always thought much about this. But in recent years, changes in my own life have led me to reflect on these issues. Let me tell you a bit about my own story.

I am a physician and the medical and health correspondent for a major network morning news show. I came to CBS News in 1995 to cover women's health, the hot new topic in medical news. Newspapers and networks began to cover this beat, launching columns and segments, working to hook the female audience.

Women's health was finally getting the attention it deserved. After years of lobbying by women's health advocates, the government and the research community were finally listening. Large medical studies of women were under way, and researchers were finally looking at the important physiological differences between men and women. I didn't cover men's health back then and didn't think a whole lot about it.

Then a few things changed. The first was the birth of my son Harry. I grew up with three sisters and no brothers. When I discovered that my baby would be a boy, I realized that I didn't know the first thing about them. Oh sure, I'd known boys as a child, had plenty of male friends, and, after all, married one. Still, I was seized with panic at the prospect of actually raising a baby boy. I was caught off guard about basic decisions, such as what to do about circumcision. And I was unprepared for Harry's amazing level of activity.

From early on, Harry was "all boy," and by the time he was fifteen months old, my husband and I had a saying: "No mere mortal can contain him." We had an adorable, squeezable, delicious little alpha male on our hands, one who seemed never to stop moving. I collapsed exhausted at the end of each day, while he rarely slept through the night.

When it came time to look for preschools, we started to hear about differences between boys and girls: that boys are behind, boys are more trouble, boys are a special challenge. This was usually accompanied by a sigh or a knowing shake of the head. The "boy thing" was going to be a challenge, and I realized I wanted to learn more about them.

The second event was more troubling. One afternoon my husband, Avery, called me at work complaining of a sharp pain in his upper back. Even though I told him that these were symptoms of a possible heart attack, I still had to convince him to go with me to the emergency room. Frankly, I had been waiting for this call. My husband is outwardly the picture of health. But as a physician I knew he was cheating the devil. High blood pressure, high cholesterol, prediabetes, and the diet of a teenage boy—all were at work inside his arteries, waiting, just waiting.

Things turned out okay that day. Tests showed he did not have a heart attack. That was the good news. The bad news: Tests showed definitively he had diabetes, with very high cholesterol and high blood pressure. The doctor told him point-blank that if he wanted to prevent catastrophe, he needed to take immediate action.

He didn't. So I did. I scheduled the follow-up appointments and made sure he went. I sat in on examinations so Avery couldn't play down his health problems as he always did. I didn't do this because I'm a physician. As any woman reading this will already know, I did it because I'm a woman, and this is what women do. We take charge of health matters, we become "Dr. Mom."

In dealing with these issues, Avery was jocular, breezy, his usual self. I was perplexed and sometimes infuriated by his lack of alarm. I could not understand why he didn't do everything in his power to prevent a disaster—read: massive heart attack. He was an Ivy League–educated lawyer who was acting like a boy.

It gnawed at me that he didn't take the whole thing more seriously. Eating a donut, he would swagger and laugh, practically taunting his body to betray him. "What are you doing?" I would screech. But then I would rationalize: "I'm overreacting. I worry too much because I'm a physician. If he were really in trouble, he would take care of himself." I did not want to be smothering or hysterical.

When I did try to start a serious discussion about his health, our conversations were, shall we say, oblique. I'd say something and get an evil look in response, a quick denial, or a long-winded rationalization. He refused to examine what was going on, and I could not break his denial. To avoid a fight I would shrug and concede, "Okay, you're probably fine."

We were getting nowhere. I love my husband and did not want to see him become ill. Plus, we had a growing family. If anything happened to him, it would devastate his son and daughters.

Around the same time, I received a letter from a viewer, a woman who wanted to know more about a prostate cancer story we had covered. By this time, I was covering general medical news on the morning show. Why, I thought, doesn't her husband ask these questions for himself? That's when it hit me: *Because that's not what men do!*

Most men do not take care of their bodies the way women do. They don't seek out health information, lay themselves bare to doctors, or recognize when they are on the brink of medical disaster until it's too late. But their mothers, partners, wives, sisters, and daughters do.

Reading this woman's letter, her love and concern came through in every line. I also realized that viewer letters and e-mails came mostly from women, even when the topic was men. I was not the only woman who was functioning as health advocate for the men in the family.

As I asked my women friends and coworkers about the roles they played in the health of their sons, partners, and fathers, things became clearer. Women were intimately involved in many aspects of boys' and men's health. The stories they told were funny, and sometimes sad.

One woman told me her husband refused to seek help though he was seriously depressed. A young mother wanted to know if her son was headed for trouble, because he insisted on sitting, rather than standing up to pee. Another friend, a single mom, was shocked to find pornography on her twelve-year-old son's computer. One woman told me her husband refused urgent coronary bypass surgery until after an important business meeting. Another friend's father is dying of colon cancer because, she believes, he ignored symptoms and refused to get checked.

These problems play out everywhere you look. During the war in Iraq, NBC News correspondent David Bloom did a brilliant and courageous job of covering the war live as it happened. But his cramped post in an armored vehicle was causing him pain in his legs. He complained to medics and consulted doctors by phone; they all advised him to seek medical attention. But he refused to leave the battlefield and died when a blood clot traveled to his lung. How terribly sad. For me, his death raises the question: If Bloom were a woman, would he have listened to those medics? Would he possibly be alive today?

No one, of course, can answer those questions with certainty. Yet it is clear that on matters of health, the gender divide operates as strongly as ever. Men do things that most women wouldn't, and they fail to do things that, for women, are routine. Scott Hensley covers health and medicine for *The Wall Street Journal* so he should, as he says, "know better." A couple of years ago, he got his cholesterol checked—"practically against my will"—by a nurse at a clinic he was writing about.

"My blood sugar was fine, but my total cholesterol and LDL [bad cholesterol] were through the roof," Hensley recalls. "Did I go to the doctor? Nope. Do I even have a primary-care doctor? Nope. Didn't then and still don't. Pathetic. For the past ten years, my trips to the doctor have been prompted by acute problems I couldn't ignore—broken bones and accidents pretty much."

Men don't act this way because they are dolts or because they have a deep-seated death wish. They don't act this way because they want to burden us with undue worry about their health. They act this way because eons of evolution and centuries of cultural conditioning make it difficult for them to act otherwise. The risks they take, their visceral fear of appearing vulnerable, their preference for "gutting it out"—all are so deeply ingrained that they're almost second nature. It's what makes them men.

As I thought about these attitudes and the issues in my own family, the idea for this book was born. I wanted to get to the bottom of what was going on in men's health, if for no other reason than to understand my own son and husband.

To get my arms around the topic was going to be a huge undertaking and one I could not do alone. So I roped my old friend Rob Waters into helping me out. As former editor of the "Men's Health" section of *Web*MD, a former writer for *Health* magazine, and a contributing editor to *Psychotherapy Networker* magazine, Rob immediately understood what I was trying to do. He's researched and written a lot about mental health and the psychological aspects of health. He's also a man, of course, and readily admits to falling into many of the attitudes and habits that are so typical of his sex. And perhaps most important, he too has a young son.

We spent a year doing research, identifying the major issues in the health of boys and men. We interviewed experts in each area, more than one hundred fifty in all. We asked medical societies, academies, and institutions to identify leading thinkers. And then we consulted more experts to hone our findings and make sure we provided the most cutting-edge and accurate information available. Each chapter has been read and vetted by experts in that field.

The result is a book that does three things: It outlines the conditions, illnesses, and health habits that are more common to males, offering tips for prevention and treatment. It looks at the biological, cultural, and psychological reasons behind men's health-related attitudes and practices. And it suggests ways that women can work with their sons, husbands, fathers, or any man they want to help to be healthier.

We've organized the book to follow the arc of the relationships with the men in your life: as the mother of a boy, the wife of a still-healthy man, and the partner of a man with health problems. We explain everything from circumcision to heart disease, and offer suggestions on what you can do if you think the man in your life eats the wrong foods or drinks too much alcohol. We weave in firsthand accounts to illustrate what happens between mothers and sons and husbands and wives. We avoid going through the usual litany of symptoms and tests, followed by treatments, but we suggest many excellent books and websites where you can find that sort of information and more. Always check our resource section for additional information. We offer concrete advice and information that helps you understand what's going on physically, developmentally, and emotionally with the men. We point out the areas of major risk to their health and tell how you can help. And we offer suggestions on how you can share your knowledge with your husband, along with some ideas about ways you can motivate him to take better care of himself and be a better health role model for your sons.

So this is a book about men's health issues—for women. Many women, including some thoughtful feminist thinkers, believe that we should not have to take care of men's health, that men should bear this responsibility themselves. On one level, I agree. We ought not to have this job. It should be enough that we take care of ourselves and our children without having to be responsible for our men's medical care as well. But the reality is that we often are. Clearly, this needs to change. Men need to feel that taking care of themselves is not a mark against their masculinity. But until this happens, we are not about to abandon the men and boys we love. Why should we? How could we?

That said, let me be clear about what this book isn't. It isn't about how to be your husband's, or lover's, or even your son's caretaker. The goal is not to make men more dependent. Rather, our goal is to arm you with information and to help you educate the boys and men in your life so that they can take care of themselves.

We hope you do enjoy this book and we offer one suggestion: After you read it, leave it around someplace obvious. Maybe he'll read it, too.

Overview:
Being a Man May Be
Dangerous to Your Health

Six years ago, after an arduous delivery, I held my newborn son Harry in my arms for the very first time. After hours of labor and a C-section, I was a total wreck. But not Harry. On that day, in the first moments of his life on Earth, he felt to me just the way I always figured a little boy would feel: full of strong, masculine energy. So confident, so sturdy, so solid. I suspect that a lot of people think as I did, that baby boys are somehow hardier and more durable than baby girls. After all, they grow up to be big, strong men. Doesn't it make sense that they should be that way from the start?

In fact, nothing could be further from the truth. Harry, I realize now, was actually lucky. Like all little boys, he started life in the womb at a distinct biological disadvantage—a disadvantage, it seems, that men face for the rest of their lives.

Here is the reality: From the moment they're conceived, males are more likely to experience a host of problems that females do not. They're more prone to birth defects, more likely to be stricken by injury or disease, and more likely to die prematurely than are women.

Actually, things start happily enough for Harry and his buddies. In fact, for one brief shining moment, they actually have a biological advantage over girls: About one hundred twenty baby boys are conceived for every one hundred baby girls. "From this point on," writes researcher Sebastian Kraemer, "it is downhill all the way."

Indeed, this fleeting numerical superiority may be nature's way of compensating for the fact that boys are more likely to be miscarried, to suffer from all sorts of medical and developmental problems, and to die in infancy and boyhood. Kraemer, a child and adolescent psychiatrist in London, recently presented the growing body of evidence about the vulnerability of males in a paper entitled "The Fragile Male," published by the *British Medical Journal*.

"The male fetus is at greater risk of death or damage from almost all of the obstetric catastrophes that can happen before birth," he writes. These include genetic abnormalities, cerebral palsy, perinatal brain damage, premature birth, and stillbirth. The result is that by the time of birth, the male advantage in numbers has dropped dramatically—to a ratio of about one hundred five boys to one hundred girls.

This pattern continues after birth and for the rest of men's lives. At every age and stage—boyhood, adolescence, adulthood, and old age—males are more likely than females to die. Indeed, for every one of the top ten causes of death in this country, from heart disease to alcoholism, from cancer to suicide, men die at greater rates than women.

LONGEVITY GAP, RACIAL DIVIDE

What all this adds up to is a pronounced difference in life expectancy between men and women, what some researchers call the "longevity gap." It's a gap that has widened over the past century.

In 1920, the life expectancy of American men and women was virtually the same: on average, 54 years. But throughout the twentieth century, life expectancy increased dramatically, especially for women. Today, women outlive men by an average of 5.5 years, with the average American man living to almost 74 and the average women to 79.5.

For African-American men, this picture is even more grave. With a life expectancy of 68, they die, on average, twelve years earlier than white women and six years earlier than white men. Part of the reason—and one that's gotten a great deal of attention—is the fact that so many black men die in their teens and twenties from violence and diseases such as AIDS. But millions of African-American men die in middle age from the same diseases that kill white Americans years later.

According to the American Heart Association, nearly 37 percent of African-American men have high blood pressure, nearly double the rate of white women, and among the highest rates in the world. African-Americans develop high blood pressure at earlier ages and die from it and related diseases at much greater rates. Compared to whites, African-Americans are twice as likely to die of heart disease, two to three times as likely to die from stroke, and four times as likely to develop end-stage kidney disease.

There are a number of factors for these glaring disparities, but one of the biggest is that many blacks have no health insurance or regular access to health care. In 1999, for instance, 23 percent of African-Americans were uninsured—compared to 13 percent of whites—and 39 percent of African-Americans didn't have a regular doctor, according to the American Medical Association. These days, thanks to the faltering economy, those numbers are probably worse.

Continuing racial discrimination also looms large. A recent report from the Institute of Medicine found "overwhelming" evidence of racial disparities in heath care that contribute to higher death rates for minorities. The report found that minorities are far less likely to be given appropriate heart medication, undergo bypass surgery, or receive proper treatment for kidney disease. They're also less likely to get the latest treatments for cancer and AIDS. And even when they have health insurance, minorities are more likely to be enrolled in lower-end plans that provide limited coverage and access to specialists.

Cultural and historical forces also play a role. Men in our culture have a tendency to deny their pain and refrain from seeking help, and for black men, many observers note, this trait is even more pronounced. Jean Bonhomme, M.D., president of the National Black Men's Health Network, calls this trait pathological stoicism. "African-American men have had to deal with tremendous hardships and not complain, because complaining didn't help," Dr. Bonhomme says. "Now we push ourselves to distorted extremes without asking for help in order to 'be a man.' It is a matter of pride to brush off pain."

In a recent conversation, Dr. Bonhomme described an incident that is typical of many men. "Several years ago, I injured my back so badly I could hardly walk. Although I was in considerable discomfort, I went in to work that day. My wife, who was employed in the same workplace, saw me drop to my knees in order to get out of a chair and said to me, 'What the hell are you doing?' I looked at myself and realized how crazy I was being. All I could think of earlier that morning was the patients I had to see, the charts I had to write. Men's traditional reluctance to slow down or see doctors even when obviously exhausted, ill, or injured understandably perplexes women. I came to realize that as men, we have been taught since childhood to downplay the signals of our own bodies. This kind of traditional male upbringing leads to attitudes that block health-conscious behavior and participation in health care among adults."

MEN'S HEALTH CRISIS

If you want to see the longevity gap in action, just visit any nursing home and you'll see at least twice as many women as men. And members of that exclusive club called centenarians—people who live to one hundred years old—are almost all women, with a ratio of four to one, according to the 2000 U.S. Census.

When you really think about it, what's going on here is nothing less than a major health crisis for men. Men are dying years earlier than they should, yet the problem receives little attention. I can't help thinking sometimes that if women were dying five or six years earlier than men, they'd be marching on Washington, demanding money for research and health programs. But most men are not up in arms about this. My guess is they're barely aware it's happening. Nor, for the most part, are they changing their behavior in the ways that would bring them longer life.

So why are men dying so much younger than women, and what can be done about it?

A FAMILY'S TRAGEDY

For one solid month in 2001, Gary Small complained to his wife, Georgeanne, that he was suffering from headaches and feeling run-down and fatigued. Gary thought it was his allergies and the fact he was working so many hours at his job as a gold electroplator at IBM. "We knew he was more tired than normal," recalls his wife Georgeanne, "but neither of us thought it was anything serious." Gary didn't seek medical attention, and in fact, had not seen a doctor in at least two years.

On April 25, 2001, Gary came home at seven in the morning after working the night shift. He passed his wife as she was leaving for work and stopped to talk with his son, Travis, who was waiting for the school bus. He told Travis, then thirteen, that he had an upset stomach and was going to rest but promised to pick him up that afternoon after Spanish class. He prepared his daughter's breakfast and got her ready for school but told her she would have to walk to the bus stop by herself because he wasn't feeling well. As she was leaving, she thought she heard him getting sick in the bathroom.

Later that afternoon, Georgeanne got a call from her son. His father had not picked him up after school as promised. She called home and talked to her daughter Heather, eleven, who told her mother "Daddy wasn't feeling too well that morning." She went to his room and tried to wake him up by jumping on the bed. But he didn't stir.

Georgeanne rushed home and found her husband dead on the bed. An autopsy revealed that he had suffered a massive heart attack.

Gary's death was a heartbreaking loss for Georgeanne and her children made all the more tragic because it was likely preventable. Had Gary Small paid attention to his body's signals and seen a doctor, there's a good chance he would be alive today. Instead, Georgeanne lost her lover and companion of fourteen years and her coparent, whose income helped support the family. Georgeanne must now care for their two children and hold the family together by herself.

OUT OF TOUCH

In 2000, a highly respected health research organization, the Commonwealth Fund, published a report on an important but little-studied issue: how men look after their health. The title of the report says a lot about what these researchers found: *Out of Touch: American Men and the Health Care System.*

For the report, the researchers surveyed fifteen hundred men about their health habits. They began their report by noting "an alarming proportion of American men have only limited contact with physicians and the health care system generally. Many men fail to get routine checkups, preventive care, or health counseling, and they often ignore symptoms or delay seeking medical attention when sick or in pain."

Specifically, they discovered:

- One man in three had no regular doctor to go to.

- One in four had not seen a doctor even once in the year before the survey.

- One third of the men over age fifty had not been screened for prostate cancer or colon cancer in the past five years, even though many experts recommend that men in that age group be screened every few years for both these cancers.

- One fourth of men said they would wait as long as possible before seeing a doctor if they felt sick, were in pain, or were worried about their health. Seventeen percent said they would wait at least a week to see if they got better.

Other studies have made similar findings. In a 1999 survey by CNN and *Men's Health* magazine, one third of men said they would not go to a doctor even if they were experiencing severe chest pains or shortness of breath, symptoms of a heart attack. And one in five men wouldn't go if they were experiencing blurred vision. Talk about denial!

Men and women deal with doctors and health care very differently. As women, we begin early on to see doctors on a regular basis for birth control, Pap smears, and other gynecological needs. For most girls, this begins at puberty, when mothers sit down with their teenage daughters to talk about their first period and get them ready to see a doctor about it. For us, making regular visits to a doctor is normal, something you do even when you're not sick. But most men never develop this habit. They see a doctor as someone you go to only when you're sick—*really* sick.

Men have lots of other bad health habits as well: They're less likely to take the medicine they've been prescribed. They sleep less than women—six hours on average, compared to eight for women. And they're much less likely to seek mental health counseling, according to an article in the September 2000 issue of the *Journal of Men's Studies.*

You may be thinking, *Sure, we go to the doctor more because we have babies.* But that's not the whole story. In 2001, the Centers for Disease Control and Prevention (CDC) showed that even when you exclude visits for pregnancy, women see doctors about 33 percent more often than do men. And women are much more likely to go for preventive care visits and annual checkups. This gap narrows as men and women age, but by then many men have missed crucial opportunities to identify problems in the earliest stages, when they can be treated most easily.

The male tendency to avoid the doctor or dally about going to see one has far-reaching consequences. Delaying seeking attention for chest pain, for example, contributes to mortality from the disease, according to the American Heart Association. More often, though, the effects are subtler. A man puts off going to the dentist and ends up with a mouthful of cavities or a tooth that needs pulling. In this way, many men allow small, manageable problems to become larger, more serious ones. How did this happen? How did men become so out of touch? Some say this is the way they are by nature, that they're a product of their hormones and centuries of evolutionary conditioning. They say men are wired to be aggressive risk takers whose body chemistry programs them to seek quick gratification and physical release. They point out that male and female brains have key structural differences, differences that begin in the womb when the developing male brain is bathed in the hormone testosterone. Add to that the centuries of conditioning that have shaped men's responses, and you end up with a creature wired to be alert to immediate dangers—like the sudden charge of a mastodon—but not built to pay much attention to more subtle, internal, or distant cues.

I believe that testosterone gets blamed far too often for male impulsiveness and aggression. Obviously, testosterone affects the behavior of boys and men, as does the evolutionary conditioning that has left males quick to jump to alert, more ready to launch into a fight-or-flight mode. But boys and men are more than the sum of their hormones, and testosterone is just one of many factors that shape male personality.

The bigger part of the answer to the question "Why are men out of touch with their health?" is that boys spend their earliest years absorbing powerful lessons about what it means to be a man in this culture. From a very young age, boys get the message they shouldn't cry or complain, that they should tough out pain and hardship. Harvard psychologist William Pollock, Ph.D., calls these counterproductive messages the "Boy Code" and notes in his best-selling book, *Real Boys: Rescuing Our Sons from the Myths of Boyhood,* that boys pick them up early on.

"Even very young boys reported that they felt they must 'keep a stiff upper lip,' 'not show their feelings,' 'act real tough,' 'not act too nice,' 'be cool,' and 'just laugh and brush it off when someone punches you,'" Dr. Pollock writes.

By the time they're teens, these messages are strongly ingrained: The "Boy Code" rules. When researchers interviewed fifteen-to-nineteen-year-old boys for the National Survey of Adolescent Males several years ago, they found that large numbers believed the notion that men must constantly prove their manhood by showing how strong and stoic they are. Here are some of the notions they subscribe to about what it means to be a man:

- A man will lose respect if he talks about his problems.
- A young man should be physically tough even if he's not big.
- It bothers me when a guy acts like a girl.

To make matters worse, the researchers also found the more boys bought into this image of manhood, the more likely they were to engage in all kinds of risky behavior, from drinking to having unprotected sex. In other words, adopting the "Boy Code" as a life philosophy leads to a double hit on the health of men and boys. First, boys are primed to ignore their bodies and their health problems for fear of being seen as "sissies." Then, these very same attitudes lead boys and teenagers to be risk takers, to engage in such potentially harmful behaviors as smoking, drinking, using illicit drugs, and driving recklessly.

These patterns continue into adulthood. Men drink and take drugs far more often than women. They're more likely to use steroids, work in dangerous jobs, and play sports where they might get injured. They're less likely to wear seat belts or bicycle helmets. They pay less attention to their diet and often eat poorly. They are three times more likely than women to drink and drive, according to the CDC. All this reminds me of the stories my father, a physician, told me about his days as a college football player. Rather than quit the game because of pain, a player would get an injection of painkiller and play on—to do anything less was unthinkable. This general recklessness is an accepted and even valued quality among men.

The Commonwealth Fund survey suggests that when men finally do get medical attention, the doctors themselves are often content to do exactly what many men probably want them to do: let them out the door as quickly as possible. Only one man in three over the age of forty reported that his doctor had ever asked about his family's medical history of prostate cancer, even though men with a family history of that disease have a greater chance of contracting it themselves.

Here's another example: Men who smoke cigarettes have a much higher risk for many problems, including heart disease. But when smokers see their doctors, do the physicians talk to them about the implications of their habits? Sadly, a lot of them don't.

Some physicians argue that there's no point in lecturing men about their bad health habits. "If we make them feel bad, they'll avoid us all the more," doctors say. It's true, most men don't want to hear finger-wagging lectures about their health. But there's a deeper problem. Many physicians subscribe to the belief that you can't get people to change so there's no point in trying.

In fact, there is growing evidence that fairly brief messages about health behavior can help people make important changes. A recent study from the National Heart, Lung and Blood Institute found that when sedentary patients—your basic couch potatoes—got just three hours of counseling from doctors and other health professionals over a two-year period, many started to exercise. Before the study, only 1 percent of them exercised regularly. After the study, 20 percent did. Bottom line: Doctors *can* have a positive influence on their patients' health habits. Maybe if most doctors did a little more nagging—in a humorous and friendly way, of course—we women wouldn't have to do quite as much.

DR. MOM

Remember this famous commercial? The members of a family are at home and in misery, sneezing and hacking away. The door swings open and in swoops Mom with a knit brow and a teaspoon of Robitussin cough syrup. The ending is always the same: Dad, kids, and finally Mom snuggle under blankets for a good night's rest. Then comes the tag line: "Recommended by doctors, pharmacists, and Dr. Mom."

At every stage of our sons' and partners' lives, women look out for their health. It starts with the kids. Mothers choose and deal with the pediatrician and take the children in for checkups and immunizations. We quiz them about how they feel and stay up with them when they're sick. It's not that husbands don't help; we need to give men credit. Most of today's dads are far more involved in caring for their kids than their fathers' generation. Still, in most families the responsibility for the health of the children falls squarely on the shoulders of Dr. Mom.

Long Island pediatrician Steven Kellner, M.D., says that mothers take the lead in dealing with their children's medical issues the vast majority of the time. If he reaches a father when he's returning phone calls to families, most will simply hand the phone over to their wife. "They'll tell me, 'Hold on a second, let me get my wife.' And you'd be surprised how often the father had no idea the mother even called."

Dr. Kellner observes that when children are born, fathers are very involved, coming with mother and baby for appointments. "But by the end of the first year, they're not coming. They fall off the wagon," Kellner says. It's not that these dads aren't involved in their children's lives, Kellner hastens to add. "They're very involved, but the way the roles are set up, the mother is the one who's taking care of the children's health."

There are, of course, some good reasons for this. Most mothers take some time off work after their children are born, while most husbands continue to work. Many families today consist of single mothers, who have no choice but to make all the family's health care decisions. And since most of today's parents were raised in families in which mothers looked after everyone's health, this kind of arrangement is familiar. So the pattern continues. And it doesn't just involve looking out for the health of kids.

In early 2001, the Bayer company commissioned a survey of some two thousand households about how they handled respiratory tract infections in the family. It turned out that women are nearly twice as likely to take care of a sick husband than men are to care for an ill wife.

"Score one for conventional wisdom," says Paul B. Iannini, M.D., a clinical professor of medicine at Yale University and scientific adviser for Bayer. "The research supports the stereotype of 'Dr. Mom' managing the health care needs for her family."

Here are a few other statistics that hint at the role women play as the medical leader of their family:

- Women make three quarters of the health care decisions for their families, according to the U.S. Department of Labor.
- Women do nearly 80 percent of the shopping in chain drugstores, according to a 2001 survey conducted by *Chain Drug Review,* a trade journal for the retail drug industry.
- Women buy most health books, and 76 percent of women use the Internet to search health-related sites, compared to 58 percent of males, according to Jupiter Consulting. Even men's health sites get a significant chunk of their hits from women.
- Women decide on their own about health insurance for their families about 40 percent of the time, more than twice as often as men do, according to the 1997 book *Marketing Health Care to Women,* by Patricia Braus.

When men do seek health information, their partner is often their primary source. A Weight Watchers survey in the early 1990s asked people about their preferred source of health and nutrition information. Women said they used physicians, health care providers, and books, while men said they used their wives. "Men are not going to go out and learn," says Karen Miller-Kovach, Weight Watchers' chief scientist. "They want to ask the wife."

The key role played by women in buying health products and making health decisions is well understood by drug companies, hospitals, and doctors, who increasingly aim their extensive marketing machines directly at women. That's what Robitussin's Dr. Mom commercials were all about.

Men benefit greatly from this medical mothering—and just from being with us. Marriage, it seems, is good for men's health. A number of studies have found that married men are healthier and live longer than unwed men. "Being unmarried can actually be a greater risk to one's life than having heart disease or cancer," claim marriage advocates Linda J. Waite and Maggie Gallagher in their book, *The Case for Marriage: Why Married People Are Happier, Healthier, and Better Off Financially.* "For example, having heart disease shortens the average man's life span by slightly less than six years. But being unmarried chops almost ten years off a man's life."

The book cites a study, coauthored by Waite, which followed some six thousand families over time, tracking their life changes and health status. It turned out that the men who stayed married lived a lot longer. Specifically, nine out of ten men who were married at age forty-eight were still alive at sixty-five, an age reached by only six out of ten men who were unmarried at forty-eight.

Waite and Gallagher, unabashed advocates of marriage, think divorce laws are too lax, and their book has drawn fire from many quarters, including feminist thinkers who believe that the benefits of marriage accrue chiefly to men. Whatever your feelings about marriage, the evidence that it protects men's health is compelling and comes from many sources. But it's hardly surprising, since being married to a woman gives most men their own personal health manager.

In the long run, however, this pattern is unhealthy—for men and women alike. Boys grow up watching Dad pay little attention to his health care or trying to tough out ailments when he's injured or sick. They learn not to talk about health problems with Dad because that's not what fathers—or men—do. So they go to the doctor with Mom and, when they're still young, discuss their health problems with her. In adolescence, they start acting more and more like their fathers, not paying much attention to medical matters and trying to ignore it when something hurts.

The result is that men of all ages learn to ignore their health, relying on mothers and wives to notice for them. Women find themselves saddled with the responsibility—and stress—of being Dr. Mom to their children, health nag to their husbands, and caregiver to their aging fathers. They may be caring for three generations of men at once.

Women have always been the caregivers in families—a role that doesn't get us much credit or reward, but one we perform anyway. But before you get the idea I'm resentful about this, let me tell you that I am proud of women's long history of being nurturing caregivers. Women like Florence Nightingale, who wrote the first book on nursing, and Clara Barton, the founder of the American Red Cross, have not only helped take care of sick and injured patients, they've also helped to bring about tremendous changes in medicine. It's fantastic that women such as Ali Torre, the wife of New York Yankees manager Joe Torre, have gotten so involved in men's health issues. After the Yankee skipper was diagnosed with prostate cancer, the couple helped create a program called Two Against One. Its goal was to reach women and men with the message that prostate cancer affects both partners and that the best way to fight it is with a team approach.

Betty Gallo takes it one step further. Since her husband, Congressman Dean Gallo of New Jersey, died from prostate cancer in 1994, she has become an advocate for men's health issues and for women's involvement in those issues. She is the cofounder of the National Prostate Cancer Coalition and a spokesperson for the Men's Health Network. Her goal is simple: "I don't want what happened to Dean to happen to anyone else."

CLOSING THE LONGEVITY GAP

Men pay a steep price for their failure to pay attention to their bodies. But so do we—their mothers, wives, daughters, and sisters. It affects our stress level, our peace of mind, and our health. When the men in our lives suffer, we do too.

Like it or not, women have a major stake in the health of men. So the question is: What can—and should—we do to help the men in our lives live longer and be healthier? This issue challenges us to walk a tightrope: We love the men in our lives and we want to help them stay healthy. But we also want them to learn to take better care of themselves—for their sakes, for our sakes, but especially for the sakes of our sons, who model so much of their behavior and attitudes on what Dad does. How do we help our husbands without letting them off the hook? And if we help them, aren't we just making them more dependent, enabling them *not* to care for themselves?

Some women argue that women should step back from their role as de facto home health aides, that we should stop being Dr. Mom—at least to our husbands. Barbara Risman, Ph.D., a professor of sociology at North Carolina State University, argues that in order to achieve greater equity between men and women, we must go through a major social reorganization in which women and men consciously move away from traditional roles. She calls this wrenching change and the dislocation it will cause "gender vertigo." As women, she says, we need to step back from our role as the nurturing caregiver so that men are forced to fill the vacuum.

While I agree with Dr. Risman's long-term goal of a more equitable social order, I disagree with her prescription for getting there, at least when it comes to our families' health. We can't stop looking out for the health of the boys and men in our lives for one overriding reason: We love them and want what's best for them. As frustrated as we are by their negligence, we want them to be healthy and to live long lives.

AN INTIMATE BOND

The health of men and women in a couple are intimately connected. Surprisingly, marriage seems to be good for our health, too. Married women live longer than their unmarried sisters: According to *The Case for Marriage,* nine of ten married women live to sixty-five, compared to eight of ten who are single or divorced. What's more, when a man's health is poor, his partner's health can suffer, too. Some surprising new research suggests that women whose husbands have heart attacks or undergo bypass surgery have a higher risk of developing the same problems. One reason is that many women share the same unhealthy diets and exercise habits of their spouses.

Plus, if men start getting sicker younger, who's going to take care of them? You know the answer to that one. We're not about to abandon our husbands when they're ill (though husbands often leave sick wives). The bottom line is that having unhealthy husbands makes our lives even more difficult.

Indeed, caring for an ill spouse is one of the most stressful of tasks. Two thirds of the women whose husbands were undergoing cardiac rehabilitation after a heart attack or heart surgery reported high levels of tension and stress, according to a 2000 study in the journal *Heart and Lung.* Many of the women said they had trouble falling asleep and were emotionally brittle. Caregivers also suffer from high rates of depression, and these feelings can last well beyond the death or recovery of a spouse.

All this means that we have plenty of reasons to help the men we love stay healthy

and to encourage them to change their habits for our own sakes. But while we're trying to get them to change their ways, we may want to look at the ways we sometimes
hold them back. It's sad but true that some women are so invested in their roles as the
family's domestic and medical managers that they resist their partners' efforts to take
on more responsibility. If we insist on always being the one to quiet a crying baby or
attend to a child's needs, we may end up discouraging the very behaviors we want to
see. Psychologists and sociologists call this "gatekeeping." Many women are not even
aware they are being gatekeepers, but their behavior builds walls between fathers and
children. Family change will require all of us to reflect, communicate, and act.

Fortunately, women are not alone in the effort to improve the health of men. There
is a growing awareness among male researchers and health advocates that American
men are far less healthy than they ought to be and that this can and ought to change.
In the early '90s, men's health activists started the Men's Health Network in Washington, D.C., to raise awareness about men's health issues. The group succeeded in getting
Congress to designate the week before Father's Day as Men's Health Week. The Network kicks off the week with free diabetes and cholesterol screenings for men who work
on Capitol Hill, from janitors to senators. Similar events are held nationwide.

The Network has also pushed for more funding for men's health problems and has
been working to establish an Office of Men's Health in the Department of Health and
Human Services—where an Office of Women's Health has existed for years.

These ideas are slowly catching on. A number of colleges and universities have men's
health clinics that offer health care and information to male students. Researchers in
the new field of gender-based medicine now devote much greater attention to the biological differences between men and women and how these differences affect responses
to medication, diagnostic tests, and treatments.

Other researchers like Tamara Sher, Ph.D., assistant professor of psychology at the
Illinois Institute of Technology, are looking closely at the role of social support in preventing illness and aiding recovery. Armed with a $2.4-million grant from the
National Institutes of Health, Dr. Sher is working with couples to see how communication and connection within a relationship strengthen health.

All this needs to be encouraged as do changes within families. More men than ever
are involved in child care. The number of hours men devote to household tasks is
slowly rising. But women are still much more likely than men to define themselves as
the caretakers of children, spouses, and parents.

In this age of managed health care, when people spend less time in the hospital
than ever before, women are being asked to take on more responsibility for the care of
ill family members. This caregiver role is unlikely to go away anytime soon. We will
continue to care for the men in our lives and for other family members. As long as
we're fulfilling these roles, we might as well do it smarter.

PART ONE

Sons

1

It's a Boy! (But First It's a Girl)

Six years ago, my coauthor, Rob Waters, attended the birth of his child. As the baby was emerging after a long night of labor, Rob let forth with that world-famous cry, "It's a girl!"—which he immediately amended (after a closer look) to "It's a boy!" In truth, all boys—or male embryos, anyway—actually do go through a sexual transformation, though it's quite a bit different from the one Rob seemed to describe. Let me explain.

The process of creating a human child begins when a man's semen—containing millions of sperm—is deposited inside the woman's vagina. Each of these sperm carries twenty-three chromosomes, as does the mother's egg. Chromosomes, found in the nucleus of every cell in our body, are tiny threadlike packages of genes and other DNA—the basic cellular blueprint for the person each embryo will become. Normally each cell of the body has forty-six chromosomes—twenty-three matched pairs, consisting of one from Mom and one from Dad.

Twenty-two of these chromosomes determine physical traits such as hair and eye color, or, say, the ability to curl the tongue. They also help shape other traits such as intelligence, personality, the ability to carry a tune or dribble a basketball. The twenty-third chromosome in the sperm is what determines the sex of the baby. That number 23 chromosome can be either an X chromosome—which will lead to a girl baby—or a Y chromosome—which will result in a boy.

The sex of the baby is determined by the father, because the mother can only contribute an X (female) chromosome while the father can deliver an X (female) or a Y (male). Pretty amazing when you think of all the pressure that queens, empresses, and czarinas have been under to bear their husbands a son. If only Henry VIII had understood this, poor Anne Boleyn might have kept her head! (Or maybe not.)

Once released by the man, sperm have some twelve to forty-eight hours to complete their mission before they die. They will cross the woman's cervix, swim through the uterus, and then into the Fallopian tubes. Most will die along the way, with only a few hundred completing the journey. Those plucky survivors then surround the egg and try to penetrate the membrane that surrounds it. Only one will succeed. Once it does, the membrane of the egg will swell, pushing away those other unlucky sperm. The nucleus of the victorious sperm will then seek the nucleus of the egg and the two will merge. The fertilized egg—now an embryo—will start to divide. Within four days, it will have about one hundred cells.

As it starts on the path of development, every embryo is essentially female. In other words, if nothing happens to alter events, its undeveloped genitals will become female. Thus, some researchers call females the "default sex." But the early embryo hedges its bets by being truly prepared for all possibilities. Amazingly, every embryo contains two sets of ducts: one that can turn into the vas deferens and seminal vesicles of a male and another that can turn into the Fallopian tubes and uterus of a female. If the embryo follows the male path, the male ducts will develop and the female ducts will fall away; if it becomes a female, the opposite will happen. And what decides all of this is the twenty-third chromosome carried on the man's sperm.

Time here for a brief word about that little Y chromosome. For decades, scientists looked upon the Y as the Rodney "I can't get no respect" Dangerfield of chromosomes, "an empty dance partner for the X chromosome" in the words of one scientist, whose sole role was determining the sex of the offspring. Just compare its gene count to that of the X. The Y possesses a few dozen genes, the X at least three thousand. To make matters worse, some new research suggests that the Y chromosome needs help from the X even on that most male of tasks—making sperm. Scientists have found that almost half of the genes connected to sperm production are found on the X.

Still, in recent years, the Y has gotten some respect as scientists, using new technology, have been able to map it and learn more about it. Experts now see the Y as critical and uniquely specialized. In addition to triggering maleness, it carries genes that focus on two other tasks: enhancing male fertility and helping cells carry out some other key chores, including building proteins.

But its most important job—turning on the boy-making machinery—is the one we've long known about. What we have found recently is that a single gene actually activates that process. Scientists have named that gene SRY for "sex-determining region Y." During the sixth or seventh week of gestation, it will switch on, starting a process that leads to the development of testes. Over the coming weeks, these tiny testes will produce and secrete that essence of maleness—the hormone testosterone—as well as other *androgens,* or male hormones. Throughout its life in the womb, the male fetus is literally bathed in testosterone, spurring its transformation from potential female into actual male.

At about nine weeks, this wave of testosterone triggers the genital tubercle, a small nodule on the surface of the groin area, to start lengthening. The genital swellings enlarge and by thirteen weeks, the *urethra*—the tube in the penis that carries urine and semen—is nearly complete. The last part of the penis to develop is the foreskin. Then at about twenty-six weeks, the testicles begin their descent into the scrotum, a process that continues until shortly before birth. Sometimes, this process doesn't happen before birth and the boy is born with undescended testicles. If this happens to your baby boy, don't worry, it's not a big problem. See page 50.

But testosterone doesn't just determine what kind of genitals the fetus will develop. It also "sexes" the brain, sculpting and organizing it quite differently depending on whether the fetus is male or female. This process shapes differences in behavior and personality that will last a lifetime. Over the last twenty years, scientists have learned a great deal about the distinctions between the male and female brains and the role that sex hormones play in shaping them. For example, some researchers have found that the corpus callosum and the anterior commissure, two nerve bundles that connect the two sides of the brain are a bit larger in females. This may help explain why, according to some studies, women tend to use both sides of their brain when they perform language tasks, while men use only their left side.

There are many mysteries and paradoxes in this process of human conception. For one thing, even though fetuses are considered to be female by default, a male is actually more likely to be conceived. As we noted earlier, researchers estimate that one hundred twenty boy babies are conceived to every one hundred girl babies. (Some experts believe that this is because sperm carrying the smaller Y chromosome can swim faster than those carrying an X.)

But this advantage is short-lived. As we've said, male fetuses are more likely to be miscarried or to die as the result of prematurity, birth defects, or delivery complications. By the time of birth, the numbers are much more even: about one hundred five boys are born to every one hundred girls. This doesn't mean, of course, that your pregnancy is likely to be anything other than normal. The vast majority of pregnancies in America, of girls and boys alike, go quite smoothly. If you are pregnant with a boy, the odds are excellent that if you take good care of yourself and get good prenatal care, you will end up with exactly what you want: a healthy, happy baby boy.

WISHING, PRAYING, AND PAYING FOR A BOY

For as long as people have been making babies, they've been trying to select the baby's sex. Anaxagoras of Clazomenae, a late fifth-century B.C. Greek philosopher, believed that baby boys were the product of sperm from a man's right testicle. So men in ancient Greece adopted the practice of tying off their left testicle before having intercourse in order to conceive a boy. A popular theory in the Middle Ages was that a woman who consumed the blood of a lion mixed with wine and had intercourse under a full moon would have a boy.

There are lots of reasons for wanting a child of a certain gender. Some parents dream of a little boy who can carry on the family name. Others already have a pack of boys and yearn for a girl for balance. And in some cases, the mother carries a gene for one of the approximately five hundred X-chromosome-linked disorders—such as hemophilia and muscular dystrophy—that are inherited mostly by boys; if they can have a girl, they know she will be safe.

Whatever the reason, literally millions of people have gotten into the game of gender selection. Internet bulletin boards are swamped with posts from women whose screen names—like 1princesswanted or coulditbeaboy4me?—make their desires quite clear. And even today, many people use techniques from old wives' tales to get the kind of baby they want. BabyCenter.com, the leading website for new and soon-to-be parents, receiving over 3 million hits per month, uncovered some of the more popular tales, and surveyed its readers about whether they would use them; 37 percent said they would. These folktales included the idea that eating lots of red meat would help produce a boy, and that having sex at night, or while standing up, or on odd days of the month would also lead to a boy.

But in this age of high technology, a growing number of Americans are looking for more scientific ways to choose their baby's sex. The Gallup organization has been asking Americans about their preference in babies since 1941 and surprisingly, the numbers haven't changed much. In its December 2000 survey, 42 percent of Americans said they would choose a boy if they could have only one child, while 27 percent would choose a girl.

It's worth noting that these numbers reflect a gaping gender gap: 55 percent of the men surveyed would prefer a boy, while just 18 percent would choose a girl. Among women, Gallup reports, the numbers were much more balanced: 32 percent prefer boys and 35 percent prefer girls. Nevertheless, there may be an unconscious preference for boys that leads to subtle but important differences in the way families operate. Research has shown when girls are the only product of a marriage divorce is more likely. But when a son is born dads will invest more emotionally and financially compared to when a daughter is born. He'll put in more work time, increase his earnings, and then reinvest that money back into the family by spending more on housing, according to research from Princeton University. Despite this, many of the clinics in the United States that offer sex selection see more of a demand for girls than boys, and much of that demand is coming from women. But more about that later.

Probably the most popular sex selection method being used today is named after its developer, Landrum B. Shettles, M.D. His book, *How to Choose the Sex of Your Baby: The Method Best Supported by Scientific Evidence*, claims that you can increase the odds of getting the sex you prefer by knowing when you ovulate and timing intercourse accordingly. This theory is built on the fact that sperm carrying a Y chromosome are smaller and swim faster, but don't live as long as X sperms. So Shettles says that if you have sex very close to the time of ovulation, a speedy Y should cross the finish line first, giving you a good shot at having a boy. On the other hand, if you have sex two to four days before you're due to ovulate, most Y sperm won't last that long, leaving X sperm with a clear field to your egg.

The Shettles method has gained a significant following. Thirty percent of people responding to a BabyCenter.com poll say they've used it to try to choose their baby's sex. But though the book has sold more than a million copies, and thousands of people swear by it, there's little hard evidence that it works. In a 1995 study on the timing of intercourse and its effect on fertility, Clarice Weinberg, Ph.D., of the National Institute of Environmental Health Sciences, looked at what happened to 221 women who were trying to become pregnant. She found that among those who succeeded, the timing of intercourse had no relationship at all to the sex of the baby.

At least the Shettles approach is relatively unobtrusive. True, you have to take your temperature a lot to pinpoint when you're ovulating, but at least you still do it—conceive a baby, that is—the old-fashioned way. That's not the case with several other approaches, which all attempt to segregate X-bearing sperm from Y-bearing sperm in the laboratory. The would-be mother can then be inseminated with semen made up primarily of the desired sperm type.

One such technique, called sperm spinning, uses a centrifuge to spin semen rapidly. Theoretically, heavier X sperms gather at the bottom while the Y sperms congregate at the top. Some reports suggested this technique has a 77 percent success rate in separating Xs from Ys, though there are no published studies on pregnancies.

Another technique, developed by a scientist named Ronald J. Ericsson, Ph.D., sends sperm swimming through a solution of albumin, a sticky protein. The idea is that more Y-bearing than X-bearing sperm will speed through the albumin, and can then be stained and segregated for use in artificial insemination. Ericsson's company, Gametrics Ltd., website (*www.gender-preselect.com*), says his technique is offered in forty-eight fertility clinics around the world; it also claims the method is "safe, reliable, and proven." That is a stretch.

In fact, these and other techniques practiced in fertility clinics and promoted in hundreds of sites on the Internet, are largely unproven and are regarded as little more than expensive snake oil by the medical establishment. Alan H. DeCherney, M.D., professor of obstetrics and gynecology at UCLA Medical School and editor of the journal *Fertility and Sterility,* put it succinctly in a 1999 interview with *The New York Times*: "They don't work, nothing works."

But there is now one exception to that blanket statement, Dr. DeCherney says today. In 1998, a Virginia fertility clinic, the Genetics & IVF Institute (IVF stands for *in vitro fertilization*) announced that it had successfully tested a new sex-selection method that was originally developed to sort the sperm of farm animals. The technique, MicroSort, makes use of the difference in the amount of DNA between X- and Y-bearing sperm to separate them. This is done by dying the DNA and separating the sperm into batches of semen that consist mostly of one or the other. This processed sperm can then be used to artificially inseminate a woman. The institute is currently using this technique in an FDA-approved trial to help couples who have a family history of genetic diseases and want to avoid passing them on to a child. But it is also being used for "family balance," meaning to conceive either a boy or a girl in a family that already has several children of the opposite sex.

So far, the clinic claims more than three hundred babies were born using this technique. It boasts a 90 percent success rate in producing girls and up to a 75 percent success rate in birthing boys. Impressive though it sounds, it gives you only a 25 percent better shot of having a baby boy than your odds with Mother Nature. Perhaps because of the higher success rate with females, most of the parents who contact the clinic— around 80 percent—are seeking girls. In any case, the procedure costs around $3,000 per treatment. Not cheap, perhaps, but much less than the cost of in vitro fertilization, which starts at about $6,000 per treatment but can run significantly higher.

What about the risks? Some experts have expressed concern that the process of dying sperm and then training a laser on them could potentially damage the sperm's DNA. To date, none of the babies born thus far through the MicroSort process show signs of genetic damage, institute representatives say.

The most sophisticated and surest way to determine sex combines in vitro fertilization (sperm and egg are brought together in a lab dish, fertilization occurs, and an embryo results) with genetic analysis in a technique called *preimplantation genetic diagnosis* (PGD). Here an eight-celled embryo is created in the laboratory and then a single cell is removed. That cell can be tested for a variety of genetic qualities including its sex. Right now reputable clinics perform PGD only in cases where there is a high risk of a life-threatening genetic disease such as sickle-cell anemia or spinal muscular atrophy.

Before trying any type of sex selection, you should think long and hard about your reasons. Say you're trying to have a boy. How will you react if you don't succeed and have a girl instead? Will you treat her any differently? Will she somehow feel or understand that she was not the "right sex"? On the other hand, the same feelings are undoubtedly experienced by some children and parents who have large families as a result of their repeated attempts to have a child of the "right" sex. They haven't made use of this technology but have simply hoped that they'd eventually have a child of a particular sex.

By the way, if you really want to have a boy, there's a simple thing you can do to boost your odds: quit smoking. A recent study from Japan found that the chances of having a boy dropped a little when one parent smoked a pack a day, and dropped a lot when both did. When both parents were smokers, only eighty-two boys were born for every one hundred girls. Another good reason to kick the habit!

GUESSING THE SEX OF YOUR BABY

If, like most people, you do leave the sex of your baby to chance, and you don't rely on technology such as a sonogram or amniocentesis to tell you, you'll still be guessing and obsessing about pink or blue just as soon as you find out you're pregnant. And again you can find no shortage of systems for divining the sex from ancient myths and old wives' tales. Some four thousand years ago Hippocrates wrote that being pregnant with a female baby made mothers look pale. In the Middle Ages, if Mom's right breast was bigger than her left, that meant a boy was on his way. And of course any woman who's ever been pregnant can tell you how other people—usually another woman—will stop you in the supermarket to congratulate you on your baby boy or girl. "Must be a boy," she'll say, "the way you're carrying low." Or "That's a girl, all right, since you're carrying so high." Or vice versa.

The Internet site BabyCenter.com looked into some of the most popular methods people use for guessing the sex of their babies. Here are a few of the surefire, can't-miss ways they uncovered:

- If your baby's heart rate is slow, you'll be having a boy; if it's fast, expect a girl.

- If you're carrying out front, it's a boy; if you're wide, that's a girl.

- If your looks improve during your pregnancy, expect a boy; if they worsen, prepare for a girl.

Source: Material from BabyCenter.com, excerpted with permission. Copyright © Baby Center, L.L.C., 2004. All rights reserved. For additional information on preconception, pregnancy, birth, or caring for a baby or toddler, visit www.babycenter.com.

I remember conducting a little study for a course in hypnosis when I was in medical school. We were testing the power of autosuggestion on pregnant women who were trying to guess the sex of their unborn baby. We used one of the oldest tests of sex determination—dangling the woman's wedding ring on a string over her stomach and seeing how it moves. If it goes in a circle, it's supposed to be a girl; if it moves back and forth, a boy. Before doing the test, we quizzed the women on whether they actually believed in it. And guess what? The women who believed the test could work had a higher rate of success in divining their baby's sex than those who didn't. Spooky.

In truth, there's almost no way to accurately guess a baby's sex. I say *almost* because there are a couple of things that happen in some pregnancies that seem to hint at a girl baby. Women who suffer from a great deal of nausea and vomiting during their first three months are more likely to have a girl, as are women whose asthma symptoms get worse during pregnancy, according to a study conducted at Guy's Hospital in London by physician Heather J. Milburn. What's more, women carrying boys seem to eat more than women carrying girls. The authors of the study in the June 2003 *British Medical Journal* theorize testosterone secreted from the fetal testicles could boost appetite. It seems that boys have higher energy requirements than girls, and that boys may be more susceptible to low energy intake.

You can, of course, get the answer through technology. These days, the way most people first find out is by looking at an image of their baby during an ultrasound examination. This procedure, usually done around the twentieth week of pregnancy, allows your doctor to diagnose certain birth defects, evaluate fetal growth, and check the position of the fetus, among other things. What it does for parents is give you your first look at your coming attraction. You'll squint and stare at the computer screen, struggling to make out what it shows. One thing you're looking for, of course, is that telltale bit of male genitalia, but it's not always easy to see, even for your OB or ultrasound technician, especially if the baby's hand happens to be in the way.

The more certain way to learn your baby's sex is to examine his or her chromosomes. Two tests—*amniocentesis* and *chorionic villus sampling* (CVS)—do this. These tests are used primarily in women over the age of thirty-five and/or those who have a higher risk of bearing children with birth defects. Amniocentesis, the more common of the two, is usually performed in the second trimester of pregnancy, while CVS can be done earlier, at the end of the first trimester. In both tests, a needle is inserted into the womb to extract some cellular material. Under a microscope, the telltale X or Y chromosomes can be seen, as can some serious problems, such as when a whole chromosome is missing or when an extra chromosome is present, as in Down's syndrome.

Do you need these tests? That depends on a number of factors, including your age and family history. Talk with your doctor about whether and when to take them.

Most people today choose to find out their baby's sex, though a significant number decide they want to be surprised. For many people, including me, it was not an easy choice. On the one hand, if you know you're having, say, a boy, you can name him, buy clothes for him, and dream about him in a deeper way. On the other hand, the months of anticipation and that moment of excitement you feel when you first find out are incredible.

For me, finding out in advance that I was going to have a boy was definitely the right thing. I'll always remember how happy I felt to be having a boy but also how anxious it made me. On the one hand, I would learn about boys and men in a whole new way. It was as if I was about to be let into some secret society that I knew nothing of, and would be able to learn their secret handshakes and rituals.

On the other hand, it terrified me. I didn't know the first thing about these strange beings and I wasn't so sure I could relate. It turns out I'm far from alone in having these worries and anxieties.

BOY ANXIETY

The more I talked to other women and looked at the postings on various websites, the more I realized my anxiety about having a boy is a common reaction among women pregnant with boys, yet largely undiscussed in professional circles. When I asked one of New York City's most popular pediatricians if any of her moms had expressed anxiety about caring for and raising boys, she literally yelled at me, "In my twenty-five years of practice I have never heard one question along these lines. This is ridiculous!"

Under the surface, however, this feeling is widespread. Here is a sampling of some of the comments found on Internet bulletin boards.

"I was afraid to have a boy," said Tina, in a story she wrote about the birth of her son, Mark. "I thought that since I was a woman, and I'd had a daughter, I wouldn't know what to do with a boy."

"When I found out I was having a boy, I was distressed, given that I come from a family of all girls and had no experience with boys," wrote Bridget, in a book review posted online. "I doubted my ability to have and maintain a close relationship with a boy-man and this was a matter of some sadness to me."

And here's what Lisa wrote in an account of the birth of her son:

Every time I was pregnant I would pray that I would have a little girl. Even after I already had two of them, I wanted another one. Why? I was deathly afraid of having a boy. What in the world would I do with one? The only little boy I have ever known was my little brother. The little brat who would pick his nose and wipe it on me, the boy who would rip the heads off of our dolls, the boy who thought it was funny to pee in the backyard and thought touching dead animals was cool. I'm sure you can understand why I wouldn't want one of those strange creatures for my own. I prayed that God would listen to my prayers and understand that I just wasn't capable of taking care of a little boy.

For some women, anxiety about having a boy comes out in dreams. For her 1985 book, *Mothers and Sons*, Carol Klein interviewed a number of pregnant women who reported dreams about their boy stretching them beyond repair or even killing them during childbirth. Hillary Grill, a New York City psychotherapist, says such dreams are far more common than we realize. Grill and two colleagues recently interviewed more than one hundred pregnant women and new mothers for their book *Dreaming for Two: The Hidden Emotional Life of Expectant Mothers*. She says that a lot of women are apprehensive about having a boy, so they express their anxiety in their dreams.

One woman dreamed of giving birth to a hairy, half-camel teenage boy who was not cute, was out of control, and decapitated her Christmas cookies. Another dreamed she gave birth to a big, unruly three-year-old. "Then," Grill says, "she comes across a friend of hers who's having this idyllic experience as a mother. She has a tiny little girl, it's only about six inches and it's really cute and she's very envious about this woman's experience."

Grill says two common themes in the dreams are giving birth to boys who are big and wild, and anxiety about birthing an unfamiliar kind of person. "It's a sense of 'How do I connect with someone who is so different? How do I take care of someone who is so different? How do I understand someone who is so different?' Women have all already been in mother-daughter relationships so they have a sense of what that relationship is and can feel more comfortable having another."

Their anxiety can be particularly acute, Grill says, if a woman has a difficult relationship with her father, especially if it involved abuse. "Girls that have been sexually abused or even physically abused by men—whether it's their father or any other man in their lives—they have a lot of anxiety about having anything to do with boys, because it brings up those feelings. They don't want to be that close to a boy."

One of the reasons their worries come out in dreams, Grill says, is that many women won't allow themselves to talk about these issues openly. It's an underground phenomenon, she says. "I have a lot of patients who say things like: 'I'm really worried that I might have a boy, and I really don't want to have a boy, and I really feel bad about this, and I really feel guilty.' I think it's something that women often feel ashamed about. I think they feel that they shouldn't have a preference, that they should only want a healthy baby and that whatever anxieties they may have are not really justified and they shouldn't really have them."

Grill tries to help these women by letting them know that their feelings aren't unique and it's okay to express them. "It's like anything else, it's important to be able to recognize that you're having them, to not feel so ashamed that you can't accept that you're feeling them. And then to work them through. Then they can look back and say, for example 'Oh, I had this really rough relationship with my father, and I'm nervous that I'm going to have a son who's like that.' Once you recognize that, you [can] say, 'Well, just because my father was that way doesn't mean that I'm going to have a son like that.' The goal is to accept that you might prefer one over the other, but then move on to the next step, which is the idea of 'I'm just happy if I have a healthy baby.' So that when the baby comes, you can treat that baby well, rather than wishing that baby was something else."

Bridget, who posted her anxiety about having a boy on a website, came to grips with her worries by reading good books on boys. "I wanted to have a friend, and I didn't think that would be possible with a boy," she said in an interview. "I felt like it was inevitable I wouldn't feel as close to my child. I started reading a lot, and that was what really changed my mind. The book that helped me the most was *The Courage to Raise Good Men,* by Olga Silverstein. When I read that book, about the very issue that concerned me, that changed my mind and helped me see it wasn't inevitable that I wouldn't be close, that I could be involved in his life.

"Christopher is now two and a half and he's wonderful. He's very sweet—and completely obsessed with tractors and trucks. I now know every kind of tractor there is. He definitely has a boy's interests. And I feel completely connected to him. I hate to see him grow up."

Like Bridget, and like most women, I fell totally in love with my son and quickly became grateful that I'd had a boy. But despite the scolding I got from the famous pediatrician—the one who called me ridiculous—I think there are plenty of women who worry about having a boy and their ability to take good care of him. I also think that when people in authority, like that pediatrician, deny this as an issue, they push many women in the closet with their feelings and fears. That's why I'm grateful that women like Hillary Grill talk about this issue and help us all realize that such feelings are quite normal, and that we can handle them so we don't deprive our boys of love.

The truth is that once these boys come into the world and into our lives, many of us begin to appreciate that we can move beyond feeling unprepared and ignorant about the male world. Now, by raising boys, we get a window into a world we've never really known before. In *Mothers and Sons,* Carol Klein expressed this idea of both great love and new insight:

> The tie [between mother and son] is stronger than that between father and son and father and daughter. The bond is also more complex than the one between mother and daughter. For a woman, a son offers the best chance to know the mysterious male existence.

And let me tell you: It is mysterious. It is strange. And I wouldn't miss it for the world.

THE WEAKER SEX

Like many boys, my first child and only son, Harry, was in no hurry to come into this world. I sometimes think he began life as a linebacker. He had broad shoulders, weighed nine pounds, and was determined to hold that line, and slow things way down. After thirty-six punishing hours of labor, he barely budged. In the end, I had a cesarean section.

My experience with Harry was typical. Of course, every child is unique, but on average, newborn boys are slightly heavier—by about a half pound—than newborn girls.

Nearly two thirds of heavy babies—those, like Harry, who weigh nine pounds or more—are boys. Since it is more dif-

> **Average weight for boys born in 2000:**
> **7 pounds, 7 ounces**
>
> **Average weight for girls born in 2000:**
> **7 pounds, 3 ounces**
>
> *Source: National Center for Health Statistics.*

ficult for larger babies to pass through the birth canal, they often take longer to be born. Which could be one reason that if you spend more than twenty hours in labor, odds are your baby is a boy! And the longer it takes to deliver, the greater the chance a C-section will be required. In fact, one large study of first-time mothers published in 1997 in the *American Journal of Obstetrics and Gynecology* found a higher rate of C-sections among women pregnant with boys: 13.2 percent for boys and 9.6 percent for girls. A more recent study, published in early 2003 in the *British Medical Journal,* found that women in Ireland who were pregnant with boys needed more medical intervention during the birth, including C-section and forceps delivery. They used oxytocin, a hormone that triggers contractions, and an epidural analgesic for pain relief more often. All of which prompted the researchers to note that when doctors joke "it's a boy" as a humorous explanation for complications during labor and delivery, they are scientifically more correct than previously supposed.

A long labor isn't only hard on the mother. It makes the birth process more traumatic for the baby and increases the chances that the baby will suffer other complications. That, in turn, can make it more likely that a baby will be fussy or have trouble sleeping in the weeks and months ahead. Several studies have found that boys are more fussy than girls during those first weeks of life. They cry more, have more disturbed sleep, and are more active, according to Carole Beal, Ph.D., a psychologist and gender researcher at the University of Massachusetts.

Other complications are also more common in the birth of boys. Women pregnant with boys face an increased risk of developing a condition called *preeclampsia,* which causes high blood pressure, fluid retention, and kidney problems. If left untreated, it can be fatal. Why is it more frequent in pregnancies of boys? No one knows for sure, but some speculate that it may be hormonal and that perhaps a woman carrying a male fetus tends to have higher testosterone and this may contribute to the development of preeclampsia.

But while some boys seem reluctant to leave the womb, others can't wait to get out. Boys are more likely to be born prematurely, about 11 percent more likely, according to the authors of one large study done in Finland in 1987. And in general, premature boys don't fare as well as premature girls. "When a premature baby boy comes in, we do worry more," says Ian R. Holzman, M.D., the head of the neonatal intensive care unit at Mount Sinai Medical Center in New York. "I worry more, the nurses worry more. Premature baby boys just don't do as well as baby girls. Boy preemies are at a disadvantage—they have more problems and get into more trouble."

The fragility of boys is not confined to preemies. Though there is no research that tells us *why* boys are developmentally behind girls at birth, it is a fact they are. So even full-term boys tend to be more vulnerable, perhaps partly because they are born four to six weeks behind girls in their development. Their relative immaturity means that boys don't weather insults in the womb as well as girls, Holzman says. When a mom smokes or has gestational diabetes, boys are more likely to suffer complications. Newborn boys are also more likely to suffer bleeding in the brain, develop an infection, or need mechanical ventilation for poor lung function.

Boys' frailty shows up even when they are born without any apparent abnormalities. Sudden infant death syndrome (SIDS) is the unexplained sudden death of a baby under one year of age. Parents often find the baby dead when they go to check on a supposedly sleeping baby. SIDS is the leading cause of death in infants between the ages of one month and one year, with most of the deaths occurring between two and four months. Once again boys are at greater risk; they are 20 percent more likely to die from SIDS. Why? No one knows for sure, but one theory is that the developmental lag in baby boys makes their sleep-wake cycle less mature and leaves them more susceptible to the breathing abnormalities that can lead to SIDS.

This fragility is seen in other ways as well. The Finnish study I mentioned earlier paints a distressing picture of the health of boys. Probably the most comprehensive examination to date of the differences in the health of boys and girls, the study looked at every baby born in Finland in 1987, then followed the children for seven years. It showed that boys had a greater risk of problems from their first moments of life. They were 20 percent more likely than girls to have low Apgar scores, the measure of a newborn's breathing, response to stimulation, muscle tone, skin color, and pulse taken at one minute and at five minutes after birth. Over the next seven years, boys were 22 percent more likely to die of various natural causes and had a 64 percent higher incidence of asthma. They would spend many more days in the hospital and need more medications. And the list goes on.

Boys also get more ear infections and have a harder time fighting them. They are much more likely to suffer from a host of developmental problems including autism, hyperactivity, stuttering, Tourette's syndrome, and a wide range of learning disabilities (see chapter 2). And if that weren't enough, they're also susceptible to diseases and birth defects that strike mostly, or exclusively, boys.

BIRTH DEFECTS AND OTHER PROBLEMS

Remember that males have only one X chromosome, and it comes from Mom. If that X has any genetic damage or irregularity, it has no "partner" chromosome that can pitch in and help by providing a healthier copy of the gene. In other words, the Y boys get from Dad can't make up for defects on the X. In contrast, girls get two doses of X chromosomes, so if there is a problem with one, the other can step in and take over. That's why so-called X-linked or sex-linked conditions such as hemophilia and muscular dystrophy strike only boys (with rare exceptions). Mothers are "carriers" of these genetic disorders, though they rarely show signs. When a carrier has a boy, there is a 50 percent chance he'll inherit the mutated X chromosome and develop the condition. If a carrier has a girl, the baby won't get the disorder but has a 50 percent chance of being a carrier, like Mom. Let's take a look at some of the birth defects and problems that disproportionately affect boys. There are more than five hundred sex-linked diseases, but just a few represent the majority of cases.

Sex-Linked Problems
Red-Green Color Blindness

The gene for the most common kind of color blindness is also carried on Mom's X chromosome and thus affects mostly boys. About 1 in 12 males (compared to 1 in 230 females) have red-green color blindness, meaning they can't distinguish between the two colors. That amounts to up to 10 percent of all men! Consider the difficulty red-green color blindness presents. Colorblind men may have trouble with traffic lights, can't appreciate red flowers, can't pick ties that match, and have trouble telling if hamburgers are fully cooked. And many careers, including fire fighting and law enforcement, require the ability to accurately perceive color.

Duchenne's Muscular Dystrophy

This, the most common form of muscular dystrophy, causes deterioration of the muscles and eventually death, usually around age twenty. It affects about 1 in every 3,000 boys worldwide. Boys with Duchenne's usually experience symptoms by age six, although symptoms can begin in infancy. As a boy's muscles weaken, he gradually loses use of them. By age ten, many need braces to walk, and by age twelve, most are confined to a wheelchair. While there is no cure or treatment, exercise and physical therapy can help maintain the use of muscles for a longer time. Since the mothers are carriers, each additional boy stands a one-in-four chance of being affected.

Hemophilia

People with hemophilia have blood that doesn't clot normally. Boys with hemophilia are missing a gene that produces clotting factors, the proteins in our blood that make it clot. Normally, a complicated cascade of proteins and cells helps to form a blood clot and prevent hemorrhaging. In hemophilia, however, the lack of an essential protein thwarts the entire process. People with hemophilia don't bleed faster, but they do bleed longer, and it's hard for their bleeding to stop. There are two kinds of hemophilia: hemophilia A, the most common type, and hemophilia B; both almost exclusively affect boys. The two genes are normally carried on the X chromosome, so if one is missing from Mom's X, a boy has no place else to get it and will have hemophilia. Although there is no cure, medications that replace the missing clotting factor can allow boys and men with hemophilia to lead relatively normal lives. Genetic tests can now determine if a woman is a carrier and whether a developing fetus has hemophilia. About 1 in 5,000 baby boys is born with hemophilia and some 17,000 Americans have the disease, nearly all men. Women sometimes develop it, but that's rare.

If you have a family history of either hemophilia or Duchenne's, genetic testing can determine if you are a carrier. Ask your physician to refer you to a genetic counselor. To find one on your own, check out the website of the National Society of Genetic Counselors, *http://www.nsgc.org*.

Fragile X Syndrome

This genetic disorder is the most common known cause of mental retardation. It results from abnormal repetitions of the genetic code of a gene on the X chromosome. Affecting approximately 1 in 3,600 males and 1 in 4,000 to 6,000 females, Fragile X syndrome is usually more serious in males, because males lack a second, nondefective X chromosome to help compensate. Most boys with Fragile X will have distinctive mental disabilities that can range from subtle learning disabilities to severe mental retardation and/or autism spectrum disorders, as well as distinctive physical characteristics, typically big ears and enlarged testicles, and behavioral problems, attention deficit disorder, and speech disturbances. There is no cure for Fragile X, but various kinds of therapy, education, and support can do much to help. Researchers at the Genetic & IVF Institute, a well-known Virginia fertility clinic, have found that about 1 in 300 women are carriers for Fragile X. They suggest that women whose sons, brothers, or maternal uncles have learning disabilities or mental retardation consider genetic testing for Fragile X before conceiving.

Chromosomal Abnormalities

Some genetic birth defects and disorders are not inherited, but arise sponta-neously as a result of onetime mutations or chromosomal abnormalities. Two condi-tions that affect males exclusively occur when an extra chromosome, either an X or a Y, appears by chance at the time of conception.

XXY Males

In the early 1940s, Dr. Harry Klinefelter and two colleagues at Massachusetts Gen-eral Hospital published an article about a group of men who had enlarged breasts, small testicles, and scant facial and body hair. The men were also unable to produce sperm. Fifteen years later, researchers discovered that such men may have an extra X chromo-some, making them XXY instead of the normal XY. Since then, large-scale studies of newborn infants have shown that the XXY pattern is one of the most common of all genetic abnormalities, affecting as many as 1 in every 500 to 1,000 newborn boys. It also turns out that XXY males vary greatly in how they express their genes. Some have the kinds of symptoms that Dr. Klinefelter described, and may also have difficulty with lan-guage and learning to read and write. But many others show very few symptoms and indeed they may go through their lives never knowing they have an extra chromosome.

"I never refer to newborn babies as having Klinefelter's, because they don't have a syndrome," said the late Arthur Robinson, M.D., who, as a pediatrician at the Univer-sity of Colorado Medical School, directed a large study of XXY males for the National Institute for Child Health and Human Development (NICHD). "Presumably, some of them will grow up to develop the syndrome Dr. Klinefelter described, but a lot of them won't." Robinson's attitude, as expressed in the quote above, published in an NICHD brochure, helped remove some of the stigma of XXY disorder. This excellent brochure can be viewed online at *http://www.nichd.nih.gov/publications/pubs/klinefelter.htm*.

Babies born with the XXY pattern show no signs of their unusual genetic arrange-ment at birth and are not likely to for several years, if ever. For those who do, the first hint is often that they learn to speak later than other children. Their language prob-lems can usually be addressed with therapy and almost all can learn to converse nor-mally. That's one reason it's important that you seek help if your child experiences these difficulties, so you can identify the problem and get the support you and your son need. For many years, XXY males were thought to be at greater risk for psychotic and even criminal behavior, but that idea has been disproved.

XYY Males

Males born with two Y chromosomes—XYY instead of the normal XY—tend to be tall and thin and often have severe acne during their teen years. But they are usually fer-tile, have relatively normal intelligence, and lead ordinary lives as adults. In fact, most

XYY males probably never know they have a chromosomal abnormality. Sixties serial killer Richard Speck's claim that he murdered eight nurses in Chicago because he was XYY, coupled with some faulty research, fueled the notion men with an extra Y chromosome were at greater risk for violent behavior and that there were lots of XYY males in prison. Years later, genetic analysis proved that Speck did not have an extra Y, and the theory that an extra Y can lead to criminality was disproved by later research.

Birth Defects That Affect More Boys Than Girls

Other problems not related to the sex chromosomes can affect boys more than girls although there is no easy explanation why.

Clubfoot

People with clubfoot have twisted feet that point down and in. It is one of the most common birth defects and affects about 1 out of 1,000 babies born in the United States every year. Boys are twice as likely to have clubfoot as girls. First described around 400 B.C. by Hippocrates, it is one of the oldest known orthopedic problems.

Clubfoot is usually evident at birth and, fortunately, is not painful. Still, treatment should begin right away. Doctors manipulate the feet to get them in the best possible position, then hold that position with a cast. For the next several months, doctors continue this process of manipulating, then placing the foot in a new cast. Sometimes, this corrects the problem and molds the bones into a normal posture. Other children need surgery, which is usually done before walking age (eight to twelve months). The exact timing varies from child to child and from surgeon to surgeon. Many kids need to wear braces for a while whether or not they have surgery. And some kids with mild forms of clubfoot may respond well to simple stretching exercises and special orthopedic shoes.

What causes clubfoot? It's not clear. Doctors used to think it had to do with the way the baby was positioned in the uterus. That may be a factor in mild forms of clubfoot, but doctors no longer think this is true for more serious cases. Rather, experts now believe that a combination of environmental and genetic factors interfere with normal development, causing problems somewhere around the tenth or twelfth week of pregnancy. Heredity is definitely a factor; a family history of clubfoot increases the likelihood that a child may have it. Some intriguing new research suggests that a mother's smoking during pregnancy increases the risk. And if Mom smokes *and* there's a family history of clubfoot, the risk can be even greater.

The good news is that the vast majority of kids with clubfoot grow up to wear normal shoes, play sports, and have full, active, normal lives. Plenty of children with clubfoot have gone on to be professional athletes, among them Troy Aikman, former quarterback for the Dallas Cowboys, figure skater Kristi Yamaguchi, and soccer player Mia Hamm.

Cleft Lip and Cleft Palate

Somewhere around the fifth or sixth week of pregnancy, the basic structures of the mouth and face are formed. Sometimes these structures don't fully close and a baby can be born with openings, or *clefts,* in the lip, the roof of the mouth (*hard palate*), or back of the mouth (*soft palate*). The opening can be a small notch in the lip or a large gap that extends from lip to hard and soft palate and base of the nostril. In the United States, cleft lip and/or cleft palate is the fourth most common birth defect, affecting 1 in 700 newborns. The condition is more common among Asian and Native American babies than whites, and less common among African-Americans. The most common form is a cleft lip combined with a cleft palate, and this affects boys more often than girls. Cleft palate alone is less common and tends to affect girls more often.

Babies born with cleft lips alone usually don't have trouble feeding, but those with clefts in their palates may. The opening in the roof of the mouth makes it hard for the baby to suck strongly enough to pull milk from the nipple. Babies with cleft palate are also prone to ear infections and sometimes hearing loss. These problems can usually be treated leaving no permanent effects.

Surgery can repair clefts, though children with more severe malformations may need more than one, even several operations. Cleft lips are usually repaired by about three months, while cleft palate surgeries are usually done between nine and eighteen months.

Research suggests that expectant mothers who smoke, take illicit drugs, or take several prescription medications, including antiseizure drugs, methotrexate (used for arthritis, cancer, and psoriasis), and Retin-A (tretinoin) or Accutane (isotretinoin) may be more likely to have babies with clefts. Very often, though, there is no known cause. Taking multivitamins containing folic acid during conception and in the first months of pregnancy seems to reduce the risk.

Protecting Your Boy

So now that you've heard all this bad news, let's try and put it in context. The vast majority of boys do not have any of the problems I just mentioned and the odds are yours won't either. Still, if you or members of your family have a history of birth defects or genetic disease, there is a chance your child could have these problems as well. Let your obstetrician know your history so he or she can refer you to a genetics specialist for counseling and testing, if necessary.

Before a pregnancy, take care of yourself. During pregnancy, get good prenatal care. See your doctor regularly. Take prenatal vitamins, especially folic acid. If you smoke, drink, or take street drugs, do whatever it takes to quit. Do these things for any child, boy or girl. But if you fail, the impact on boys can be especially harsh. Smoking during pregnancy, for instance, is more likely to cause boys to be born with a low birth weight. Smoking also triples the risk of SIDS—and we know that boys are more susceptible. To reduce the risk of SIDS after your baby is born, do not allow someone to smoke around him or in your home. And above all, always put him to sleep on his back. A national effort educating parents to put their babies to sleep on their backs has cut the number of SIDS deaths by half in recent years. Be sure to include plenty of "tummy time" when he's awake to help develop all muscles. Check out this website from the American Academy of Pediatrics for a summary of tips on putting baby to sleep: *http://www.aap.org/new/sids/reduceth.htm.*

THE CIRCUMCISION DECISION

Looking back I can hardly believe that we never talked about it. After all, Avery, my husband, and I had known for weeks our first child would be a boy. We talked about names. We talked about what he might be like and who he might become. You'd think that as a doctor, I would have thought about it. I didn't. I was too exhausted from the pregnancy and a bout of the flu to think about anything but the day when I would finally see my baby and the ordeal of pregnancy would be over.

Forty-eight hours later, the trauma of a difficult delivery all but forgotten, I sat upright in bed, the sun streaming through the windows of my hospital room, my miracle, my perfectly formed son, Harry, cradled in my arms. Avery sat in a chair next to me. "I think we better ask the doctor to perform the circumcision before we leave the hospital," he said, not quite looking at me.

I looked at him blankly, exhausted but awash in postdelivery hormonal bliss. "What?" I asked. When it hit me what he meant, I was horrified and angered. "Are you *crazy*?!" I screamed. "You want to *cut* my brand-new baby boy? This is insane. Just look at his little body! It's perfection. Why would anybody want to change it? Who in their right mind does such things to tiny babies?" I burst into tears and clutched Harry tighter. I was not going to let anyone hurt my baby.

Poor Avery. He hardly knew what hit him. I think he was as taken aback by my reaction as I was by his announcement. Avery is Jewish; I'm not. *Circumcision*—the surgical removal of the foreskin around the glans, or head of the penis—was a foregone conclusion to him, a ritual as old as his faith. It had never occurred to us to discuss it. Now here we were: He was astonished; I was outraged. With me in tears, round and round we went, and slowly I came to realize that I wasn't just dealing with my husband and my son; I was dealing with human history.

No one really seems to know when circumcision started or why. In the Old Testament, God tells Abraham he will create a great nation if Abraham obeys His covenant. The covenant includes circumcision. The penalty for not being circumcised was severe: Uncircumcised men were "cut off" from their people, cast out. But the practice did not begin then, ritual male—and female—circumcision dates to prehistory. Male circumcision is evident in Stone Age cave drawings. Ancient Egyptian mummies are circumcised. The practice is widespread not just among Jews but also Muslims, many African cultures, and even Australian aborigines.

While many ancient practices—such as the Jewish (and Muslim) prohibition against eating pork—arose from legitimate health concerns, it's less clear if removal of an infant's foreskin was justified medically. Some theorize that circumcision arose amongst desert-dwelling people because sand, trapped under the foreskin, caused irritation and infection. There is some modern backing for this theory. According to historical documents published by the Office of the Surgeon General and Center of Military History, United States Army in 1987, American soldiers fighting in the North African desert during World War II experienced this problem because of sand and poor hygiene in combat conditions. As a result almost 150,000 of them were hospital-ized with infections of the foreskin and many ultimately underwent circumcision in the field. There were probably other reasons our ancestors practiced circumcision—something far more compelling, far more primitive. It was as a way to distinguish friend from foe and keep members of one tribe from deserting to another.

When the anger, misunderstanding, confusion, and fear settled in that hospital room years ago, I understood finally what my husband wanted: He wanted his son to look like him. It was that simple, that tribal, that deep. And when, in the end, I agreed and the doctor took my son away to be circumcised, I felt I'd somehow failed him, right at the start. I feel that way still and suspect many mothers feel the same. We were both wounded that day.

Is there any medical justification for circumcision today? That depends on whom you ask. What moved male circumcision from religious ritual to a common lay prac-tice by the nineteenth century—at least in some Western societies such as the United States—was its alleged medical benefits. The natural, intact foreskin was blamed for an incredible array of maladies for which there was no known cause, from eczema to tuberculosis, even paralysis. But one of the main targets was masturbation, the great demon of the nineteenth century, the purported cause of epilepsy, blindness, and madness.

By the mid–twentieth century, the practice was widespread in this country. After the experience in WWII and because of a better understanding of the relationship between certain diseases and lack of circumcision, the practice became an article of faith, and the majority of baby boys underwent circumcision. It also became a social marker since, before the advent of medical insurance, only those with money could afford the additional surgery.

Then, in 1971, the American Academy of Pediatrics announced that there was no clear medical or hygienic benefit to circumcision. In the years that followed, a growing and vocal anticircumcision movement arose, with advocacy groups like the National Organization of Circumcision Resources Centers (NOCIRC), Mothers Against Circumcision, and Infants Need to Avoid Circumcision Trauma (INTACT), crusading against the procedure. Even Dr. Benjamin Spock reversed his position on circumcision in the 1970s and recommended that parents leave baby boys alone.

Some of these groups see circumcision as a savage violation of children's human rights in which innocents are subjected to a barbaric procedure without any say in the matter. It's not harmless surgery, they say, it's mutilation because it removes healthy tissue. Some men have even attempted to restore foreskin by hanging weights from the remaining skin or trying other ways of stretching it back over the glans. Some report that the glans becomes moist again and their sexual sensitivity increases, though there is no scientific documentation for this.

The debate rages, with the staunchest opponents arguing that the trauma of circumcision may be related directly to male defensiveness, even aggression. But wait. Is there any evidence that these are characteristics or attitudes shared only by circumcised men? Hardly. Personally, I find it a bit of a stretch to attribute such complex lessons to an admittedly painful experience during an infant's first days of life.

On the other hand, it's also far from clear that routine circumcision provides any definitive health benefits to infant boys or the men they become. The latest statement from the American Academy of Pediatrics (AAP), issued in 1999, says that although there may be *potential* medical benefits, the evidence is not enough to recommend routine neonatal circumcision. In other words, they take no firm stand for or against. Data from 1999 shows that about 65 percent of American boys were circumcised, but also finds great geographical variation. In the western states (with their higher Hispanic and Asian population), only 37 percent of newborn boys were circumcised, whereas in the Midwest, 81 percent underwent the procedure, an increase over 1971. There is also a great deal of international variation. In Britain, for example, circumcision rates are estimated at 5 percent or less.

Many parents feel that since the AAP does not endorse circumcision, it is unnecessary. Several new parents told me just that. But I think the real point of the AAP position is that there is no overwhelming medical rationale for performing or not performing a circumcision. It remains a personal choice—not of the infant, of course, but the mother and father. To help with that decision, here's a rundown of the pros and cons of circumcision followed by some advice on when and how to make the decision. Good luck.

CIRCUMCISION RATES IN OTHER COUNTRIES

Britain: 3.8 percent of boys are circumcised.
Canada: 48 percent of boys are circumcised.
United States: 65 percent of boys are circumcised.

Circumcision: The Pros and Cons
Infant Urinary Tract Infections (UTIs)

Dr. Tom Wiswell was a skeptic when he set out to look at the evidence that circumcision would reduce the risk of UTIs. As a researcher at Walter Reed Army Medical Center, with access to a database of 200,000 boys, he reasoned that if there were any evidence of a link between being uncircumcised and UTI, he would find it there. What he found surprised him: Boys with foreskins were much more likely to develop a UTI than those without. Since Wiswell's research first appeared in the journal *Pediatrics* in 1986, at least nine other studies have confirmed the connection. Some research also suggests that UTIs can contribute to scarring of the kidney, leading to a risk of high blood pressure and severe kidney problems later in life.

UTIs are a less than compelling reason for circumcision, though, because UTIs in boys are relatively rare, circumcised or not. They're just less rare in boys without foreskins. According to the AAP, a review of the literature finds 1 of every 100 uncircumcised baby boys will develop a UTI by age one, which adds up to about 20,000 cases a year in the United States. Among circumcised baby boys, 1 of every 1,000 boys will develop a UTI.

Sexually Transmitted Diseases (STDs)

A number of studies suggest that uncircumcised men have a higher risk for STDs, possibly because the foreskin provides a moist environment for bacteria and viruses, but the increased risk is relatively small. In fact, many experts argue that behavioral factors, such as safer sex practices, are more important risk factors in STD prevention. What is becoming increasingly clear—largely from research in other countries—is that uncircumcised men may have a dramatically higher risk for contracting HIV. Some researchers believe that circumcision is the key to the huge difference in infection rates in parts of the world that are otherwise similar. A case in point: The rate of HIV infection is 25 times higher in Thailand than in the Philippines. Both countries have lots of prostitution and STDs. The big difference: circumcision is routine in the Philippines (98% of men are circumcised), but rare in Thailand. Interestingly, Thailand has more HIV infection even though it also has a much higher rate of condom use.

In 2000, the *British Medical Journal* reviewed more than forty studies conducted over the past decade. All of them showed a strong connection between lack of circumcision and transmission of HIV. So why would having a foreskin increase the risk of contracting AIDS? The authors of the *BMJ* review outlined three possible reasons. First, the foreskin is specialized tissue with a high concentration of immune cells that can act as entry points for the AIDS virus. Second, the foreskin tissue is delicate and more likely than other parts of the penis to be torn or scraped during intercourse.

Finally, the intact foreskin can be a common site for other STDs. Since STDs can cause open sores or lesions, they give HIV a way to enter the body.

The research is so compelling that some health experts have suggested circumcision should be used as a way to combat the AIDS epidemic, especially in those African countries where circumcision is rare and AIDS is all too common. What the research doesn't explain is why AIDS is not raging through the heterosexual population of say, Europe, where circumcision is also rare. Perhaps, says researcher Daniel Halperin, Ph.D., it takes a combination of factors including a high level of untreated STDs and numerous sexual partners to create an AIDS epidemic among heterosexuals.

Perhaps the most compelling evidence that circumcision can reduce HIV transmission comes from a study of couples in Uganda. In one group, women were infected with HIV but men were not. Over a thirty-month period none of the men who were circumcised contracted HIV, while 29 percent of the uncircumcised men did. In couples where the man was HIV positive and the woman not, circumcised men were less likely to transmit the virus to their partners. Interestingly only those circumcised men who also had the highest amount of virus in their bodies transmitted the virus to their partners.

The latest research on the issues comes in a 2003 report from the U.S. Agency for International Development (USAID), which found that circumcised men are at least 50 percent less likely to contract the AIDS virus than uncircumcised men. But the authors point out that advocating circumcision in developing countries may send the wrong message: that circumcised men are invulnerable to the AIDS virus. They, of course, are not.

Penile Cancer

This is a rare disease. An estimated 1,400 cases are diagnosed each year in the United States, according to the American Cancer Society. That's about 1 in 100,000 males annually in the United States. It is, however, more common in developing countries, where hygiene is poor. When it does occur, it is always in uncircumcised men.

Infections

Infections or inflammations can occur in both circumcised and uncircumcised boys and men. However, uncircumcised males of any age can get *phimosis,* a condition in which the foreskin cannot be retracted over the head of the penis. Up to 7 percent of uncircumcised boys and men will have to have a circumcision later due largely to recurrent foreskin infections. It is the leading reason to circumcise older boys and adults. Both problems are discussed more extensively in chapter 6; the point here is that some problems happen only to uncircumcised males. One reason many urologists (though by no means all) lean toward circumcision is that they see these problems in boys and adults every day. The poor men who suffer these illnesses are not happy campers, so it's hard to blame urologists for wanting to eliminate these problems completely.

A Possible Benefit for Women

The newest wrinkle on the health effects of circumcision relates to women. A recent study in the *New England Journal of Medicine* found that women with circumcised partners may be less likely to get cervical cancer because men with intact foreskins are more than three times as likely to harbor certain strains of the human papilloma virus (HPV). In the study, women whose partners were uncircumcised and had more than six sexual partners were at greater risk of developing cervical cancer. This is probably not as big an issue in the United States, where most women get regular Pap smears. It could be a factor in poorer nations, where access to Pap smears and medical care is limited.

Sexual Response

One of the central arguments against circumcision is that the removal of the foreskin deprives a man of a certain type of sexual pleasure. Circumcision opponents point out that foreskin contains sensitive nerve endings that are lost when removed, and argue that if the head of the penis is not covered and protected, the skin can become tough and desensitized. This is hard to prove, although anecdotally some men who were circumcised as adults report lost sensitivity. Doctors from Montefiore Medical Center in New York presenting at the 2003 American Urological Association meeting in Chicago actually tested penile sensitivity in circumcised and uncircumcised men and found there was no difference in the two groups in penile sensation to a variety of measures such as vibration and pressure.

As for women, one survey by Williamson and Williamson published in the *Journal of Sex Education* in 1988 suggested they prefer a circumcised penis by a margin of three to one. Sex researcher Dr. Edward O. Laumann in *Sex, Love, and Health in America: Private Choices and Public Policies* says circumcised men report more oral and anal sex than uncircumcised men.

Concerns About the Locker Room

Some parents worry that if their son is the only one uncircumcised, he will look different. That may be true in certain geographical areas but in others there will be lots of boys with intact foreskins sharing benches and showers. Kids will tease about many things, but I don't think fear of teasing should weigh heavily in a decision about circumcision.

Looking Like Dad

For many men this is a big factor in the circumcision decision. After weighing benefits and downsides, it may come down to this: They'd like their sons to look like them, and that may or may not mean circumcision. This, obviously, is a question for you and your husband to resolve.

Hygiene

Many people say a circumcised penis is easier to keep clean. The truth is that good hygiene can be taught to uncircumcised boys easily and should avoid problems down the road (see below and chapter 6).

The Procedure

Circumcision takes no more than five minutes in skilled hands. After an analgesic cream is applied or pain-numbing medicine is injected into the penis, a small slit is made in the foreskin. A clamp is placed around the tip of the penis to protect the glans. Then using a scalpel, the foreskin is removed. The most commonly used devices for neonatal circumcision are the Gomco clamp, the Mogen clamp, and the PlastiBell. No one method has been proven better by any scientific study. The most important thing is that the person performing the circumcision is skilled and has done it many times.

The procedure is normally performed by obstetricians or pediatricians, usually before the family leaves the hospital. For people of the Jewish faith, circumcisions are performed by a trained religious practitioner called a mohel during the Bris Milah, a ceremony that occurs eight days after the birth. Some mohels are also licensed physicians. When selecting a practitioner, find one with a lot of experience and make sure pain medicine is administered and has a chance to work prior to the procedure.

Risks and Pain

So how risky and painful is circumcision? Experts once argued that infant boys did not feel pain during circumcision. How could anyone believe that? No one really argues that anymore. These days, pain is a legitimate concern. The American Academy of Pediatrics states that all boys undergoing circumcision should have some anesthetic. Pain control methods include a topical analgesic cream called EMLA and the injection of pain medicine such as lidocaine. This recommendation only came in 1999! Research shows that newborns circumcised without analgesia experience pain and stress that is reflected in their heart rate, blood pressure, oxygen saturation, and stress hormone levels.

Circumcision complications are uncommon and rarely serious. According to the AAP, research suggests that complications occur in one in two hundred to one in five hundred circumcised males. Bleeding and infection were most common. Foreskin can also be cut too long or too short. Over time the bare glans (tip) can become irritated and cause the opening of the penis to become too small or constrict, leading to urination problems and sometimes requiring surgery.

For many couples, circumcision is a nonissue. They are for or against based on religious, cultural, scientific, or moral grounds. For others, the decision can be harder. Before you decide, it's worth doing what we *didn't* do in my family: take time to investigate medical research and the arguments for and against. I'll always remember those moments of decision in the hospital as unhappy ones. I believe that if my husband and I had discussed circumcision earlier, much unhappiness would have been avoided.

Here's another reason to decide ahead of time. If you delay the procedure, there is some evidence it becomes riskier. A 2001 study in the journal *Pediatrics* found that many parents delay the circumcision decision until the baby is two to four months old. The reason, according to the authors, is that many parents do not discuss circumcision with their doctors in advance. While 36 percent were asked about their decision before, 14 percent were not asked until they were in the delivery room—not exactly a place conducive to clear thinking. Big mistake. If a baby weighs more than fifteen pounds, the risk of bleeding during the procedure goes up says Phillip Nasrallah, M.D., pediatric urologist at the Children's Hospital Medical Center of Akron. In order to best control any bleeding, doctors will use general anesthesia rather than simple local anesthesia. If general anesthesia is necessary, it will increase the risk of a medical complication and will cost thousands, rather than hundreds of dollars. According to the same study, many parents were swayed initially not to circumcise their sons because insurance did not cover it.

As you investigate the circumcision debate, and it is a lively one, try not to be swayed by the overheated passion of either side. Talk it through and think as calmly as you can, and do it long before the baby is born. Whatever decision you make, your son will thrive and enjoy his penis, circumcised or not.

Caring for the Uncircumcised Penis

A lot of people believe—mistakenly—that the uncircumcised penis of a baby needs to be scrupulously cleaned and cared for. Perhaps the biggest misconception is that you have to retract the foreskin and clean underneath it. "This is completely false," says Dr. Nasrallah. "You will only cause more problems."

The foreskin of an uncircumcised baby stays connected to the glans, or head of the penis for months or years. Though most often the foreskin separates and can be retracted by age five, some boys won't be able to retract their foreskin until they reach puberty, and it's not a problem. Until it disconnects from the glans, there's no reason to pull back the foreskin. Cleaning beneath it can cause a child pain and the risk of bleeding, irritation, or skin damage.

How should you care for an uncircumcised penis? Just gently wash the outside with soap and water, and dry it as you would any part of the body. Beyond that don't do anything. No need to use a Q-tip. No need to scrub vigorously or to use an antiseptic. Dr. Nasrallah's advice is clear: "Leave it alone."

Unfortunately, this advice is not widely known, even among many physicians. In years past, most American boys got circumcised, so pediatricians had little experience with uncircumcised penises. Now more parents are leaving their boys uncircumcised and some health care providers are giving them bad advice, urging mothers to push back the skin and clean thoroughly, Dr. Nasrallah says.

"I would say in my practice the most irate parents are those who come in and have had their little kid tortured because of improper advice regarding the care of the foreskin," Dr. Nasrallah says. "The pediatrician has yelled at the mother for not pulling it back far enough and not keeping it clean and then I tell them, 'No, you don't have to that.' And they want to know, 'Well then why did my pediatrician order me to?'" Good question.

If your baby is uncircumcised, you should occasionally watch him urinate to make sure the opening at the tip of the foreskin is big enough for a normal stream of urine flow. If it comes out in a slow trickle, that's something to talk to your doctor about.

TIPS FROM THE AAP

Here are some tips from the American Academy of Pediatrics information sheet on caring for an uncircumcised penis:

- Never force the foreskin to retract over the head of the penis!
- Wash the penis with soap and water as you would any other body part. When the foreskin begins to naturally separate, it is okay to retract it to a comfortable level for washing.
- When the foreskin separates from the glans, skin cells are shed. These may look like white lumps, resembling pearls, under the foreskin. These are called smegma, and it is normal and nothing to worry about.
- When your son is able to wash on his own, teach him to gently pull back the foreskin to wash with soap and water and then pull the foreskin back over the glans.
- Things to watch out for in an uncircumcised baby: a stream of urine that is never more than a trickle; the baby appears to be uncomfortable during urinating; the foreskin becomes considerably red or swollen.

Later, once the foreskin has separated from the tip of the penis on its own, then it's okay to gently pull down the skin and clean underneath. When he's old enough, teach your son to clean it himself. He should also learn to keep the foreskin dry, since skin that's chronically wet with urine may become irritated.

Caring for the Circumcised Penis

Usually a penis heals in seven to ten days after a circumcision. During that time, the tip may look quite red and there may be a yellowish secretion. This is normal. After circumcision, a small bit of foreskin often remains. Once the wound from the circumcision heals, gently push down the skin and clean around it. But as with an uncircumcised penis, you should not force the remaining foreskin back.

WHEN TO CALL A DOCTOR AFTER A CIRCUMCISION

- If your baby doesn't urinate normally within four to six hours after circumcision.
- If his penis bleeds steadily, oozes blood, or forms large blood clots. (There should be no more than a drop or two of blood for a day or two.)
- If redness around the tip of the penis grows worse after three to five days.
- If the normal yellow discharge or coating around the tip of the penis lasts longer than a week.
- If your son's doctor applied a PlastiBell and the plastic ring does not fall off after a week to ten days.
- If the baby develops a fever.

THE FAMILY JEWELS
Some Things to Know About the Family Jewels

It's inevitable. One of the first things that many moms and dads really notice about their newborn boy is his genitals. For many parents, those first looks can bring quite a shock, and while they may have questions or concerns about their new baby's genitalia, they are often embarrassed to ask doctors or male relatives. When a boy is born, his penis and testicles are often very red and large. This can be striking, like your boy is some kind of oversexed superstud. But don't worry. The redness and swelling is caused by exposure to female hormones from the placenta and fades in a few days or weeks.

It's important to remember that the genitals of baby boys, like those of adult men, do not all look alike. There's variation from penis to penis, as well as a number of

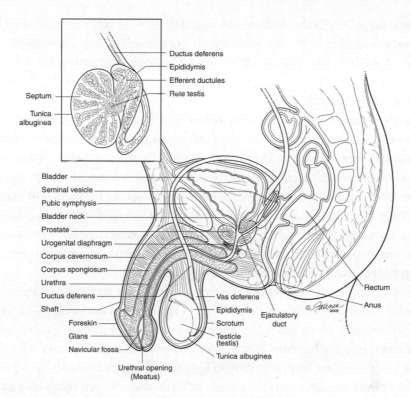

problems that can affect the genitals. Most are easily solved, and many aren't really problems at all, though they can be quite alarming to parents.

Some parents worry their son's penis appears extremely small. Most of the time, a small-looking penis is actually normal in size but partially hidden inside a pad of flesh around the pubic bone in chubby babies and in young boys. In these cases, a "buried penis" or "inconspicuous penis," as it is called, will fully emerge as the boy grows. Sometimes, though, the problem persists beyond childhood, especially in overweight children. In this case, some experts recommend surgery to give the boy a more normal-looking penis, but this is controversial. Doctors can usually determine early whether a buried penis will unbury; the physician simply pushes on the baby fat and sees if the penis projects forward.

In rare cases, a boy can be born with an extremely small penis, which doctors call *micropenis.* Doctors define micropenis as about three quarters of an inch in length stretched at birth. This is usually the result of a testosterone deficiency during fetal development and is normally treated with testosterone and other male hormones. Most boys who get hormone treatments end up with a penis of normal length.

A couple of other things often surprise or worry parents. Baby boys, even young infants, get erections. This is completely normal and nothing to be concerned about.

Even more surprising is that babies—boys and girls—can have firm, swollen breasts for several weeks after birth. Sometimes their breasts will release a few drops of milk, the result of the big dose of Mom's hormones a baby gets in the womb.

Troubles with Testicles

A baby's *scrotum*—the sac of skin below and behind the penis that holds the testicles—can be wrinkly and red or small and smooth. The testicles can move around in the scrotum, but sometimes after about six months of age they may move up so far they seem to disappear. Doctors refer to this as *retractile testicles.* It usually happens in response to fear and cold. Sometimes the mere act of looking for them will make them retract. They come back down into the scrotum just as rapidly when in a warm, safe situation. Fortunately, there are no medical problems associated with retractile testicles. The real problem with retractile testicles is they are often confused with a more serious problem, undescended testicles (*cryptorchidism).*

To understand undescended testicles, let's look at how testicles are formed. They form inside the abdomen when a male fetus is six or seven weeks old. Shortly before birth, they migrate down from the abdomen, traveling through a tube called the *inguinal canal* into the scrotum. Sometimes one or both testicles don't start or complete the journey before birth and remain lodged in the abdomen. About 3 percent of boys have at least one undescended testicle at birth, and it's even more common with premature boys.

The good news is that in most cases, the testicles come down by themselves in the first three or four months after birth without treatment. If, however, the testicles have not dropped by the time the boy turns one—and they don't for about 35 percent of boys with undescended testicles—then it makes sense to help get them where they ought to be. Why does it matter? There are several reasons.

First, testicles are in the scrotum and not the abdomen for a reason: Sperm don't like it hot. It's several degrees cooler in the scrotal sac, which hangs free from the warmth of the body. Testicles that aren't in the scrotum simply can't make many sperm, and that can greatly reduce a man's fertility.

The other reason to seek treatment is that undescended testicles are at a higher risk of developing cancer. Further, it's difficult to detect testicular cancer when the testicle is not accessible and can't be examined.

Then there's what may be, for your boy, the most important reason: The scrotum of a boy with undescended testicles looks different, and that can result in anxiety or expose him to teasing.

The most common treatment is a minor outpatient surgery called an *orchiopexy.* A small incision is made in the groin that allows the surgeon to move the testicle down. This procedure works best if the testicle is in the groin area, not higher up in the abdomen. A more complicated surgery with a laparoscope, a kind of surgical telescope with tiny instruments, can be used when the testicles are in the abdomen. An alternative to surgery is hormone injections, which may stimulate the testicle to move down on its own.

Sometimes doctors find the testicle is either abnormal or missing. In that case, the abnormal testicle can be removed and a prosthetic inserted in the scrotum to simulate the appearance of normal genitals. For more on this in older boys and teens, see chapter 6.

Swollen Testicles

Besides being bathed in mother's hormones, a baby's scrotum may be swollen for other reasons. Fortunately, most are not serious. Here are some of the most common causes:

Hernias and Hydroceles

The most common cause of swollen testicles in young boys is a *hydrocele,* which means "water sac" in Greek. When the inguinal canal—the opening that allowed the testicle to drop down—doesn't close, fluid leaks into the scrotum. Usually hydrocele happens to only one testicle, but occasionally, both sides are affected. Usually it's painless and it generally disappears within a year without treatment. If not, outpatient surgery can take care of it.

A doctor can identify a hydrocele by shining a light on the scrotum, in a procedure called transillumination. An area of the scrotum will glow red when a hydrocele is present because the light can shine through. A solid mass, such as a tumor, blocks the light.

A hydrocele is often accompanied by an inguinal hernia, though hernias also happen on their own. Between 1 percent and 3 percent of full-term babies are born with hydrocele and hernia, though the rate is higher in premature babies. A hernia is a piece of intestine that bulges through the wall of the abdomen or slips down into the groin, often creating a painful swelling in the scrotum. Sometimes, the bit of intestine slides into the scrotum when a boy is standing and moves back out when he lies down. A hernia can also appear when the baby strains or cries, or anytime there is increased pressure from the abdomen that makes the bulge grow. It usually recedes again when pressure subsides. As long as the bulge can be pushed back in, there is no danger.

Occasionally, the intestine gets stuck in the groin and kinks. This can be painful and cause fussiness and vomiting. It can also cut off the blood supply to this part of the intestine. The bulge will then become red, hard, and cannot be pushed back. This is a medical emergency and the doctor should be called, since immediate surgery is needed.

To avoid these complications, inguinal hernias should be repaired surgically. The operation is routine, but it does require general anesthesia. Hernias can run in families, and girls can be born with hernias, too. Most inguinal hernias are found on the right side, and they are nine times more common in boys. Another type of hernia is called an *umbilical hernia,* and this happens to both boys and girls. Here a piece of intestine pushes through the abdominal wall near the navel. It usually closes on its own and rarely needs treatment.

Testicular Torsion

Testicular torsion is rare, and that's a good thing. It's painful even to talk about. When the *spermatic cord* gets twisted, it cuts off the blood supply to a testicle and other connecting tissues in the scrotum (see diagram on page 49). It most often occurs during puberty, although in about 5 percent of cases, testicular torsion occurs before birth or shortly after, according to Dr. Nasrallah. At birth, the doctor may feel a firm mass in the testicle rather than the typical spongy, soft consistency. In older babies, it can be hard to recognize. Parents often see their boy in distress—crying a lot and perhaps vomiting—but have no idea where the pain is coming from. That's one reason it's important to undress a distressed baby and look for signs in the groin. Here's what to look for:

- swelling on one side of the scrotum, most often the right.
- one testicle that is elevated in the scrotum.
- extreme tenderness in the whole area.

Testicular torsion is a serious medical emergency. It's extremely painful, and if not treated in a few hours, the testicle will be seriously damaged and need to be removed. Get to the doctor immediately. In some cases, a doctor may be able to manually untwist the cord. If not, surgery is required. (For more about torsion in older boys, see chapter 6.)

Problems with the Penis
Hypospadias

Hypospadias is a condition in which the opening of the urethra is not located on the tip of the penis, as it should be, but at the bottom of the shaft, somewhere between tip and base. As a result, urine flows out from the middle of the penis instead of the tip. As a boy grows and potty trains, hypospadias may make it difficult for him to stand while urinating.

A few years ago, I met a young couple who had just given birth to a boy we'll call Jacob.* Jacob was a beautiful, healthy child but he had hypospadias and his parents were beside themselves. Like most people, they had never heard of this problem before, and were embarrassed and afraid about the future. Fortunately, this is one problem that can be corrected quite easily.

There appears to be a wide variation in where the opening of the urethra occurs, even in "normal" males. One 1995 study, in the *Journal of Urology,* found that of five hundred "normal" men only 55 percent had an opening exactly at the tip of the penis. Even men with hypospadias reported no cosmetic or functional problems.

No one knows exactly what causes hypospadias, but it seems to be on the rise. The Centers for Disease Control reports that it is the most common congenital anomaly of the penis and has more than doubled over the past thirty years; it now affects almost one in one hundred newborn boys. Not all experts are convinced this represents a real increase in the number of cases. They argue that hypospadias is more likely to be reported today than it was in the past. It sometimes runs in families and if a child is born with hypospadias, there is a small chance of finding it in another family member. Nevertheless, many experts believe that the dramatic increase of hypospadias may have environmental causes. They believe that exposure to pollutants that mimic estrogen may impede the circulation of testosterone in the developing male fetus.

Testosterone is essential to the formation of the urethra, which occurs somewhere between the eighth and twelfth weeks of gestation. Triggered by testosterone, two folds of tissue fuse together leaving a tube between them, which forms the urethra. If they don't fully fuse, a hole may be left anywhere from the base of the penis to the area near the tip.

Hypospadias is sometimes accompanied by another problem, called *chordee,* which causes the penis to bend downward when erect. If the bend is significant, it can be corrected surgically. Boys born with hypospadias should not be circumcised at birth because the foreskin may be needed later to correct the problem.

The most important thing about hypospadias is this: As alarming and strange as it may seem, it can usually be solved easily. Jacob's family is a good reminder. Although families are understandably upset about the condition and worried about what it will mean for their son, surgery to repair hypospadias has improved dramatically in recent years. Rather than multiple surgeries starting at age two, today just one procedure performed by six months is typically needed. Jacob had his when he was three months old. It was quick and easy, and now at age five, it is almost impossible to tell there was ever anything unusual about his penis.

Epispadias

A similar but rarer condition is called epispadias. In boys with epispadias the opening to the urethra is on top of the penis instead of on the tip. In some cases, these boys may also have a serious malformation of the bladder called *bladder exstrophy,* where the bladder is outside the abdomen and actually exposed to the air. Once again, these extremely rare problems can normally be corrected with surgery.

A Tight Squeeze

Another occasional problem occurs when a hair (a loose hair from a parent or even the child) gets wrapped tightly around the penis. This can be very painful, and if it happens to a baby, you may be mystified about the cause of his discomfort. This is another good reason you should undress an inconsolable baby and check his whole body, including his penis.

For more on genital conditions that affect older boys and how to recognize them and their treatments, see chapter 6.

IS IT A BOY OR IS IT A GIRL? THE INTERSEX CHILD

Discovering the sex of a newborn child as it emerged from its mother's womb used to be one of life's great dramatic moments. These days, few parents leave this discovery to the day of birth, and even those who do usually know for sure within a minute of birth whether to paint the nursery pink or blue. However, in some births a baby's gender is unclear even after it emerges from the womb. Few things are more confusing and frightening to new parents.

Babies of unclear gender are more common than most people think. Approximately 1 in every 2,000 to 3,000 newborns comes into the world with "ambiguous" genitals; that is, their genitals differ in size or shape from what is considered "normal" for the child's genetic sex. These intersex babies, as they are known, may have no evident testicles but seem to have a penis. Or they may have a penis so small that it appears to be a clitoris, but they also have testicles. Intersex babies are the result of a number of hormonal or, more rarely, chromosomal variations from the normal pattern. Here are some of the main causes of intersexuality and the ways children express them:

Congenital Adrenal Hyperplasia (CAH)

By far the most common cause of intersexuality, CAH is a disorder in which either an XX (chromosomally female) or XY (chromosomally male) child has an enzyme deficiency that causes the adrenal glands to enlarge and function abnormally, producing too little corticosteroid (cortisone) and too much androgen (such as testosterone.) When a female fetus gets bathed in excess testosterone, it triggers the clitoris to grow larger and can cause the *labia,* or vaginal lips, to partially close. Her internal organs (the ovaries, Fallopian tubes, and uterus), however, remain normal. An XY (male) fetus with CAH will not have ambiguous genitals. He may have early puberty or he may have no symptoms at all.

The most severe form of this disorder, known as *salt-wasting CAH,* is life-threatening. It disrupts the adrenal gland's production of the hormone aldosterone, which maintains the balance between salt and water in the body. Boys or girls with this problem can go into shock and die unless treated promptly. Children with severe CAH must take medication daily, and missing even a day or two may prompt a life-threatening adrenal crisis. The condition can be detected with a blood test and can even be diagnosed prenatally in affected families. Prenatal treatment of the mother with corticosteroids can minimize the effects on the newborn.

Androgen Insensitivity Syndrome (AIS)

This genetic condition leaves the cells of an XY (chromosomally male) baby either partly or completely unable to respond to androgens, or male hormones. An XY fetus with complete AIS will develop testes and release a hormone that prevents development of a uterus and other internal female structures, the same as any other normal XY baby. However, because the cells fail to respond to testosterone, the baby will be born with external genitals that are female and not male, along with undescended testicles, giving the baby the appearance of a normal girl. In some cases, the problem goes undetected until adulthood, when a woman fails to have menstrual periods. Because her internal structures are undeveloped she is infertile.

Partial AIS (PAIS) expresses itself in a variety of ways, some more obvious than others. Affected babies may have slightly impaired, greatly impaired, or almost no response to androgens. As a result, babies with PAIS can look like females with slightly enlarged clitorises or like boys with small or average penises. In most cases, the problem is obvious at birth.

Klinefelter's Syndrome

(See page 36.)

Controversy Brews

At one time people born with ambiguous genitalia, now called intersex, were called hermaphrodites or pseudohermaphrodites. The change in terminology in many ways mirrors the revolution in knowledge about and attitudes toward this very sensitive condition. The dilemma for the parents begins the day they find out their child is intersex. Parents are typically shocked, afraid, and desperate for answers, which doctors scramble to provide. The American Academy of Pediatrics calls such births a "social emergency" that requires "urgent medical attention." Since the late 1950s, the practice has been for a team of pediatricians, endocrinologists, and psychologists to assess the baby's chromosomal gender, hormonal balance, and anatomical structure, and to advise the parents on whether to raise the baby as a boy or girl. Then, with the parents' consent, they assign the baby a sex, and surgically remove or alter sexual organs that do not fit that choice.

That means in practice that in girls with CAH, for example, doctors may recommend surgically reducing the size of a significantly enlarged clitoris. Doctors have argued that this surgery should take place in the first year or two of a child's life in order to minimize psychological distress to the child—and to the parents—of growing up with genitals that are markedly different from other children's.

But what if it's not clear what the right decision is? What if the sexual organs are surgically removed, and that later turns out to have been a mistake? What if the surgery to reduce the size of the clitoris disrupts important nerves impairing the person's ability to enjoy genital stimulation or reach an orgasm? For many years, leading experts didn't worry about the sexual or psychological consequences of making a "wrong" decision because they assumed that the child's sexual identity was malleable. If the parents, the professionals, and the world at large treated a child as a boy, then "he" would come to identify himself as a boy, since that's all that he knew. Unfortunately, there has been little scientific follow-up in most cases of infant genital surgery and it is hard to draw any broad conclusions about what happens to these children as adults. It has been generally assumed that most do okay, but without studies proving this, there is really no way to know with any certainty. This issue came to national attention following journalist John Colapinto's profile of David Reimer in *Rolling Stone* magazine and then in a full-length book, *As Nature Made Him*. Though David was not, in fact, born with ambiguous genitalia his story is a cautionary tale of what can go wrong when assumptions about an individual's gender are made in infancy.

The David Reimer Story

The David Reimer story begins when he was eight months old, when David and his identical twin were being circumcised. During David's circumcision the doctor made a horrible slip and destroyed his penis. His horrified parents turned to John Money, a psychologist and renowned sexuality expert at Johns Hopkins University in Baltimore, who had become an outspoken champion of the possibilities for sexual transformation. He believed that children were born, psychologically speaking, without a fixed gender identity and developed one only through their experiences growing up.

Babies born with ambiguous genitals could, in Money's view, be made into either sex. At the time, penile reconstruction was not feasible, and surgeons were better able to fashion genitalia resembling a vulva than an appendage resembling a penis. Hence, most babies with ambiguous genitals were destined to become girls. That was the case for David, who would be renamed Brenda.

Though David was born a boy with unambiguously male genitals, Money advised David's parents to turn him into a girl, through reconstructive surgery, female hormones, and raising him as they would a girl. They debated and agonized briefly, then decided to follow the advice of this famous and supremely confident man whom they "looked up to like a God," as David's mother later told Colapinto. At twenty-two months, David's testicles were removed and he began his life as Brenda.

Money wrote about the case in papers and books; discussed it in lectures and media interviews. He portrayed the treatment as a great success that had left "Brenda" a normal girl, interested in dolls and feminine clothes, while her twin brother played with cars and gas pumps. "Her behavior is . . . that of an active little girl," he wrote in one paper, "clearly different by contrast from the boyish ways of her brother."

Money's claims were, in fact, completely inaccurate. "Brenda" was wildly unhappy. She got into fights frequently, refused to play with dolls, and insisted on urinating standing up. She flunked first grade, was miserable and virtually friendless at school, and, when she hit puberty, resisted taking estrogen and refused to have surgery to create a vagina. When she eventually learned the truth about her history, she insisted on a very different kind of surgery—surgery that would return "her" to being a male.

For many years, Money's theories, bolstered by the supposedly successful adjustment "Brenda" had made as a girl, were the principal rationale for the standard method of treating intersex babies with surgery and hormones. But some of these intersex children have now grown up and, as adults, are outraged by what was done to them. Some have even undergone surgery to reverse the sexual assignment given by doctors.

Activists Fight Against Shame, Secrecy, and Surgery

One of these adult children, Cheryl Chase, was born in 1956 with ambiguous genitals including what could have been interpreted either as a large clitoris or a small penis. At eighteen months, she underwent a clitorectomy and was raised as a girl, leaving her no way to have an orgasm and no knowledge of her true history. In her early twenties, she gradually uncovered the truth of her birth and began to contact other intersex adults. Her efforts bore fruit and, in the early 1990s, she and others founded the Intersex Society of North America (ISNA.) Today, the group works to change the way intersex children are treated, campaigning against the standard practice of performing irreversible surgery on intersex children, then concealing the truth as they age. Says Chase: "Every child should be allowed to grow up free of shame, secrecy, and unwanted sexual surgery."

The group argues that children born with ambiguous genitals should be evaluated at birth and given a preliminary sex assignment. The medical team, in consultation with the parents, should try to make the best choice they can at that moment. They should raise the baby accordingly but refrain from genital surgery unless necessary for the health of the child. Once old enough to make the decision, the child can then determine whether he or she wishes to change the preliminary gender assignment given at birth.

As these children age, they should be informed about the situation and encouraged to explore their feelings and attractions. They can contact other intersex children or adults to learn from their experiences. At puberty, they should be allowed to make their own decision about whether to have surgery or hormone treatments that would shape future sexual identity.

ISNA's call for avoiding surgery until the children themselves can make informed decisions is controversial. No doubt there are people who have undergone "traditional" treatment and done well, but there have been no long-term studies on these patients. Only now are these studies being done to evaluate long-term outcomes and assess the impact of traditional recommendations. ISNA's call for a moratorium on gender surgery goes against many medical experts who argue that failing to correct genital abnormalities at an early age can negatively affect a child's body image and self-esteem and subject the child to teasing and rejection by peers. But a growing number of doctors now question the rush to surgery and endorse ISNA's call for waiting until the child can decide. All this of course leaves many parents in a difficult place. The best advice is to get as much information as possible before making a decision. See the Resources section for more information.

Boys Versus Girls

So you've made it through your pregnancy and are heading home with your new boy. You have, no doubt, spent time picking out the perfect baby outfit for the ride home and can't wait to finally get to know the new guy in your life. Coming from a family of three sisters, I was probably more excited than most to be the mother of a son. I remember bringing Harry home as one of the happiest days of my life. Some people think I am crazy, but I enjoyed every single moment of taking care of him, including changing dirty diapers. I was so thrilled and proud and so hopeful for the future. I was and still am wild about Harry!

I breast-fed my son and recommend that you do the same. There's a mountain of research that shows that breast milk is healthier than formula and contains antiviral and antibacterial substances that protect babies against a variety of infections and illnesses. Breast-fed babies have a lower incidence of many problems, including infection, anemia, diarrhea, meningitis, diabetes, gastroenteritis, asthma, constipation, and allergies.

Then there's the issue of when he sleeps—and how little you do. Some say that boys are worse sleepers than girls, and one recent study seems to bear that out. Researchers at the Debrecen Medical University surveyed one thousand mothers of newborns in Hungary and asked them about their babies' sleeping patterns. It turned out that girls established a pattern of sleeping mostly at night more quickly than boys, and they tended to sleep about thirty minutes longer at night.

I can tell you this much, as the mother of three small children: None of them let you sleep nearly enough. In my case, my daughters did seem to learn more quickly than my son how to sleep through the night. But to be fair, I have friends who claim the opposite: Their boys slept like angels and their daughters kept them up all night. Individually, babies vary enormously in their fussiness, sleeping patterns, personalities, and physical development. Still, when you look at large groups of babies, some differences between the sexes do emerge, differences in their physiology and level of development. Boys are less developed at birth, about four to six weeks behind girls, according to some researchers. Their brains and nervous systems are a bit less formed. They also tend to be slightly larger than baby girls, especially in head and chest size.

Baby boys have lower baseline heart rates and are more reactive than girls. In one recent study, the heart rates of two-day-old boys jumped when doctors startled them by slapping the table; the heart rates of baby girls barely changed.

There are a number of other biological differences between boys and girls. Perhaps because of their head start in development, girls tend to walk a bit earlier than boys. Girls also tend to mouth their first words at a younger age and develop language mastery sooner. Boys catch up later, but in the early years, girls are generally more verbal. Boys, on the other hand, are more physically active, as anyone who's spent time at a preschool notices. Most boys are racing, zooming, jumping—virtual motion machines next to impossible to slow down.

Conventional wisdom to the contrary, testosterone levels do not differ much between boys and girls in the years before puberty. The hormone is detectable in the blood of both (as is estrogen) but at extremely low levels. Estrogen levels are higher in girls, however, which may have something to do with the fact that girls tend to begin puberty earlier than boys.

MEDICAL PROBLEMS MORE COMMON TO BOYS

A number of medical problems are more common in young boys. Some may show up in the first few weeks or months after birth. Others may not be apparent for several years. Young boys, for instance, are more likely to have respiratory problems and gastroenteritis, and to suffer accidental injuries. Boys are more likely to suffer from asthma, although that changes around puberty when girls begin to suffer in greater numbers. Older boys are more likely than girls to wet their beds and have the bowel problem *encopresis* that causes them to soil their pants (see chapter 4). Here are a few of the medical problems that affect boys more frequently.

Gastroenteritis

This is a big word for a severely upset stomach that causes diarrhea and vomiting. Virtually every child gets it, usually once or twice a year during the first few years, but boys tend to get it more often. It can be very serious. More than 200,000 American kids under five are hospitalized with it every year, and some three hundred die, according to *American Family Physician* (1999). Usually caused by a virus or bacteria, gastroenteritis normally goes away in a few days. The most serious possible complication is dehydration. The diarrhea and/or vomiting rids the body of critical fluids. If your child has gastroenteritis, the most important thing is to make sure he gets lots of fluids. The American Academy of Family Physicians has suggestions for coping with gastroenteritis:

- If you're breast- or bottle-feeding your baby, keep doing it, and try to do it more often.
- If an older child has diarrhea but isn't vomiting, he can eat regular food. Encourage him to drink as much liquid as possible. Most food and drinks are okay, though fatty foods and sugary drinks might make the diarrhea worse. Noodles and rice are good choices, as are fruits, vegetables, and yogurt.
- If he's nauseated but not vomiting, give him small sips of liquid every few minutes. Frequent sips will keep him hydrated and are less likely to cause vomiting than drinking a lot at once.
- If he's vomiting repeatedly and can't keep solid food down, give him an oral rehydration solution. These drinks (such as Pedialyte, Infalyte, or Rehydralyte) contain a mix of water, sugar, and mineral salts and are available at your local grocery or drugstore. They all work the same and are safe if you follow directions. Begin with one or two teaspoons every one or two minutes. This adds up to over a cup an hour. Even if he vomits again, a lot of this fluid will stay down. If he does well, give him bigger sips a little less often, every five minutes or so.
- Take your child to the doctor if he's under two years old and his vomiting and diarrhea last more than twelve hours. This is important if he's vomiting often, has a lot of diarrhea, or has a fever.
- Call your doctor right away if your child:
  - Has pain in the stomach along with the vomiting.
  - Has blood in the diarrhea.
  - Is under six months of age.
  - Has any of these signs or symptoms of dehydration: He has dry lips and mouth; is passing little urine or urine that's dark in color or strong-smelling; has little or no tears when crying (babies), or has sunken eyes (babies or toddlers). Also if he's dizzy, pays no attention to toys or TV, is hard to wake up, or vomits up everything he eats and drinks.

Other Woes That Boys Are Prone To

In babies with a condition called *pyloric stenosis,* a muscular valve doesn't open as it should and the contents of the stomach can't pass into the small intestine. Babies with this problem usually start to vomit quite forcefully during their second or third week of life. They may also lose weight and seem listless. See a doctor right away. Surgery may be needed to spread open the valve. This is one of the most common surgeries performed on newborns.

Babies with *Hirschsprung's disease* have problems moving digested food through their colons because they are missing nerve endings that direct the gut muscles to contract. If this causes an obstruction, the baby may start vomiting and his stomach can become bloated and painful. Surgery to empty the gut and remove a portion of the colon seems to solve the problem 90 percent of the time. The problem can be genetic in nature, but the cause can also be unknown.

A boy is much more likely than a girl to show symptoms of a rare genetically induced enzyme deficiency called *glucose-6-phosphate-dehydrogenase* (G6PD). African-American males have an especially high risk. It doesn't usually cause problems, but if a person with G6PD takes medications such as antimalarial drugs, sulfa drugs, or aspirin, they can become anemic. If your son has symptoms of G6PD such as fatigue, pale or yellowing skin or eyes, shortness of breath, rapid heart rate, or dark urine, see the doctor right away.

DEVELOPMENTAL, PSYCHIATRIC, AND NEUROLOGICAL PROBLEMS

In almost every psychiatric or neurological condition that begins in infancy or early childhood, boys predominate. Boys are more likely than girls to suffer from mental retardation, autism spectrum disorders, stuttering, Tourette's syndrome, oppositional defiant disorder (ODD), attention deficit hyperactivity disorder (AD/HD), and bed-wetting, among others. Males are also more likely to develop brain tumors, leukemia, and cerebral palsy, and to have several other neurological abnormalities. Some problems, such as dyslexia and other learning disabilities, may not become visible until school age. Other disorders, including the following, may become apparent sooner.

Autism and Other Pervasive Developmental Disorders

Autism hampers normal brain development and hinders a child's ability to interact with others. It is one of the most common of all developmental disabilities; somewhere between half a million and 1.5 million Americans have it or a related form of pervasive developmental disorder (PDD). Fully 80 percent are boys. The most recent statistics from the Centers for Disease Control (CDC) (2003) indicate that autism spectrum disorders occur in 3.4 children per 1,000.

Children and adults with autism have trouble speaking, playing, or relating to others. They may make unusual movements, called stereotypies, such as flapping their hands or rocking, and interact in unusual ways with objects and people. They may be easily overstimulated from things they see, hear, touch, smell, or taste. And some autistic children, though not most, can be aggressive or injure themselves.

Many autistic children might seem normal in their development for the first two years. Then, around two and a half, parents may begin to notice delays in language, play, or interaction with others. The symptoms and severity of autism can vary greatly—in some children it can be mild; in others, severe.

People with autism respond to their environment in different ways. Some have trouble controlling their physical and mental reactions. They may, for instance, find it too stimulating to maintain eye contact, be touched by other people, or be close to them. As a result, some people with autism withdraw from social contact, even with family members.

Autism can be difficult to diagnose. If your son is having any of these problems, check out the list of symptoms below. If he exhibits seven or more of these behaviors, get a full evaluation.

Signs and Symptoms of Autism

- Inappropriate laughing and giggling
- Lack of speech, impaired speech, or "lost" speech (i.e., child loses words he once had)
- Does not respond to name being called or orient in the speaker's direction
- Appears to have no fear of typical dangers
- Apparent insensitivity to pain or extreme sensitivity to pain
- Repeats words or sounds in place of normal language
- Spins objects repeatedly
- Not interested in cuddling and may resist it as well as other physical contact
- Ritualistic behaviors
- Uneven motor skills. For instance, he can't kick a ball but can stack blocks
- Doesn't make eye contact
- Difficulty in mixing with other children
- Resists change in routine or changes in environment or changes in people he is familiar with (for example, upset over new furniture or Mom's new haircut)
- Marked physical overactivity or extreme passivity
- Crying tantrums and extreme distress for no discernible reason

People with autism seem to be more prone to allergies or food sensitivities, possibly because their immune systems are somehow impaired. Wheat and dairy sensitivities seem to be especially common. If you suspect your son has allergies, or is sensitive to certain foods, talk to a doctor. You may want to try eliminating suspect food from his diet and see if his symptoms change.

While autism is a lifelong condition that can't be "cured," many people with autism learn to function quite well and lead full and independent lives—going to college, marrying, having a career. They may have trouble communicating and interacting socially for the rest of their lives, but with support and assistance, many people with autism are able to cope with their disability quite well.

The incidence of autism has risen sharply in recent years, alarming many parents and public health researchers. Several years ago, British researcher Andrew Wakefield, of the gastroenterology unit at the Royal Free Hospital in London published a paper about a group of twelve young patients with autism who had been immunized with the measles, mumps, and rubella (MMR) vaccine. The paper's suggestion of a possible connection touched off public concern that the vaccine might cause autism. Since then, additional studies have found no evidence of any connection between the vaccine and autism, and public health officials in many countries continue to recommend the MMR vaccine and believe it's safe.

But that didn't end the worries about vaccines. In 1999, researchers discovered that vaccines contained greater quantities than previously realized of thimerosal, a preservative that contains ethylmercury—a compound related to mercury. Mercury is a known neurotoxin; a different form, methylmercury, has been shown to lower the IQ of children whose mothers ingested it in contaminated fish or grain. Thimerosal has now been removed from all vaccines. At the end of 2002, in a move that enraged many consumer advocates, Congress passed a law (Vaccine Provision in the Homeland Security Act of November 2002) that shielded vaccine makers from liability for any health problems the vaccines may have caused.

Tourette's Syndrome and Other Tic Disorders

People with tic disorders exhibit repeated involuntary movements or sounds, known as tics. They may, for instance, jerk their head, shrug their shoulders, blink their eyes, clear their throat, sniff, thrust their arm, kick, or jump. These are known as motor tics. They may also exhibit vocal tics, unusual sounds or noises such as grunting, barking, coughing, humming, whistling, or honking. A surprisingly large number of children (as many as 20 percent, according to a 2001 study by researchers from the University of Rochester Medical Center) develop a mild tic disorder at some point. Far fewer, around 8 percent, according to the Rochester neurologists, develop Tourette's syndrome (TS), the best-known kind of tic disorder.

People with Tourette's syndrome have motor tics and at least one kind of vocal tic. Roughly three fourths of people with Tourette's are male. Their symptoms begin during childhood, almost always by age fifteen. The motor tics tend to start around age seven, and the vocal tics may begin a year or two later. The most famous symptom of Tourette's, repeated swearing, is actually quite uncommon, occurring in only 10 to 15 percent of patients. The severity of symptoms varies from one child to another and can also depend on the amount of stress a child is under, as well as the presence of conditions commonly seen with Tourette's such as obsessive-compulsive disorder, attention deficit hyperactivity disorder (AD/HD), and anxiety. When a person with TS is under a lot of stress, their tics may increase; when relaxed or focused on an absorbing task, they often decrease.

Fortunately, most people with TS have relatively mild symptoms that are not disabling, so medication isn't needed. For those with more serious symptoms, there are a variety of medications to help control tics. But medicating people with TS and AD/HD is an imperfect science. Boys with both conditions are often put on stimulants that improve their attention problems, but this can increase their tics.

Various kinds of therapy can also be helpful. Family therapy can help the whole family deal with problems posed when one member has TS. Behavioral therapy can sometimes help patients manage their tics. And biofeedback and relaxation techniques can help reduce stress and minimize tics.

Obsessive-Compulsive Disorder

Some people, children and adults alike, worry a lot, but people with obsessive-compulsive disorder seem to worry all the time. Their thoughts get stuck on certain fears, which repeat endlessly like a record stuck in a groove. They may worry about catching germs, whether they turned off the stove at home, or whether they're making the right choice in even the most minor of decisions. They cope with these fears by continuing to repeat certain actions: They wash their hands repeatedly, or return home several times to check the locks and windows or to make sure the gas is turned off. These behaviors can take up a lot of time, and interfere with a person's life.

In adults, slightly more women than men are believed to have OCD. But in children just the reverse is true, researchers say: Nearly twice as many boys have OCD as girls. It can begin as early as preschool, but the peak age for OCD symptoms to begin is around ten. Half of all adults with OCD say their symptoms began before they turned fifteen. OCD is usually treated with antidepressants, cognitive-behavioral therapy (in which children learn to reframe and redirect their obsessive thoughts), or both. As always, if children are prescribed antidepressants, they must be monitored very closely for side effects. One rare risk that researchers were again looking into as this book went to press was the possibility that antidepressants could cause some children to become so agitated that they consider committing suicide.

Epilepsy

Epilepsy is the third most common neurological condition and is believed to be more common among males. People with epilepsy have repeated, unprovoked seizures. These seizures can begin any time, but about 20 percent of epileptics have their first seizure by the age of five, and half by age twenty-five. Some 2.5 million Americans have epilepsy; one third are children.

The causes of epilepsy are not well understood. In fact, in most cases, no one cause can be clearly identified. Young children are believed to develop epilepsy as the result of a virus, their oxygen supply being cut off during pregnancy, or as a result of trauma to the head. Older people may develop it as a result of car accidents or strokes.

Epilepsy cannot be cured, but it can usually be controlled with medication, which can prevent seizures or greatly reduce their frequency. There are a number of different drugs used to treat epilepsy, and it often takes some trial and error to find the best drug, with the fewest side effects, for each person.

A seizure, of course, is a medical emergency. If someone you know has one, try to clear a space around the person so they won't hurt themselves by bumping or crashing into things. Call 911 immediately. Do not stick anything in the mouth of the victim.

EMOTIONAL DIFFERENCES BETWEEN BOYS AND GIRLS

Most children, of course, don't get any of the aforementioned physical or neurological problems. So for most parents, any differences between their sons and daughters will mostly be matters of individual personality. Still, there are some subtle differences in the emotional responses of boys and girls. A number of researchers have noticed that baby boys, in general, seem more sensitive. Harvard researchers Edward Z. Tronick, Ph.D., and M. Katherine Weinberg, Ph.D., have spent many years comparing baby boys to baby girls and have observed that, in general, "infant boys are more emotionally reactive than girls . . . and display more distress and demands for contact than do girls."

In one recent study, Weinberg put six-month-old babies through some mildly upsetting events, then had their mothers stand by, stone-faced and unresponsive. After a short time, the moms were asked to reconnect with the infants in a normal way. The boys tended to fuss, cry, and squirm and to try hard to get attention from Mom. The girls, on the other hand, were much more able to soothe and calm themselves, by sucking their thumbs or distracting themselves by looking away. "The boys had much greater difficulty regulating their emotional states on their own," Weinberg noted.

This difference in sensitivity doesn't evaporate right away. When researchers at the University of Arizona played tapes of a crying baby to kindergarten and second-grade children, the boys became more upset. Some became quite agitated and their heart rates jumped—they were the most likely to rush over and turn off the speakers. The girls, on the other hand, stayed calmer and were more likely to try to soothe the baby.

Somewhere along the line, though, these patterns start to shift and boys begin to express less emotion than girls. Why? That issue is at the heart of a great debate over the differences between males and females, a debate that has raged for centuries, most recently with renewed vigor.

The Great Gender Debate

Nature or nurture, biology or culture, genes or socialization: What are the key factors that go into making up a child's personality and disposition? The debate on this question swings like a pendulum. In the 1960s and '70s, researchers began to question the notion that the roles and personalities of males and females in our culture were shaped solely by biology. The belief that males were "wired" for aggression and dominance and that females were wired to be maternal, emotional, and nurturing came under fire.

The '90s saw a major swing back toward the primacy of biology and genetics. Scientists mapped the human genome. Genes that influence personality were identified. Researchers identified key differences in the brain structure of men and women.

These gender debates reverberate loudly in the arena of child rearing. As parents striving to raise boys who will pay attention to their health and bodies, and who will develop healthy and respectful attitudes and behaviors toward themselves and others, these are important questions we grapple with daily. Many of us who believe in progressive child rearing are amazed to discover that no matter how much we strive to raise kids in an atmosphere that doesn't restrict them by gender, boys and girls quickly show fundamental differences in behavior.

My cowriter, Rob Waters, and his partner, Lenore, are raising their son in Berkeley, California, as progressive, sexually diverse, and gender-neutral a place as probably exists on the planet. Their son, Josh, now seven years old, had trucks and dolls, baseball uniforms and dress-up dresses to play with and wear as a toddler. But by age three, he was picking up sticks and turning them into guns (he's never had the "real" item), destroying blocks, and delighting in play with his bow and arrow, rockets, and anything that flew. He also loved to "battle" and play superhero games. As he grew, he was friendly toward girls but rarely sought them out as playmates. My own son, Harry, raised in New York City, acts in much the same way. He will play with girls but prefers boys and roughhousing. He spends hours wrestling, chasing, and tackling his male friends, shooting hoops, and throwing a football.

Is this just boy nature, the imprint of biology? It's not that simple. Josh watches little TV, but he has gone to school since he was two. Even in a Berkeley preschool, it's impossible to escape from the subtle—and not-so-subtle—influences of other children with older siblings and more exposure to television. So maybe when boys and girls act like, well, boys and girls, they're imitating the behaviors of other children of the same sex or picking up on signals from their own parents. Maybe they sense, a lot sooner than we might suspect, how they're supposed to act if they want to be "real" boys or "real" girls.

Most people would probably agree that boys and men in our culture express a more limited range of emotions than girls and women. But they don't start out that way. A number of different studies have found that infant boys are actually more emotionally expressive than infant girls. One study, by Dr. Weinberg, found, for instance, that six-month-old boys showed a wide range of feelings, from anger to joy, more often than girls. Another found that baby boys cry more when they're frustrated.

As children age, however, these patterns reverse, and boys express less emotion than girls, a trend that, for most, endures for the rest of their lives. "There seems to be a developmental shift in which males become less intensely facially expressive of emotions with age, whereas females become more so," writes Leslie Brody, Ph.D., an associate professor of psychology at Boston University and an expert on gender and emotions. But why?

One theory, proposed by Doris Silverman, Ph.D., an adjunct professor of psychology at New York University, is that male babies get so aroused and overstimulated that they can't make prolonged eye contact with their mothers and often cry and look away. The result, Silverman believes, is "diminished social interchange . . . and increasing separation . . . between mother and infant."

Brody thinks that mothers and daughters may develop a deeper pattern of interaction because moms have to work harder to read their less demonstrative girls. Whatever the process, boy and girl babies soon pick up cues from parents, teachers, and others about which behaviors and emotional expressions are acceptable and which are not.

Mothers, for example, flash smiles and positive expressions to girls more often than to boys. They also speak to preschool children differently, using a greater variety of emotion words with their daughters than with their sons. Even preschool teachers were found by one researcher to smile more and be more physically affectionate with girls than with boys.

But let's not just pick on moms and teachers. Dads also use more emotion words with daughters than with sons and use demands, teasing, and threats more often with boys. Men also tend to express feelings less frequently and less intensely than women. Leslie Brody points out that this kind of modeling by fathers is absorbed by sons, perpetuating the male tendency to suppress emotions. The result of all this conditioning is that by the time they're in preschool, children associate emotions such as sadness, fear, love, and warmth with females. One study in which preschoolers were observed as they talked found that girls were six times more likely to use the word *love* and twice as likely to use the word *sad*. Two other studies found that mothers didn't speak about *anger* or use the word *angry* in creating a storybook for their daughters, but did so with their sons.

A number of researchers have observed that boys are steered away from expressing or dwelling upon feelings of sadness but given license to express anger. Anger, these experts suggest, becomes the one emotion that is generally acceptable for them to express. Here's how Dan Kindlon, Ph.D., and Michael Thompson, Ph.D., put it in their best-selling book *Raising Cain*.

> When boys express ordinary levels of anger or aggression, or they turn surly and silent, their behavior is accepted as normal. If, however, they express normal levels of fear, anxiety, or sadness—emotions most often seen as feminine—the adults around them typically treat them in ways that suggest that such emotions aren't normal for a boy.

Boys are thus placed in what William Pollack, Ph.D., the Harvard child psychologist and author of *Real Boys,* calls "emotional straitjackets," their range of emotional expression sharply curtailed. As they grow, they are indoctrinated into a set of rules and behaviors Pollack refers to as the "Boy Code." "Boys learn the 'Boy Code' in sandboxes, playgrounds, schoolrooms, camps, churches, and hangouts, and are taught by peers, coaches, teachers and just about everybody else," Pollack writes.

At the heart of the "Boy Code" are four highly stereotyped ideas of how "real" boys and men should behave. These models were named by two masculinity researchers, Deborah S. David and Robert Brannon. They are:

The sturdy oak: Men should be independent and stoic and never show weakness.

Give 'em hell: The mantra of coaches throughout the land, this teaches boys that they should be macho, take risks, and use violence.

The big wheel: Men should be powerful and dominant and act like everything's under control—even if it isn't.

No sissy stuff: Real men should never cry or show feelings like warmth or empathy that might be seen as feminine. If they do, they get ridiculed as "sissies" or "fags."

What does all this have to do with health? That question is perhaps best answered by the title of a paper published twenty-five years ago by James Harrison of the Albert Einstein College of Medicine, "Warning: The Male Sex Role May Be Dangerous to Your Health." Harrison examined why men die earlier and are less healthy than women and concluded that much of the reason had to do with men adopting traditional male roles. They deny their feelings, keep problems to themselves, ignore the signals their bodies send them, and don't seek health care when they need it. "Sex-role socialization," he wrote, "accounts for the larger part of men's shorter life expectancy."

Long before adulthood, when men pay the price of poorer physical health and shorter longevity, the negative consequences of adopting the "Boy Code" begin in ways large and small. We'll discuss those problems as we explore some of the social, emotional, and psychological issues that our boys grapple with and which profoundly affect their ability to learn, love, and find happiness and health.

IS THE ENVIRONMENT DAMAGING THE HEALTH OF OUR CHILDREN?

Taken by themselves, recent findings about health problems in men and boys don't seem especially earth-shattering. The incidence of testicular cancer grew by more than 100 percent over a recent forty-year period, but it is still a rare disease. The number of U.S. boys born with hypospadias is believed to have doubled, but it can usually be treated quite effectively. The number of boys born with undescended testicles has also risen sharply. And then there were those reports that started emerging a decade ago about men's declining sperm counts, and the growing demand for fertility treatments from couples having trouble conceiving a baby, often because the man is infertile.

What do these problems have in common? Obviously, they all involve the male reproductive system. What's not so obvious is that all could have a common cause. That, at least, is what a growing number of scientists now suggest. "These conditions do not occur at random," a Danish researcher, Dr. Niels Skakkebaek, told a European conference on reproduction recently. "They may all be symptoms of an underlying problem." Skakkebaek and his colleagues have even coined a new name for this cluster of conditions, *testicular dysgenesis syndrome* (TDS). Their theory is that chemicals in our environment that pregnant mothers are exposed to may disrupt the normal development of their sons' urinary, genital, and reproductive systems.

The culprits, they believe, are a group of chemicals that interfere with or block normal hormonal processes. These so-called endocrine disruptors are found in such commonly used substances as paints, pesticides, plastics, and detergents, as well as computers, toys, and compact discs. Some endocrine disruptors contain compounds that mimic estrogen. Others are not estrogenic per se, but they block the action of testosterone and other male hormones.

Because the male sexual organs begin to develop as early as the seventh week of gestation, when the young male fetus is bathed in its own testosterone, could maternal exposure to endocrine disruptors possibly block the release of testosterone or interfere with the ability of fetal cells to respond to hormones as they should? Though this theory has not been proven in humans, some laboratory evidence in animals suggests that it might.

Could endocrine disruptors be a factor in undescended testicles, hypospadias, low sperm counts, male infertility, and related problems? Experts point out that this is still only a hypothesis that requires further testing before it can be validated. It is, though, based on several observations. Skakkebaek and his colleagues note that men with testicular cancer have higher than normal incidence of hypospadias and undescended testicles. They point out that rats and other animals exposed to endocrine disruptors in utero develop both of these problems. And they point to the Florida alligators with the "teeny weenies."

In 1980, a chemical company's waste pond overflowed, spilling large amounts of chemicals, including DDT (dichlorodiphenyltrichloroethane), into Lake Apopka near Orlando. The gators were largely wiped out; more than 90 percent died soon after the spill. But a few survived and continued to breed. Fifteen years later, a researcher noted that surviving alligators had penises that were 25 percent smaller than normal and their testosterone levels were as low as females'. They also had high levels of a DDE, a breakdown product of DDT known to suppress testosterone, in their tissues.

DDT is no longer used in this country, but it is still present in many lakes and waterways, since it can take at least fifteen years to break down, and continues to contaminate some fish populations. It also continues to be used in many developing countries to combat malaria. Many other chemicals have similar anti-androgenic properties. Environmental scientists are especially worried about a family of compounds knows as phthalates, used to soften plastics and make them flexible, as well as in solvents, detergents, and other products. A study by Harvard researchers in the May 2003 issue of *Epidemiology* found that among men being treated at a fertility clinic, those with the highest levels of two phthalates in their urine had the lowest sperm counts.

A number of medical products such as IV bags, plastic tubing, and catheters contain one widely used phthalate, DEHP (di-ethylhexyl phthalate). In July 2002, the FDA issued a public health notification urging doctors performing certain medical procedures, especially those involving infants and pregnant or lactating women, to substitute products made with other materials whenever possible. "Exposure to DHEP has produced a wide range of adverse effects in laboratory animals, but of greatest concern are effects on the development of the male reproductive system and production of normal sperm in young animals," the notice said. The agency acknowledged that there had been no reports of problems in humans but urged precautions "to limit the exposure of the developing male to DEHP."

Because of these concerns, European regulators banned the use of phthalates in some products, including baby toys. Here, phthalates have been voluntarily removed from pacifiers, bottle nipples, and toys intended for the mouths of babes. In June 2003, the American Academy of Pediatrics issued a report on phthalates that noted that "the most sensitive system is the reproductive tract of immature males." It called for more research into the effect of phthalates on children, and suggested that hospitals look for alternatives to devices containing DEHP.

Another notorious chemical that was banned in the United States more than twenty-five years ago but still contaminates many waterways, may also have unique effects on males, though this is debated amongst scientists. In a 2002 study in the *Lancet,* researchers from Taiwan showed that adolescent boys who had been exposed to high levels of PCBs (polychlorinated biphenyls) in contaminated cooking oil were significantly less likely to father a son in adulthood. They speculate that PCBs damage sperm carrying Y chromosomes. A dioxin spill in Italy in 1976, according to a group of Italian and American scientists, produced similar results: In the years after adolescent males were exposed, they fathered far more female than male children.

Finally, while the effect of the drug diethylstilbestrol (DES) has been well documented in the daughters of women who took it during pregnancy, we have heard less about its effect on male children. The drug, used to prevent miscarriages, was withdrawn from the market in 1971 after it was linked to genital abnormalities and rare cancers in the daughters of women who used it. But there is also evidence that women's use of DES may lead to a number of genital and reproductive problems in their sons, including testicular cancer, epididymal cysts, and reduced fertility. A 2002 study in the *Lancet* reported that the risk of hypospadias increased twenty-fold in boys whose maternal grandmothers took DES. Yet many people, including many doctors, are unaware that DES can affect male offspring.

If you want more information on DES, contact DES Action by phone (510-465-4011) or at this website: *http://www.desaction.org.* Also check out a new CDC website with good info: *http://www.cdc.gov/DES.*

What to Think

Our purpose is not to scare or frighten you about the environment. There are many questions that remain and many things scientists aren't sure of. Studying cause and effect of environmental toxins is complex, fraught with difficulty, and controversial. Scientists have many hurdles to clear before they can say for sure what a certain chemical will do to humans. For example, just because a particular chemical is in the environment does not necessarily mean it will affect humans. Just because a particular chemical is on a foodstuff does not mean that it will be absorbed by the body and distributed to target tissues. Just because a certain chemical affects animals does not mean it will affect humans in the same way or at all. Just because more cases of a certain disease are being reported does not always mean there are actually more cases; it could merely show that more people are aware of the problem and are therefore reporting it. Scientists will continue to examine these complex questions, so stay tuned.

Other Environmental Hazards

Reproductive problems are not the only environmental threats our children face. Some childhood diseases have risen over recent decades, and some experts believe that children's exposure to environmental toxins is a factor. Asthma rates among children tripled in the 1980s but seem to be holding steady now, according to the Centers for Disease Control. So do childhood cancer rates, though they grew by 33 percent from 1975 to 1998.

While the cause of these increases is far from clear, children are generally more vulnerable than adults to pollution and environmental toxins. That's because pound for pound, kids eat, drink, and breathe more than adults, which leads to a greater, more concentrated exposure. And because their bodies and nervous systems are still developing, toxins can interfere with their normal development. Here's a look at some of the most serious environmental threats to children based on the National Resources Defense Council's list of the top five environmental threats.

1. **Lead poisoning.** It's been known for decades that high levels of lead can cause serious problems, including seizures, coma, and even death. But in the past ten years, scientists have learned that much lower levels can cause serious long-term effects such as learning disabilities, behavioral problems, and decreased intelligence. Today, according to the CDC, some 430,000 children younger than six have elevated lead levels. Because it often occurs with no obvious symptoms, lead poisoning frequently goes unnoticed.

   The biggest source of lead exposure comes from paint and from dust contaminated by flaking, peeling paint. Millions of homes and buildings built before 1978, when lead paint was banned, contain lead. It is also found in dust, soil, and drinking water.

   Contaminated drinking water is the source of about 20 percent of Americans' lead exposure, according to the Environmental Protection Agency. Lead can leach into water from old lead pipes and solder. Though lead pipes and leaded solder were banned some years ago, leaded solder is still sold in some hardware stores, and even today, faucets and plumbing fittings may legally contain up to 8 percent lead. The biggest risk is to babies who drink formula made from water laced with lead.

According to the EPA, you can reduce the risk of drinking leaded water by flushing out the faucet: Run the water for fifteen to thirty seconds, especially if you haven't turned on the tap for a few hours.

2. **Air pollution.** In 1995, nearly 18 million children under ten lived in areas where air quality flunked federal standards. Many experts believe that air pollution is a significant factor in the soaring rates of childhood asthma; almost five million children under eighteen have this respiratory disease. Breathing polluted air also causes kids to have more, and longer-lasting, respiratory infections. Over time, the cellular damage caused by air pollution can adversely affect children's immune systems.

3. **Pesticides.** Ten years ago the National Academy of Sciences issued their findings on pesticides: They pose a greater risk to children than to adults. One reason is that children are exposed to much higher levels of pesticides because they eat, drink, and breathe proportionately more than adults relative to their body weights, and consume more fruits and juice as well. As a result children may be at risk for a variety of cancers, neurological diseases, birth defects, and immune system problems. In 1995, officials from the Department of Agriculture tested some seven thousand fruit and vegetable samples, finding residue on 65 percent. The ten most pesticide-laden fruits and veggies, according to the Environmental Working Group, are: strawberries, bell peppers, spinach, cherries, cantaloupes grown in Mexico, apples, apricots, green beans, grapes grown in Chile, and cucumbers. For more on this, see the Environmental Working Group's newsletter at *http://www.foodnews.org/highpesticidefoods.php.*

4. **Secondhand smoke.** We all know by now how bad cigarette smoke is for our health. Yet millions of children under five are exposed to cigarette smoke in their homes. A 1999 study found that 43 percent of babies younger than one year old live in homes with at least one smoker. Exposure to secondhand smoke can double or triple the risk of SIDS (sudden infant death syndrome) in babies and increase the incidence in children of asthma, respiratory infections, pneumonia, and ear infections, as well as the long-term risk of cancer.

5. **Contaminated water.** America's drinking water supply has improved greatly in recent years, and is better than that of most countries. Yet microbial contamination of water causes periodic outbreaks of illness such as the one in Milwaukee in 1993 when the microbe cryptosporidium sickened hundreds of thousands and killed dozens when water purification failed to kill the bug. Other toxins—such as pharmaceuticals, phthalates, and arsenic—may also pose risks to children.

What does all this mean for you and your family? Hard to say. Exposure to many of these products may be difficult or impossible to avoid, and scientists continue to debate the levels at which various toxins are actually dangerous. Still, if you're pregnant or have children, you might want to do a few things to protect your children. A few suggestions:

- Don't let young children (those who are still putting things in their mouths) use toys that are made with phthalates. Any soft plastic toy may pose a hazard unless marked as "PVC-free" or "phthalate-free." Call the manufacturer to find out if the toy contains phthalates or PVC. Check this website for a list of banned toys: *www.toysafety.net*. You can also go online to the U.S. Food and Drug Administration, *www.fda.gov*.

- Go organic. According to the U.S. Department of Agriculture, 73 percent of conventionally grown produce contains at least one pesticide residue, while only 23 percent of organic produce does. That's an excellent reason to shop for organic fruits and vegetables whenever possible, since they're grown without using pesticides or chemical additives. If you can't find organic, or it costs too much, be sure to thoroughly wash or peel all fruits and vegetables. You can wash fruits and vegetables in a highly diluted solution of liquid soap and water, then rinse thoroughly.

- Go easy on the fish. Some, especially big predatory fish that live a long time, can contain high levels of mercury, PCBs, dioxin, and other chemicals and pesticides they picked up in the environment. The FDA advises pregnant women to avoid eating shark, swordfish, king mackerel, and tilefish. It is prudent for nursing mothers and young children to avoid them as well. Many other groups say canned tuna is also a source of mercury in the diet and recommend it be avoided by pregnant women and that others should avoid eating it in large quantities. Bottom line: Obey fish advisories regarding sport fish.

- Don't use pesticides around the house. If you must use them, consider a natural alternative by checking out either of these websites: *http://www.clickondetroit.com/landscaping/1199678/detail.html* or *http://homeandgarden.nzoom.com/cda/printable/1,1856,147561,00.html*. Also don't use pesticides that are no longer approved for home use, such as organophosphates. Many people have stored these in garages for years not realizing they are not safe and should no longer be used in homes.

- Keep kids inside as much as possible on days when air pollution is bad.

- If you live in a house built before 1978, test it for lead paint. You should also have your children's blood tested for lead.

- Wash your kids' hands often, especially before they eat.

- Don't smoke, especially around kids!

2
Snips and Snails

For years, many pediatricians pretty much ignored the descriptions parents gave of their infants' early behavior. Mom and Dad might have thought their days-old babies were fussy or placid, easygoing or irritable, but most experts thought that all newborns were pretty much the same—little bundles of nerves that acted on reflex but lacked individual personalities. Personality, the experts believed, would develop later, in response to environment and rearing.

Then, in the 1950s, a groundbreaking project called the New York Longitudinal Study turned that notion on its head. Starting in 1956, researchers followed the lives of 133 newborns, interviewing parents about their babies' patterns of sleeping and eating, toilet habits, levels of activity, and social interactions. The children were interviewed intermittently throughout childhood, adolescence, and early adulthood so researchers could assess the course of their lives and the relationship between their characteristics as babies and the people they became.

What emerged from this study was a basic theory that's widely accepted by personality researchers today: Every child comes into the world with a distinct personality and way of interacting with others, what psychologists call temperament. Is he quiet and retiring or active and gregarious? Is she intense and dramatic or low-key and laid back? We're all born with these kinds of characteristics, and some stay with us for a lifetime. Certainly, these traits will shift over time and be influenced by our life experiences, but their congenital basis is present at birth and they'll start showing themselves in a matter of weeks or months as the nervous system matures.

Stella Chess, M.D., and Alexander Thomas, M.D., the leaders of the New York study and the godparents of temperament research, identified nine different characteristics that combine to make up each child's temperament. These include a child's activity level, emotional intensity, sensitivity, response to strangers or new situations, adaptability to change, general mood, attention span, distractibility, and the regularity of his or her sleeping and eating patterns and other daily routines.

It's important to understand that temperament, like many other traits of biology, is not destiny. "You can't take that biology, isolate it, and say just because it's present at birth that it's going to stay stable," says Jacqueline Lerner, Ph.D., a professor of psychology at Boston College who worked on the New York Longitudinal Study in its later years. She says that while the temperament of most babies remains relatively stable from one year to the next, "you occasionally see total reversals—very difficult babies becoming easy and vice versa. It all depends on the context"—meaning the circumstances under which children live and the kind of parenting, support, and assistance they get at home, in school, and in other settings.

But if researchers have found that people's temperaments change a great deal over time, they have also found that a child's early temperament can provide important clues about his or her future personality and life course. A longitudinal study in New Zealand that has followed more than a thousand youngsters from the age of three looked at children classified into three categories: undercontrolled, inhibited, and well adjusted. Most kids fit into the well-adjusted category and were the most likely to grow up to be friendly, optimistic adults. But the kids classified as undercontrolled were likely as young adults to be unreliable, impulsive, and antisocial. Those termed inhibited were prone to be cautious, unassertive, and depressed.

Chess and Thomas realized that to understand the meaning of a child's temperament they also needed to look at something else: the way that child's temperament fit with the demands, expectations, and temperament of his or her parents, and of his or her child-care providers and teachers. If there's a good match between a boy's temperament and his environment—what researchers call "goodness of fit"—things often go smoothly. If not, life can be trying. A boy may struggle to meet the demands placed upon him, or he may rebel. "Babies with a temperament become kids with a temperament and eventually become parents with a temperament," says Robin Goodman, Ph.D., clinical associate professor of psychiatry at New York University School of Medicine and director of AboutOurKids.org. "So parents have their own temperament that may or may not match that temperament of their child."

The point for parents is to understand that every child is unique and may have different likes, dislikes, styles, and interests than you do. You may make friends easily and like having other people around; your son may be on the shy side and prefer the solitude of his room. You may like doing things spontaneously, while he wants to know what's coming, to never be taken by surprise. Bottom line: Get to know your son for who he really is and try not to project your own preferences and proclivities on him.

"Understanding a boy's temperament is important because more temperament issues and temperament-related 'difficulties' occur for boys," says James Cameron, Ph.D., a psychologist who worked with Chess and Thomas and now runs The Preventive Ounce, a California group that contracts with health-care providers to evaluate children's temperaments and counsel their parents. "Perhaps the cause is genetic, linked to testosterone levels early in life. Perhaps it is because boys seem to encounter more intrauterine problems and birth difficulties that could later affect temperament.

We simply don't have clear answers here. But we do know that parents of boys bring more temperament complaints to the attention of pediatricians than parents of girls."

The more you understand about your boy's temperament, the better you'll be able to protect him from undue stresses and to love and discipline him in the most effective way. If you know that he's basically primed to react in a certain manner, that it's part of who he is, you won't have to feel guilty or surprised when he acts or responds in those ways.

"Parents who understand how their son's temperament 'works' are better able to work *with* their child's temperament, rather than fight against it," says Cameron. "A parent of a novelty-approaching, active, but easily frustrated boy could learn ahead of time that saying 'no' and 'stop' all the time won't work. They could learn that telling their son what *to* do, rather than what *not* to do, allows them to go with their son's temperament, not against it. The result: a more positive parent-son relationship."

Good parents modify their parenting style to fit the temperament of their child. That doesn't mean that your boy rules the roost, says William Carey, M.D., director of behavioral pediatrics at Children's Hospital of Philadelphia, and a leading authority on child temperament. "On the contrary, it means there should be minor adjustments in the parents' management that recognize the child's temperament."

To help professionals and parents understand more about children's individual temperaments, Carey designed a series of questionnaires that rate children on their habits and patterns. You can find and take a parent-friendly temperament questionnaire for your infant, toddler, or preschooler, modeled on Carey's work, at the Internet site of The Preventive Ounce (*http://preventiveoz.org*). You can also read more about temperament issues in Carey's 1997 book, *Understanding Your Child's Temperament*, available through Behavioral-Developmental Initiatives (*www.temperament.com*).

The Preventive Ounce questionnaire has been tested extensively in families who are members of Kaiser Permanente, a large HMO. It asks more than fifty questions about your child; for example, how likely he is to fall asleep and wake up at the same time each day? How likely he is to withdraw from a new person? Take the test when your baby is between four and eight months old and again when he's a toddler and a preschooler. You'll get predictions, based on the surveys and the known behavior of other children, of how likely your boy will be to have, say, frequent temper tantrums or how prone to injuries and accidents he's likely to be. You'll also get advice on how to deal with problems that seem likely to arise.

BOYS, GIRLS, AND TEMPERAMENTAL DIFFERENCES

Overall, boys and girls fit into most temperament categories in roughly equal numbers. But there are some important differences. Thanks to whatever combination of genes and socialization is at work, boys tend to revel in physical play, to be in per-petual motion. They're also more likely than girls to act aggressively, to snatch toys from their pals and classmates, and to wrestle and fight. And because boys also tend to be impulsive, to have trouble sitting still, and to jump from one idea and activity to another, many adults worry about their ability to focus attention.

"Girls have more problems with overinhibition—shyness and perfectionism," says Cameron. "Boys have more problems with underinhibition—uninhibited curiosity, aggression, defiance, noncompliance."

These traits can be trying, but they certainly aren't all bad. In fact, harnessed pro-ductively, they can help boys be creative, daring, and resourceful. Unchanneled, how-ever, these attributes can cause boys big problems at home, in school, and with relationships. They can prevent a boy from achieving academically and land him in trouble with authority figures such as parents, teachers, and principals.

One temperament trait that's found in nearly identical numbers of girls and boys is shyness. If anything, girls may be a bit more likely to be born with what psychologists call an "inhibited" temperament. But the impact of having such a temperament can be greater on males. Shyness in females is considered "acceptable" and "appropriate"; not so among boys. Just as girls (and women) who are active and assertive can be judged harshly in our culture, so too can boys and men who don't conform to the ideal model of confident, outgoing maleness.

SHY GUYS

Brian, a friend's son, would have to be called painfully shy. He hangs back from the crowd, almost never makes eye contact, and speaks in a voice so hushed you have to struggle to hear him. He is reluctant to go to birthday parties and is the only child I have ever known who did not want one himself; he doesn't like to be the center of attention, his mother says. He has a few friends, and other kids like him, but he's much quieter and more reserved than other boys. If not for his mother's efforts, he would probably never have friends over to his house. In some ways, Brian's shyness may be harder on his mother than on him. As she watches him get left out of the rowdy, phys-ical activities of the other boys, she worries. She worries that his shy nature won't change, that he won't learn to be assertive, that he'll have trouble succeeding in the world because of it. Is she right to worry? That's not an easy question, but the way she and her husband raise Brian, along with other experiences he has, will have a lot to do with what happens to him later. Environment, or nurture, is a big factor.

Shyness is a complicated and often misunderstood trait. There's a popular notion that shy people are born that way, that shyness is contained in a gene. It's not that sim-ple. Researchers generally describe two different kinds of shyness: one, an inhibited temperament present at birth; and the other, which develops later, usually around the age of four or five. "An inherited temperament is not the same as shyness nor does it guarantee that an inhibited infant will be a shy adult," says Bernardo Carducci, Ph.D., a psychologist who directs the Shyness Institute at Indiana University.

Jerome Kagan, Ph.D., a psychologist and temperament researcher at Harvard University, has found that up to 20 percent of children are born with a clear aversion to new people and new situations. In a series of now classic studies, Kagan tracked the reactions of four-month-old babies to sensory stimulation—lights, sounds, and smells they had never experienced. He also looked at their response to new situations, such as their mothers leaving the room, being left with kids they didn't know, and being faced with tasks they had never encountered. Twenty percent of these babies—Kagan calls them "high reactors"—responded by becoming upset and agitated. Their hearts raced, and they shook their tiny limbs, arched their backs, and wailed. Others responded more calmly or not at all.

Kagan's research strongly suggests that this kind of temperament is inherited. He found that twin babies tend to have similar reactions to this stimulation. And he has shown that the brains of high-reactive and low-reactive babies respond differently and may even be structured differently. Now he and researchers from the Brazelton Institute in Boston are trying to see if these temperamental traits can be found and assessed even earlier, in the second and third days of life.

But remember: Biology is not destiny. By the time the children he studied were four and a half, Kagan found, 87 percent of the highly reactive ones had become less fearful. True, none of them would become an extrovert at four, and they were unlikely to do so as adults either. But most of them were functioning fairly normally at four; and odds are, they will in the future as well.

Many shy children, perhaps most, don't start out with this kind of inhibited temperament. They become shy a little bit later in response to various stresses and worries. Arnold Buss, Ph.D., a researcher now at the University of Texas, describes a later-developing shyness that may first show itself around four or five and grow stronger in later years as children learn to compare themselves to others. Not surprisingly, the worst and most painful years for this kind of shyness can come during adolescence.

The things that trigger this kind of shyness often happen at home. "About forty percent of the people I survey cite such factors as a lack of family support, parental absence, parents not teaching social skills, overprotective parents, parental neglect, and other family-related issues for their shyness," Carducci says. "Obviously, these are not characteristics that people are born with."

Whether they were born with shy tendencies or developed their shyness during early childhood, it is, for some, an enduring and problematic trait. In that longitudinal study that followed children in New Zealand, around 8 percent of the three-year-olds were classified as inhibited. They were timid, uneasy, and easily upset around strangers. At age eighteen, they were more likely to be cautious and unassertive with little desire to take on leadership roles. And as twenty-one-year-old adults, they were more likely to be depressed and had few friends or other social supports.

The trouble with this study is that it tells us nothing about these children's families and the environment they are being raised in. Are they uncontrollable or inhibited at age three because that is their innate temperament? Or are there things going on at home that contribute? If their family life was difficult at age three, it was likely to be difficult throughout their childhood and adolescence. So what, exactly, is being measured here?

If your son is showing signs of great shyness and timidity, you need to figure out why. If his shyness seemed to develop at four, five, or six years of age, it may have something to do with things going on at home or in school. Children whose parents divorce, for instance, can become clingy and withdrawn. The loss of a beloved caregiver or an upsetting situation at preschool or school may be a factor. Or perhaps you're protecting him from the world too much, not giving him enough of a chance to meet and interact with other people, to take risks. These kinds of triggers, if you can figure them out, can often be addressed successfully.

It may be harder to overcome true temperamental shyness that's been there from his earliest days. With shy toddlers, avoid the tendency to explain "He's just shy" when your son hides behind your skirt or buries his face in your shoulder. Labels have a way of sticking and becoming self-perpetuating.

For children of any age, reduce stress and conflict in your own home; family fights, for instance, can be scary for shy kids. Try to protect him from being criticized, shamed, or pushed around by older siblings and peers. Be calm, affectionate, and supportive as you try to gently nudge him into play dates and other social contacts.

William Carey, M.D., author of *Understanding Your Child's Temperament*, says parents of shy kids should avoid overloading them with new experiences, and instead, prepare them for new situations slowly. "That doesn't mean you don't allow new experiences," he stresses. "Just avoid overload. Don't push too hard. Praise them for overcoming their fears of novelty." As the child gets older, encourage him to be more independent.

Parents of shy kids have to walk a bit of a tightrope, encouraging kids to come out of their shells while not pushing them too hard, supporting them as you also let them find their way. "Parents—without being mean or cruel—need to let kids experience anxiety [because] there's something about that experience that teaches them how to handle it," says Robin Goodman. "Parents can stand by and be supportive and comforting, without being overprotective. Because if they're overprotected, it reinforces the pattern of a kid needing help, a kid being insecure, a kid not being able to do something on his own, a kid needing to be taken out of the struggle. You don't want to restrict them totally and manage their environment, because then they never learn how to handle it."

Perhaps the most important message to get across to your child is acceptance. Let him know that he is loved unconditionally, that he doesn't have to earn love by doing anything, including being more social than he's ready to be. You'll need to work at this kindly and patiently, and understand that it may be a long haul. Shyness rarely goes away by itself.

SOCIAL ANXIETY DISORDER (SAD)

Some children and adults are so painfully shy that they're afraid to talk to other people or go to public places where they might have to interact socially. They worry people will judge or criticize them, and they fear being embarrassed or the center of attention. A child may be afraid to raise his hand in class, play, or even talk with other kids. For some, the anxiety is so strong that it causes physical reactions such as tremors, sweating, or even vomiting. In its most severe form, known as *selective mutism*, children simply can't or won't speak to anyone other than, perhaps, members of their own family and sometimes only under particular conditions.

About 3 percent of children and up to 5 percent of adults suffer from social anxiety disorder (SAD), says Deborah Beidel, Ph.D., a psychologist and codirector of the Center for Anxiety Disorders at the University of Maryland. Boys and girls are equally likely to have this problem, but boys may be more likely to deny it, Beidel says. And since these children are so quiet and withdrawn, their troubles are often ignored. That's a problem, Beidel says, because the disorder doesn't usually go away without treatment and can lead to depression in adolescence and adulthood.

Back in 1980, psychiatrists decided that these symptoms defined a unique disorder and social anxiety disorder, also known as social phobia, was born. Until a few years ago, few people other than psychiatrists had ever heard of this disorder, and it was rarely mentioned in the press. This ended in 1999, when this little-known disorder suddenly came out of the closet and became the subject of literally millions of media reports describing the misery and pain of people who suffered from it. The reason for this sudden rush of attention: a massive public relations campaign, orchestrated by a PR firm working for Glaxo SmithKline, manufacturer of the antidepressant Paxil.

In May of that year, Paxil became the first medication approved by the FDA for treatment of social anxiety disorder. According to *PR News,* an industry newsletter, the disorder was mentioned in media accounts more than 1 billion times in 1999, up from just fifty two years before. Virtually all the new stories mentioned Paxil, but in case people missed them, the company spent millions more on ads, many of which asked: "What if you were allergic to people?" and targeted young adults.

Despite all the hype, Paxil is only moderately effective, helping a little more than half of patients in studies feel more relaxed and less paralyzed in social situations. Paxil is not approved by the FDA for use by children, but many doctors prescribe it and other medications to children anyway, a common practice known as "off-label" prescribing. Because of studies linking Paxil to an elevated risk of suicide in children and teenagers, the FDA recently issued a warning against the use of Paxil by children and adolescents.

At the University of Maryland, Beidel and her colleague Samuel Turner, Ph.D., are using a form of behavioral therapy to help children with SAD. Working slowly, they focus on helping the children learn basic social skills such as talking on the telephone or greeting people. They trained other children who don't have social phobia to work with those who do in group sessions. According to Beidel, nearly 70 percent made significant strides in overcoming their fears and interacting socially.

ACTIVE BOYS OR "HOW DO YOU MANAGE?"

As the mother of a boy, I was completely unprepared for the level of activity that my sweet and wonderful son, Harry, could maintain for hours on end. From the earliest age, he seemed to be the most active kid around. With a huge grin on his face, he whooped, hollered, and generally raised hell from the moment he could walk.

Mothers of little girls were often horrified by my son's behavior. With hair bows never out of place, their little girls would sit serenely in the sandbox, quietly shoveling sand as my son ran and screamed and jumped. On more than one occasion, a mother sniffed, "How *do* you manage?" or worse, "I feel *so* sorry for you." Indeed, several implied he had AD/HD. Boy, did that make me angry!

Then again, I worried, maybe he did. I wasn't so sure back then, and such comments kept me up at night. Was my son somehow "abnormal"? If I knew then what I know now, I would not have spent one second worrying. Of course, I was a new mother without much experience with boys. Now I understand that just because my son is active and sometimes kind of wild, it means only one thing: He's a boy—a healthy, active, normal boy.

Boys' greater activity levels are observed from their first days. In one study, researchers watched newborns for eight hours during their first two days of life, recording how much and how often they yawned, waved, cried, turned, startled, kicked, and grimaced. In each category, the boys were slightly more active than girls; they were also awake more of the time.

By the time they become toddlers, these differences become more apparent. Data from a longitudinal study of children in Quebec released in 2002 found 36 percent of seventeen-month-old boys often fidget and 25 percent are often restless or hyperactive, 6 percent more than girls in each of those categories. Things haven't changed much, apparently: When twenty-one-month-old children born in Berkeley, California, were assessed back in the 1920s, 29 percent of the boys and 17 percent of the girls were reported by their mothers as overactive or restless.

Most likely, both genes and culture are at play in perpetuating these motion machines: Young boys start out more active and physical, and they are encouraged to keep it up. Dads tend to bounce baby boys more on their knees and roughhouse with them in ways they don't with girls. Moms tend to do more arts-and-crafts activities with their daughters than their sons.

By the time they get to preschool and elementary school, this higher level of activity among boys has become more pronounced, especially when boys are in groups, stimulating and egging each other on. "By school age, the average boy in a classroom is more active than about three fourths of the girls, and the most active children in the class are very likely to be boys," write Dan Kindlon and Michael Thompson in *Raising Cain.*

So how do you decide if your boy's activity level is a problem? That is an increasingly difficult decision, and one of the most pressing behavioral issues boys and their parents face.

ROUGH BOYS

Quick, take a guess: At what age are people the most aggressive? Nineteen, perhaps? Or seventeen? Or fifteen? Or twelve? No, it's not any of these. The age when people commit the greatest number of aggressive acts is around twenty-four *months.* Hour by hour and day by day, the average two-year-old commits far more aggressive actions than the typical teenager. For many years, Richard Tremblay, Ph.D., a psychologist at the University of Montreal and one of the world's leading experts on childhood aggression, has been surveying mothers in Quebec province and asking about their toddlers' behavior.

Most children sometimes push, bite, kick, or hit other children in order to get what they want, the moms report. And, not surprisingly, boys tend to commit these transgressions more often. At twenty-nine months, 41 percent of boys (and "just" 27 percent of girls) sometimes kicked other children; 33 percent of boys (and 23 percent of girls) bit other kids; and 24 percent of boys (and 15 percent of girls) hit other kids. Toddlers—in case you didn't already know this—can be tough. Why do you think they're called the "terrible twos"?

Experts stress that this kind of aggressive behavior is a normal part of growing up, one of the ways children develop a sense of their own identity and learn the limits of acceptable behavior. During those wonderful years, boys generally throw more tantrums and lash out more at their parents, says Carol R. Beal, Ph.D., a child psychologist at the University of Massachusetts and author of the book *Boys and Girls: The Development of Gender Roles*.

But if boys are more physically aggressive from the start, they also learn aggression on the playground, from older brothers, and from men they see around them or on TV. In one study, kids who didn't hit or fight at the beginning of their first year of preschool were joining in the melee by year's end.

Most research in the United States and other societies comparing boys and girls has found boys to be more aggressive. This is true for both verbal and physical aggression and among all social classes. One reason is that boys are simply more physical, and their style of play leads to more bumping, shoving, and the inevitable retaliation. Also, Beal points out, "boys are more concerned with dominance relations, and . . . aggression is often the means by which dominance is established and acknowledged."

The good news for most parents is that children's tendency to smack and shove declines pretty steadily during their elementary school years. Another Canadian study found that levels of physical aggression among both boys and girls declined slowly but steadily between the ages of four and eleven.

But for those children who continue to be physically aggressive in elementary school—and again, this is mostly boys—aggression can become a habit that leads to lifelong problems. An aggressive child is far more likely to become an aggressive teenager and, ultimately, a violent adult. Virtually every violent adult was once an aggressive child.

Case in point: A recent Australian study found that children who were aggressive at five years of age were nearly three times as likely as other kids to be suspended from school, five times as likely to be delinquent, and almost seven times as likely to be physically aggressive at age fourteen. And a long-term study conducted by researchers at the University of Michigan followed 850 children to adulthood and found that one out of every four boys who were highly aggressive at eight had a criminal record by thirty.

Such outcomes are not inevitable, experts say. Children may be born with a predisposition to aggression, but the way parents respond and behave can have a major impact on their kids.

"The biggest predictor of whether a kid is going to have aggression problems is whether there's violence in the family," says Kurt Fischer, Ph.D., an education professor at Harvard. And by violence, Fischer means parents spanking or beating their children as well as fighting with each other.

Fischer and a team of researchers from Harvard and Brandeis spent several years interviewing mothers and their children, aged seven to thirteen, in Springfield, Massachusetts. Two key findings emerged from their research. One, that family violence led to future aggression, was hardly surprising. There is a mountain of research showing that children who are punished physically or who live in homes where physical violence occurs frequently are more likely to be violent themselves.

But the researchers also found that children who had inhibited temperaments—kids who were socially withdrawn, uncomfortable in new situations, or anxious about making new friends—were also more likely to be aggressive in later years. "These kids hold things in to try to control the situation and to control themselves," Fischer says. "They withdraw, they inhibit, and they shut down to try and reduce their emotionality." Then, at some point, these bottled-up emotions come bursting out—in angry and violent action.

The worst combination, of course, was when inhibited kids lived in families that experienced a lot of violence. That was the case for two boys in the study who ended up in jail for violent behavior, one for murder.

There are two lessons here for parents. One is obvious: They should do everything they can to refrain from using violence or harsh physical punishment against their children or other family members. The other is a bit more subtle: Parents need to notice what's going on with their children and help inhibited kids find ways to express the feelings they lock up inside.

Perhaps the more common and vexing question for so many parents of boys is how to distinguish between normal playground roughhousing and unacceptable violence. When should you "let boys be boys" and when, and how, should you intervene? It's not an easy issue.

"The problem is most people chalk up behavior like hitting, biting, or tantrums to the terrible twos," Richard Tremblay said in a 1998 interview with *Parenting* magazine. "They don't take it seriously. Most of those kids will turn out all right. But in some cases, ignoring such behavior, treating it as 'cute,' or responding with aggression in kind—like spanking—can have bad consequences."

HELPING YOUR CHILD AVOID VIOLENCE

The American Psychological Association and the American Academy of Pediatrics put together a useful guide for parents on how to help children avoid aggressive and violent behavior. The guide is called "Raising Children to Resist Violence: What You Can Do" and it's available on the APA website at *http://www.apa.org/pubinfo/apa-aap.html*. Here are some key points:

Show Your Children Appropriate Behaviors by the Way You Act

Children learn by example. The behavior, values, and attitudes of parents and siblings have a strong influence on children.

Most children sometimes act aggressively. Be firm with your children about the dangers of violent behavior. Praise them when they solve problems constructively without violence. Children are more likely to repeat good behaviors when they are rewarded with attention and praise.

Teach your children nonaggressive ways to solve problems by:

- Discussing problems with them,
- Asking them to consider what might happen if they use violence to solve problems, and
- Talking about what might happen if they solve problems without violence.

Parents sometimes encourage, model, or sanction aggressive behavior without realizing it. For example, some parents think it is good for a boy to learn to fight. Teach your children that it is better to settle arguments with calm words, not fists, threats, or weapons.

Don't Hit Your Children

Hitting, slapping, or spanking children as punishment shows them that it's okay to hit others to solve problems and can train them to punish others in the same way they were punished.

Be Consistent About Rules and Discipline

When you make a rule, stick to it. Children need structure with clear expectations for their behavior. Setting rules and then not enforcing them is confusing and sets up children to see what they can get away with.

Make Sure Your Children Don't Have Access to Guns

Guns and children can be a deadly combination. Teach your children about the dangers of firearms or other weapons if you own and use them. If you keep a gun in your home, unload it, hide it, and lock it up separately from the bullets.

Try to Keep Your Children from Seeing Violence

Violence in the home can be frightening and harmful. A child who has seen violence at home may be more likely to try to resolve conflicts that way. Discourage violent behavior between siblings. Keep in mind that hostile, aggressive arguments between parents frighten children and set a bad example. If people in your home physically or verbally abuse each other, try to get help from a counselor and stop it. Children who can't avoid seeing violence in the street, at school, or at home may need help from a psychologist, counselor, or clergy.

Keep Your Children from Seeing Too Much Violence in the Media

Seeing a lot of violence on TV, in the movies, and in video games can lead children to behave aggressively. As a parent, you can control the amount of violence your children see.

- Limit television viewing to one or two hours a day.
- Make sure you know what shows and movies your children watch, and what kinds of video games they play.
- Talk to your children about the violence they see in the media and help them to understand how painful it would be in real life.
- Discuss with them ways to solve problems without violence.

Teach Your Children Ways to Avoid Becoming Victims of Violence

- Teach them safe routes for walking in your neighborhood and to walk with a friend at all times—and only in well-lighted, busy areas.
- Stress how important it is for them to report crimes or suspicious activities to you, a teacher, another trustworthy adult, or the police. Make sure they know how to call 911.
- Make sure they know what to do if anyone tries to hurt them: Say "no," run away, and tell a reliable adult.
- Stress the dangers of talking to strangers. Tell them never to open the door to, or go anywhere with, someone they don't know and trust.

Help Your Children Stand Up Against Violence

Teach them to respond with calm but firm words when others insult, threaten, or hit another person. Help them understand that it takes more courage and leadership to resist violence than to go along with it.

Help your children accept and get along with others from various racial and ethnic backgrounds. Teach them that criticizing people because they are different is hurtful, and that name-calling is unacceptable.

Could Your Child Be Violent?

If your child is acting in some of the ways described in this list, you may want to talk to a doctor, counselor, or other professional who is experienced in dealing with behavioral issues.

Warning Signs in the Toddler and Preschool Child

- Has many temper tantrums in a single day or several lasting more than fifteen minutes each, and often cannot be calmed by parents or other caregivers.
- Often yells, screams, or hits in an aggressive way, for little or no reason.
- Is extremely active, impulsive, and fearless.
- Consistently refuses to follow directions and listen to adults.
- Frequently watches violence on television, engages in play that has violent themes, or is cruel toward other children.

Warning Signs in the School-Aged Child

- Has trouble paying attention and concentrating.
- Often disrupts classroom activities.
- Does poorly in school.
- Frequently gets into fights with other children.
- Reacts to disappointments, criticism, or teasing with intense anger, blame, or revenge.
- Watches many violent TV shows and movies or plays a lot of violent video games.
- Has few friends and is often rejected by other children because of his or her behavior.
- Makes friends with other children known to be unruly or aggressive.
- Consistently does not listen to adults.
- Is not sensitive to the feelings of others.
- Is cruel or violent toward pets or other animals.
- Is easily frustrated.

Warning Signs in the Preteen or Teenaged Adolescent

- Consistently does not listen to authority figures.
- Pays no attention to the feelings or rights of others.
- Mistreats people and seems to rely on physical violence or threats of violence to solve problems.
- Often expresses the feeling that life has treated him or her unfairly.
- Does poorly in school and often skips class.
- Misses school frequently for no identifiable reason.
- Gets suspended or expelled from, or drops out of, school.
- Joins a gang, gets involved in fighting, stealing, or destroying property.
- Drinks alcohol and/or uses inhalants or drugs.

Source: From Raising Children to Resist Violence: What You Can Do. *Copyright © 1996 by the American Academy of Pediatrics and American Psychological Association. Adapted with permission.*

SCHOOL DAYS
Helping Your Boy Get Ready for School

Before you know it, and often before you feel ready, it's your little boy's first day of kindergarten. It's the beginning of his entry into a whole new world, one that will be the focus of his life for the next thirteen years. But before that day comes, there are some things you can do to help prepare him for it. Most of them you'll probably do without even thinking about it.

The field of brain science has exploded in recent years with new information about how the brains of young children are stimulated. There are now brain-stimulating videos and interactive computer programs to teach three-year-olds their letters and numbers. Many parents research the latest high-tech learning toys and tools and work with their kids using flash cards like those from Baby Einstein and Baby Webster.

The advice of most child development experts—with which I fully agree—is simple: Relax. Play with your child. Enjoy him. Read to him as much as you can. Let him socialize with other kids. Rather than trying to "teach" him, help him to have interesting, fun experiences. Let him dance, sing, and draw. Give him drums. Take him to museums and performances. Read to him some more. Talk to him—and listen to him—a lot. If he makes up stories, write them down in books that he can illustrate.

If he goes to a preschool, be sure it's one that focuses on supporting his social and emotional growth and lets his cognitive growth occur mostly through appropriate play. If he doesn't, make extra efforts to provide other chances for him to play and interact with other children.

What you don't want to do is push him to read and write before he's ready. A two-year-old who memorizes his ABC's or can count to twenty may not start reading or adding any earlier than one who learns at age four. Children may recite the alphabet or a series of numbers, but until they are developmentally ready, they do not understand what they "mean" or that letters and numbers are symbolic.

After you've done all these things, how will you know if your boy is ready to start school? In 2000, the Child Mental Health Foundations and Agencies Network (FAN) released a report on school readiness that identified social and emotional readiness as the key. "A socially and emotionally healthy, school-ready child has many, though not necessarily all, of the following characteristics," the report said. "He or she is confident, friendly, has good peer relationships, tackles and persists at challenging tasks, has good language development, can communicate well, listens to instructions, and is attentive." If you think he's not doing well in several of these areas, talk to your pediatrician or family physician about whether he might need some special help.

One question you'll need to think about is when you want him to start kindergarten. These days many parents choose to delay their son's entry so that he starts at five and a half or six instead of four and a half or five. Many parents and educators now believe that because boys tend to be less mature and school-ready than girls at age five, it makes sense to wait a little longer. Leonard Sax, M.D., a physician and psychologist from Poolesville, Maryland, argued in a recent article in the journal *Psychology of Men and Masculinity* that the kindergarten curriculum tends to emphasize girls' strengths and boys' weaknesses.

In the article, Sax suggested that at the age of five, boys should enter an alternative kindergarten that focuses on group activities and nonverbal skills instead of early reading and mathematics. At six, they could start regular kindergarten, one year after the girls. Such an approach makes sense, he says, because "the average five-year-old boy is performing at a level of verbal skill that is, on average, at least one year behind the average five-year-old girl."

There is some evidence that delaying the entry of children who are not quite kindergarten-ready helps them succeed. A 1997 report from the U.S. Department of Education found that children who entered kindergarten a year later than normal performed as well or better than kids who entered at the standard age. The late entrants were also less likely to receive negative comments from their teachers.

The key question you'll need to answer if you're considering holding back your five-year-old is what to do with him during that year. Is there a high-quality preschool where he can enjoy himself as he gets ready for next year?

Race and class have a lot to do with who goes to kindergarten when. White, middle-class parents who have better preschool options are more likely to exercise them and hold their boys back. Low-income minority families are much less likely to do so. Consequently, their children may come to kindergarten at age five, ready or not. One result, according to a 1997 report from the U.S. Department of Education: African-American children are more likely to be required to repeat kindergarten, a trend that will continue throughout the school years. Not surprisingly, boys are much more likely than girls to repeat kindergarten; they make up two thirds of the repeating class.

Another approach aimed at addressing the differences in maturity and in learning styles between boys and girls is single-sex education (teaching boys and girls separately). Leonard Sax has come to believe that is a better solution than delaying boys' entry into kindergarten. He recently helped found, and is the executive director of, the National Association for Single Sex Public Education, which advocates the creation of single-sex schools in public school districts. "Many parents choose to send their children to single-sex private schools," he says. "This option should be available to parents who want it, but who can't afford private school tuition."

At last count, fifty-six public schools around the country offer single-sex education; seven of these just became single sex in the fall of 2003. There are a number of variations on the single-sex theme. Some schools are only for boys or girls but the more common variation is to maintain separate-sex classrooms and bring boys and girls together for lunch, music, art, and other electives.

Dr. Sax argues that single-sex education is most effective for boys in the early elementary years, kindergarten through grade four. "It dramatically expands educational horizons in that age group," he says. "Boys in single-sex classes are much more likely to pursue interests in art, music, dance, drama, and cooking, than are boys in coed classes. The great majority of boys benefit from access to single-sex educational opportunities."

Boys and School: An Often Uneasy Match

Walk into a typical kindergarten or first-grade classroom and you'll see a buzz of activity. You may see kids sitting on the floor in a circle as the teacher reads a story, stopping every so often to tell a child to stop bothering his or her neighbor or to ask another to sit back down. You may see kids at groups of tables—stations, in the education jargon of the day—working on art projects or math or reading while the teacher circulates, corralling kids who can't stay in their seats, breaking up tugs-of-war over markers or books. In almost any coed class in America, most of the kids jumping out of their seats, or pushing, shoving, and sitting in the time-out area are boys.

Stroll to the principal's office and notice the students sent there by teachers because of discipline problems. Drop by the detention room or where kids serve out their in-school suspensions. Then check who's in line at the nurse's office, waiting for their daily dose of Ritalin. The odds are that in all these cases, you'll see a lot more boys than girls.

This is not an easy time for boys in American schools. Many experts feel that boys are in crisis, that they're failing in school and being failed by schools, that they're pressured and anxious, and that they're resorting, increasingly, to violence. A spate of books and studies have focused attention on "the boy problem," shining the kind of spotlight on boys that books such as *Reviving Ophelia* shined on girls ten years ago.

Whether or not it constitutes a crisis, it is clear that many boys are having a wide range of academic and social problems and are falling behind girls in a number of critical areas. *Raising Cain* authors Dan Kindlon and Michael Thompson argue that the school culture is biased against boys. "Grade school is largely a feminine environment, populated predominantly by women teachers and authority figures, that seems rigged against boys, against the higher activity level and lower level of impulse control that is normal for boys," they write. "Many boys face a steady diet of shame and anxiety throughout their elementary school years. From it, they learn only to feel bad about themselves and to hate the place that makes them feel that way."

Behind from the Start

In the fall of 1998, the U.S. Department of Education assessed 19,000 kindergartners around the country as they entered school. Researchers, who will follow these kids for the next five years, looked at their skills and school-readiness and found some important differences between boys and girls. Overall, the differences in academic skills were fairly small, but the gap in behavior and social skills was greater. Here are some of their findings:

- Seventy percent of girls knew the letters of the alphabet when they entered school, but just 62 percent of boys. Twice as many boys as girls (14 percent versus 7 percent) had difficulty clearly articulating words and communicating.

- Twice as many boys as girls (18 percent versus 9 percent) had difficulty paying attention for sustained periods. Boys are also more likely than girls (20 percent versus 16 percent) to be much more active.

- Teachers reported that more boys than girls angered easily (14 percent versus 9 percent) and argue with others (13 percent versus 8 percent). Teachers also said that 60 percent of girls—but only 43 percent of boys—often comforted or helped their classmates.

The report's authors offered the following observation: "The higher frequency of behavior and adjustment problems that males exhibit when entering kindergarten foreshadows the greater number of males who experience conduct and disciplinary problems later in elementary and secondary school."

Another dynamic is emerging strongly with the nationwide push for standardized testing and stricter, more uniform standards in schools: Children are expected to study more, to learn more, and to do more homework at an ever-earlier age. Most veteran teachers would probably agree that kindergarten today is the equivalent of first grade a decade or two ago. The trouble is that kids today, and especially boys, are not developmentally different than they were a few years ago, no matter what's now expected of them.

"Kindergarten is a whole other experience compared to twenty years ago," says Lawrence Diller, M.D., an author and behavioral pediatrician with a large practice in the affluent suburbs east of San Francisco. "It has become a much more academic experience, and the demands on younger children have absolutely created some behavioral problems. In preschool, it's the same—we're suddenly asking three- and four-year-olds to learn their letters and numbers. I'm a much busier guy because of the increased expectations on children."

School Behavior and Discipline Problems

Most children start their school careers with wonderful optimism and great hope. But because boys are less ready developmentally and less able to control their bodies and impulses, they have more behavior problems from the start. As they work their way through school, they continue to get in trouble more often, earning more time-outs and trips to the principal's office, and more school suspensions than their female peers.

- Parents of elementary school boys are about twice as likely to be contacted by a teacher or principal about problems with their schoolwork or behavior, according to a report from the Department of Education.

- Boys are far more likely to be disciplined by school authorities. For example, 66 percent of in-school suspensions, 70 percent of out-of-school suspensions, and 79 percent of expulsions in Florida schools during the 1998–99 school year were given to male students. This pattern is repeated in school districts throughout the country.

- At least twice as many boys as girls get special education services for students with learning disabilities. In Florida schools, boys are twice as likely to be diagnosed with a learning disability, speech impairment, or developmental delay, and they are four times as likely to be classified as having autism or emotional disturbance. Many of these disabilities—autism, for example—are biological problems. But many experts contend that one of the reasons there are so many boys in special education classes is that their unruly behavior simply attracts more attention. Bad behavior may also spur some teachers to exile boys they can't manage from their classrooms. African-American boys are especially likely to be put in special education classes.

"The kids who have problems with impulse control are primarily boys, and they get in a lot more trouble in school," says Harvard's Kurt Fischer, Ph.D. "Girls don't get in trouble as much because they're less physical. They may have trouble attending in the classroom, but they're not bouncing around the classroom and throwing spitballs at other kids. So they don't get identified by the teacher as being a behavior problem, they don't go to the counselor, they don't get assessed, and they don't get diagnosed."

The Performance Gap

For many years, feminist researchers have been concerned with disparities that leave women earning less money and wielding less power than men, and they point at school as a starting point for these inequities. Researchers such as Carol Gilligan, Ph.D., theorized that during adolescence, girls lose their voice and their self-confidence. They worry over test scores that show boys outscoring girls in math and science and doing better on the SATs.

In recent years, however, many education researchers have shifted their attention to boys and noted a growing performance gap that is the exact opposite of what many educators once feared. These observations have kicked off an ideological gender war. Critics on the right, such as the conservative writer and commentator Christina Hoff Sommers, author of *The War Against Boys,* argue that boys are now suffering precisely because of the extra attention paid to girls in an effort to redress past wrongs. Others, like Harvard's William Pollack, contend that boys are doing poorly not because schools spend too much effort addressing girls' needs but because they ignore the unique needs and issues of boys. Whatever the case, there's little doubt about the result: Boys are performing more poorly in school than girls, and the gap seems to be widening. Consider these findings from reports released by the U.S. Department of Education:

- Boys trail girls in their reading and writing skills at every age and stage. In the year 2000, 36 percent of fourth-grade girls and just 27 percent of fourth-grade boys were rated as proficient readers. Twelfth-grade boys went from scoring 10 points behind girls in reading in 1992, to trailing by 15 points in 1998. In the writing department, eleventh-grade males were writing at the level of eighth-grade females in 1996.

- Boys are more likely to be held back and to drop out of school. In 1995, 8 percent of elementary school boys and 5 percent of girls were held back to repeat a grade. In 1997, 11.9 percent of males and 10.7 percent of females dropped out of high school.

- In 1984 equal numbers of male and female high school students took advanced-placement examinations, which can lead to college credit. By 1997, more females were taking and passing the exams.

- Among high school seniors, 60 percent of females are confident that they will attend and graduate from a four-year college, compared to 49 percent of men; 22 percent of females say graduate school is "definitely" in their future compared to just 16 percent of males.

Learning Disabilities

A learning disability is a neurological (brain-based) problem that causes difficulties with processing information. It has nothing to do with intelligence; in fact, a learning disability is usually suspected when a child's difficulty in learning seems at odds with his or her intelligence. In general, boys are more likely than girls to be diagnosed with learning disabilities. Is that really because they're more susceptible to them? That's possible; it may be the case with the most common learning disability, dyslexia. But there is also little doubt that some boys may draw more attention to themselves because of their active and impulsive behavior.

In recent years, some educators and child development researchers began to question the use of terms like *dyslexia* and *attention deficit disorder,* because they see them as pejorative labels that can humiliate children but aren't good at describing either the problems or skills of an individual child. Mel Levine, M.D., is a professor of pediatrics at the University of North Carolina and the founder of All Kinds of Minds, a nonprofit institute that develops programs to help parents, teachers, clinicians, and children address differences in learning. Dr. Levine believes that "different minds learn differently," as he writes in his book *A Mind at a Time,* and that many children are ill served by a one-size-fits-all education philosophy. In a recent video, he explained his disagreement with such labels.

> The model we're describing is one that avoids labeling kids. So we don't use terms like, "LD," "ADD," . . . (or) "dyslexia," . . . We set aside all the labels and say, "Instead of labeling the kids, why don't we label the phenomena? It's much more precise. It's much more specific. It's much less stigmatizing." . . . Labels . . . reduce kids. [They] can be stigmatizing, pessimistic, and they can become self-fulfilling prophecies. . . . I kind of find it dehumanizing when a kid says, "I'm an ADD kid." I keep saying, "Anything else?" That's what we mean by reductionism. You've reduced somebody. You've lost all the richness as a human being, in a sense, by saying that. And so we favor description over classification and try to get by without any categories, without any labeling, but focusing on the phenomena, the profile, the breakdowns, the strengths . . .

With that in mind, we're going to discuss some of the most common learning disabilities. And while I agree with Dr. Levine, we're going to use the old terms because they are still in wide use. They're also the terms that are used by school officials and that enable kids to obtain access to special education and related services or accommodations when they need it.

Reading Disabilities

Reading disability, or dyslexia, is the most common of all learning disabilities, affecting between 5 percent and 12 percent of children, according to a recent study by researchers at the Mayo Clinic. People with reading disabilities have a neurological impairment that makes it hard for their brain to readily understand and process the most basic element of spoken language, the phoneme. Phonemes are the individual sounds within syllables and words formed by letters or blends of letters. As a result, they have trouble reading, writing, and spelling.

Some studies have found that boys are four or five times more likely than girls to have reading disabilities. Recent studies came to differing conclusions. One, from Connecticut, found that boys and girls are equally likely to have dyslexia; another, from the Mayo Clinic in Minnesota, found more boys than girls with the problem. Whatever the actual numbers, it's clear that lots of boys have dyslexia and that the earlier it's diagnosed, the better.

Dyslexia has long been known to run in families. Experts say people with dyslexia nearly always have at least one relative with the condition as well. In early 2001, British scientists reported they had tied the disorder to chromosome 18. If researchers succeed in identifying the precise genes on the eighteenth chromosome responsible for this problem, a genetic test might someday let parents know their child's risk while he or she is still very young.

If the answer to most of these questions is yes, talk to your pediatrician or local school district about getting a fuller assessment. If your son is dyslexic, don't worry or panic. It's important to understand that having dyslexia does *not* mean that he is cognitively impaired, "slow," or mentally retarded. In fact, the term is only applied to people with at least normal intelligence. There are many famous and brilliant people who have had dyslexia, including Albert Einstein and Thomas Edison.

Dyslexia does not mean that your son will not learn to read. By using a combination of special teaching techniques in the classroom, behavioral therapy to teach good study habits, and intensive instruction from a reading specialist, kids with dyslexia can and do learn to read. They may not do it as quickly as you do; indeed, they may always read a bit slowly. But many adults with dyslexia learn specific coping strategies so thoroughly that their dyslexia stops being a disability.

The Dyslexia Institute, a British organization, developed the checklist below to help parents identify kids who may have a reading disability.

All Ages
- Is he bright in some ways with a "block" in others?
- Is there anyone else in the family with similar difficulties?
- Does he have difficulty carrying out three instructions in sequence?
- Was he late in learning to talk or in speaking clearly?

Ages Seven to Eleven
- Does he have particular difficulty with reading or spelling?
- Does he put figures or letters the wrong way, e.g., *15* for *51, 6* for *9, b* for *d, was* for *saw*?

- Does he read a word, then fail to recognize the same word farther down the page?
- Does he spell a word several different ways without recognizing the correct version?
- Does he have a poor concentration span for reading and writing?
- Does he have difficulty understanding time and tense?
- Does he confuse left and right?
- Does he answer questions orally but have difficulty writing the answer?
- Is he unusually clumsy?
- Does he have trouble with sounds in words or a poor sense of rhyme?

Source: Reprinted with permission of The Dyslexia Institute.

Other Learning Disabilities

Dysgraphia

This neurological problem causes people to have difficulty writing. They may have trouble with the physical aspects of writing such as holding a pencil or they may find it difficult to spell or put thoughts on paper. As a result, they may avoid tasks such as writing school papers and they may have trouble fleshing out their ideas on paper even though they can explain their ideas verbally.

Dyscalculia

This neurological problem causes difficulty organizing and processing information related to math or numbers. It affects between 2 percent and 6 percent of U.S. elementary-age school children. Making change or balancing a checkbook can be extremely difficult. People with dyscalculia may also have a poor sense of direction, and difficulty reading maps or following directions.

Dyspraxia

This interferes with the sending of messages from the brain to the body, causing trouble with certain movements or with speech. It affects around 2 percent of the population; most are male (see page 131, "The Clumsy Child").

Sensory Processing Disorders

These disorders are problems in the way the brain receives and processes sensory information from our senses of sight, smell, hearing, taste, and touch. People with this kind of disorder may have trouble distinguishing letters, figures, or sounds from each other. They may also struggle with spatial relationships and have trouble reading maps or navigating. This can obviously interfere with someone's ability to learn, solve problems, and complete tasks.

If you suspect that your child has a learning disability, talk to your pediatrician about getting an assessment, or request one from your local school district, which is required by law to provide it. If the school district psychologist diagnoses a learning disability, the district must prepare a treatment plan that may include special classes. This won't cost you anything.

Boys and AD/HD

Boys are generally more active than girls and they tend to have less control over their impulses. They're also far more likely than girls to be diagnosed with attention deficit/hyperactivity disorder (AD/HD) and four times more likely to be prescribed stimulant medication to treat it. Are these two trends related? As anyone who has children, or who follows the news, is aware, the number of kids (mostly boys) put on medication over the last twenty years has exploded, and the drug of choice—Ritalin—has become a household word.

The AD/HD-Ritalin explosion has kicked up furious controversy, and raises important questions for the parents of boys. Critics contend that AD/HD has become a trendy, overused diagnosis, fueled by the marketing efforts of pharmaceutical companies, the frustration of harried teachers and parents, and the acquiescence of physicians who, far too often, prescribe stimulants to children when asked, without attempting other interventions first. They suggest that boy nature—the fact that boys tend to be rambunctious, impatient, and have trouble staying in their seat—has been turned into a disorder requiring medical treatment.

Others counter that AD/HD is a legitimate neurologically based condition that is widespread and sows misery into the lives of children and their families. They say that stimulant medications can be effective in helping distracted, impulsive children focus their energy, and that these medications are, if anything, underused.

So how can parents sort through this minefield and figure out what's best for their child? That's not an easy task. Let's begin by talking about the disorder and how it's diagnosed.

Attention deficit/hyperactivity disorder is a behavioral problem with two basic elements. Children with AD/HD have a hard time focusing their attention or concentrating. They may also be excessively active or restless. As a result, they have trouble completing tasks, can't sit still, have trouble paying attention, and are easily distracted and forgetful.

Many experts consider AD/HD a neurological condition. In one recent study, researchers at New York University found that brains of people diagnosed with AD/HD are 3 percent smaller, on average, than the brains of people who are not. That's a fascinating finding from a research perspective but the differences in brain volume are too small to be helpful in diagnosing the disorder. There is still no blood test or brain scan that can detect whether a child does or does not have AD/HD. Instead, clinicians look at a child's symptoms and how he functions at home and in the classroom. And they look to the bible of the psychiatric profession, *The Diagnostic and Statistical Manual of Mental Disorders,* fourth edition (DSM-IV), published by the American Psychiatric Association.

The DSM-IV recognizes two kinds of AD/HD—inattention and hyperactivity/impulsivity. Here is the manual's checklist of symptoms used to diagnose these conditions.

Inattention
For at least six months, a child often exhibits six or more of the following symptoms:

- Fails to give close attention to details or makes careless mistakes in schoolwork, work, or other activities.
- Has trouble keeping attention on tasks or play activities.
- Doesn't seem to listen when spoken to directly.
- Doesn't follow through on instructions or finish schoolwork, chores, or other tasks (and not because he or she is rebelling or doesn't understand what he or she is supposed to do).
- Has a hard time organizing tasks and activities.
- Dislikes or avoids tasks that require sustained mental effort (such as schoolwork or homework).
- Loses things needed for tasks or activities (school assignments, pencils, books, tools, or toys).
- Is easily distracted by things around him or her.
- Is forgetful.

Hyperactivity/Impulsivity
For at least six months, a child often exhibits six (or more) of the following symptoms:

- Squirms or fidgets in seat.
- Has a lot of trouble staying seated.
- Runs around, jumps, or climbs at times when it's not appropriate.
- Has trouble playing quietly.
- Acts driven or "on the go."
- Talks excessively.
- Blurts out answers before questions have been fully asked.
- Has trouble waiting his or her turn.
- Interrupts or intrudes on others.

These symptoms must begin before age seven, be present in two or more settings (such as school and home), and clearly impair the child's ability to function at school or in social situations. Finally, they should not occur as a result of other disorders or mental illness.

Source: Adapted with permission from the Diagnostic and Statistical Manual of Mental Disorders, *4th ed.,* © 1994, American Psychiatric Association.

Are We Overdiagnosing and Overmedicating Our Kids?

The trouble with the list of symptoms above is that it reads like a basic definition of childhood, especially for boys. How many kids *don't* squirm or fidget in their seat? How many kids *don't* run around or play when they shouldn't? And how many actually *do* listen to what grown-ups tell them to do? "I find the diagnosis so hopelessly vague that maybe it should be abandoned and we should get another diagnosis to replace it," says William Carey, M.D., director of behavioral pediatrics at Children's Hospital of Philadelphia.

Most studies have found that 3 percent to 5 percent of children have AD/HD; a recent study of children in Minnesota found that roughly 7.5 percent of children there fit strict definitions of the disorder. What distresses Dr. Carey and others is that in some places, more than one quarter of boys are being diagnosed with AD/HD. That's what Gretchen LeFever, Ph.D., a clinical psychologist at Eastern Virginia Medical School, found when she tracked AD/HD diagnoses in three Virginia schools for a recent study. She sent surveys to parents of children in these three schools and found that 28 percent of boys and 11 percent of girls had been diagnosed with AD/HD. Nearly 85 percent were taking medication. Of those taking medication, 37 percent got no other help, such as behavioral therapy. Incredibly, in one school 63 percent of students who were young for their grade were taking medication for AD/HD.

Other experts feel that numbers like these are aberrations, that while there may be overprescribing, the real problem is exactly the opposite. "It would be erroneous to conclude that there is overdiagnosis and overtreatment of AD/HD," wrote Rachel G. Klein, Ph.D., a longtime AD/HD researcher and director of research training at the New York University Child Study Center, in a recent Center newsletter. "There is overwhelming evidence that stimulant medications are the treatment of choice for children with AD/HD . . . (Yet) many if not most children with AD/HD are not receiving adequate treatment."

Clearly, there are degrees of inattention, distractibility, and impulsive behavior. As your child ages, he should develop more ability to sit still and focus for longer periods of time. He should develop a greater capacity to control his impulses and refrain from blurting things out or running around the classroom.

If your son's teacher expresses concern or irritation with his behavior, that's obviously a problem you'll want to pay attention to. But it doesn't necessarily mean that he has AD/HD, even if the teacher says he does. "I've had numerous examples of kids who had normal nervous systems but were just kind of feisty and temperamentally difficult," says Dr. Carey. "Many teachers jump to the conclusion that he must have AD/HD and send notes home to the parents recommending stimulant medication to make the child easier to manage. Unfortunately, an overworked pediatrician or family doctor with only a few minutes per patient may take the teacher's word for it and prescribe medication without doing a full evaluation."

As we've noted, a problem in too many schools is that classes are not set up for high-energy, impulsive boys. Too many classrooms are run in a boring, repetitive style that doesn't capture the interest or imagination of children or allow for the movement and stimulation they need.

The key question, really, is how much of a problem your son's behavior poses for him, for you, your family, teachers, and classmates. Do his impetuous actions or his inability to follow directions keep him from getting along with others? Does he get in trouble at school? Does his behavior cause him unhappiness?

If you find yourself answering "yes" to these questions, you should talk to your pediatrician or family physician. He or she should make a preliminary assessment of the problem and refer you to someone—a child psychologist, psychiatrist, or behavioral pediatrician—who can make a full multidisciplinary evaluation of your son. Such an evaluation should include conversations with and rating scales completed by your child's teachers, counselors, and other important adults in his life, like coaches or recreation leaders. The psychologist or pediatrician should also consider other reasons why children are restless or inattentive in school: undetected learning problems, difficult temperaments, undiagnosed perceptual or processing problems, lack of sleep, hunger, depression, or abuse in the home. "All kids who are having trouble paying attention in school should also have a thorough psychoeducational evaluation by a qualified psychologist to discover cognitive strengths and weaknesses," says Dr. Carey. Based on all this, your pediatrician or psychologist, in consultation with you, can make a diagnosis.

Treatment Options

There are three basic approaches to helping children with AD/HD—parent education, behavioral therapy, and, most common of all, medication. In many cases, a combination of these approaches may end up working the best.

Parent Education

Parent education programs teach parents about AD/HD and help them adjust their expectations and the way they manage their children. The idea is that many parents raising children with AD/HD get locked into patterns of interacting with their kids that make it more likely that they won't comply. The classes help parents learn to focus on family interactions and to adjust expectations and discipline to accommodate—rather than fight against—the disorder.

These programs teach parents, for instance, not to overwhelm an already overstressed child with multiple demands. They help parents recognize the most problematic settings and situations for a child, to learn how and when to monitor a child closely, and when to allow a kid more freedom and room. Example: It can be hard for children to go from an activity they're interested in (computer game) to one they're not (homework or housework). In that situation, parents may need to be physically close to the child and to actively help him make the transition, rather than shouting directions up the stairs and then getting angry when those directions are not followed.

Parent education classes are often offered through local hospitals, health maintenance organizations, or parenting organizations. Many parents find them quite helpful but they are often not enough to help families in which a child has clear and persistent AD/HD. These families will need to consider trying behavioral therapy and/or medication.

Behavioral Therapy

Behavioral therapy programs are designed to train parents (and sometimes teachers) to use behavior management techniques with their children. They help parents establish incentives to encourage appropriate behavior and consequences to discourage inappropriate behavior. They focus on many of the same issues and ideas as parent education classes but with more depth and detail. Behavioral therapy sessions generally involve parents, not children. (They are not to be confused with cognitive behavioral therapy, which aims to help children change their thought patterns. This kind of therapy, while very useful for some problems, has not been found effective for children with AD/HD.)

Behavioral training programs normally begin with eight to twelve weekly group sessions with a trained therapist. The therapist teaches parents ways of managing the time children spend at home, along with techniques for giving directions to children and for reinforcing good behavior, while discouraging problematic behavior. Trainers also focus on techniques that can help teachers and parents build more structure into a child's time in the classroom. One example: Parents can ask teachers to send home frequent, even daily, reports or notes so they find out how things went at school that day and can reinforce the teacher's efforts and offer rewards or consequences.

Most behavioral therapy training also counsels parents on how to prevent children from relapsing into old ways and how to handle these relapses when they occur.

Medication

By far the most common way of treating AD/HD is with stimulant medications, which have been used to treat attention problems since the 1930s. The first drugs used for this purpose were amphetamine and dextroamphetamine, both of which are still used today. Methylphenidate was developed in the 1940s and marketed under the name Ritalin in the 1960s. But it wasn't until the 1980s and '90s that the use of Ritalin and other stimulants really soared. Today the hottest stimulant medication for AD/HD is Adderall, a form of amphetamine which is growing in popularity largely because it is not yet available in generic form and is being heavily promoted by its manufacturer, Shire Pharmaceuticals. There is no evidence that it works any better than different formulations of Ritalin, which is available as a lower-cost generic.

Stimulants have been found by numerous studies to reduce hyperactivity, impulsiveness, and distractibility in most children—for as long as they're actually taking the medication. One of the largest studies of treatment for children with AD/HD, organized by the National Institutes for Mental Health, was reported on in 1999. The Multimodal Treatment Study (MTA study) followed nearly six hundred children aged seven to nine—80 percent of them boys—for fourteen months. The children were treated with stimulants, intensive behavior therapy that included both parent and teacher training, or they were treated by the family's pediatrician in whatever way he or she decided. Some children got both behavior therapy and medication. All approaches helped reduce the children's symptoms at least somewhat, but the researchers found medication to be the most successful single treatment in reducing symptoms.

The MTA study's lead investigator, Peter Jensen, M.D., a Columbia University child psychiatrist, reported that 56 percent of the children who took stimulants experienced a reduction or complete discontinuation of their behavioral problems. But the most successful approach, the study found, was to combine medication and behavioral therapy. That combination helped 68 percent shed their symptoms.

"Medication is the most effective treatment," says Jensen. "But it is not a substitute for effective parenting methods based on behavior therapy principles. Both together are a good package, and should be augmented by extra school supports as well, such as tutoring if needed, [and] school classroom accommodations."

What about side effects? In the short term, stimulants seem safe. The most common side effects are nervousness, difficulty sleeping, and appetite loss. Less common are skin rash, nausea, dizziness, headache, weight loss, and blood pressure changes. Perhaps the biggest problem is that many who take stimulants become irritable or depressed as the medication wears off. The long-term picture is less clear. Though a growing number of children take stimulants for years, the MTA study lasted only fourteen months, and few studies have followed children for longer. In late 2002, a new medication, Strattera, was approved by the FDA for children and adults with AD/HD. The first nonstimulant drug approved for AD/HD, Strattera increases the amount of a neurotransmitter, norepinephrine, available in the brain.

SCHOOLYARD BULLIES

The neighborhood or schoolyard bully is nothing new. The sad truth is that few of us go through childhood without being bullied. Ironically, kids who become bullies are often picked on or abused by someone bigger or more powerful than they are, frequently their own parents or older siblings. But while many adults tend to downplay the seriousness of bullying, it frightens and scars many children. The following discussion on bullying was adapted from an article in *Reader's Digest* written by my coauthor, Rob Waters.

Bullying: Zak Hollis's Story

Zak Hollis is a large, soft-spoken boy and because he has Tourette's syndrome, a neurological disorder, he sometimes jerks his head and body in uncontrollable ways. Being different from other children made him a target. In 2000, when Zak was ten and a fourth-grader in Albuquerque, New Mexico, other kids would walk up to him, jerk their heads back and forth, and laugh. They'd call him "dork," "tic-boy," and "retard," and, when he complained to teachers, "tattletale." Sometimes, he says, even teachers told him to stop tattling.

"The kids would tease me and mimic me. They made fun of me every day," Zak says. "I wouldn't cry at school, but I would at my home. I hated that school. I felt so stressed out there, I felt sick all the time."

Of course, it's not just kids with neurological problems or special needs that get treated this way. Every year, millions of American children are victimized by bullies at school. Indeed, a survey of 15,000 sixth to tenth graders published in the *Journal of the American Medical Association* in 2001 found that 30 percent were involved in bullying—as perpetrators, victims, or both. Nearly half of sixth graders reported being bullied, and 13 percent said they were bullied at least once a week.

Children who are taunted and abused by classmates do different things with their pain and anger. A few—like the school shooters in Littleton, Colorado, or Jonesboro, Arkansas—strike back with deadly fury. A report released in 2001 by the Secret Service looked at forty-one children involved in recent school shootings and found that two thirds felt they had been "persecuted, bullied, threatened, attacked or injured" prior to attacking their classmates.

Another response, equally tragic but far more common, is to turn this anguish violently inward. In 1999, more than 1,800 children and teenagers took their own lives, many out of despair at the way they were treated by their peers and classmates.

Of course, most kids who are bullied don't shoot up their schools or commit suicide. But they may go through school feeling like Zak Hollis—miserable and afraid. Experts say that children victimized by bullies are more likely than other kids to be lonely, depressed, anxious, and angry. "When kids are picked on throughout elementary school, they're really struggling by the time they get to middle school," says Laurie Austin, a social worker and former coordinator of violence prevention programs for the Albuquerque schools. "School becomes a place of anger and victimization. They're more likely to drop out. A lot of them just disappear."

The young victims of bullies often turn into depressed adults, says Dan Olweus, Ph.D., a Norwegian psychologist who pioneered research on bullying. And bullies themselves have problems. One study by Olweus found that 60 percent of kids who were defined as bullies in middle school years had criminal records by the time they were twenty-four. And many continue to gravitate toward violence. "Often bullies in school are like domestic violence offenders in training," says Austin.

But schools don't have to be this way. In 2001, Zak Hollis transferred to Chelwood Elementary School. He's found a home there, a haven from teasing and unhappiness where the whole community—students, teachers, and parents—became part of an effort to deal with bullying.

In the fall of 2000, Chelwood began a program known as bully-proofing. First developed by Dan Olweus, and refined by a group of psychologists and school counselors in the Cherry Creek, Colorado, school district, it is based on the idea that bullies are a small minority who gain power over other children only because no one stops them.

In most schools, around 10 percent of kids act as bullies and another 15 percent play the victim, says Chelwood's former principal, Jack Vermillion. "The other 75 percent just want to stay out of it so they don't get picked on. Our philosophy is you get that 75 percent who are not being bullied standing up with the 15 percent who are. Now you've got 90 percent against 10 percent saying, 'No, you're not going to do that at our school.' "

Starting in kindergarten, the school trains children who are being bothered by another child to ask that child to stop and then, if necessary, get help from an adult. Children who see an incident are urged to help, again, by asking the bully to stop and getting adult help if needed. Says Vermillion: "We're trying to get kids to become people who stand up and get involved."

In elementary and middle schools in Norway, such programs led to a 50 percent drop in bullying behavior, vandalism, fighting, and truancy, according to studies conducted by Olweus. Similar, though less dramatic results came out of a study of middle schools in South Carolina.

If there's a problem with bullying at your child's school, you might want to tell the principal or other school officials about the bully-proofing program. To get more information, contact the people at Cherry Creek or visit their website at *www.bullyproofing.org*.

DON'T BE A VICTIM: HELPING YOUR BOY DEAL WITH BULLIES

What should you do if you think your child is being victimized at school? Here are some suggestions from Carla Garrity, Ph.D., a child psychologist in Cherry Creek, Colorado, who helped develop the "bully-proofing" program and wrote the book *Bully-Proofing Your Child.*

Listen to Your Child

If your son says he's getting picked on, believe him. Don't diminish his experience. Let him know you're concerned and will help. Ask questions that help assess the situation: Is this transient or minor teasing that's likely to blow over? Is he mildly bugged, or scared and distressed? Has he asked the child to stop? Has he told a teacher and has the teacher responded?

Be Ready to Act

Go to school and talk to a staff member about the situation if the bullying is serious or continues for several weeks. Start with your child's teacher, but be prepared to go to the counselor or administrator if the teacher doesn't respond.

Don't Call the Bully's Parents

This rarely helps matters, since parents tend to defend their own child.

Enlist an Assist

If your child's being bullied, he's going to need help. A friend or two who look out for your child can make a big difference. If he has trouble getting help on his own, ask a teacher or counselor to recruit help from other kids. A friend can accompany a bully-prone kid when he goes to the bathroom or during recess. And a friend can also remind a boy who provokes the wrath of others to cool down and withdraw from a brewing fight—before it starts.

Stay on Top of Things

Keep talking with your child and the school about how things are going. If necessary, try to meet with the principal and teacher regularly. In the end, if the school fails to respond or help, you may need to consider changing schools.

COULD YOUR BOY BE A BULLY?

It may be hard for you to believe that your own angel could be a bully. But bullies are *somebody's* children, so you might want to take a closer look.

The main thing about bullies is that they like to be in control. They act tough and cool, as if they can't be hurt and are never sad, or scared. Boy bullies try to dominate with their bodies and fists; girls by using their wits and words to hurt or exclude. They don't generally show regret, compassion, or empathy. "Bullies are quite smug and unrepentant," Garrity says. If you want to assess whether your kid is a bully, Garrity suggests asking two questions:

"Do others sometimes pick on you?" If the answer is no or never, you may have a child who bullies. Bullies rarely admit to having problems with other kids.

"How do you feel when you see someone else getting picked on?" If the answer is along the lines of "He got what he deserved," watch out.

If you think your child is acting like a bully, don't let it go or dismiss it. The most important thing you can do is to teach your child to have empathy—and model it yourself. "You draw their attention to the pain they have caused another child," says Garrity. "Make them look at the fact that someone else is bleeding or hurt."

The best time for kids to learn empathy is before they get to sixth grade, when kids are quite amenable to change. After that, Garrity says, it gets tougher, but it's more important than ever to try.

Source: Reprinted with permission of Sopris West Educational Services, from Bully-Proofing Your Child *by Carla Garrity. Copyright © 2000.*

3

Boys and Accidents and Injuries

From the moment he could walk by himself, my son Harry was nearly unstoppable. He would climb on everything, jump on anything, and run ahead when the spirit moved him. And let me tell you, the spirit moved him a lot. By the time he was a year old, my husband had made up Harry's motto: "No mere mortal can contain him." He was nearly four before we were comfortable letting him out of his stroller to walk with us on the streets of New York. If he wasn't restrained, he would take off running or veer abruptly toward the street with gleeful abandon.

Some years before, early on in my medical career, I was working at a small clinic on Manhattan's Lower East Side, making house calls to homebound elderly people. One day as we strolled down the street going from one building to the next, we passed a place where flowers, small candles, and condolence cards written in Spanish were placed along the street. I asked the nurse, Cookie, what had happened. She told me that a boy of six was riding a skateboard and had been hit by a taxi and killed. She knew the family and their heartbreak. Shaking her head with a heavy sigh, she said to me, "As a mother of a boy, you have to be prepared to lose him. This is what I told his mother." I have not forgotten her remark.

Cookie's words were a trifle dramatic, but they weren't far from the truth. Boys are far more likely than girls to suffer accidents and injuries. As a mother, I think about this every time we leave the house and my son wants to ride his bike or skateboard. I watch my two girls closely, but I almost don't need to. When we go out, they stay close by my side without me having to shout. My son, on the other hand, rarely misses a chance to dash ahead.

Statistically speaking, accidents and injuries are the biggest threats to a child's life. Bigger threats than cancer, pneumonia, meningitis, and heart disease combined. Nearly half of all childhood deaths result from unintentional injury. And boys are far more likely than girls to be injured or to die. In 1999, nearly 3,600 boys aged fourteen and under died from an accidental injury. Among girls, the number was substantially lower, around 2,200. Boys had a death rate that was almost 50 percent higher, a pattern that begins at age one and continues to old age.

The irony of these numbers is that injuries are not the problems we tend to worry about most as parents. And we do worry about so many things: Are they eating right? Are they getting enough sleep? Could a stranger kidnap and kill them? Could they contract a terrible disease?

The National SAFE KIDS Campaign, a research and advocacy group dedicated to preventing unintentional injuries in kids under fourteen, has surveyed parents about their worries. Their responses include things like AIDS, drive-by shootings, and crime, says Angela Mickalide, Ph.D., the group's program director. "Unintentional injury is not on the radar screen for most parents," she says. Yet one in five children are injured seriously enough to require medical attention, according to SAFE KIDS. SAFE KIDS prefers to call accidents "unintentional injuries" because they believe the word *accident* implies an unpreventable occurrence when in fact more injuries can be prevented.

Leading Causes of Death for Boys and Girls, 1 to 14, 1999

Cause of Death	Boys	Girls
Auto accidents	1,290	929
Drowning	585	274
Fires or burns	325	246
Suffocation	197	97
Pedestrian injuries (including by motor vehicle traffic and other)	447	273

Source: Centers for Disease Control and Prevention.

Take a look at the list above. In every category, more boys die than girls. In some cases boys are 50 percent more likely to die than girls!

Of course, most injuries are not fatal. For every kid who dies from an unintended injury, many more are hurt but alive. In the year 2000, 4.2 million boys aged fourteen and under were treated in hospital emergency departments for unintentional injuries, a number 50 percent higher than for girls.

Many things can injure children, and nearly all happen more often to boys than girls. Here are some examples, drawn from CDC statistics for 2000, and from other sources:

- More than one third of all injuries that required a child to go to the ER—2.4 million in all—were falls. Boys fourteen and under were more than twice as likely to die and 40 percent more likely to be injured in a fall as were girls of the same age.

- Almost 1.6 million children aged fourteen and under were injured when they were accidentally struck by a person or object. Two thirds—more than 1 million—of them were boys.

- Boys fourteen and under were five times as likely to die and two and a half times as likely to be injured in bicycle accidents as girls the same age.

- Boys fourteen and under are six times more likely than girls to be killed by an accidental gun shot, according to SAFE KIDS.

- When children die in residential fires, the most common cause of the fire is children playing with matches or other incendiary material. One study found that boys aged six to fourteen are nearly twice as likely as girls to have played with fire at least once.

- In 1998, more than 75 percent of children under fifteen injured or killed in farm accidents were boys.

BOYS AND BODIES OF WATER

For children, the second most common cause of injury-related death is drowning, and boys are two to four times more likely to drown than girls. My friend Mary McGorry learned this in a frightening way. She was putting on her bathing suit upstairs in a rented beach house on the Maryland shore when she gazed out the window and saw her six-year-old son Patrick in the water.

Just seconds before, Mary had cautioned Patrick, his four-year-old brother, and their cousin to wait at the door while she went upstairs to change. She also told them not to go to the water, which was a mere fifty feet from the house. But the boys didn't listen. They ran to the water's edge, where the waves were deceptively calm, and Patrick dove in. Mary ran down to the beach and sat for a minute watching the kids. With a big wave about to break on him, Patrick dove into it. Within seconds, the current was pulling him far from the shore.

Mary charged into the water, screaming for help from lifeguards far down the beach. She reached Patrick and struggled desperately to keep him above the water and tow him toward shore. But the current was strong and she made no progress. Finally, the lifeguards reached them and threw a flotation device. They hung on for more than five minutes before they were able to swim to shore.

A few months later, Mary still cries when she talks about it. "Every time I close my eyes at night I see Patrick's little head bobbing in the water," she says. Patrick, on the other hand, seems unfazed, with little apparent grasp of the danger he was in.

In 2000 more than nine hundred children under age fifteen drowned in the United States, making drowning the second leading cause of injury-related deaths for kids in that age range. It is an especially big threat to young children—25 percent of kids under five who die from an injury die by drowning. And once again, two thirds of drowning victims under fifteen are males. It's also important to point out that for every child who drowns, four more almost drown and need hospitalization. Some of these survivors end up with serious neurological problems because their brains were deprived of oxygen.

Kids drown for different reasons at different ages. Infants and babies under one year of age most often drown in the bathtub or a bucket. Kids from one to four usually drown in swimming pools, while those from five to nineteen may drown in lakes, ponds, rivers, or pools.

"Why are most drowning victims men?" That was the title of a recent study in the *American Journal of Public Health.* The authors conclude that males tend to overestimate their swimming abilities and place themselves in riskier situations than females. Older teenagers and adult males were also a lot more likely to drink alcohol when swimming or around water. Among teenaged or young adult males, there is a risk not only of drowning, but of injuries from diving into water that is too shallow. Diving accidents are the most common recreational injury that causes spinal cord damage.

BOYS ON BIKES

Whether it's the thrill of speed, the sense of independence, or the feeling of power it gives them, boys love to ride bicycles. As little guys, they cruise around on their trikes and Big Wheels, then graduate to two-wheelers ASAP. Many boys are really into their bikes and spend a lot of time riding them. Unfortunately, they can get seriously hurt in the process. When it comes to bicycling, boys suffer more injuries and deaths than girls, by a long shot. According to the CDC, in 2000, nearly 370,000 kids under age fifteen were injured while cycling seriously enough to be treated in an ER; 70 percent of them were boys. The National Highway Traffic Safety Administration reports that in 2001, 176 children under sixteen were killed in bicycle crashes; about 90 percent of them were males.

The vast majority of these injuries could be minimized or prevented by wearing a bicycle helmet. According to the CDC, wearing a helmet can reduce the risk of head injury by 85 percent and brain injury by 88 percent. If all bike riders wore helmets, the CDC says, 500 deaths and 151,000 injuries would be avoided each year. That's more than one death per day and one injury every four minutes. (For more information, see *www.cdc.gov.ncipc/factsheets/bikehel.htm.*)

In recent years, campaigns to promote helmets have been successful, especially among children. A survey conducted for the Consumer Product Safety Commissions found that helmet use among riders increased from just 18 percent in 1991 to 50 percent in 1998. According to parents surveyed, 69 percent of kids under sixteen wore helmets regularly, though some safety experts doubt those figures. Too many children and teenagers resist wearing helmets because they think they're not cool or they find them uncomfortable. As of 2000, only twenty states and the District of Columbia had passed laws making helmet use mandatory for children.

Helmets, of course, are not just for bike riders. Skateboards, in-line skates, and scooters can all result in head injury. In fact, as these sports become more popular, more and more kids are treated in emergency rooms for injuries sustained on skateboards or roller-blades.

Here are three good ways to encourage your boy to wear a helmet:

- Wear one yourself whenever you ride a bike or strap on skates.
- Explain—repeatedly—how important it is.
- Let your child pick out his own helmet. If a kid thinks his helmet is cool, he's much more likely to wear it. It's well worth spending extra dollars to buy one he really likes.

Be sure you buy a helmet that fits well and that he wears it properly. The helmet should be snug on the head and not move around easily. Wear it well forward, not pushed back, so it covers the top of the forehead. The chinstrap should fit snugly under the chin.

BOYS, CARS, AND CROSSING THE STREET SAFELY

The bells of an ice cream truck ring out and kids come running from every direction. A child darts out between parked cars and is struck by a moving vehicle. Such accidents happen far too often: According to the CDC in 2000, of the 534 pedestrians under fourteen killed by car, 329 were male. Males made up more than two thirds of the 44,593 pedestrian injuries in kids under fourteen (30,039).

When kids between five and nine are hit by vehicles, it's often because they dart out into the street. This is an age when many kids are starting to assert their independence—they often think they know just about everything and can take care of themselves. Unfortunately, children, especially boys, can be impulsive and they lack the cognitive skills and experience to judge a vehicle's distance and speed.

"There is clear research suggesting children ages five to six don't have cognitive skills to judge the speed of traffic and the size of traffic gaps," says David Schwebel, Ph.D., an injury researcher at the University of Alabama, Birmingham. "I am currently doing a study on this by having children cross a pretend road immediately adjacent to an actual street. The children use the cars on the real road to cross our pretend street on the grass. Almost all six- to seven-year-olds dart across when a car is coming, presumably because they don't have the cognitive skill to judge the traffic."

The rule here: Kids under ten should *never* cross the street by themselves.

The National SAFE KIDS Campaign has a number of suggestions on how to teach children about pedestrian safety.

Set Limits

- Require children to carry a flashlight at night, dawn, and dusk. Add reflective materials to children's clothing.
- Prohibit play in driveways, unfenced yards, streets, or parking lots.
- Walk with your child to find the safest route to school and other common destinations. Look for the most direct route with the fewest street crossings. Make sure he or she walks that way every time.

Teach Your Child Safety

Give your child some practical training in traffic safety; it can make a real difference. Teach your child to:

- Look left, right, and left again before crossing the street. Cross when the street is clear, and keep looking both ways while crossing. Walk, don't run.
- Understand and obey traffic signals and signs.
- Cross at corners, using traffic signals and crosswalks when available. Do not enter the street from between parked cars or behind bushes or shrubs.
- Stop at the curb, or at the edge of the road if there is no curb, before crossing the street. Never run into a street without stopping—for a ball, a pet, or any other reason.
- Walk facing traffic, on sidewalks or paths. If there are no sidewalks, stay as far to the left as possible.
- Watch for cars that are turning or backing up.

Practice these skills with your children over and over again. Supervise them until they show you they know how to be safe.

Source: Reprinted from "How to Teach Kids Pedestrian Safety," with permission from National SAFE KIDS Campaign.

Falls

Every year, more than 2.3 million kids in the United States under fifteen hurt themselves badly enough in falls to be treated in a hospital emergency room. Young children are at the greatest risk; about half of all deaths and injuries from falls happen to kids under five. They fall from windows or balconies; they tumble down stairs. According to the American Academy of Pediatrics, older boys are more likely to fall from dangerous areas such as fire escapes and roofs.

Some 200,000 preschool and elementary schoolchildren get treated in an ER every year after being hurt in an accidental fall on a playground. Most of these injuries happen when kids fall off swings, monkey bars, climbing structures, or slides. More than one third of the injuries are severe, causing fractures or internal injuries, according to the CDC. Make sure you have appropriate window guards on your windows, gates on stairs, and have childproofed your home to prevent falls.

Dog Bites Boy—Often

Most parents don't think much about a dog bite, but every day, about 914 people are bitten badly enough to be treated at a hospital emergency room. That's more than 300,000 serious dog bites a year—more injuries than from skateboards, baby walkers, and in-line skates combined! In addition, another 4 million people suffer less serious bites, and half of them, according to the CDC, are children under twelve. A few people each year—fifteen to twenty—are killed when mauled by a dog or dogs.

What group is the likeliest to get bit? Boys between five and nine years old. They get treated in the ER for dog bites nearly 60,000 times per year, according to researchers at the University of Pittsburgh. Of nine activities examined in the study, only baseball and softball injuries accounted for more ER visits than dog bites.

What's especially troublesome about dogs biting children is that more than 70 percent of the bites are to the child's face, neck, and head. Larry R. Schmitt, M.D., a child psychiatrist in La Jolla, California, says the experience can traumatize children. In a letter to the *Journal of the American Medical Association*, Schmitt wrote that for a child, the experience of being attacked by a dog was the equivalent of an adult being mauled by a bear. And yet, Schmitt says, many of these kids suffer emotionally in silence, not talking about or processing the terrible fear they continue to feel. Why? Schmitt says many kids don't want to upset their parents, who may act guilty or anxious when the attack is mentioned. And boys, Schmitt says, may feel it's unmanly to speak about their fears. He treated one boy who broke down in tears more than one year after he was badly bit in the ear.

Most dogs who bite children are familiar; they belong to neighbors or even to the child's family. For that reason, it's important to teach all young children to be careful around dogs. Here are a few suggestions:

- Never leave a child under five alone with a dog, especially if one of them is eating. No one should approach a dog that is eating or caring for puppies.

- Teach children to be cautious with dogs. That means they shouldn't pet strays or unfamiliar dogs, climb fences into areas occupied by dogs, or tease a dog. Approach all dogs with care, even the family pet. And always ask an owner's permission to approach or pet a dog.

- Be sure you supervise and restrain your dog properly, especially when children are around.

- If a dog approaches or bites, teach children to remain motionless. If they're knocked down, they should curl into a ball and lie still.

- If your child is bitten, let him talk about it later, so he can heal emotionally as well as physically.

BOYS AND GUNS

Go to the website of the group Stop Handgun Violence, look at the faces, and read the stories. It will break your heart.

Twelve-year-old Brian Crowell was at a friend's house, talking on the phone with his sister when his friend showed him a gun he had found in his mother's room. Thinking he had removed all the bullets, the friend pulled the trigger. Brian was hit in the neck and died a few hours later.

Phranquee Binkerd was at her boyfriend's house when they found a gun. They were looking at it, thinking the chamber was empty, when it discharged, killing Phranquee. She was fourteen years old.

Andrew Papen and a friend found an old handgun while playing at Andrew's house. His father had forgotten it was there. The gun went off, killing Andrew, who was twelve years old.

These are the faces, the flesh-and-blood children behind some grim and hard-to-fathom statistics:

- From 1995 to 2000, an average of four children age nineteen and under were killed every day in gun-related accidents and suicides. And nearly 85 percent of children killed in unintentional shootings are boys.

- In 2000, according to the CDC, 3,888 American children and teenagers under eighteen were injured in the accidental firing of a gun. Nineteen of them were female; 3,870 of them were male.

- American children between five and fourteen are nine times more likely to be killed in the accidental shooting of a firearm than children in twenty-five other industrial countries combined.

- According to a new Harvard University study, children who live in the five states with the highest levels of gun ownership (Louisiana, Alabama, Mississippi, Arkansas, and West Virginia) are sixteen times more likely to die in an accidental shooting than children who live in the five states with the lowest levels of gun ownership (Hawaii, Massachusetts, Rhode Island, New Jersey, and Delaware).

- Some 40 percent of U.S. households have guns, and 22 million children live in households with guns.

- A gun in the home is twenty-two times more likely to be used in an unintentional shooting than in self-defense.

The bottom line here is that in addition to deliberate, violent shootings, guns kill lots of children because so many Americans keep guns at home. And because boys, when they find guns, find it almost impossible to resist the urge to look at them, handle them, and play with them.

Researchers at Emory University conducted an experiment not long ago that quickly hit the front pages. They recruited a bunch of eight- to twelve-year-old boys, separated them into groups of two or three, and turned them loose in a room where a real gun had been hidden. The researchers watched through a one-way mirror. Of the groups that found the gun 75 percent of the time at least one kid in the group actually handled it. In half the groups, one or more members pulled the trigger. This happened despite the fact that more than 90 percent of the boys who handled the gun or pulled the trigger had previously received gun safety training.

When ABC News repeated this experiment, planting hidden cameras in the room, the boys who found guns became so excited they could scarcely contain themselves. One fifteen-year-old boy was so drawn to the gun that he kept going back to it to handle it, again and again—a total of nine times. "Something in my head was just telling me to touch it and play with it," he later explained.

Guns, Gun Play, and Your Boy

The best way to address boys' overwhelming attraction to guns—both toy and real—is an issue parents have grappled with for years. Some aspects of this issue are complicated, but others are—or ought to be—incredibly simple. Let's start with the easy part.

Don't Keep Guns in Your Home

If you keep a gun in your home for self-defense, take a few moments and think about what you're doing. A study in the *New England Journal of Medicine* created controversy when it found the risk of getting killed was 2.7 times greater in homes with guns as opposed to homes without them. The National Rifle Association did not like this study, naturally. Nevertheless, a gun in the home is far, far more likely to hurt or kill a family member or friend than to be used against a threatening stranger in self-defense.

If You Must Have a Gun, Lock It Up

If you (or your spouse) feel that you absolutely *must* keep a gun in the house, keep it locked up and unloaded, with the ammunition hidden and stored separately. Just think for a moment how you'd feel if your child found your loaded gun and played with it. Think how you'd feel if your child or a friend was injured or killed. It happens every day. Don't let it happen in your home.

The trickier issue is figuring out how to deal with boys' overwhelming interest in playing with toy guns. My own belief is that giving my son "real" toy guns and weapons amounts to an endorsement of violent play. I've learned firsthand, though, that not having actual toy guns doesn't keep a child from engaging in gun play. Like most parents of boys, I've watched with a mixture of amusement and horror as my son and a pack of his little friends turned sticks, Tinkertoys, even pieces of bread into guns with which he could shoot me, his sisters, his father, and the doormen at our building. In Harry's world, we've all died a thousand deaths.

The reality is that little boys want to feel powerful and to conquer their fears. Playing with toy guns is a way to do that. According to Laura Davis and Janis Keyser, parenting educators and authors of a column on the Internet site ParentsPlace.com, boys—especially those around the age of four and five—become fascinated by toy guns. Don't worry about this. It's developmentally normal and doesn't mean your son will grow up to be a violent person.

How should parents deal with our boys' interest in gun play? Here are Davis and Keyser's guidelines for responding to your son's fascination with guns while encouraging nonviolence.

Set Parameters for the Play

When we forbid a form of play, that play often goes underground and we lose an opportunity to help our children figure out answers to their questions. Make it clear to children that any play that intimidates, hurts, or frightens another child is unacceptable. Then clarify the rules about toy guns at your house: "In our family, you're not allowed to point guns at any people without their permission." Or, "I want you to keep your gun play outside."

Provide Props for Play That Have Multiple Uses

Giving children open-ended props encourages flexibility and creativity. When a child makes a gun out of plastic blocks, ten minutes later, those plastic blocks can be transformed into a container ship. However, when children play with highly realistic guns, those guns can only shoot and kill.

Make Your Values Clear

Children care deeply about how we see the world. Share your perspective with your son: "When I see you playing with guns, it really upsets me because people can be hurt by real guns."

Help Children Deal with Their Fears

Often gun play increases when children are feeling fearful. Children look for symbols of power (such as guns and swords) to help them feel more secure. Helping children deal with their fears can take some of the intensity out of their gun play.

Let Your Kids Know That People Are Working to Stop Violence in the Real World

Kids sometimes use gun play to cope with fears about violence in the real world. If your child seems scared of real violence, talk about people who are working to stop fighting and end war. This can help kids feel safer and, therefore, less driven to engage in gun play.

Provide Kids with Alternatives to Gun Play That Help Them Feel Powerful

Four- and five-year-olds love to be competent. Providing them with real work experiences such as carpentry, cooking, and gardening can channel some of the energy being directed into gun play in a new, more creative direction.

Source: Reprinted with permission from an article entitled "Little Boys Who Love Guns: Encouraging Nonviolent Play," written by Janis Keyser with Laura Davis for ParentsPlace.com, an iVillage website.

WHY BOYS?

This section of the book is filled with scary statistics and anecdotes aimed, primarily, at pointing out one thing: Boys, for some combination of reasons, tend to live on the edge, take risks, and seek thrills more than girls. In the process, they get hurt much more often than girls. I don't raise these issues to scare you. There's enough fear going around these days. I hope to raise your awareness, point out some of the major risk areas, and suggest simple steps that help reduce your boy's chances of becoming a statistic. The question is, why? Why are boys so much more likely to get injured?

Barbara A. Morrongiello, Ph.D., a psychology professor at the University of Guelph in Ontario, Canada, has shown that boys tend to downplay their chances of getting hurt. "Boys tend to believe that they're not as vulnerable to injury," she says. "They think 'It's not going to happen to me' more often than girls seem to." If boys do get hurt, they're more likely to attribute it to bad luck, rather than something they did. Girls, on the other hand, tend to be more realistic about dangers and more likely to take the blame if injured. "Girls seem to proceed more cautiously than boys," Morrongiello says. "A boy is thinking, 'I won't get hurt—or if I do it won't be too bad. Or it won't be my fault.'"

Of course, these tendencies emerge in studies of large groups of children; the way any individual child acts is much less predictable. "You'll certainly see boys that are very cautious and girls who are risk takers," she says.

Still, on balance, Morrongiello has observed that these differences in thinking result in substantial differences in risk taking. She found that even boys as young as two are more likely to approach hazardous things in a laboratory and to interact with them. Girls, on the other hand, are more tentative. They may approach an object, but will look back to see if Mom is watching. "Boys were quick to get in there and interact with the hazard, making it a little more challenging for moms to keep boys safe," Morrongiello says.

David Schwebel, Ph.D., is a pediatric psychologist at the University of Alabama, Birmingham, who studies how and why kids get injured. Boys, he says overestimate their abilities: "Boys think they can do more than they can." In one study, Dr. Schwebel had kids reach for an object on a shelf. Sometimes the object was within their grasp, sometimes not. Boys, more often than girls, tried to reach higher than they actually could. "Translate that into trying to climb a tree and you can see how injuries happen," he says. Though he points out that this overestimation of ability is broad generalization (that is, some girls overestimate too), "There's something going on that in general makes boys more likely to overestimate."

So what is it about boys that causes them to be risk takers, that leads them into harm's way so much more often? The knee-jerk reaction that "boys will be boys" doesn't really explain much. Christine M. Kennedy, R.N., Ph.D., a child development expert and associate professor at the University of California, San Francisco, says parents tend to see boys as being more physically capable than girls and treat them accordingly. "Based on these perceptions," she says, "they encourage their young boys to do things that they really aren't quite ready for."

Morrongiello concurs. "Studies we have done show that moms and dads seem to be more tolerant of risk taking by sons than by daughters. They [tend to] focus on mastery and independence as good goals for how they want their son to be." What's more, points out Schwebel, the more impulsive a boy is, the more likely parents are to believe the child is more capable than he actually is.

It's not that parents are forbidding their girls doing things, but rather they caution girls more with subtle and not-so-subtle cues they're frequently not even aware of delivering. In one study, parents were asked to teach their two- to four-year-olds how to slide down a fireman's pole. Morrongiello found that parents urged their boys to complete the task 65 percent of the time, compared to 19 percent of the time for girls. They helped the boys get down 17 percent of the time and assisted the girls 67 percent of the time. And when a boy resisted completing the task, 58 percent of parents continued to insist that he do so, much more than they did with girls. And here's the part that really surprised me: It didn't matter which parent was supervising the child. Mom was just as insistent as Dad was.

In exploring this issue, I'm not suggesting that you keep your son from taking appropriate risks. Learning new skills and overcoming physical and mental challenges are part of the joy of growing up. It's also part of what makes boys boys, and I wouldn't want to change that for the world. What you can do is be aware that with a young boy, you may need to be more vigilant, supervise him more closely, and review carefully the rules you set up to protect him from injury. As he gets older and more cognitively capable, your goal should be to help him think about the risks involved in different activities and to find strategies to minimize them.

It's also important to follow through with consequences when he does risky or forbidden things. If he rides his bike without wearing his helmet, a logical and appropriate consequence is to forbid him from riding for a while. If he climbs a tree higher than you've told him he could go, bar him from climbing for a spell.

Teaching your child to exercise good judgment sounds like obvious advice for parents, but you have to think through how you are going to do that. "Instilling good judgment involves talking about why certain activities could be dangerous and also discussing why it was a bad idea to do something that resulted in injury," says Jodie Plumert, Ph.D., an injury researcher at University of Iowa. "It's critical for parents to provide children with a causal explanation rather than just saying 'Don't do that.' It's like a doctor explaining to patients why it's important to take the full course of antibiotics rather than just saying 'You should take all the pills.'"

In the end, the best thing you can do is appreciate his energy and enthusiasm as you try to moderate his more reckless impulses. Help him become aware of the risks and dangers of the activities he loves, but don't be afraid to impose limits. Boys will be boys—but parents must also be parents.

4

Boys and Body Control

It seems rather ironic: Boys, those running, swooping, jumping creatures who seem unable to sit still, are more likely to have problems with what I'll call, for lack of a better term, body control. They take longer to toilet train, and they're more likely to wet their beds, stutter, and be clumsy. No one is really sure why. Boys start out several weeks behind girls in neurological development at birth. But many experts suspect there's more to the story. Genetic and hormonal factors combined with how we socialize boys probably delay some basic developmental skills. The following is a discussion of a variety of things that boys are more likely to confront during development than are girls. Not to say that girls avoid all these issues—they certainly don't!

TOILET TRAINING

It's true: Boys on average finish toilet training at thirty-nine months while girls get it done four months earlier. Why are boys so slow in this department? That's a question many weary moms and dads ask themselves as they watch little girls dance around in flowered underpants while their boys are still wrapped in diapers.

"There's probably some delay in the maturation of the nerves that help sense when the bladder is full," speculates Robert Needleman, M.D., an expert in behavioral and developmental pediatrics and a vice president of Dr. Spock Company (*www.drspock.com*). "But nobody probably really knows." One thing that is not responsible, Needleman and other experts say, is bladder size. Boys' bladders are no smaller than girls.

Whatever the reason, it's probably best not to ask your mother or father about this one. They're liable to go into one of those "when you kids were raised, we didn't put up with this kind of behavior" speeches and insist that you should just strip off that diaper and park him on the potty.

They're right about one thing. One and two generations ago, parents were indeed potty training their children much earlier. A 1957 study from Stanford found that 50 percent of parents began toilet training when their babies were around nine months old and that 90 percent were fully trained by the time they were eighteen months.

Things began to change a few years later. In 1962, T. Berry Brazelton, M.D., the famous Harvard Medical School pediatrician, published a hugely influential paper in the journal *Pediatrics*. The paper was based on a study of over 1,000 babies and found that kids who were potty-trained at two or three had fewer toileting problems later in life than kids who were trained earlier. The early trainers, Dr. Brazelton found, were more likely to wet their beds later and to have problems with constipation because, in their anxiety, they withheld their poop.

Brazelton argued that parents should follow their children's lead when it comes to toilet training, waiting for signs of interest from the child and not pressing them before they appear ready. Pediatricians and parents alike took Brazelton's advice to heart and in the years that followed, the toilet training age got steadily older. Today, according to a recent study from the Medical College of Wisconsin, 60 percent of children are trained by around age three; by four years 98 percent of kids are out of diapers. For some kids, the process happens even later, which is why Pampers and Huggies now come in size 6 for kids as big as thirty-five pounds. Not surprisingly, two thirds of Huggies size 5 and 6 diapers are sold for boys.

Dr. Brazelton's go-slow advice and the trend toward later toilet training is not without critics. Psychologist and "traditional parenting" expert John Rosemond ridicules the notion parents should wait for signs of readiness from a child as "psychobabble." Rosemond, who delivers more than two hundred lectures a year and hawks T-shirts that say BECAUSE I SAID SO, advocates what he calls the "naked and $75" method for children under two. "Let the child walk around the house naked from the waist down, put the potty where it is easily accessible, and correct mistakes matter-of-factly," he writes. The $75 pays for carpet and furniture cleaning.

I didn't train my kids that way, and few mainstream pediatricians concur with Rosemond's approach, but I'm sure it can work for some kids. I'm partial to Brazelton's technique because I think it carries less risk of problems later—problems that could be a lot more bothersome than your kid still being in diapers at the age of three. My feeling is that if you push kids to train before they're ready, you're setting them up to fail.

I'm not going into great detail about the method Dr. Brazelton and others espouse since it's available in so many places for you to read. Try "Successful Toilet Training for Boys" on the parenting website BabyCenter.com. A great book to check out is *Potty Training the Brazelton Way* by Drs. Brazelton and Joshua Sparrow.

Here are a few suggestions:

- Potty train your boy sitting down since pee and poop often come out at the same time. Once he's mastered his sit-down technique, he can rise whenever ready. He'll probably want to anyway, especially if he's got a dad or older brothers to watch. This can be messy at first, since good aim comes with practice. Little boys in a hurry often don't wait for the last drops of urine to hit the toilet. This leaves either the floor or their pants wet.

- If Dad or an older brother can get involved, take advantage of it. Your little man can watch the big guys and see how it's done, without much need for verbal instruction. This can really speed up the process. And here's another trick for improving his marksmanship: A good friend taught her son by floating a colorful paper circle in the toilet and having him take aim. It works great.

- Beware though, if you also have daughters. When my twin girls were learning to potty train, they watched their older brother standing up. At three, my daughter Ruby went through a phase where she liked to stand over her little potty and pee like her big brother. Sometimes her aim was better than his!

- One word of caution with boys: You might want to help them raise and lower the toilet seat. Though there is usually a little space between lid and bowl, many a little penis has no doubt been hurt when the toilet seat crashed down on it. Also, urine guards on training toilets can get in the way so you may want to get a toilet that doesn't have them.

- Finally, be patient. You can expect the process to take eight to ten months, according to that study from the Medical College of Wisconsin.

NIGHT TRAINING

Once your boy has gained control over his bodily functions during the day and he no longer wears diapers, the next challenge is for him to stay dry during the night. This can take a while. Be prepared and don't try to rush it.

To start, put him to bed in training pants or pull-ups—"like bigger boys wear"—and encourage him to get up during the night to change if he wakes up wet or needs to pee. Have him pee before he goes to bed so it becomes a habit. When you notice that his pull-ups are rarely wet in the morning, retire them. Praise him for his great progress and for how big he's become.

Be ready, though. This process is rarely a straight dash to the finish line. In all likelihood, wet nights are not yet a thing of the past. Use a plastic liner to protect the mattress. Let your son know he can call you if he wakes up wet. When it happens, gently sponge him off so his skin doesn't become irritated, change his pajamas and bedding, and get him back to sleep. Be calm and matter-of-fact. It's no big deal.

Exactly how long this next phase takes varies greatly. Some kids, especially boys, continue to wet their beds on occasion long after they've finished toilet training. If this happens once in a while, don't worry about it. But if it happens frequently, you'll want to develop a strategy to deal with it. Don't get upset. Bed-wetting—or nocturnal enuresis—can be frustrating for both parent and child.

BED-WETTING

Twice as many boys as girls have problems with bed-wetting, according to the National Institute of Diabetes and Digestive and Kidney Diseases, which reports that, overall, about 10 percent of five-year-olds, 5 percent of ten-year-olds, and 1 percent of eighteen-year-olds wet the bed.

So why do more boys have this problem? And why do they take longer to get over it? No one knows for sure, but many experts think it's a part of the general trend of boys lagging behind girls developmentally. Because of this lag, doctors tend not to worry about or treat bed-wetting boys before age six, though they may treat girls at age five.

Bed-wetting seems to have a strong genetic component. A child whose parents both wet their beds is very likely—with a 77 percent chance—to have the problem as well. If only one parent was a bed wetter, the odds drop down to a still-high 44 percent. In 1995, Danish researchers actually found a gene located on chromosome 13 that is at least partly responsible for nighttime bed-wetting.

In some children, bed-wetting is related to the body's levels of antidiuretic hormone, or vasopressin, a hormone that normally rises during sleep and reduces the kidney's urine production. If nighttime levels of this hormone fail to rise as they should, too much urine can be produced, filling the bladder as if it were daytime.

Bed-wetting may be annoying to you, but for children it is embarrassing and miserable. A poll taken in 1996 found that 21 percent of parents punished their children for wetting the bed.

"It is important that parents have compassion and care when dealing with a bedwetting child so as to avoid feelings of shame," says Brian F. Greer, M.D., a child psychiatrist in private practice in Boca Raton, Florida. "There is absolutely no role for punishment in the treatment of bed-wetting."

Studies confirm that kids who wet their beds often feel so bad about it that it negatively affects their self-image and even their academic performance. Research also shows that bed-wetting is not generally caused by any behavioral or psychological problem. It is not an act of defiance or lack of will on the part of a child. We now know that:

- Bed-wetting is not related to small bladder size.
- Bed-wetting is not caused by drinking too much liquid before bed, though that might make things worse.
- Bed-wetting is not generally caused by emotional problems, though punishing a child who wets his bed can lead to them.
- Bed-wetting is not the result of laziness or manipulation and is not something a child can control.

In treating bed-wetting, doctors classify it in two different ways. The vast majority of kids who wet their beds have never been able to keep dry at night. They are said to have *primary enuresis.* A few kids get through toilet training and learn to stay dry at night, but then wet their bed later. They have *secondary enuresis.* This second form can be related to a urinary tract infection or to the onset of a more serious problem such as diabetes. But it can also be related to a child going through intense stress or emotional trauma—anything from being sexually abused or bullied at school to the birth of a new sibling, a death in the family, or the parents' divorce.

If Your Boy's a Bed Wetter

The most important thing is to do nothing that's likely to make him feel worse than he already does. Don't shame, criticize, or punish him. Don't even show your frustration or disappointment. If he's under six years old, you may not want to do much of anything. Few pediatricians, in any case, will treat a five-year-old boy for bed-wetting, and many believe six-year-old boys are too young for treatment.

If a boy is still not dry by age six or so, then it's time to check in with the pediatrician. Often reassurance is all that's needed. Remember, bed-wetting is embarrassing and uncomfortable for your son and can limit his social life, which means he should be eager to control the problem. Don't keep him from overnight activities because of it. A thick pair of pajamas and his own sleeping bag can usually save him from embarrassment. Here are a few things to do at home to try to prevent or stop bed-wetting.

- Remind him to pee before going to bed. If he says he doesn't need to, make him try anyway.

- Limit his intake of liquids in the last two hours before bed, especially of caffeinated sodas and other drinks. While drinking before bed is not the cause of bed-wetting, drinking less might give his body a bit less in the way of raw materials to process.

- Talk to him and let him know that bed-wetting is not his fault. If you or your husband were bed wetters, tell him. If he understands that it's a genetic problem, he's likely to feel less ashamed.

- Try waking your child once a night for a bathroom trip. Set an alarm near your child's bed or your own.

- Try a moisture alarm that goes off when he starts to urinate so he can jump up and finish in the toilet. This trains his body to recognize the signs of a full bladder and can be quite effective—if child and parents are motivated and patient. It can take months to work but is one of the most effective methods to help train the sleeping brain to respond to a full bladder.

Medications are sometimes prescribed for bed-wetting. The antidepressant imipramine has been used for years, but has fallen out of favor recently because of potential side effects. These days a synthetic hormone called desmopressin acetate (DDAVP), which is similar to the body's own hormone vasopressin, is administered as a nasal spray or a pill before bedtime, usually for three to six months. If it works to keep your son dry, you can gradually taper off the drug. It can also be used as a stop-gap measure for camp or overnights. However, kids who stop taking it often start wetting the bed again.

Bed-wetting can be a frustrating hassle, and in some kids it lasts far too long. But if it happens to your son, stay calm and be compassionate. You, and he, will get through it eventually.

ENCOPRESIS

A messier and often more intractable potty problem—though, thankfully, a much rarer one—happens when children out of diapers soil their pants on a regular basis. This problem, known as *encopresis,* happens to between 1 percent and 2 percent of all children and is four times more common in boys than in girls. About 80 percent of the time, it's related to a child being constipated.

In those cases, a child doesn't have regular bowel movements, or doesn't fully empty his bowel of feces, which build up in his colon. The resulting fecal mass can become large and hard, making bowel movement painful. Liquid feces may leak out around the hard stool, soiling a child's underwear. Over time, the large, hard stool stretches the muscles of the colon and rectum, causing them to become less sensitive. The stretched muscles and nerves stop signaling the brain to go to the bathroom.

At first, the leaks are small, showing up as streaks or stains in the underwear. Lots of parents figure their child just isn't doing a good job wiping. But over time, the intestine stretches further, and the amount of leakage increases. Eventually the child is having major accidents and passing whole bowel movements in his underwear.

For the most part, encopresis is not a behavioral problem; children aren't pooping in their pants because they're lazy or angry. But the underlying constipation may be related to a child feeling anxiety for some reason and withholding his poop.

A study several years ago at the University of Pennsylvania looked at children who withheld their poop and found they were often kids whose toilet training was late. In fact, when children didn't become toilet trained until after three and a half, they became "stool toileting refusers" (as the researchers called kids who wouldn't poop) half the time. So did three quarters of kids who weren't trained by their fourth birthday.

An occasional accident is probably nothing to worry about. In fact, doctors only use the term encopresis when a child is regularly soiling his or her underpants for a period of at least six months. You may not want to wait that long to deal with it, though. Talk to your pediatrician if you notice your boy has more than an occasional accident.

Treating encopresis is not quick or easy; it often takes six months or longer to get the problem under control. He may need to use enemas to get those hard, compacted stools out of his colon, as well as laxatives to soften them. Many doctors will wait to use enemas because some kids experience them as punishment. To help get things moving you'll want to make sure he eats lots of fiber (fruits and vegetables), drinks plenty of liquid, and gets regular exercise. These things help soften his stools and help him poop more regularly. Doctors also recommend that a chronically constipated child be put on a schedule where he sits on the toilet after meals. The body's own reflexes generally make it easier to poop after a meal.

If the underlying problem is that he's withholding his stool, he may need to return to wearing diapers. That was the approach Bruce Taubman, M.D., of the University of Pennsylvania used with great success in his study of "toileting refusers." He instructed parents to tell their children that they couldn't wear underwear until they were pooping and peeing in the toilet. They were also told to make no efforts at all to toilet train these boys and girls.

"Many of the parents were very reluctant to do this," Taubman wrote in his study. "They considered it going backward, negating all they had achieved, and worried it would confuse the child." But when they followed Taubman's instructions, it worked. Within three months, twenty-five of twenty-eight refuseniks were back on the potty again, doing their business as they should.

STUTTERING

As they learn to speak, many children have trouble getting out words or they repeat syllables or sounds. Their minds are swimming with questions, ideas, and fragmented thoughts, and they are just beginning to figure out how to turn them into speech. Mistakes are bound to happen. They may throw in lots of fillers like "um," "er," and "uh," or repeat syllables or words once or twice *li-li* like this. For a child under five, this mild stuttering is normal, and most children outgrow it.

But some children have a more serious stuttering problem that endures beyond their early years. These kids may repeat the sound at the start of a word three or more times, more *li-li-li-li-like* this. They may elongate certain sounds like *mmmmom*, speak quickly, or pause for a long time in the middle of a sentence or even a word. Many kids do a combination of these things, and they may also seem nervous or distressed as they struggle to speak.

Stuttering is a common problem. About 3 percent to 5 percent of preschool-aged children stutter, and the ratio of boys to girls is about the same. But by fifth grade, for reasons no one really understands, 80 percent of stutterers are male, a ratio that persists into adulthood. The good news is that almost 80 percent of kids who stutter will overcome their speech problem, either on their own or with the help of a speech therapist, by the time they're sixteen. The bad news is that kids who stutter, whether they overcome their speech problems or not, are often teased and humiliated by other children. This is probably the most difficult part of stuttering.

All together, some three million Americans stutter, including such celebrities as actors Bruce Willis and Julia Roberts, former basketball star and current sports commentator Bill Walton, and ABC-TV news reporter John Stossel, who has become a spokesperson for stutterers. James Earl Jones stuttered so badly that he passed through his early and middle childhood scarcely talking. In high school, he discovered that he could read Shakespeare aloud—if he was alone at his family farm.

No one knows exactly what causes stuttering, though there have been plenty of different theories. Hippocrates wrote that stuttering was caused by dryness of the tongue. Others suggested that it stemmed from anatomical defects in the mouth, and this led to useless and sometimes mutilating surgical procedures. Stuttering is not caused by bad parenting or hidden psychological problems, and it has absolutely nothing to do with intelligence. Stressful events, such as parents divorcing or changing preschools, can make stuttering worse, but they don't cause the problem.

The current thinking is that stuttering stems from a neurological problem that causes glitches in the timing and rhythm of speech. Researchers at the University of Toronto have used PET scans to examine the brains of stutterers and non-stutterers and have found that people who stutter make greater use of the right side of their brain when they speak, while non-stutterers use their left brains more. The left side is more effective at directing speech, the researchers say.

Ways to Help Your Child with Stuttering

If your child stutters, there's a lot you can do to help him. The most important thing is a calm, uncritical attitude. Let him know you accept him as he is, whether he stutters or not.

- Speak to your child in a slow, relaxed way and encourage other friends and family members to do the same. Do your best Mr. Rogers impression.

- Encourage all members of the family to take turns talking and listening. Children who stutter find it much easier to talk when there are few interruptions and they have the listeners' attention.

- Make it a point to spend some stress-free, relaxed time each day with your child. Let him talk about whatever is on his mind.

- When conversing with a child who stutters, pause a second or two before you respond or answer a question. This keeps things relaxed and unhurried.

- If he's talking to you and he stumbles, keep normal eye contact and calmly wait for him to finish. Don't tell him to slow down or relax. It rarely helps. And don't finish his sentences.

- Don't act annoyed or impatient if his stuttering worsens. He's doing the best he can, and your acceptance can help him a lot. Use facial expressions to let him know that you're listening to what he's saying, not how he's talking.

- When he gets upset, reassure him in whatever way seems most helpful to him. For some children, it feels good to hear a message like "I know it's hard, but lots of people get stuck on words." Other kids are more reassured by a touch or a hug. Don't act as if nothing happened, though. That can make him think stuttering is so bad it can't even be mentioned. Instead, encourage your child to talk about his stuttering if he wants to.

Get Professional Help

If your child stutters on more than 10 percent of his words, stutters with great effort and tension, or avoids stuttering by changing words and using extra sounds to get started, he probably needs speech therapy. Look for a speech and language pathologist with a certificate from the American Speech-Language-Hearing Association. There are several places you can turn for this help.

Your local school district is required by law to provide speech therapy to children in the community who need it. Some school-based speech therapists have experience with stuttering, others may not. Find out if your school district has a specialist. Or look for one at a speech clinic, university, hospital, or in private practice. If you fight, you may get the school district to pay, but you'll need to become knowledgeable about the law and how the system operates.

The Stuttering Foundation of America (1-800-992-9392), *www.stutteringhelp.org*, can provide you with the name of a speech-language pathologist in your area who specializes in stuttering.

There are a number of other advocacy organizations that maintain websites that can be great sources of information and can help you get in touch with experts and other parents and children who are grappling with the same issues.

SNORING

Things aren't going so well for your child at school. He's having trouble paying attention, he doesn't seem to be remembering things, and he isn't performing well academically. He's got a lot of energy—too much, in fact. The teacher complains that he's "bouncing off the walls." Sounds like classic symptoms of attention deficit disorder, right? Well, not so fast. The problem could actually be something altogether different, and quite unexpected. Your child could have sleep apnea.

Sleep apnea? Since when do children get sleep apnea? If you've heard of it, you may know that it's primarily a disorder of overweight adults. But it turns out that children can get it too. Timothy Hoban, a pediatric sleep specialist at the University of Michigan, says sleep apnea affects 1 percent to 3 percent of all children. It causes a child to stop breathing during sleep for anywhere from ten seconds to one minute. And it can happen many times a night. Each time breathing is interrupted, sleep is too, because the brain has to wake the sleeping child so he or she can start breathing again. A lot of times, the kid will startle awake momentarily, and make a loud gasping or snorting sound before falling back to sleep.

Sleep like this would leave adults yawning and feeling groggy during the day. Not so with kids. "It's surprising to learn that sleepiness is not one of the common symptoms in children," says Hoban. "In fact, many kids may be inattentive, energetic, or even hyperkinetic." Kids under eight who snore seem to be the most likely to be hyperactive. In one recent University of Michigan study, 30 percent of kids who snored—but only 9 percent of kids who didn't—had high hyperactivity scores. Kids with sleep apnea are also more likely than other kids to wet their beds, be behind on growth charts, and, in rare cases, have high blood pressure.

My neighbor Geri's identical twin sons snored so loudly it kept the rest of the family awake. She mentioned this offhandedly to their pediatrician, not thinking it was a "real" problem. Luckily for her, the pediatrician realized her boys might have sleep apnea and ran tests. It turned out they did. Now they've been treated successfully and the boys—and the rest of the family—are getting a good night's sleep.

In adults, the cause of sleep apnea is usually obesity—excess fatty tissue around the throat can literally obstruct the air passage. That can also happen in kids, but it's much more common for kids with sleep apnea to have enlarged tonsils and adenoids. And that brings us to the good news about children's sleep apnea: Surgery to remove tonsils and adenoids solves the problem for most.

In years past, like when I was a kid, a lot of kids got tonsillectomies if they had frequent sore throats with tonsillitis, enlarged and infected tonsils. The procedure fell out of favor because doctors realized that for most kids with sore throats, tonsillectomies were not really necessary. More recently, however, the T&A (tonsillectomy and adenoidectomy) has made a comeback as a way to treat sleep apnea. These days, it is normally done as an outpatient procedure. A simple operation, it does require general anesthesia and that's usually the scariest part for kids and parents.

Many kids with sleep apnea outgrow it, especially if they're younger than six when they develop the problem. Kids between two and six tend to have especially large adenoids, compared to the size of their airway. In many cases, as they get older, the airway will grow more than the adenoids, and the problem eases or disappears. Until things change, these kids can get a better night's sleep by wearing a mask that pumps oxygen into their nose and mouth.

If your child is snoring a lot, talk to your pediatrician, especially if he's having problems in school. Treating the sleep apnea just might resolve troublesome daytime behaviors.

NIGHT TERRORS AND SLEEPWALKING

Boys are more likely than girls to have night terrors. These are much worse—and scarier—than regular nightmares. Your child, who was sleeping peacefully, suddenly sits up and starts screaming in the middle of the night. He's utterly terrorized and may keep hollering for up to thirty minutes. During that time, nothing you say helps comfort him; in fact, it makes things worse.

Unlike nightmares, which take place during the REM (rapid eye movement) stage of sleep, night terrors take place during deep, non-REM sleep. They usually happen to children between three and eight and generally begin about ninety minutes after a child falls asleep. It's hard to believe but even though his eyes are open and he's screaming to wake the dead, a child who's having a night terror is actually still asleep. He probably won't remember a thing in the morning.

If your son has night terrors, don't try to wake him, as many parents do. This usually just makes him agitated. Better to help him lie back down so he can continue sleeping. If night terrors become a pattern, you may be able to prevent them by waking him up about thirty minutes after he's fallen sleep, breaking up the first hour of really deep sleep. Fortunately, night terrors do go away on their own.

One other sleep disorder that occurs more frequently in boys—though thankfully it's less common than night terrors—is sleepwalking. Sleepwalkers face the potential for real harm. Parents may need to set up gates or barriers to prevent a child falling down the stairs or off a balcony. Parents should avoid shaking, slapping, or shouting at the child while he's sleepwalking. Usually kids outgrow this by adolescence.

THE CLUMSY CHILD

Some boys really do have two left feet. Steven* is a sweet six-year-old boy so lacking in coordination the other kids disperse when they see him coming. Running is a contact sport for Steven. His arms flailing in every direction, he smacks kids in the face, falls on them, or trips them. The result: Kids get angry and Steven is excluded. It's heartbreaking to watch and even tougher for Steven, who must confront not only his physical failings, but social ones as well.

Years ago the term "clumsy child syndrome" was coined to describe kids like Steven. It is also called *dyspraxia, developmental dyspraxia,* or *developmental coordination disorder.* Children with this problem are of normal intelligence and apparently healthy but have coordination difficulties severe enough to interfere with their socialization or academic performance. It is usually diagnosed between the ages of six and twelve and is more common in boys. Learning disabilities, AD/HD, poor handwriting and drawing skills, as well as social immaturity are more likely to occur in kids who lack physical coordination. Clumsiness was once believed to be a phase that kids outgrew. Newer research shows the opposite. Clumsy kids often have problems that continue into adolescence and adulthood. Parents must understand that a clumsy child is not lazy or sloppy, and the problems are not likely to disappear. If your son fits this description, have a discussion with your pediatrician. Family physician S. Sutton Hamilton, M.D., of the Virginia Commonwealth University School of Medicine, has studied clumsiness in kids and says the single most important thing for parents is to recognize it is not the child's fault. "These kids really are doing the best they can," he says. He also advises parents to be sure their child is evaluated for co-existing conditions such as learning disabilities. Occupational therapy can help some children improve some motor skills and self-esteem. Finding the right activity, such as swimming or horseback riding, can help a clumsy child achieve athletic success.

5

The Care and Feeding of Boys

Most teenagers are in the prime of good health. They're young, they're strong, and they feel invincible. Yet, as we all know, there are reasons to be concerned about the health of our teenagers, especially boys. The two biggest worries are that many teen boys do risky things, and that they're learning the same bad health habits that harm the health of many men and cheat them of years of life.

Some risky behavior exacts a stiff price in a hurry. Up to 80 percent of what kills teens is the result of risky behavior—reckless or drunk driving, violence, and depression. Others—like smoking or drinking—may take their toll over time.

There's another risk males seem especially prone to taking. It's a form of neglect—macho neglect—and it's been honed to an art form by generations of men. They learn to ignore their pain, to pay little attention to their body, and avoid seeing doctors whenever possible.

The teen years are a time when health habits really take shape. The health messages boys absorb during these years, and the habits they develop can easily become lifelong patterns. Much as we'd like to think things have changed, the "tough guy" messages so common in our culture still hold sway, especially with adolescent boys trying to prove their manhood.

Young boys are still hearing "big boys don't cry." Coaches still exhort older boys to "suck it up" and play through pain or embarrassment. Males of all ages hear sports announcers gush over the courage and strength of a football player who's playing with a broken hand or is back on the field, taped up, after an injury. Or a vice president who's back at work a day or two after a heart attack or an angioplasty.

Sadly, a lot of boys also hear the men in their lives—their fathers or uncles or big brothers—insist that an injury or ailment is no big deal and they don't need the doctor. "When the going gets tough, the tough get going," doesn't mean going to the doctor.

These lessons take their toll and perpetuate a male behavior pattern that damages the health of men. These are the reasons males of every age are more likely to die than women, and that men's average life span is five years shorter. The time to change this pattern is during a boy's youth, when his attitudes and beliefs are still being formed.

BOYS AND DOCTORS

Because they tend to be healthy, adolescents are less likely to go to the doctor than people of any other age group. Not surprisingly, teenage males are even less likely to go than females. The not-so-funny joke among doctors is that from last childhood vaccination, until their arrival by ambulance gurney after their first heart attack, the male of the species is not seen in the doctor's office.

A couple of years ago, a team of researchers, including adolescent medicine specialist Gail Slap, M.D., reviewed data on the doctor visits of thousands of children and teenagers. They found that in the years before age eleven, boys were slightly more likely than girls to visit the doctor, probably because boys are more likely to be injured in accidents. Then, during puberty, when girls start menstruating and dealing with gynecological issues, they begin visiting the doctor much more often; by the late teen years, nearly 70 percent of all doctor visits are made by young women. Not surprisingly, the researchers were alarmed by this trend.

"The declining utilization of non-emergency health services by males during adolescence is particularly disturbing given their simultaneously increasing rates of injury, homicide, suicide, sexually transmitted disease, and substance abuse," wrote Slap and her colleagues. "The older adolescent male is at high risk for morbidity and mortality, challenges the health care system with costly and often irreversible crises, yet provides limited opportunity for preventive counseling or early detection."

This gap between males and females is not just a result of girls needing gynecological care. Many boys, by late adolescence, have developed a resistance to doctors. "Boys hate to go to the doctor because they have to drop their drawers and they don't want to do it," says Jonathan Trager, M.D., an adolescent medicine specialist in Great Neck, New York. "I think that keeps a lot of young men away."

This is a problem for several reasons. If boys only go to the doctor when sick, doctors have little chance to get to know their patients. Doctors can't ask questions and learn about a boy's life and habits. And boys don't have the chance to get accurate information and work with the doctor on issues they are concerned about, such as sexuality or puberty. Surveys of adolescents by the Commonwealth Fund show 58 percent of adolescent boys wish doctors would talk to them about preventing sexually transmitted diseases, but only 24 percent of the doctors did.

Most experts, including the American Academy of Pediatrics, recommend that all adolescents—males and females—visit a doctor annually. Yearly visits allow doctors to keep up with their young patients at a time of rapid change and provide timely information and advice as they go through puberty and become sexually active, explains Martin Fisher, M.D., the chief of adolescent medicine at North Shore University Hospital in Manhasset, New York.

"The annual checkup is meant to pick up the psychosocial issues and risks of adolescence even more than the straight medical issues," Fisher explains. "The idea is to get them in once a year and ask them important questions including questions about sexual activity and substance abuse." This is not always easy to do with boys. "A lot of the psychosocial issues of adolescence affect both boys and girls, but the girls are more willing to talk about those issues and to come back for [follow-up] visits," he says.

Regular visits also allow doctors to intervene with teenagers about other bad health habits that often start in the teen years, such as smoking, being overweight, and not exercising.

Bottom line: Be sure your son has a doctor he likes and can talk to, and make sure he sees him—or her—once a year. As Jonathan Trager put it: "Don't assume that because your son is healthy he doesn't need to go to the doctor."

The Right Doctor for the Right Boy

If you're like a lot of mothers, you may have put a lot of energy into choosing your child's pediatrician—back when he was still in your womb. If all goes well, your son may want to stick with this doctor all the way through adolescence. Some teenagers, however, no longer want to go to a "baby doctor" or sit in a waiting room filled with toys and crying infants. So whom should he see now?

Some family physicians or adult internists see adolescents, and there are a growing number of doctors trained in the relatively new field of adolescent medicine. Adolescent medicine specialists are pediatricians or internists who have more in-depth training on issues that affect adolescent health.

What qualities should you look for in a doctor for your adolescent son? The most important quality is the ability to relate to the patient. Some pediatricians—like the wonderful doctor my son sees—can transition from treating young children to adolescents quite nicely and are comfortable with both age groups; others are uncomfortable with teens and talking about the issues that affect them. The solution is simple: Ask your son's doctor if he or she works with teenagers and feels at ease dealing with the issues that are summed up in the acronym SHADESS—for school, home, activities, drugs, emotions, safety, and sexuality. Ask your son about his preferences. After all, it's his doctor.

But remember this: Just because a doctor asks questions doesn't mean he or she will tell you how your son responds. In fact, in most states, doctors are forbidden from doing so by confidentiality laws. Legally, a doctor can't report back to the parents what the child says unless the child is in danger or is being abused. This can be a very touchy area, so everyone—parents, teenage patient, and doctor—should understand the ground rules. Sit down and clarify them before your son and his doctor delve into these areas. Your son is entitled to confidential care and that is good. Too often teens don't seek help at all because they mistakenly believe the doctor will tell their parents.

One last point: Many parents instinctively assume that boys are more comfortable with male doctors, but that is not always so. "They may in fact prefer a female doctor," says Jonathan Trager, M.D. "They may be comfortable with the female doctor they've had since childhood. It all depends on the relationship with that doctor, and if the doctor is sensitive to their needs."

Teach Your Child a Little Family History

One way to help your adolescent take a bigger role in managing his own health care is to acquaint him with your family tree and family's medical history. "Teenagers need to start to know about their family history," says Jonathan Trager. If there's a history of diabetes, heart disease, or cancer in your family, your children need to know and understand the implications.

What About the Sports Physical?

If your child is an athlete and wants to play organized sports, he'll need to get a physical before he can play. In many states, he'll need to get one each year. So what exactly is a sports physical, and how does it differ from a standard one? And does getting a sports physical satisfy the need for an annual physical? That can be a tricky question.

"A sports physical is specific for sports; you're checking the overall child's health, but you're asking questions specifically," says Eric Small, M.D., assistant clinical professor of pediatrics and orthopedics at Mount Sinai School of Medicine in New York, and author of *Kids & Sports*. "If they have asthma, how is that going to impact their sports? Have they had a history of concussion?" Unfortunately, Dr. Small says, "Much of the time the exam offered during a 'sports physical' is so cursory that it has little value."

What a good sports physical can do is focus on things that can affect athletes during play. For example, sudden death in an athlete, thankfully a rare event, is almost always due to an undetected heart abnormality. The challenge is to find that abnormality before it causes serious trouble. Using sophisticated screening tests for heart problems in every athlete is simply not cost effective. Critics of sports physicals often point out that "clearing" a kid to play gives a false sense of security, since a problem is unlikely to be detected during an exam.

So what can you do? Have your son answer the questions below. If the answer is yes to one or more, then a more involved evaluation of a boy's cardiac system might be in order and you should mention this to his doctor. These key questions, according to

Randy Eichner, M.D., professor of medicine at Oklahoma University Health Sciences Center, can help identify boys at risk.

- Have you ever fainted during exercise?
- Have you ever had chest pain during exercise?
- Has anyone in your family died suddenly under the age of forty?
- Has anyone in your family been diagnosed with a thick heart or Marfan syndrome?
- Have you ever used cocaine or anabolic steroids?
- Has any doctor ever disqualified you from sports?

Of course, many boys live in fear of the sports physical because they don't want the doctor to find anything that would exclude them from play. The good news is that this rarely happens; less than 1 percent are disqualified from play, according to the *American Family Physician* in 2000. Nevertheless, boys are often reluctant to check problems on the sports questionnaire, according to Dr. Small. "They're less likely to give you a medical history, especially if it's not the family doctor. The doctor doesn't know them, so they check off everything as 'no.'"

The goal of the sports physical is not to exclude kids from sports but to help them play safely. Here are other aspects of a boy's health history that should be discussed during a sports physical.

- A history of asthma.
- A history of breathing problems during exercise.
- A history of concussion.
- A history of trouble concentrating in school.
- A history of headaches.
- A history of problems in the heat.

The bottom line, however, is that a sports physical does *not* automatically take the place of annual contact between a teenager and a doctor who knows him well.

TESTICULAR SELF-EXAM

One important skill young boys should be taught early on during a regular physical is the testicular self-exam. Too few boys are aware that this simple test can help save their lives. Testicular cancer is the most common form of cancer in young men between the ages of fifteen and thirty-five! Make sure the doctor or other health provider has informed your son about the testicular self-exam.

HOW TO PERFORM A TESTICULAR SELF-EXAM

All males age fifteen and older should perform a monthly testicular self-exam. The National Cancer Institute recommends the following:

- Stand in front of the mirror and check for swelling of the scrotal skin.
- Examine each testicle with both hands. Place the index and middle fingers under the testicles with the thumbs placed on top. Roll the testicle gently between the thumb and the forefingers. Don't be alarmed if one testicle seems slightly larger than the other. That's normal.
- Find and familiarize yourself with the *epididymis,* the soft, tubelike structure behind the testicle that collects and carries sperm. If you know what it feels like normally, you won't mistake it for a suspicious lump. Cancerous lumps usually are found on the sides of the testicle but can grow up front.
- Other signs which should be checked by a doctor include: enlargement of a testicle, a heavy feeling in a testicle, or an accumulation of fluid in the scrotum.
- If you find a lump or anything that you are uncertain about, see a doctor right away. The abnormality may not be cancer, but if it is, chances are great it can spread if not stopped by treatment. Only a physician can make a correct diagnosis.

Remember, testicular cancer is highly curable!

THE FEEDING FRENZY: WHAT'S ON THEIR PLATE?

As a doctor and a mother, I'm concerned about the epidemic of childhood obesity. I want my kids to eat a healthy, well-balanced diet and avoid junk food. Unfortunately, like most working mothers, I don't have time to tend an organic garden or cook a perfect meal every night. But I know what my children should eat: A lot of fresh fruits and vegetables, whole grains, and healthy types of protein and fat.

The most important thing we can do for our children's eating habits is to make sure they learn about good nutrition. That means teaching kids about the foods that are all around them, that are advertised heavily on TV and that are unhealthy and harmful. I give my kids this message almost every day. It's a constant battle and one I resent having to fight. You can't just walk down the street without the kids constantly begging to stop in every store with a Coke or candy machine. But that's the reality we live in. (I'll talk more about what you should feed your whole family in chapters 11 and 15.)

TEENAGE MALE: BOY OR HORSE?

Adolescent boys are notorious for eating a family out of house and home. Not since the first year of his life will your son go through a more dramatic growth spurt than the one during puberty. In roughly a two-year period—between about twelve and fourteen for most—the mass of an adolescent boy's body nearly doubles. This requires a great deal of fuel, which is why you'll want to start getting frequent flyer miles on your grocery purchases.

Even before then, boys tend to eat more than girls. The average ten-year-old boy downs about 200 calories more than girls the same age. As boys age, this gap tends to widen so that by eighteen, the average male is consuming some 900 calories more than the typical young woman of eighteen. Teenagers' need for protein rises along with their need for calories.

Though most people are aware how important adequate calcium intake is for females, many do not realize that it is also critical for healthy bone development in males. And the adolescent years are when the process of bone development, and the need for calcium, are at their peak. Unfortunately, this increased need for calcium, along with a sudden growth in your son's appetite, is likely to happen at about the time he stops coming home for many of his meals. Thus, his dietary mainstays are likely to turn into french fries, sodas, burgers, and onion rings and he's getting more of his calories from between-meal snacks. He's also more influenced by his pals and less heedful of your ideas about what makes a healthy diet.

FOOD FOR JOCKS

If your son is an athlete, he should consume plenty of carbohydrates—not excessive amounts of protein, as many parents think. Carbs are the key source of fuel for brain and body. For athletic kids, calories and nutrients should be obtained from a diet that emphasizes nutrient-dense complex carbohydrates (50 percent to 55 percent) and adequate amounts of protein (12 percent to 15 percent) and fat (25 percent to 30 percent) to support growth and physical activity. Variety, balance, and moderation in food choices should be promoted, says Suzanne Nelson Steen, R.D., director of a sports nutrition service at the University of Washington and the coauthor of *Ultimate Sports Nutrition*.

Finally, athletic kids should drink plenty of liquid to avoid dehydration. Steen recommends 5 to 9 ounces for every twenty minutes of play. The idea that kids should just drink when thirsty is absolutely wrong, she says. Rather, they need to drink so they don't become thirsty. Dehydration can carry serious consequences.

6

When Things Go Wrong

THE FATTENING OF THE LAMBS

One day not too long ago my husband and I took our children to a shopping mall in western Massachusetts. This mall looks like thousands of malls all over the country. It has a Sears and a JC Penney's, athletic shoe shops, and bookstores. It also has a food court, that convenient collection of fast-food emporiums that graces hundreds of malls.

If you want to see America's obesity epidemic in action, just sit at a food court for half an hour. You'll see shoppers standing in line, choosing between burgers and burritos, pizza and fried chicken, french fries and 64-ounce super-sized sodas.

Many of the people—probably most—lining up at the food court would qualify as overweight or obese. And sadly, it's not just adults. Look at the hefty kids, huffing and puffing as they carry trays filled with fries and shakes.

This is the face of overweight America, the reason for the seemingly endless pronouncements and reports that emanate from health experts and bureaucrats. The latest word, from a national health and nutrition survey conducted in 1999 and 2000, is that 10 percent of two- to five-year-olds, and more than 15 percent of children and teenagers six and older, are overweight. That's more than twice the number of overweight kids measured in the late 1970s. It is truly a staggering problem, so staggering that in 2001, then Surgeon General David Satcher called obesity in children an epidemic.

The implications are huge. Fat kids, not surprisingly, are more likely to grow into fat adults, with all of the health problems of obesity. But long before they reach adulthood, overweight children face greater health risks than children of normal weight. More children than ever are being diagnosed with type 2 diabetes, which used to be found only in adults. Childhood asthma rates are rising steadily, and some researchers believe there may be a connection to obesity. And the early warning signs of heart disease are now found in the arteries of teenagers. Consider this observation from William Klish, M.D., chief of gastroenterology and nutrition at Texas Children's Hospital in Houston and the former chair of the Nutrition Committee of the American Academy of Pediatrics. "I think childhood obesity is the single most serious health problem in the United States today," Dr. Klish said in a lecture to pediatricians at Baylor College of Medicine. "If an answer to this obesity epidemic is not found, the present generation of children will not live as long as their parents." The biggest threat is the explosion of type 2 diabetes among young people. But that's not the only one. Here are some of the many health risks overweight kids may face.

Diabetes

Twenty years ago, type 2 diabetes among children was so rare that only 2 percent of all new cases of type 2 diabetes—the one strongly connected to obesity—occurred in people aged nine to nineteen. In fact, until recently, type 2 diabetes was known as adult-onset diabetes because it so rarely appeared in the young.

A disease that was once seen almost exclusively in adults is now being seen in younger, fatter people. "Twenty years ago I never saw a case of type 2 diabetes in a child at Texas Children's Hospital," says Dr. Klish. "Now more than one third of the children with diabetes that we're treating at TCH have type 2, and the percentage is rising rapidly."

What's more, many overweight children and teenagers who don't yet have diabetes are on the road to developing it. In one recent study, researchers at Yale School of Medicine tested the glucose levels of 167 obese children and adolescents and found that nearly one quarter of them had blood sugar high enough to be classified as prediabetes.

"Most of these children are at high risk of type 2 diabetes," said Sonia Caprio, M.D., an associate professor at Yale and senior author of the report. "And if they develop diabetes before the age of twenty, they face a lifetime of being at very high risk for complications from

TYPES OF DIABETES

Type 1 Diabetes

This results from the body's failure to produce insulin, the hormone that "unlocks" the cells of the body, allowing glucose to enter and fuel them. It is estimated that 5 percent to 10 percent of Americans who are diagnosed with diabetes have type 1 diabetes.

Type 2 Diabetes

This form results from insulin resistance (a condition in which the body fails to properly use insulin) combined with relative insulin deficiency. Approximately 90 percent to 95 percent (16 million) have type 2 diabetes.

Prediabetes

Prediabetes is a condition that occurs when a person's blood glucose levels are higher than normal but not high enough for a diagnosis of type 2 diabetes. It is estimated that at least 16 million Americans have prediabetes, in addition to the 17 million with diabetes.

Gestational Diabetes

Gestational diabetes affects about 4 percent of all pregnant women, about 135,000 cases in the United States each year. It usually resolves after pregnancy but many women will develop type 2 diabetes later on.

diabetes." Indeed, four of the teenagers had full-fledged diabetes at the start of the study but didn't know it, and three others went from having prediabetes to diabetes during the four years of research.

The study shows that one fourth of kids and teenagers who are now obese may spend their adult years struggling with diabetes, and the risks that it brings—of heart disease, kidney disease, blindness, and loss of limbs.

So should your child or teenager be checked for diabetes? The American Diabetes Association has developed guidelines for screening children. The guidelines are a bit complex, but the best advice is speak to your doctor if your son (or daughter) of ten or older is significantly overweight and has a close relative (parent, grandparent, sibling, first cousin, aunt, or uncle) with type 2 diabetes. Overweight African-American, Hispanic, American Indian, Asian, or Pacific Islander kids have an especially high risk.

Heart Disease

Over the past fifty years, the overall death rate from heart disease has dropped in the United States. But, according to the CDC, the rate of sudden cardiac death among young people has gone up. In 1996, more than three thousand teenagers and young adults aged fifteen to thirty-four died suddenly from heart attacks, a 10 percent increase over seven years. More than two thirds of those who died were young males. Many of these heart attacks result from coronary artery disease, meaning the arteries to the heart are blocked by fatty plaque (the accumulation of cholesterol and fats inside artery walls).

Of course, most kids are not going to drop dead of a heart attack. But there's plenty of evidence that dietary habits today can affect them later in life, even while they are still young. French researchers examined the blood vessels of forty-eight obese children and compared them to of kids of normal weight. They found that the obese children were more likely to have blood vessels that were stiff and unable to easily respond to changes in blood flow, signs of an emerging risk for heart disease.

In another study, researchers reviewed the autopsies of 856 young people who died in car accidents, from homicide, or from suicide. They found that even in people as young as fifteen, fatty streaks and plaque could sometimes be found in the arteries leading to the heart. Not surprisingly, smokers were the most likely to have these early warning signs of heart disease. But next on the risk list were males—but not females—who were obese. These overweight boys were four times more likely than slim ones to have the advanced plaques that can cause a heart attack by blocking the flow of blood to the heart.

High Cholesterol

It used to be people didn't pay much attention to their cholesterol levels until middle age. Do we now need to measure the cholesterol levels of our children and worry about what they spread on their toast?

The answer, according to the American Academy of Pediatrics, is maybe. It depends largely on your family history. The AAP recommends checking the cholesterol of children over two if either their parents or grandparents had a heart attack, stroke, or were treated for heart disease before age fifty-five. You should also test if you or your child's biological father has a total cholesterol level of 240 or higher. Even if there's no known family history of high cholesterol or heart disease, it's a good idea to watch cholesterol levels of kids who are overweight or eat a lot of foods high in fat, especially saturated fat, because they're likely to have high cholesterol. If the mainstay of your son's diet is burgers and fries, you may want to check his cholesterol.

If this seems like it's going too far, you should know that heart disease can actually have its roots in childhood, and that cholesterol is part of the equation. According to the American College of Cardiology, one third of adolescents have elevated cholesterol levels. Yet surveys show that few Americans have any idea that heart disease can start that early.

If you have your son's cholesterol level checked, look for numbers a bit different from the ones you watch for yourself. In children, total cholesterol levels under 170 are optimal. Levels between 170 and 200 are considered borderline, and anything 200 and over is considered high. If your son has borderline or high numbers, you and he should talk to the doctor. Together, you'll want to work out a plan for him to cut the fat and exercise more.

High Blood Pressure

High blood pressure is known as the silent killer because it has no symptoms, even as it increases the risk of heart attack, stroke, and kidney disease. Children and teenagers are probably not going to have a heart attack or stroke, but having high blood pressure at a young age can set the stage for problems later. Teenagers with high blood pressure are likely to be adults with high blood pressure. And the damaging effects can be see in the blood vessels and hearts of people as early as in their twenties.

Kids who are overweight, have high cholesterol, or get little exercise may all be at risk of developing high blood pressure. And because there is a hereditary component, people whose parents or grandparents had high blood pressure are more likely to develop it too. High blood pressure is especially common among African-Americans. If your child falls into this risk category, be sure you help them maintain a healthy weight.

And the Threat of Social Stigma

School can be a cruel place for overweight kids. Even though more children than ever are overweight, the attitude toward them seems to grow increasingly harsh. In a famous experiment from the 1960s, a group of children were shown drawings of kids who were obese, deformed, disabled, or apparently healthy and were asked to rank the figures by how much they liked them. The majority of children ranked the obese kid last. When that study was recently repeated, middle school children and college students still ranked the obese child last.

Numerous other studies show that children develop strong negative ideas about overweight kids at an early age. While we may shake our heads at the meanness of children, grown-ups set the stage. I'm embarrassed to say that some of the most negative attitudes toward overweight people come from those in the medical profession. In surveys, 39 percent of doctors said their obese patients were lazy, and 87 percent said they were indulgent. In another study, 24 percent of nurses said they were repulsed by caring for obese patients. When teachers were surveyed, 28 percent said that obesity was the worst thing that could happen to a person.

The embarrassment that overweight kids feel as a result of these attitudes can't be overstated. In one study, 90 percent of overweight kids between nine and eleven felt ashamed of being fat.

Sadly, overweight children often get teased the most during sports or physical activity. And what happens when kids who are taking part in gym classes or after-school recreation programs get picked on? Not surprisingly, it turns them off sports and physical activity, one of the things they most need to shed pounds and get healthy. In some sports such as football, very heavy kids may be excluded from play for fear they will hurt other children.

Teasing, meanness, low self-esteem—all these can have a lasting effect on an overweight child. Kids who are teased about their weight are prone to developing eating disorders, British researchers have found.

Why Are Kids So Fat Today?

Many factors contribute to a child becoming overweight. The problem in America today is that a number of these factors are coming together at the same time. You know many of them: more high-calorie, low-nutrition junk food, less exercise, more time spent sitting in front of the TV or a computer, drastic cuts in physical education classes in schools. Genes also play a big part, as do the dining habits that children develop at home. In fact, if you want to see the single biggest influence on your child's future weight, you need only look in the mirror. Most overweight kids have at least one overweight parent.

Like it or not, we bequeath to our children not only our genes, but also our eating and exercise habits. If we munch on junk food and eat high-fat meals, why wouldn't our children? And since most adults don't get enough exercise, should it surprise us that half our kids don't get enough vigorous exercise and 14 percent are completely inactive, according to the CDC?

Of course, we parents are far from the only influence. Kids today spend hours sitting in front of the TV or playing video games. When they watch, of course, they get no exercise, and are likely to eat high-calorie snacks. The result is that the more TV children watch, the more likely they are to be overweight, according to a recent study in the *Journal of Developmental and Behavioral Pediatrics.*

One of the problems for overweight kids is what Melinda Sothern, Ph.D., an exercise physiologist at Louisiana State University and the author of *Trim Kids,* calls the "vicious cycle" of obesity: First, a kid starts to gain weight because of his genes or because he gets high calorie/low nutrition foods at home or at school. Then, when he runs around and plays, he finds himself short of breath and sweating heavily. He feels discouraged and self-conscious, and gradually participates less, spending more time instead watching TV or sitting behind the computer. Then, of course, he's likely to gain more weight. One, two, or all of these factors can lead to a child gaining excess weight.

Schools, increasingly, are part of the problem. School cafeterias offer high-fat fare such as pizza and french fries, ice cream and candy, often courtesy of fast-food purveyors. A nationwide survey taken in 2000 for the Centers for Disease Control and Prevention found that more than 20 percent of schools were selling brand-name fast foods. In California, another 2000 survey found, 95 percent of high schools were selling à la carte fast foods from Taco Bell, Pizza Hut, and Domino's as well as other big-name franchises. Walk down the hall, just outside the cafeteria, and you may find soda vending machines lining the hallways. Meanwhile, gym classes are becoming things of the past. According to the Centers for Disease Control and Prevention, in 1995 only 25 percent of U.S. high school students get a daily fix of exercise from physical education classes. Compare that to 1991 when 42 percent of high school students participated in PE classes.

People often wonder why government-sponsored education programs designed to teach the importance of healthy eating aren't more effective. One reason is that they're vastly outgunned. The food industry spends billions to promote high-calorie foods of little nutritional value. Meanwhile, the Agriculture Department devoted all of $10 million to Team Nutrition, its program to get health information into American classrooms, and the National Cancer Institute spent $1 million a year to promote the Five-a-Day message—that kids should eat at least five servings of fruit and vegetables a day.

Yale obesity researcher Kelly Brownell, Ph.D., gets to the root of the problem in his book *Food Fight: The Inside Story of the Food Industry, America's Obesity Crisis & What*

We Can Do About It. He states it clearly: Parents must protect their kids from an increasingly toxic environment! Read this book and you will see why we as mothers need to think seriously about what we feed our children and how we can stop the fattening of the lambs.

Weight Gains and Growth Spurts: What to Look For

Many parents think and hope their child will grow out of a weight problem. That sometimes happens, especially to boys, who may get chubby, then suddenly shoot up and trim down. Toddlers and preschoolers often look plump, but as they grow in height, things often even out. The same thing often happens just before puberty, a time when many boys put on a few pounds.

"Right before puberty hits, boys will gain a little bit of fat," says Melinda Sothern. "But then once his testosterone kicks in, he'll greatly reduce his fat." For that reason, she says, it's difficult to diagnose overweight in a boy who's in puberty. If your son puts on a few pounds during these years, talk to your pediatrician and watch what happens over the course of a year. If he drops some weight, you don't need to worry. If his weight stays high, relative to his height, then it may be time to intervene.

For most boys, the big growth spurt of adolescence comes between twelve and sixteen, when the typical boy gains around a foot of height and thirty to forty pounds of weight. Put another way, boys gain about 15 percent to 20 percent of their adult height and much of their adult body weight during those years. No wonder teenage boys eat like horses. That's the only way to meet the huge demand for energy and nutrients this massive growth spurt requires.

One common problem though is that many parents don't recognize when there is a real problem. A 2003 study in the journal *Pediatrics* showed one third of mothers surveyed did not realize their child was overweight. Those who did realize their child had a weight problem perceived it to be a problem for girls much more often than for boys.

Preventing Obesity: A Family Affair

The best way to help your children stay healthy and control their weight, experts say, is to make healthy eating and exercise habits a family effort. The first step is for parents to examine their own patterns.

"Children closely model their parents," says Leonard Epstein, Ph.D., a childhood obesity researcher and professor of pediatrics at the State University of New York at Buffalo. "It is very hard to eat healthy and be active if other family members are eating potato chips and ice cream and watching a lot of TV."

If you want your kids to eat veggies, you need to eat veggies in front of them yourself. If you want them to exercise, they need to see that you're not a stranger to sweat. And if you want them to avoid junk food, don't supply it. Children can learn to like and eat a wide variety of foods, if exposed to them early in life. Leann Birch, M.D., a nutrition researcher at Penn State University who studied children's food preferences, says that even when young children initially reject a new food, they often learn to accept it over time if given many opportunities to try it.

One way to make healthy eating a family goal is to involve the whole family in putting good food on the table. Eat as many meals together as possible, and eat them at the table, not in front of the TV. According to Leonard Epstein, the average child eats 600 calories a day in front of the TV. Cut that in half, he says, and you'd eliminate 25 pounds a year!

Involve your children in the shopping, planning, and preparation of meals and encourage them to try new foods. My son, Harry, is thrilled to help me cook dinner. Ask them to help prepare food or set the table and allow them to choose some of the food served. When you present something new, tell them they have to try a little, but you won't make them eat it if they don't like it. Don't punish your child or yell at him for failing to eat something healthy. And when he does eat healthy food or tries something new, praise him for his healthy habits.

Should I Put My Child on a Restrictive Diet?

In a word, no. In two words, absolutely not. Putting your child on a restrictive diet—one where certain foods are forbidden—can have all kinds of negative effects. It can interfere with your son's growth and development. It can deprive him of nutrition he needs. It could cause him to obsess about the foods he's forbidden to eat. And even more fundamentally, putting a child on a diet sends a message to kids that they've failed, leading them to feel guilty or ashamed—exactly the kinds of feelings that kids soothe by eating more.

Diets can backfire, says William Dietz, M.D., Ph.D., the director of Nutrition and Physical Activity at the CDC. "When foods are put off limits for young children, they become much more desirable, and they are likely to overeat them when they're offered."

There are, of course, some children whose medical problems—such as food allergies or diabetes—require they adhere to a special diet, which your child's doctor should supervise.

Instead of putting your child on a restrictive diet, teach him about the differences between healthy and not-so-healthy foods. One approach is Leonard Epstein's Stoplight Diet, which links different kinds of food with the colors of traffic lights.

Focusing on yellow- and green-light foods will increase your nutrient density, lower dietary fat, and reduce intake of simple sugars:

- Red-light foods include candy and soda, fast food and pizza, cakes and cookies, full-fat cheese, fatty meats—anything with a lot of sugar or fat and low nutrient density (nutrients per calorie). They should be eaten rarely.

- Yellow-light foods are more nutritious than red-light foods and can be eaten in moderation. Examples of yellow food include whole-grain breads, 2 percent milk, pork, tuna, or chicken without the skin. Portion size matters; take small servings.

- Green-light foods, such as vegetables and fruit, are nutritious, contain very little dietary fat, and can be consumed often. Also includes fat-free dairy products and baked or broiled fish and lentils.

Here are some other tips for helping everyone in your family keep their weight at healthy levels:

Don't Recruit for the Clean-Plate Club

This may go against what your grandmother taught, but it's a bad idea to guilt-trip or otherwise convince your child to clean his plate. What can we say? Grandmas are great, but they don't know everything. We should all learn to stop eating when full. Pushing a kid to finish what's on his plate sends the opposite message and teaches him to ignore the signals that he's had enough.

One of the reasons kids overeat is because we teach them to. We don't mean to, of course, but a recent study in the *Journal of the American Dietetic Association* found that preschool children around three and a half eat what they want, regardless of how much food offered. But by the time they turn five, the amount they are served influences how much they eat. If you put food on a child's plate and encourage him to eat it, he's likely to eat more whether he really wants it or not. If you dish out small portions, they're more likely to eat the quantity that they want.

Don't Ban It, But Don't Bring It Home

Taking a hard stance on junk food is always a tricky proposition. Banning all sweets and junk food may seem attractive, but research shows that it's likely to backfire. Leann Birch found that restricting unhealthy foods often causes children to obsess over those items and eat all the more when they're not being watched. Besides, you know kids—they usually do the opposite of what you tell them.

A more effective approach is to teach—and model—healthy habits, and let your kids make their own choices about what they eat, especially when out of the house. Kids should eat what they want at birthday parties and other special occasions. They'll learn that cake, cookies, and soft drinks can occasionally be part of a diet that's healthy overall. If your child is already overweight, though, you should urge moderate portions. At home, lead by example and bring nothing into the house that you don't want them to eat.

Don't Use Food As a Bribe

All right, let's be honest: What parent among us has not, in a desperate moment, offered ice cream or cake as trade for something we want our kids to do? We know it's wrong when we're doing it, and yet in the heat of the moment, we resort to food bribery.

According to surveys, some 60 percent of mothers (the honest ones) admit to using food as a reward. It's nothing to be ashamed of, but it's nothing to be proud of either. Using food as a reward sends the wrong message: that sweets and treats are special and "worth more" than other types of foods. It also teaches kids an easy way to manipulate: refuse to do something unless they get a sweet reward.

Remember: Food Is Not Love!

Few things evoke more pleasant feelings than the smell of pot roast simmering on the stove or a pie baking in the oven. Is there any greater symbol of a mother's love than the way she feeds her family? It's natural to get satisfaction from watching your family enjoy something delicious you have cooked. But if the food that earns you all this adulation is high in fat and loaded with calories, then it can become a problem.

Ask yourself if food is your love connection to your family. If it is, you need to take a hard look at what you feed your family and how they respond. If serving unhealthy food earns you love, you are definitely not helping your loved ones, and you may want to examine your motives. Many women I know say "This is what they like," and "This is all they'll eat." They're afraid that their families will reject *them* if they don't cook the expected foods. If you're in that trap, you need to make some changes. But do it slowly. Don't go from steak and potatoes to tofu and brown rice overnight. In the long run, though, you want to create a new definition: Real love for your family means helping them eat healthier food, live healthier lives, and hang around to a ripe old age.

Here are some other nutrition tips drawn from the book *Trim Kids,* by Melinda Sothern and her colleagues from the Committed to Kids weight management program at Louisiana State University. The program has helped over two thousand children lose weight by developing healthy eating and exercise habits.

NUTRITION TIPS FOR PARENTS OF YOUNG CHILDREN

1. Discourage kids from drinking sugary beverages like soft drinks. If your child is thirsty, give him water.
2. For treats, choose healthy fruits and vegetables such as grapes, raisins, strawberries, and carrots.
3. Put out the message that all food is okay, though some foods are healthier than others. Encourage kids to pick more of the healthy foods and never give food as a reward.
4. Require kids to take at least three bites of each food you serve. Have them grade the foods: A, B, C, D, or F. Serve A, B, or C foods again.
5. Keep nutritious foods low in fat and sugar within easy reach.
6. Allow kids to eat non-nutritious foods away from home infrequently. *Gradually* reduce fast-food consumption to less than once per week.
7. Provide healthy, attractive snacks in the morning and afternoon.
8. Make sure children eat a healthy breakfast and discourage snacking after dinner. If children aren't hungry when they wake up, they may be eating too late at night.
9. Don't give negative attention to unhealthy eating. Focus instead on praising your child when he chooses healthy foods.

Source: Copyright © 2001 by Melinda S. Sothern, Ph. D., M.Ed., C.E.P., T. Kristian Von Alman, Ph.D., and Heidi Schumacher, R.D., L.D.N., C.D.E. Reprinted with permission of HarperCollins Publishers, Inc.

Get Help If You Need It

If your child is seriously overweight or seems to be heading in that direction, ask your pediatrician, family physician, or call the local hospital to get numbers for programs in your area for overweight children. Programs such as Committed to Kids are successful in helping children lose weight. Good programs emphasize three things above all: getting kids off the couch to exercise, helping them learn healthy eating habits, and including the whole family in the program.

In general, boys are more successful in weight-loss programs than girls, according to Leonard Epstein. Perhaps the biggest reason is that boys tend to be more physically active and less resistant to exercise.

That's the experience of Melinda Sothern as well. She says it's usually easier to motivate boys into sports, especially if they're making a little progress shedding weight. "Once they get some of that fat weight off, they get motivated because their speed picks up and their skills improve pretty quickly," says Sothern. "That motivates them to join a team and once they get into sports their physical activity is built in."

Kids, Exercise, and Obesity

It's sad but true that American kids are more sedentary today than at any time in our history. Of course, we adults are more sedentary than our parents and grandparents, so why should this be surprising? Here are a few sobering facts from the 1996 report on Exercise and Health by the U.S. Surgeon General:

- Half of young people between twelve and twenty-one don't get vigorous exercise on a regular basis, and some 14 percent reported that they had no recent physical activity.

- Only 19 percent of all high school students are in physical education classes where they get twenty minutes of exercise or more.

- Between 1991 and 1995, the number of high school students taking part in daily PE classes dropped from 42 percent to 25 percent.

So What Is a Parent to Do?

If we want our children to stay healthy and keep off extra weight—and we want the same thing ourselves—we must think about calories burned and calories consumed. We need to help them get moving, and to get moving ourselves.

The best and most enjoyable way to do that is to make physical activity a normal part of family life. According to government guidelines, kids ought to get at least thirty minutes of activity a day, and we should be a part of that. There are dozens of activities a family can do together: bike riding, in-line skating, hiking, jogging, soccer, and baseball, to name just a few. Make it a habit after dinner to go for a walk as a family. If you have a choice between driving and walking, set a good example and walk. If you live within bike-riding distance of school, pedal to school with your child.

Encourage Your Boy to Get Involved in Sports

Sports are a great way for kids to stay fit, have fun, and maintain health. But no single sport or exercise routine is right for every child. Let your boy try different sports and discover what he likes and what he's good at. Pay attention to his interests, his aptitudes, and his body type. Forcing a child into a sport is a terrible idea, one that's likely to make him resentful and possibly to reject sports altogether.

There are many different kinds of sports. Team sports are the most common, and they're good for lots of kids, but some kids can feel pressured or nervous if they're afraid of letting down their peers or their parents. Others may feel ashamed or embarrassed if their skills are less developed than others.

Melinda Sothern says many kids do better when they get involved in individual sports such as swimming, martial arts, or tennis. For overweight kids, martial arts can be especially good, she says, because "they set their own goals and don't have to compete against others."

One of the biggest mistakes a parent can make is to push a child into a team sport that's not a good match for the child. "Where a lot of parents go wrong," Sothern says, "is they'll take a child who's sedentary and maybe a little overweight and who doesn't have the physical prowess or technique, and they'll put them in a team setting and it'll turn them off. Because they will get teased and they won't get picked and they'll sit on the bench and be waterboy."

... But Don't Push Him Too Hard

Many parents think the best way to get an overweight kid into shape is to take the "no pain–no gain" approach. "Make 'em sweat," they figure. "That will help them build character." But, according to Sothern, pushing kids that way is one of the worst mistakes a parent can make. "A child who's overweight, who's already being teased, may also be getting negative reinforcement from peers and teachers because they can't keep up," she says. "Those children shut down when pushed too hard."

Sothern's program for overweight kids is designed to build mastery and self-confidence by helping them taste success. "The best thing that parents can do is give them a goal for physical activity that they can actually reach," she says. Only then, when the child feels comfortable, should you encourage him to go to the next level.

Sothern advises parents to play sports with kids from an early age. The earlier, the better, because the older kids get, the harder it is to train their muscles. Start young, she says, and build slowly. She also has a special message for fathers:

"Dads, it's not going to build character to scream at your kid, to yell at your kid, to push your kid, to tell him he's slow, or to beat him. Let him win," she says. "Let your kid beat you."

Unplug Your Child

They don't call this the wired generation for nothing. Consider these numbers for a moment: One third of American children between the ages of two and seven have TV sets in their bedrooms. Sixty percent of American children live in homes with three or more TVs. Fifty-eight percent of American kids live in homes where the TV is usually on during meals. Result: The average child or adolescent spends more than three hours a day watching television, and 17 percent watch more than five hours a day.

Then there's the time kids spend on their computers—playing games, surfing the Internet, or e-mailing their friends. Kids between two and seven log about forty minutes a day at the keyboard, while kids from eight to eighteen spend 1 hour and 40 minutes. In case you were wondering, only about a fourth of that time is spent doing their homework. Boys, by the way, spend twenty minutes more watching TV and thirty minutes more on their computers and video games than girls. This worries Melinda Sothern. "Young boys in this country are getting very good at computer games very young," Sothern says. "Then because they're sitting in front of the computer, and they're less physically active, they put on a couple extra pounds. So their exercise tolerance and their heart and lung function are low because they don't exercise regularly. Then, when they do go outside and go into a team setting, they fail. So they go home, back to the computer, where they can be anybody."

Boys used to focus most of their competitive urges on sports, Sothern says. These days, however, a lot of kids aim that energy at their computers instead.

For all of these reasons I like the recommendations made by the American Academy of Pediatrics in 2001. They suggest that parents allow their children to spend no more than one or two hours per day watching television programs, playing video games, or logged on to their computers. Help boys break away from these armchair pursuits and they have lots of time for riding bikes, shooting hoops, and other exercise.

Teach Media Literacy

When they do watch TV, kids—like all consumers—are bombarded with advertising, aimed at getting them to consume unhealthy foods and drinks. They'll see sodas guzzled by cool kids (not fat ones) and burgers devoured by basketball stars. Children are especially vulnerable to these images. Help your children understand and resist advertising messages by watching with them and discussing what you see. Make a joke of how silly the ads are and how ridiculous their claims. Let them know that commercials are not to be believed, and remind them what they are—ways of getting people to buy things they don't need and eat food that's not healthy.

Here are some other exercise tips from Sothern and her colleagues, as adapted from their book *Trim Kids*.

TIPS TO ENCOURAGE YOUNG CHILDREN TO BE PHYSICALLY ACTIVE

1. Ask your child to walk briskly whenever he walks.
2. Create an environment for active play both inside and outside the home.
3. Limit time spent watching TV and playing computer and video games. Remove TVs, computers, video games, and game systems from the child's bedroom.
4. Expose your child to as many different kinds of physical activity as possible in a nurturing, nonintimidating environment.
5. Give your kids plenty of chances to safely climb, run, and jump. It's good for developing muscle strength and bone density.

6. Reserve at least one day each weekend for fun fitness activities the whole family can enjoy.
7. Avoid drawing attention to sedentary activities. Instead, praise your child when he chooses to be active and play.
8. Encourage physical play for thirty minutes before homework. TV should come last, after play, homework, and dinner.
9. Offer choices: vacuum your room or walk the dog; shovel snow or dance in your room; rake the leaves or go for a bike ride.

Source: Copyright © 2001 by Melinda S. Sothern, Ph.D., M.Ed., C.E.P., T. Kristian Von Alman, Ph.D., and Heidi Shumacher, R.D., L.D.N., C.D.E. Reprinted with permission of HarperCollins Publishers, Inc.

STATURE AND STATUS

Teenage boys have lots of worries, and one of the biggest is height. Height, for boys, is a very big deal—a much bigger deal than for girls, though some experts think that might be changing a bit. Tall boys are viewed as handsome and cool; short boys are often overlooked. Even before the teen years, boys who are smaller than their peers are sometimes treated as if they are younger and they may be teased or bullied. For many boys, how tall they are has a great deal to do with how they feel about themselves, at least for a while.

The good news is that most of these problems and concerns diminish with time. Many boys are simply late bloomers. They spend two or three years nervously looking up at their classmates (including, most painfully, those early-blooming girls). Then, in the span of a few months to a year, they grow six inches or more. Other boys never have that big growth spurt, but they realize that, while they may never play center on the basketball team, their life can be just fine. And if they enjoy basketball, they can look at these guys as role models: Mugsy Bogues, the five-feet-three-inch former star, or five-feet-five-inch dynamo Earl Boykins, now the NBA's shortest player.

For a few boys, though, neither their shortness nor their shame ever disappear. They grow up feeling vaguely inferior or resentful that others treat them that way. Many physicians—pediatricians, psychiatrists, endocrinologists—assume that many, if not most, short boys meet such a fate, and they have searched for medical interventions that would allow them to help boys avert it.

Part of the reason for this assumption is that many studies of short children were based on kids referred to pediatric endocrinologists (specialists who deal with hormones and growth issues). These studies found that very short children are at increased risk for behavior problems because they are stigmatized, have low self-esteem, and don't cope well with these issues. But the children in these studies are the ones with the most serious problems, or they have parents who *think* they have serious problems and may treat them accordingly. That's how they ended up in a specialist's office. And that raises questions about whether the research is truly representative. Put simply, if you study short kids with problems, it may seem like *all* short kids have problems.

Other research has come to different conclusions. One study in England, the Wessex Growth Study, followed over one hundred short children drawn from a community rather than a clinic, and compared them to one hundred other children of normal height. It found no difference between the groups in their self-esteem or likelihood of behavior problems. Another study, from the University of Florida, found no significant differences between short kids and kids of normal height in their intelligence, behavior, and ability to focus attention.

Ora Pescovitz, M.D., a pediatric endocrinologist at Indiana University School of Medicine, sums it up this way: "Many short children do extremely well without any major psychosocial problems related to their stature. But there are children for whom this becomes the focal point of their lives and it is truly handicapping. So there is a spectrum, and I don't think it is fair to say that short stature is a problem for everybody because for a lot of kids it's not."

So what do we mean by "short," and why do some kids end up that way? First of all, we're not talking about people who have genetic abnormalities such as dwarfism, but rather about otherwise typical children who, for no apparent medical reason, are much shorter than other kids their age. The Endocrine Society, a doctor's association, uses the term "short stature" to refer to people who are shorter than 97 percent of others of the same age and sex.

Short—and Normal

These are normal healthy kids who have inherited genes for short stature from their parents. Short parents tend to have short kids, and tall parents tend to have tall kids—no surprise. Children who are genetically short grow at a normal rate, have no underlying medical problems, and enter puberty about the same time as everybody else. In the end, they are somewhere around their parents' height, which means they are shorter than most. Because most parents are comfortable with their height, they're unlikely to see their children's height as a problem or seek treatment. This attitude often transfers to the child, helping him accept his stature.

The best thing you can do for genetically short kids is to love them, support them, and help them to be comfortable with their size. If you have a short child and are concerned about his health, talk to your doctor. Odds are, he is completely healthy. "Just remember," says Edward Reiter, M.D., a pediatric endocrinologist at Baystate Medical Center Children's Hospital in Massachusetts, "we're talking about height—not life-threatening disease."

Late Bloomers

We all remember a guy like this: In ninth grade, he's short and skinny with a baby face and a squeaky voice. By senior year, he's as tall as the others, with a mustache growing in. Late-blooming boys basically start adolescence well after most other boys—doctors call this a *constitutional delay*—then have a big growth spurt and catch up. Until they do, it can be tough socially and psychologically.

In some cases, kids who have emotional trouble as a result and are motivated to seek help are given testosterone injections to push puberty along. But even without treatment, these kids will eventually reach the promised land of puberty and grow to normal adult size. The cause is often genetic; late bloomers are often the children of late bloomers.

If your son is concerned, or if you are, about whether he'll ever catch up to the pack, speak to his doctor. It's usually easy to determine if he's a late bloomer or likely to remain short. X rays can assess what doctors call the bone age. If a boy's bones appear less mature than what would be normal for his chronological age, that's a strong hint that he'll keep growing after other boys slow down. My cowriter, Rob Waters, used to beg his pediatrician to tell him if he would ever catch up to his peers. His doctor, a sweet and reassuring man, gave him the news he wanted to hear: "Just be patient. You'll grow six inches in a single year." It finally happened—when he was sixteen.

Hormone Deficiencies

Some children are deficient in human growth hormone (HGH), a hormone released by the pituitary gland, which stimulates tissues to grow. A few children are even born completely lacking growth hormone or the ability to make it. They're born small, often less than five pounds after a full-term delivery. Doctors can treat these children with injections of synthesized growth hormone and believe the treatment may add as many as four to eight inches to eventual adult height. Few experts would disagree with this course when there is clear evidence the child has a hormone deficiency. However, determining whether a child is deficient in the hormone is not straightforward. Human growth hormone, like many hormones, circulates at varying levels in children and not everyone agrees on what level warrants treatment.

Some researchers advocate giving the synthetic hormone to short kids who are *not* deficient in HGH. This is controversial. Giving the child this drug, they argue, will make it more likely that he will grow to "his full genetic potential" and help protect him from teasing, low self-esteem, and various emotional or behavioral problems. In one recent study published in the *New England Journal of Medicine,* short children with no hormone deficiency were given growth hormone for between two and ten years. Boys gained an average of 2 inches and girls about 2.3 inches over their natural expected heights. In July of 2003 the Food and Drug Administration approved growth hormone (Humatrope) for use in healthy but abnormally short kids—that means boys whose expected adult height is shorter than five feet three inches.

Critics argue that putting children on growth hormone who are not lacking it, except in the rarest of cases, is unnecessary and provides only modest gains. They contend that there is no good evidence that short kids will have emotional or psychological problems, and they point out that synthetic HGH may have adverse side effects. Finally, they raise the question of whether the urge to put kids on these hormones may be driven by pressure from parents who want taller kids, or pharmaceutical companies who want to sell drugs.

Should You Consult with a Doctor?

The Human Growth Foundation, a nonprofit research and advocacy group, suggests that any child who is no taller than kids two years younger, or whose growth rate has dropped off significantly, should be evaluated by a doctor. Usually, that means seeing a pediatric endocrinologist who checks the child's height and growth rate, assesses family history, measures bones in the hand and wrist, and takes X rays to assess bone development and blood tests to check for growth hormone deficiencies. Then, together, you can decide what to do.

Guys Who Are Tall—Way Tall

Being tall can have its advantages, especially when running for president. Since the beginning of the television age, 1952, the taller presidential candidate has always won, with two exceptions: Carter versus Ford, where Carter won, though he was half an inch shorter, and Nixon versus McGovern. McGovern was nearly two inches taller than Nixon but lost anyway. If you are still confused about who really won the presidential election of 2000 after the balloting snafu in Florida, it may help to know that Gore is six feet one inch and Bush five feet eleven and a half inches. Presidential aspirations aside, being too tall can be a problem for some boys. Though most tall boys are completely healthy, there are sometimes underlying medical conditions.

Precocious Puberty

Boys normally start puberty around twelve, but the process can begin quite normally at any point between nine and fourteen. Precocious puberty means it begins to happen earlier—before age nine for boys. There are a few known causes of precocious puberty. It can be inherited. It can be caused by head trauma or a tumor in the pituitary gland, the hypothalamus or a nearby part of the brain that impinges on those areas. It can be caused by an untreated thyroid condition, and it is sometimes related to being overweight. Most of the time, however, the cause is not known.

Going through puberty early can be difficult and embarrassing. Though it's usually tougher on girls, whose breast development is more obvious, it can subject boys to teasing. And let's face it—most boys are not ready at fourteen or fifteen, much less at nine, to handle the emotional impact of puberty. In the long term, there's another problem: These early bloomers often have their adolescent growth spurt early but then stop growing prematurely as well. The result is that while they're taller than their peers for a time, they can end up being quite short. When kids seem to be hitting puberty too early, doctors may recommend a class of drugs known as GnRH (gonadotropin-releasing hormone) analogs, which can stop the early release of hormones and slow down the process of maturation. Fortunately, these drugs seem to have few side effects.

Kids who start going through puberty prematurely should see a doctor for evaluation so that a tumor, thyroid condition, or other problem can be detected and treated if possible.

Marfan Syndrome

Chalk one up to mother's intuition. Karen Murray, president of Liz Claiborne's Menswear Division, knew almost from the day her son, Michael, was born that something was not quite right. When she gazed at him in the nursery, he looked somehow larger and longer than the other babies. Friends and relatives commented on his long fingers. As he grew, he seemed different from other babies: He flopped over in his high chair and walked with a tilt. His chest was indented, and it was hard not to notice how fast he grew.

Despite repeated reassurances from her husband, her pediatrician, and numerous other specialists that Michael was perfectly normal, Karen had a nagging suspicion that something was wrong. Eventually she became so preoccupied with her suspicions it began to interfere with her marriage. Her husband accused her of "looking for something that wasn't there." Even her son's pediatrician labeled her "a neurotic mother." Eventually the marriage dissolved under the weight of her obsession with her son's health.

On her son's fifth birthday, Karen, now a single mom, bought him a computer that came with a free CD-ROM called *Family Doctor*. As her son slept quietly, she turned on the computer and loaded the CD-ROM. In minutes, Karen finally discovered what no doctor had been able to tell her: Michael had Marfan syndrome, a rare genetic condition that weakens the connective tissue that holds together blood vessels and other structures of the body. These weaknesses can result in sudden death from a ruptured aorta.

The next morning, she rushed her son to the hospital and demanded that they give him an echocardiogram. Sure enough, Michael's aorta was twice the normal size. When her husband heard the news, he was devastated, and contrite. The couple was soon back together. Karen used her son's story to get the word out on national television about Marfan syndrome, resulting in hundreds of calls to the National Marfan Foundation from people who never knew what was wrong with them. Michael's story no doubt saved lives.

People with Marfan syndrome have disproportionately long limbs and tend to have loose joints and ligaments. Symptoms can also include an indented or protruding chest bone, curvature of the spine, flat feet, nearsightedness, and dislocated lenses. The most famous person with Marfan syndrome is thought to have been Abraham Lincoln.

The syndrome is no more common in boys than girls, but boys may be at heightened risk because people with the disorder are frequently tall and tall boys are more likely to play sports, especially basketball. The fast pace and physical contact can put great stress on the aorta, making basketball potentially deadly. A number of people with Marfan have died while playing. Unfortunately, because the disease has subtle symptoms, many people don't know they have it and many physicians are unaware of the telltale signs. There is no blood or laboratory test for Marfan syndrome.

If your son is unusually tall and is interested in playing basketball or other fast-paced contact sports, he should have a thorough sports physical, which should pay special attention to the systems affected by this syndrome.

Treatment for Marfan syndrome consists mainly of close monitoring. People with the disorder generally have annual heart exams, including echocardiograms; careful monitoring of the skeletal system, especially during childhood and adolescence; and medications to lower blood pressure and ease the stress on the aorta. People with the syndrome often need to avoid strenuous exercise and contact sports to protect the aorta, the joints, and the eyes.

EATING DISORDERS—NOT JUST FOR GIRLS ANYMORE

Over the last few decades, the Barbie doll has come to be a potent symbol of the ideal feminine body type for girls and young women. It is, of course, unattainable. If Barbie were life-sized, she would have an 18-inch waist, a 39-inch DD bust, and 33-inch hips on her 110-pound frame. Nonetheless, millions of American girls literally made themselves sick trying to twist their bodies into this unachievable and unnatural shape. Today, American males have their own icons, as Harvard professor of psychiatry Harrison Pope, M.D., recently discovered.

His fourteen-year-old daughter was busy on the Internet, doing what she called her "Barbie project"—observing how the doll was shaping the body image of American females. It struck Pope that there might be a male equivalent, and he began to do his own research. He soon discovered that GI Joe had done some serious bulking up. When the action figure was introduced in 1964, he was in good but normal shape: with the equivalent of a 32-inch waist, 44-inch chest, and 12-inch biceps. Fast-forward three decades and check out GI Joe Extreme, introduced about eight years ago. Were he life-sized, Pope figures, he would have a 55-inch chest and bulging 27-inch biceps—an absolute impossibility unless he were popping steroids. Batman, Luke Skywalker, and Han Solo figures are all similarly ripped—with bulging pecs and washboard abs even bigger than the touched-up models on some men's magazine covers.

These are the new images of American masculinity. Many young men try their hardest to achieve the look, to mold their bodies into these impossible shapes. To do it, they're spending endless hours at the gym and taking dangerous anabolic steroids and supplements, all in pursuit of a physiological impossibility. Many parents, pleased their son is doing something "healthy," never consider he may take steroids or other substances to get this beefed-up look.

Studies show that when boys are shown images of male bodies and asked to pick their ideal, they choose images of men who could look that way only through the use of anabolic steroids. Of course, it's also worth noting that when girls are asked about their ideal body shapes for men, they pick more normally proportioned fellows. The result of this new preoccupation with muscular bodies is an emerging epidemic of eating and body image disorders among boys. Indeed, one in four children with anorexia who is referred for treatment is now a boy, according to the Office of Women's Health of the National Institutes of Health. Eating disorders include anorexia (and bulimia), once seen as the almost exclusive province of females.

Teenage boys and young men are also being seen for some new conditions. Together, Pope and his colleagues have dubbed these male disorders the "Adonis Complex" and have written a best-selling book by the same name. Among the new disorders are these:

- **Bigorexia,** also known as muscle dysmorphia, is a new term for men who try to make themselves look buff, with bigger biceps, bigger chests, and bigger muscles of every kind. Boys and men with bigorexia somehow believe that they are too small, despite the hours they spend pumping iron. According to Roberto Olivardia, Ph.D., a clinical psychologist at Harvard Medical School and coauthor of *The Adonis Complex: The Secret Crisis of Male Body Obsession,* the typical case of bigorexia is a man who is very fit, very lean, and muscular. Yet despite all that muscle mass, he believes that he is small.

- **Body dysmorphic disorder (BDD)** leads people to be preoccupied or obsessed with an imagined defect in their appearance. Men with BDD may stare at themselves in the mirror for hours and be repulsed by their nose, their arms, their skin, or their waistline. They may obsess about losing their hair, even though others see a full mane. For some people, this obsession becomes disabling and depressing, and sometimes even leads to suicide attempts. "If you notice that your son is saying, 'Oh I'm so fat' or 'I'm too skinny' when he's of perfectly normal weight, then that's a red flag to wonder what's going on with this kid that he doesn't see himself in the way that other people see him," says Olivardia.

- **Anorexia** and **bulimia** have become increasingly common in boys for much the same reason as girls: low self-esteem, emotional pressures, and family and relationship problems. Some experts think homosexuality can put boys at higher risk, but Olivardia doesn't agree. "We believe that gay men are more likely to discuss such issues and seek treatment for them, while heterosexual men are too ashamed," he says. Because gay men are more open, he adds, many professionals conclude that these problems are more common among gay men.

As with girls, boys with eating disorders are also at risk for anxiety, depression, and substance abuse. One difference in the way girls and boys present with these disorders: Girls may just *feel* overweight when they begin obsessively dieting, but boys usually *are* overweight. Pope and his colleagues estimate that 25 percent of high school boys have tried unhealthy ways to lose weight such as fasting, crash dieting, or diet pills. That amounts to some 1 million boys.

The National Eating Disorders Screening Program recently conducted a survey of 5,700 high school students in thirty states and found that 17 percent of boys showed signs of eating disorders including binge eating or vomiting to control weight. Roughly 90 percent received no treatment for the problem.

Sadly, it's not surprising. One of the difficulties with boys is that they are often reluctant to talk about what is normally seen as a female problem. This silence, says Olivardia, "gives people the illusion that men or males don't suffer with these problems when in fact they do. But they suffer in secrecy because they fear that they might be labeled as feminine or gay or not masculine." Indeed, one study of males hospitalized for an eating disorder found they felt ashamed because they had a stereotypically "female" disease.

WARNING SIGNS OF AN EATING DISORDER IN BOYS

- Excessive dieting, fasting, or a severely restricted diet.
- Difficulty eating with others, lying about eating.
- Frequently weighing self.
- Focus on certain body parts; e.g., buttocks, thighs, stomach.
- Disgust with body size or shape.
- Distortion of body size—a boy feels fat even though others tell him he is already very thin.

Steroids and Supplements

Surely the most dangerous part of this obsession with body image is the willingness of growing numbers of boys to use anabolic steroids and various nutritional supplements in an effort to build up muscles or improve athletic performance. These performance-enhancing substances have become a national craze among young males and expose millions of them to uncharted side effects and risks.

About 5 percent of children and teenagers from ten to seventeen say they've tried steroids or other performance-enhancing supplements, according to a nationwide survey taken for the Blue Cross and Blue Shield Association in 2001. Twenty percent of the children surveyed said they personally know someone who takes these substances.

Another study, published in the *Journal of the American Academy of Pediatrics,* found that 5.6 percent of middle-school and high-school students—and a whopping 44 percent of high school seniors—use creatine, an over-the-counter supplement said to provide quick energy to boost athletic performance. Boys were four times more likely to take it than girls.

The pressure to bulk up in unhealthy ways comes from many sources and is especially intense among young male athletes and bodybuilders. Coaches press high school players to add muscle mass and weight. Weight lifters at gyms seek an edge as they compete with each other. Athletes on varsity squads search for ways to improve their performance—and share their secrets-in-a-bottle with each other. In the competitive world of high school and college sports, these pressures can be hard to resist.

Recently, former baseball star Ken Caminiti admitted that he was using steroids during the 1996 season, when he won the Most Valuable Player award. He estimated that half of Major League Baseball players were also taking steroids. He quickly retracted that statement, but another recently retired player, slugger Jose Canseco, put the number even higher.

And who could forget Mark McGwire's admission that he was using an over-the-counter steroid, androstenedione, in an effort to improve his performance as he chased Roger Maris's home run record in 1998. McGwire's public use of andro, as it is commonly known, suddenly made these substances "acceptable" and sent sales of andro soaring.

What are these substances and how do they work? And, most important, what risks do they pose for kids that take them?

Anabolic Steroids

These synthetic substances are derived from the male hormone testosterone. Testosterone performs two functions. It is androgenic—that is, it spurs the creation of masculine characteristics such as facial hair and a deep voice—and it is anabolic, which means it builds muscle mass. Anabolic steroids are an attempt to separate these functions and stimulate the muscle-building part only. They are prescription drugs sometimes used medically to replace testosterone in men with inadequate levels, but are mostly used illegally by people who want to bulk up. When they are taken in combination with physical training and a high-protein diet, they can indeed increase muscle size and strength.

The exact risks of steroids are still in dispute, though experts agree they are dangerous to adolescents and children, mostly because they can disrupt the body's own production of hormones and trigger an early end to growth. They can also push up blood pressure and cholesterol levels, trigger severe acne and premature balding, and cause testicles to shrink and breast tissue to grow. Many experts also fear they can cause long-term damage to the cardiovascular system, the liver, and the reproductive organs. They are also known to cause irritability and even severe aggression among some—" 'roid rage," as it is known.

"We're going to be seeing a whole host of health problems amongst males about twenty years from now," predicts Roberto Olivardia. "People are going to wonder where all this is coming from, and it's because of this silent thing called anabolic steroids."

Androstenedione

This steroid is a testosterone precursor. It readily converts to testosterone in the body, but unlike other steroids, is legal and easily available over the counter. Like most dietary supplements, it is not regulated by the Food and Drug Administration. The question for many researchers is just how anabolic, or muscle-building, it is. And, more important, does it have side effects similar to those of testosterone?

Andro has been banned by several sports organizations (the International Olympic Committee, the National Football League and the National Collegiate Athletic Association), though not professional baseball, and its popularity seems to have waned somewhat. But it has been replaced as the hot substance by another supplement, creatine.

Creatine

This amino acid produced naturally in your body helps deliver energy to your cells. Because it's considered "natural," creatine is unregulated and is easily available in health food stores, where it does a brisk business among young athletes. People who take it say it gives them quick bursts of energy and helps them build muscle and strength. But that is far from clear, experts say.

When people first start taking it, they may gain five pounds in as many days, but this extra weight is from water, not muscle. Thus far, there is little hard evidence that it actually boosts the power of weight lifters or the performance of sprinters or ballplayers.

The most common side effect of creatine is nausea and it can be quite severe, causing long bouts of vomiting in some users. The extra water the muscles accumulate can also cause cramping, muscle strains, and dehydration. The University of Tennessee recently banned creatine after fourteen of its football players had cramping episodes during a game. No one knows the long-term effects of creatine.

Ephedra

Also known as ma huang, this herbal stimulant is found in dozens of energy-boosting sports drinks, supplements, and appetite-suppressing diet pills with names like Ripped Force, Ripped Fuel, Stocked, and Ripped to the Max. Its active ingredient, ephedrine, is found in many prescription and over-the-counter medications such as decongestants and allergy medications. A chemical cousin of amphetamine, it stimulates the central nervous system and can boost blood pressure and heart rate to dangerous levels. It has been linked to many reports of heart attacks, strokes, seizures, high blood pressure, and chest pain. A number of these cases led to deaths, including that of Baltimore Orioles pitcher Steve Bechler, who died in February 2003 less than twenty-four hours after a spring training workout. The medical examiner found that ephedra, contained in an over-the-counter supplement Bechler had been taking, contributed to his death from heatstroke. Since this death and other deaths linked to ephedra, in 2003 the U.S. government banned the sale of ephedra.

Diuretics

Athletes use diuretics to lose weight quickly. These powerful and potentially dangerous medicines tell the kidneys to eliminate water, and with the water goes weight. Rapid weight loss may alter the critical sodium and potassium balance and this can disrupt the heart's electrical activity and lead to cardiac arrest. Wrestlers have died trying to drop weight through diuretic abuse. Signs of diuretic use include frequent urination, rapid weight loss—sometimes in just a few days—and fatigue.

What Can a Parent Do?

First of all, pay attention. Many parents have almost no idea what their children are doing with their time and what pressures they are under. Understand that the teenage years can be challenging and that teenage boys and girls alike worry and obsess a great deal about their bodies. Notice your son's habits and moods. Be sympathetic. If he wants to talk, listen to what he has to say. True, if you ask him questions, he may not answer, which means you need to know some of the other people in your son's life—his friends, his teachers, his coaches. Get to know them, and you'll have a better sense of what's going on with him and possibly a heads up on problems. For example, when kids take steroids or supplements, they often do it together. If teammates are doing it, it's more likely your son is too.

You also need to bring up these issues yourself and talk to him about eating disorders, body image problems, steroids, and supplements. Let him know how dangerous they can be, but encourage him to work out, play sports, and do other things that are important to him.

Try to counter the images of absurdly buffed bodies in the media by talking realistically about what is possible. Don't criticize, belittle, or demean his concerns about his appearance, no matter how exaggerated or untrue they may be. Help him broaden his horizons so his world does not end up revolving around the way he looks or his athletic performance. If you think he needs it, get professional help.

If you're concerned about your son, look out for the following clues and warning signs, as described in *The Adonis Complex.*

CLUES TO THE ADONIS COMPLEX IN BOYS

1. Does your son work out excessively (for example, more than two hours a day in the gym)? Does his time in the gym seem out of proportion to what he needs for his athletic activities at school? Do his workouts constantly take precedence over other important activities, such as studying, hobbies, or other healthy activities with peers?
2. Does your son seem preoccupied with looking like extremely muscular men in bodybuilding magazines, comic books, television, or movies?
3. Does your son use large quantities of dietary supplements, such as creatine or protein powders, hoping to build up his body and become more muscular?
4. Does your son use drugs found in health or nutrition stores like ephedrine, DHEA, or androstenedione in an attempt to become more muscular?
5. Are there any clues that your son is using steroids? Has he grown more muscular than appears naturally possible? Has he developed a physique that raises the suspicion of steroid use? Has he abruptly developed acne or mood changes during a time when he was rapidly gaining muscle size?
6. Does your son have sudden, sharp fluctuations in weight? Does he suddenly gain or lose large amounts of weight?
7. Does your son use dangerous techniques to lose weight? For example, does he fast or go on extreme diets? Does he refuse to eat with the family because he's on a special diet? Does he use laxatives or diuretics?
8. Does your son spend a lot of time examining himself in the mirror or reflecting surfaces like store windows?
9. Does your son spend a lot of time grooming and still feel he doesn't look good enough? Does he spend a lot of money on appearance-enhancing

products (hair gel, skin products) or spend lots of time in the bathroom trying to make himself look better?

10. Does your son use any type of body camouflage? For example, does he often wear a baseball cap, even indoors or when it doesn't fit the occasion? Does he wear bulky clothes that cover him up, even in the heat of summer?

11. Does your son frequently ask you or other people if he looks okay? When told he looks fine, does he still think he doesn't?

12. Is your son reluctant to go to school or participate in social activities for no apparent reason?

Source: Adapted with the permission of The Free Press, a division of Simon & Schuster Adult Publishing Group, from The Adonis Complex: The Secret Crisis of Male Body Obsession by Harrison G. Pope, Jr., M.D., Katharine A. Phillips, M.D., Roberto Olivardia, Ph.D. Copyright © 2000 by Harrison G. Pope, Jr., M.D., Katharine A. Phillips, M.D., Roberto Olivardia, Ph.D. All rights reserved.

THINGS ONLY BOYS GET

Earlier, we talked about the genitalia of newborns and baby boys. Some of the same problems are encountered in older boys, but the way these problems present is often different. In addition, there are conditions that affect boys as they get older that moms should be aware of. Of course, as women we know little about the male anatomy and even less about what can go wrong.

Don't for a minute think your son knows more than you do about his own anatomy. He's probably more clueless than you are. Phillip Nasrallah, M.D., says it's amazing how little teenage boys know when it comes to their own bodies. A 1984 survey in the journal *Pediatrics* revealed a big gap between what girls understood about breast cancer and what boys knew about testicular cancer. Dr. Nasrallah wanted to see if things had improved over the years, so in 1998 he surveyed more than three hundred male athletes between the ages of twelve and eighteen who were undergoing sports physicals. Surprise! Almost nothing had changed between 1984 and the late '90s. Boys were still largely ignorant of basic information regarding male reproductive health. Why? The reason, the authors speculate, is that, "Mothers are usually charged with child rearing and issues of health education fall on their shoulders. A mother's knowledge of male health issues is typically limited." They go on to point out that there is little media attention on issues specific to boys and, worse still, there is almost no formal education for boys about their own health. What's more, as boys get older, their contact with the health care system becomes less frequent. Clearly, boys need the chance to become better educated about their own bodies.

In this section, we're going to talk about some of the problems boys can have with their genitals. There's a good chance you will never have to deal with these. Still, it's not a bad idea to at least be familiar with them, so you can recognize them early and get help if they appear. Educate yourself and pass this information along to your son—and even to his father.

Uncircumcised Boys, Unnecessary Worries

A few years ago, when I was working in a clinic, a young mother came in with her six-year-old uncircumcised son. She was concerned because his foreskin did not completely retract over the head, or glans, of his penis. He wasn't having any problems, but she was worried because when he was first born, a doctor told her if the foreskin did not separate from the head of the penis by the time he was five or six, he would need to be circumcised. Now here he was—a healthy six-year-old boy—but his foreskin moved only slightly. She told my colleague in Spanish that she couldn't afford surgery but was afraid her son would get ill without it. A quick inspection revealed nothing abnormal about the child's penis; he could urinate normally and there were no signs of infection. All she really needed was a little reassurance that her son's penis was normal.

As we explained in chapter 1, when a boy is born, his foreskin (if he doesn't get circumcised) does not usually pull back. Over time, it will naturally separate from the glans, usually between the ages of four and seven. But for some boys it just takes longer, and that's okay—as long as the tight foreskin doesn't obstruct the flow of urine or cause pain or swelling.

Many parents worry unnecessarily when their son has a tight foreskin that does not retract to expose the tip of the penis. Doctors call this *phimosis,* but it's really not a problem unless there are other symptoms. Unfortunately many parents and even some doctors think they should force the foreskin over the head of the penis to get it to separate or to keep the penis clean. This is not only painful, it can cause scarring or other damage. Don't do it! Phimosis can also result from an infection underneath the foreskin, known as *balanitis,* or from other medical problems such as diabetes. This type of phimosis usually happens in older boys or adult men.

You don't need to do anything about phimosis that is not causing problems. If your boy feels discomfort, hot soaks and improved hygiene (for example, making sure the tip of the penis is dry after urinating) may help. Doctors used to recommend circumcision routinely for boys or men with phimosis that caused problems. This may be necessary as a last resort, but there are newer, less drastic kinds of treatments that doctors use to separate the foreskin from the penis such as applying steroid cream to the area several times a day.

The following problems can arise in an uncircumcised penis. If you notice any you need to take your son to the doctor.

Paraphimosis

This problem is essentially the opposite of phimosis. Instead of being unable to retract the foreskin, an uncircumcised male with *paraphimosis* can't get the foreskin to return to its normal position covering the glans. Instead, it remains pulled down and literally gets stuck. When this happens, the head of the penis and the foreskin may swell and become painful.

This problem can occur after a boy has pulled the foreskin down and doesn't pull it back up again. A doctor or nurse may do the same thing during an exam or if they're placing a urinary catheter. However it happens, if the foreskin is left in this position too long it may start to swell. This usually causes pain, but not always. Whether it's painful or not, this is a medical emergency and you need to get your son to the doctor (preferably a urologist) or the hospital.

Doctors will try to reduce the swelling so that the foreskin can be pulled back over the tip of the penis. They may use ice packs, apply gentle pressure, or wrap the penis in a tight gauze dressing to decrease swelling. If needed, pain medication can be given by injection or topically. Once the swelling is down, the doctor will pull the foreskin back into place.

If these techniques fail, doctors may try to drain fluid from the swollen foreskin with a needle or they may make a small slit in the foreskin to open the tight ring of skin that has formed like a small tourniquet. In rare cases, an emergency circumcision may be performed.

The main thing to remember is not to leave the foreskin pulled down. Teach boys to put their foreskin back where it belongs! If they gently pull it back over the glans each time they pull it down, you'll avoid this problem.

Balanitis

If the head of the penis become red, itchy, and inflamed, it may be caused by an infection called *balanitis.* It's more common in uncircumcised boys and men because of warmth and moisture under the foreskin, which can promote the growth of infectious organisms.

Balanitis can be triggered by a variety of things including irritation from soaps, bubble baths, or detergents. Sexually transmitted diseases can also cause it, or it can be associated with an underlying problem such as diabetes or drug allergies. It can also be caused or compounded by poor hygiene. Gentle cleaning, antibiotic cream, and if necessary, an antibiotic medication can usually take care of the problem. Patients who suffer repeated bouts of balanitis might be candidates for circumcision.

Normal Issues for Uncircumcised Boys

Other things can cause uncircumcised boys or their parents to worry even though they're perfectly normal.

Ballooning

Uncircumcised boys often experience a ballooning of the foreskin when they urinate. The urine is momentarily trapped beneath the foreskin, pushing it out. As long as there is no pain or sign of infection, there's no problem. This usually disappears as the foreskin begins to separate from the glans. In fact, ballooning may speed up this process by stretching the foreskin a bit.

Spraying

Uncircumcised boys sometimes spray when they urinate, rather than peeing a neat stream. Nothing to worry about here (though you may object to the mess). If he retracts the foreskin, this usually stops the spraying.

White Pearls

As they get older, some boys discover little white "pearls" that collect under the foreskin. The "pearls" are dead skin cells called *smegma*. This is a normal part of maturation that occurs as the foreskin detaches from the glans (tip). This does not require any treatment although they may spontaneously open and the "cheesy" material may drain out. This process actually helps the foreskin separate from the glans.

A Clean Bill of Health

If your son is uncircumcised, you—and he when he's old enough—need to know how best to clean his penis. It's not difficult. Just gently wash and dry the accessible areas. Do not force the foreskin to retract further than is comfortable. Once the foreskin has separated on its own from the glans, gently pull the skin down and clean the exposed area with a little soapy water. Pat it dry and pull the foreskin back up. That's all you need to do.

Testicular Emergencies

A painful or swollen testicle is a medical emergency. If your child or teenager has these symptoms, get medical attention right away. This is not always as easy as it sounds. With baby boys who cannot yet speak, detecting the problem can be difficult. You may have a sense that something is wrong, but you can't tell what it is. One sign is a baby who cries uncontrollably; he may even vomit from the pain. If this happens and you don't know why, undress him and look at his groin. A discolored scrotum is a sign that something is wrong, as is tenderness or discomfort when the scrotum is touched (see chapter 1).

The problem with many older boys and teens is they may be reluctant to tell you they have a problem. They just don't like to talk about their testicles with Mom, or even, in many cases, with Dad. Let your son know that if he ever has any medical questions or problems, he can always talk to you about it. It can help prevent a serious problem.

Testicular Torsion

We talked about testicular torsion in the newborn section but it's more likely to happen to older boys or teenagers. If it happens, it's a serious medical emergency.

Torsion occurs when the spermatic cord becomes twisted, pinching off the blood vessels that supply the testicle. In teens and older boys, torsion sometimes happens after a workout or some kind of strenuous activity or trauma. But in a lot of cases, there is no inciting event. Older boys are sometimes reluctant to mention that their testicle is swollen or painful, and minimize symptoms or say they have a bellyache rather than discuss their testicles. In some cases, boys have waited to get help—with disastrous results. The testicle can be badly damaged or lost in as little as six hours. Getting to a doctor immediately is essential so that surgery can be performed as soon as possible. According to Richard Schlussel, M.D., chief of pediatric urology at Mount Sinai, says few kids get help early enough to save the testicle. "Most of the time the parents say to me 'He never told me. This started a few days ago.'" Most parents have never heard of testicular torsion, Dr. Schlussel says.

The most common complaint is sudden, severe pain in a testicle. The testicle can become swollen and discolored—bluish or reddish—and may be pulled high in the scrotum, near the abdomen. It often causes stomach pain and vomiting and is sometimes confused with other problems like gastroenteritis. No matter what other symptoms are present, scrotal pain must be evaluated immediately!

Doctors can sometimes untwist the spermatic cord manually, easing the pain and restoring blood flow. But in most cases, surgery is required—and promptly. One thing that won't help is antibiotic medication, though sadly it's sometimes prescribed. Torsion is not an infection, though it may sometimes look like one to an inexperienced doctor.

Epididymitis

When a boy or man complains of pain in his scrotum, the most common reason is an infection of the *epididymis*, a long coiled tube that connects to each testicle and leads to the urethra. It's the place where sperm goes to mature after it is produced in the testicle. About 60,000 males end up in the emergency room each year with symptoms of epididymitis. (See diagram of male anatomy, page 49.)

Epididymitis is caused when bacteria, a virus, or another infectious agent spreads in the urinary tract. The infection may also involve the testicle and is then know as *epididymo-orchitis.* Less commonly, there can be an infection of the testicle alone, called *orchitis.* Years ago, before the mumps vaccine, orchitis was more common, a symptom of the mumps virus. Today, it is very rare.

Symptoms of epididymitis include pain, tenderness, or swelling in the scrotum, usually only on one side. Often the pain starts in the back of the testicle and quickly radiates to the entire testicle and then into the groin. The scrotum may be red and hot, and there may be burning during urination. Fever is common.

How do you tell the difference between epididymitis and torsion? It's not always easy. The main difference is that in epididymitis, the symptoms tend to come on slowly while with torsion the symptoms are abrupt, though by the time they get to the hospital, most are feeling terrible.

In boys who are not sexually active, the cause of epididymitis is usually a bladder infection that has spread to the testicles. It may be a signal of an anatomical abnormality of the urinary tract. It can also occur after tests or surgery in which a catheter is inserted into the bladder through the penis. In sexually active males, the cause is most often a sexually transmitted disease, usually chlamydia or gonorrhea. In fact, sexually active men in their twenties and thirties are the most frequent sufferers of epididymitis.

Whatever the cause, the symptoms of epididymitis require immediate evaluation by a doctor. Treatment depends on the cause and can include antibiotics, ice packs, pain relievers, and bed rest.

Testicular Injury

Sooner or later, most boys and men will get kicked, kneed, or otherwise smacked in the groin. The real problem comes when they try to tough it out and avoid seeking help.

If your boy gets struck in the genitals, the pain can be pretty intense. He may also experience nausea, dizziness, lightheadedness, and sweating. Many testicular injuries are relatively minor and the pain, although intense initially, will often subside in less than an hour, along with the other symptoms. But if the pain lasts longer, or if the testicles become swollen or discolored, he should get to a doctor right away. The doctor will look for signs of testicular torsion, a ruptured testicle, or possibly, a hernia. All three can require surgery.

For testicular injuries that don't require surgery, the best treatment is ice, rest, and antiinflammatory medication. Wearing underwear that gently supports the testicles can also help.

Studies have shown a relatively high number of infertile men had at least one injury to their testicles when they were young, usually around the age of fifteen.

The best way to prevent testicular injuries and avoid later problems is for boys and teenagers to wear athletic supporters and cups when playing sports (see chapter 9).

Testicular Cancer

Alex Johnson* was relaxing in bed one night when he reached down to do what men do—scratch his scrotum. That's when the thirty-three-year-old writer and new father discovered a firm, painless lump in his right testicle. The worst-case scenario quickly flashed through his mind.

"I remember thinking, 'I've got cancer, I'm going to die, I will never see my son grow up,'" Johnson recalls. "But then I did the strangest and dumbest thing. I rationalized that it was probably nothing and pretty much forgot about it until three weeks later when I mentioned it to my wife and she freaked out."

Their worst fears came true. An ultrasound showed he most likely had cancer. A few more tests and a chest X ray later, he learned it had spread to his lungs. So far, there's a happy ending to this story: After surgery and extensive treatment, Alex is now cancer-free. And because he froze sperm prior to treatment, he is even the father of a baby girl.

Still, his worries aren't completely over. Every six months, for at least two more years, he must return to his doctor for more tests. "Those are the toughest days. I am able to put it in the back of my mind except when I have to go in for follow-up. Then it's almost like the first day all over again."

Alex's case is classic in every respect, not very different than that of the most famous testicular cancer survivor—bicyclist Lance Armstrong, who denied his symptoms and kept riding for *six months* until he was nearly incapacitated by headaches, blurry vision, and testicular pain. He was even coughing up blood. When Armstrong was finally diagnosed, his situation was grim, an aggressive cancer throughout his body.

But as the whole world knows, Armstrong fought back and beat his cancer, going on to return to racing and win the Tour de France five times—as of this writing. Comedian Tom Green was the next celebrity to go public with his testicular cancer. Green even made it the focus of a special on MTV, in which he encouraged boys of the MTV generation to remember to check their "nuts."

Almost overnight, celebrities like Armstrong and Green have pushed testicular cancer into the spotlight. The increased attention comes at a good time. In 1999, researchers from Cancer Care Ontario and the U.S. Centers for Disease Control and Prevention reported a sharp jump in the incidence of testicular cancer. They found the number of men diagnosed with testicular cancer—mostly in their twenties and thirties—has increased almost 60 percent over the past three decades.

The good news about testicular cancer is that despite the increase, and the fact that it's the most common cancer among young men, it's still quite rare and highly curable. Some seven thousand American men are diagnosed with the cancer each year, and more than 90 percent will beat it. When men do die from testicular cancer, it's often the result of inadequate follow-up after treatment. That's too bad, because even when testicular cancer does recur, it is still highly treatable.

What's behind the increase in testicular cancer? Some experts think it may be related to chemical exposure during pregnancy (see chapter 1). A few other factors seem to increase risk as well. Men born with an undescended testicle (*cryptorchidism*) have a much higher risk. Men infertile from other causes also seem to have a slightly higher chance of developing this cancer; Caucasian men are at greater risk than Asians and African-Americans.

Men like Tom Green and Lance Armstrong hope that by making their battle with testicular cancer public they'll encourage other men to give their "nuts" a gentle squeeze every month or so. Every guy over fifteen should learn to perform this test and should do it every month. If he feels any unusual lump, swelling, or an area of hardness, he should get the area checked by a doctor. (For more on how to do a testicular exam, see page 137.)

Non-Emergencies
Hernias

Hernias are common in newborn boys, as we discussed back on page 51, but they also happen to older boys and adults. Women and girls get hernias, too, but they're far more common in males.

Like all organs of the body, the intestines are surrounded and held in place by a thin layer of tissue. When a bit of intestine protrudes through a weak area in the abdominal muscle, it's called a hernia. In males, the most common place for the intestine to poke out is through the inguinal canal, the opening that the testicles of a developing male fetus passed through to get from the abdomen into the scrotum. The canal usually closes before the boy is born or during his first two years. But not always. If it doesn't, the intestine can pop down into the scrotum (an *indirect hernia*).

Hernias can also occur in older males (and females) as a result of strenuous activity like lifting a heavy object and are usually easy to diagnose. Doctors can feel the protruding tissue manually using the old "turn-your-head-and-cough" procedure. Older boys and men tend to get *direct hernias* where a weakness of the groin tissues allows the intestines to protrude into the groin.

Most hernias cause few symptoms, but because they can "grow" in size as more intestine bulges through, there is a risk of the intestine becoming strangulated, or squeezed so tight its blood supply is cut off. Hernias can often by pushed back into the abdomen, but chances are high it will pop back out later. For that reason, it is almost always a good idea to repair the hernia surgically.

Surgery for most hernias is a simple outpatient procedure. Occasionally, a more complicated surgery may be performed and will keep a patient in the hospital overnight. Hernia surgeries are one of the most common surgical procedures performed—700,000 a year.

Varicocele

A varicocele is multiple enlarged or varicose veins in the spermatic cord leading to the scrotum. In boys, it can interfere with the normal growth of the testicle if not repaired. Most varicoceles appear on the left side. They are thought by many experts to be a common cause of infertility, perhaps because they interfere with the normal circulation of blood. This keeps the scrotum too warm, and excess heat damages or destroys sperm.

Varicoceles are quite common—10 percent to 20 percent of men past puberty have them. Most have no symptoms, though some will notice an ache or heavy feeling in their testicles. If there is no pain, and, in adults, if the varicocele is not interfering with fertility, treatment may not be necessary. In teenagers, operations for varicocele are generally done when there is a significantly smaller left testis. If surgery is needed, there are several options, but all methods are successful.

Spermatocele

These are small growths inside the scrotum. They happen when the epididymis gets obstructed and the sperm builds up inside, ballooning out and forming a small cyst. They are usually painless and don't generally need treatment, but they can sometimes grow quite large—up to five or six inches. If this happens, or if a spermatocele is painful, doctors may need to remove it surgically. In most cases a spermatocele causes no problem and does not need treatment.

Undescended Testicles

As we mentioned earlier, many boys are born with one or two undescended testicles. Usually, this is detected early on (see discussion of retractile testicles on page 50) and doctors then help the process along by hormone treatment or surgery. But occasionally, a boy can have an undescended testicle that doesn't get discovered until he reaches puberty. In other rare cases, a testicle that descended normally at birth can migrate back up into the abdomen. This is known as an *ascended* testicle.

In either case, if your teenage son has a testicle in the abdomen instead of in the scrotum, you'll need to consult a urologist. There are several issues to consider. The testicle can be brought down, but if it has been lodged in the abdomen since birth, it may be incapable of producing sperm. It's also at higher risk of developing testicular cancer. This is true whether it is brought down or not. But if it is in the scrotum it can be examined regularly so that a cancerous mass can be detected. The other option is simply to remove the testicle, which will prevent the possibility of cancer. If it is removed, a prosthetic testicle can be inserted so the boy's scrotum looks normal.

Sometimes even when the testicle is brought down in infancy it does not develop normally and is smaller than the other. This bugs some men and is associated with a higher rate of cancer developing. This could be another reason to remove the testicle and insert a prosthesis.

If a boy has had an undescended testicle, he'll need to pay special attention, as this increases the risk of testicular cancer. Fortunately the chance of this happening is still less than one in one hundred. Nonetheless, he'll need to learn how to perform a testicular self-exam and do it monthly. Let him know that this is essential.

The Breast Kept Secret of Boys: Gynecomastia

Of all the changes that boys go through during puberty, the most unwelcome is surely the growth of breast tissue. Doctors call it *gynecomastia* from the Greek words *gyne* for "women," and *mastos* for "breasts." It happens far more than most people think—as many as 70 percent of boys will have some enlargement of their breasts during puberty. Fortunately, it is only temporary for most, and the breasts disappear in a matter of months.

But that is not always the case. Merle James York founded the website Gynecomastia.org five years ago as a way to help and support others experiencing one of the most common but rarely discussed issues of male puberty. Merle knows about gynecomastia only too well. As a skinny 70-pound teenager he suffered endless ridicule because of his own gynecomastia. The kids in junior high nicknamed him "tits," and girls offered him their bras. But unlike most boys, his breast growth did not regress after puberty. He was thirty-three years old when he finally underwent surgery to remove them. "I was doing it for my thirteen-year-old self and all the torture he went through," he says. Things may even be worse for boys today as social pressure to achieve a perfect male image continues to mount. Many of the e-mails to Merle's website reflect these boys' anguish. The good news is that there are treatments and surgeries that can help.

What causes the male breasts to grow? Hormones. In males, the normal ratio of testosterone to estrogen circulating through the bloodstream is around 100 to 1. During puberty, this ratio can sometimes be disrupted and a higher level of estrogen may circulate for a while in the body. Since both male and female breast tissue responds to estrogen, they begin to grow. Usually, after a few months, this ratio corrects itself and the breast tissue recedes.

Gynecomastia can also result from medications that inhibit testosterone or contain estrogen or promote its synthesis. Amazingly, a boy may not even take the medications himself to experience this effect. If another person or family member is using estrogen creams, for instance, and the boy has prolonged contact with that family member, some of the estrogen can be absorbed into his body and cause gynecomastia. This, however, is quite uncommon.

Body-building drugs such as steroids and androgens can also have this effect, and with more teenagers and men than ever using steroids, lots of men of all ages are at risk of gynecomastia. Abuse of anabolic steroids by body builders can lead to "bitch tits" as they are called in those circles. Marijuana smoking is also thought to cause breast enlargement in males. And finally, breast enlargement in males can also be related to chromosomal problems such as Klinefelter's syndrome (see page 36).

Obesity is also a problem, and a confusing one. Many obese boys appear to have enlarged breasts. Often the extra fat makes it look like they have breasts. But in some heavy men, the breast tissue really is enlarging, and researchers who have studied large numbers of men with gynecomastia have found that they are much more likely to be overweight.

Once again, the issue is hormonal. When the body is housing higher than normal levels of fat tissue, it can accelerate the body's conversion of testosterone precursors—hormones that normally would turn into testosterone—into estrogen instead. Exactly how this happens is not known. For some overweight teenagers, a condition that begins in puberty may continue into adulthood, causing them tremendous shame and embarrassment.

Boys who develop gynecomastia during puberty usually notice a small firm mass under the areola on one side. It normally progresses to involve both sides but can also stay lopsided. Their prominent nipples are not only embarrassing, they can also be painful. The combination of discomfort and embarrassment often keeps boys from engaging in sports, partly because they're embarrassed to take off their shirt. Some boys won't take their shirts off to swim either.

For many boys, this deep shame translates into a fear that they are turning into a girl or will be homosexual. It is sad that such a common problem causes boys so much distress. If more boys understood how normal the problem is—and talked about it—perhaps they would not feel so tortured.

Boys going through this need your understanding. They may be so immobilized by fear and embarrassment they won't bring it up and may resist your attempts. But you'll do them no favors by avoiding the topic. If you can see they feel ashamed and withdrawn, or you find out they are being teased, try to get them to talk with someone who can help them understand how normal this is. I knew a very kind and understanding pediatrician who gave these boys notes to get out of gym because he had the problem as a kid and fully understands the panic they feel about being "found out" and teased. Most adolescent boys who develop gynecomastia will see their unwanted breasts disappear in a few months, or sometimes a year or two, without any treatment. But if it lasts more than a year or so, it may not go away on its own and treatment may be necessary.

A doctor, usually a pediatric endocrinologist, will check testosterone levels and thyroid function, and do other tests. The doctor may also check the size of the boy's testicles using a small device called an *orchidometer,* which looks a bit like egg cups. Even though there is absolutely no physical pain involved, boys *really* don't like this test. But it helps the doctor tell if the testicles are normal size, which is important in finding out if there is an underlying problem such as Klinefelter's syndrome (see page 36). In fact, Klinefelter's is often not discovered until puberty, when these classic signs and symptoms begin to appear. In rare cases, gynecomastia can be related to a tumor or overactive thyroid gland, another reason why it's important to check with a doctor.

Once unusual problems such as thyroid malfunction or Klinefelter's are ruled out, options for treating the problem become clearer. If the boy is significantly overweight, a major weight loss effort is a good idea in any case, and it may correct the hormonal imbalance in his body. If not, medications that block the action of estrogen may help. The last option is plastic surgery to remove the offending breast tissue.

THE THINGS BOYS WORRY ABOUT

Everyone worries about sexual matters, but part of what makes the teen years so intense, and can make teenagers feel so insecure, is the fact that they don't realize how universal their worries are. Here are some things in the sexual realm that teenage boys worry about.

A Matter of Size

Not long ago, a good friend of mine told me she wanted to ask an embarrassing question. Then, as delicately as possible, she told me that her son's penis seemed unusually small. Lots of parents worry about this, but often they're too embarrassed to ask even the pediatrician. Boys, as they grow older, also worry about the size of their penis, as do grown men. Unfortunately, for some boys and men, their mistaken belief that their penis is too small is a source of great embarrassment and shame.

It's important to understand that penises, like people, come in many shapes and sizes. There are very, very few men whose penises are too small to function sexually. It's also true that penises, like feet, tend to look smaller when you look down at them. Plus, most men tend to look at and compare their penis to others when it's not erect.

Mention these facts to your son if he asks you questions or expresses concern about his penis size. If he doesn't want to talk about it with you, get his father to talk to him. Or suggest he talk with his pediatrician, especially if the pediatrician is male.

In rare cases, a boy may have an extremely small penis. There are a couple of reasons why this can happen and we discussed them back on page 49.

Retracting Testicles

Testicles sometimes pull a disappearing act and slip up into the abdomen. It's actually quite natural, part of a mechanism designed to protect the testicles from injury. A muscle—the *cremaster* (suspender) muscle—is the force behind the cremasteric reflex. It pulls the testicles toward or into the inguinal canal, a cavity just inside the abdomen, when a man is cold, scared, or sexually excited, or when he's exerting himself physically. As long as they descend again when the excitement ends or the temperature warms up, there's no reason to be concerned. If a testicle fails to descend again, check with a doctor to make sure there isn't a problem.

The Problem of Blue Balls

It sounds rather ominous and it can be uncomfortable, but it's really nothing to worry about. In case you've never heard the term—or haven't heard it since you were a teenager—let me tell you about blue balls.

When men get sexually aroused, blood flows into the genitals. Some blood enters the penis and stays there, causing an erection, and some flows into the scrotum. If arousal lasts a long time—from a prolonged makeout session, for instance—then the blood stays put. New blood is red but older blood, which has less oxygen, is bluish. After a while, the skin of the scrotum takes on a distinctly bluish tinge.

The intense discomfort is a result of all that blood that's coursed into the groin getting trapped there, putting pressure on the blood vessels that service the area. The engorged area impinges on the nerve endings around the testicles. The result: aching testicles, though it has nothing to do with a buildup of sperm, as many mistakenly believe.

So how can men relieve this discomfort? Ejaculation is the quickest way. But the truth is that when the arousal and erection subside, and the blood flows out of the groin, the ache will fade as well. If the subject comes up with your son (or daughter), let him know that blue balls are not going to injure him or cause anything more than lingering discomfort.

7

Sturm und Drang? The Teen Years

Put mildly, teenagers don't have a very good rep—especially not teenage boys. Spend a little time watching TV or browsing through titles at your local bookstore and you'll probably be convinced that adolescence is a pathological condition and that teenage boys are surly, gun-toting belligerents who are threats not only to themselves, but to the rest of us as well. School shootings like the one at Columbine High School have become the defining image of a generation, covered regularly in specials, daily news reports, and best-selling books.

Check a few of the books released in the last few years. My favorite title had to be *Unglued and Tattooed: How to Save Your Teen from Raves, Ritalin, Goth, Body Carving, GHB, Sex, and 12 Other Emerging Threats.* Then there's *Yes, Your Teen Is Crazy: Loving Your Kid Without Losing Your Mind,* and *Difficult Teens: A Parent's Guide for Coping.*

With these teenage portrayals predominating in the media and on bookshelves, it's no wonder so many parents of young children look ahead to the teen years with fear and dread. Teenagers are "in crisis," the cliché of the day goes, and it's getting worse.

You may be surprised to learn that much of the bad rap teens get is undeserved. There is evidence that teenagers today may be doing a bit better than just a few years ago in terms of what researchers refer to as "health-risk behavior"—drug use, drunken driving, suicide. That's the view that emerges from the Youth Risk Behavior Survey (YRBS), a national survey of ninth- to twelfth-grade students commissioned by the Centers for Disease Control and Prevention. In 2001, the survey found:

- Twenty-nine percent of high school students smoked cigarettes occasionally, down from 36 percent in 1997. The number of regular smokers dropped from 17 percent to 14 percent.

- Seventeen percent of students said they carried a weapon, down from 22 percent in 1993.

- Nineteen percent said they seriously considered suicide, down from 24 percent in 1993.

- Thirty-one percent of students said that in the previous 30 days they'd been a passenger in a car with a driver who'd been drinking, down from 35 percent in 1993.

Now, no one would say these numbers are anything to feel great about. And the fact they are moving in the right direction cannot take away from a sobering reality: Millions of American teenagers are stressed out, struggling, and at great risk. Easing their pain, and helping them avoid these perils and pitfalls, is the most important work we can do for our teenage sons.

The teen years are a time in people's lives when they tend to take risks, push the limits, and act impulsively. It's an age when they're old enough and strong enough to do real damage. In a culture in which risk taking can involve substance abuse and violence, the combination can be toxic.

The Real Health Issues for Teenagers

The vast majority of teenagers and young adults are in good physical health. The biggest health problems in these years—being overweight or smoking—generally don't exact a toll for many years. The two diseases that cause the most deaths among teenagers—cardiovascular disease and cancer—account for only a small percentage of those who die. About 75 percent die as a result of behavior, their own or someone else's.

The biggest threats to the health and well-being of adolescents, especially boys, are not physical but behavioral: injuries from drunk or careless driving, assault or violence, and suicide. No other health issues even come close.

If you want to help your adolescent boy stay healthy and avoid risky, dangerous behavior, your most important task is to spend time with him, stay connected. He needs to know that you care—even when he acts like he doesn't. He needs you to ask him about his life—even when his response is a one-word grunt. He needs your help thinking ahead about the risks and pressures he is likely to experience. The moment he's deciding whether to get into a car with a pal who's had too much to drink may be too late.

When parents spend time with their children and have close connections with them, when they've developed relationships with open communication, children are more likely to internalize their parents' advice. They're also more likely to have a sense of their own value and to have confidence in their ability to make good decisions. In this chapter, we'll talk about the risks today's teenagers face and how you can help your boy navigate them. Let's begin, though, by talking about the process of puberty.

Help! My Baby Is Growing a Beard

Let's admit it. As we go through our child's early years, that all-too-short period when they're cute, cuddly, and affectionate (much of the time, anyway), we sometimes wish we could stop them in their tracks. "If only he could stay as he is now," we sigh (unless, of course, he's throwing a tantrum or waking us for the fourth time that night). We can't, of course. The day will come when our little boy starts to become a young man.

Puberty brings more change than a person will experience at any stage of life other than infancy, and it happens at breakneck speed. In a matter of a few years, most children grow a foot in height, become adult-size, and develop the ability to reproduce. The maturation process is a product of complex interactions between brain, testicles, pituitary gland, and hormones that cascade through the body. These biological processes don't exist in a vacuum, though; they are influenced by the environment in which our children live.

For most boys, puberty begins somewhere between the ages of nine and fourteen, with the average around twelve. That's about two years later than most girls—two years that can stretch into three, four, or even five for some late bloomers. The process of sexual maturation follows a sequence described in detail by Dr. James Tanner, a British pediatrician, and his colleagues, and known as the "Tanner stages." While the timing of this process can vary a great deal, the sequence is predictable.

The first signs of puberty come when a boy's testicles grow a bit larger and a sparse growth of downy pubic hair appears. Soon, his penis will grow larger and the pubic hair will get thicker and curlier. Hair grows in his armpits. In many boys, a small amount of breast tissue may develop at this time. This is completely normal and will usually go away within a year or so. (See chapter 6 for more about boys with breast tissue.) Then his voice breaks and deepens, and his muscles get bigger and more defined. The final changes rewrite boy's faces, giving them that most grown-up of features, facial hair, as well as those dreaded zits. This whole process usually takes about three years, which means it's usually completed between twelve and seventeen.

We're all familiar with what I've just described. One thing that's new, however, is that researchers are learning more about what's happening inside the brain during puberty. Scientists once believed brain development and the growth of neurons was a process that happened in utero and during a child's earliest years. But new technologies, including sophisticated scans that provide a glimpse at what's going on inside the brain, have shown that brain growth continues into adolescence.

The timing of puberty varies greatly from child to child. In recent years, doctors have been paying a lot of attention to the age children start to mature, as a result of a 1997 study by Marcia Herman-Giddens, M.D., and her colleagues at the University of North Carolina. She found that girls appeared to enter puberty much earlier than in the past. More recently, Dr. Herman-Giddens found a similar though less pronounced trend in boys. For reasons beyond the scope of this book, both of these studies are controversial, and some experts question her findings. Whatever the truth, if your boy shows signs of entering puberty before he's nine, or if he hasn't started to mature by age fourteen, have him evaluated by a doctor. (See pages 156–57.)

Scientists have been trying to figure out what triggers puberty to begin and why it appears to begin at younger and younger ages. There are a number of unproven theories, ranging from improved nutrition and health care to exposure to chemicals that mimic the action of hormones. Some researchers have even suggested that exposure to stressful events can accelerate the onset of puberty.

One problem with early puberty is that people often assume that a child's intellectual and social development keeps pace with their physical development. In other words, they may assume that a kid who looks older will be better able to think through the consequences of his actions, while a young-looking kid may not understand consequences as fully. In fact, researchers say there is no relationship between cognitive and physical development.

The underlying message is that if your son enters puberty so early or so late that he's significantly out of step with most kids in his peer group, he may have a hard time. He may feel isolated or disconnected, and he may suffer in silence. Your job is to pay attention, notice what's going on, be there to offer help and encouragement, and get other help if he needs it. Even if he goes through puberty at a normal time and pace, it can be a jarring transition, one that you can help him get through with a little advance planning and some timely conversations.

PREPARING YOUR SON FOR PUBERTY

If you think your husband is oblivious and unaware of his body, talk to a teenage boy. *Clueless* is the word that comes to mind. To give you a sense of how little boys know about their bodies, when middle school, high school, and college athletes from twelve to twenty-five were surveyed by researchers from Children's Hospital Medical Center of Akron (as reported in the *Journal of Urology* in 2000), more than half had no idea why a genital exam was included in a sports physical. Over 90 percent of those surveyed could not correctly answer three basic questions concerning the most common testicular conditions in their age group, such as testicular loss and testicular tumors. Only 38 percent knew that males in their late teens and early twenties have an increased risk of testicular cancer. And most couldn't recognize the signs and symptoms of serious problems in their testicles. They also had little idea about how to protect themselves from genital injuries.

Prepubescent boys are just as ignorant about the dramatic changes that lie ahead for them. You can help by letting them know what's in store: how their genitals will grow, about wet dreams and masturbation, growth spurts and acne, romance and sexuality. They should understand the basic sequence outlined above.

There are a number of good books on these issues, some written for parents, some for teenagers. In the Resource section, we list a number of titles in age-appropriate categories. You may want to purchase one and leave it around for your son to "find." For more on puberty and sexuality, see chapter 8.

Not All Teen Spirit Smells Bad!

Nearly one hundred years ago, G. Stanley Hall, one of the fathers of American psychology, popularized the term "adolescence" in a 1904 book by the same name. He described adolescence as a time of *sturm und drang*—storm and stress—and of unavoidable turmoil and pain that was "strewn with wreckage of body, mind, and morals." Teenagers, he wrote "are emotionally unstable" with "a natural impulse to experience hot and perfervid psychic states."

Hall's view became the received wisdom among researchers and the general public, who largely accepted the idea of adolescence as an inherently tumultuous time when raging hormones take control of teenagers' brains and bodies, causing them to lash out at their parents and themselves. Today, those views continue to hold sway, reinforced by the recent work of neurobiologists who contend that the teenage tendency to act out, take risks, and think irrationally is caused by sweeping changes in the brain.

The neurobiologists' views were on display in a recent series on PBS called *Inside the Teenage Brain,* which showed how imaging technology has allowed scientists to look into adolescent brains. They discovered that just before puberty, teen brains go through a growth spurt in which neurons and the connections between them are overproduced, then must be pruned like the branches of a tree. "In many ways, it's the most tumultuous time of brain development since coming out of the womb," Jay Giedd, M.D., a brain researcher with the National Institute of Mental Health, says during the program.

Most of this growth and pruning happens in a part of the brain just above the eyes, the prefrontal cortex. This area is the command center of the brain, responsible for coordinating many activities, including planning and organizing, as well as inhibiting impulses and regulating verbal expression.

The result of these changes in the brain, says Charles Nelson, Ph.D., director of the Center for Neurobehavioral Development at the University of Minnesota, is that "once [a] kid becomes a teenager, for a brief period of time, it's as though [he's] been invaded by another body."

But many social scientists and public health researchers dismiss such language as overheated and reject the notion that the teenage years are inherently a time of crisis, or that teenagers pass through some kind of biologically driven psychotic break. The report from a recent forum on adolescence convened by the Institute of Medicine made the following observation:

Adolescence continues to be seen as a period of time encompassing difficult developmental challenges, but there is wider recognition that biology is only one factor that affects young people's development, adjustment, and behavior. . . . There is now greater recognition that most young people can move through the adolescent years without experiencing great trauma or getting into serious trouble. . . . In fact, there is mounting evidence that parents, members of the community, service providers, and social institutions can both promote healthy development among adolescents and intervene effectively when problems arise.

In this more nuanced view, adolescence is seen as a time of great change, but one that most teens can navigate, especially if they have some help. Daniel Offer, M.D., a professor of psychiatry and behavioral science at Northwestern University, spent some forty years collecting data on thousands of adolescents in long-term studies. He argues that the vast majority of teenagers are satisfied with their lives and their relationships with their parents, and that they are quite capable, thank you very much, of making good decisions. "The normal American teenager sees him- or herself as a competent individual who is able to resolve the problems that come his way during the adolescent years, without too much pain, suffering, doubt, or indecision," Dr. Offer wrote in a 1981 book.

This doesn't mean, of course, that the teenage years aren't stressful and trying, and, for a significant minority of kids, traumatic, depressing, and even dangerous. That said, trauma and depression are not inevitable. The quality of most teenagers' lives has as much to do with what's going on in their homes and relationships as in their genes or biology. Indeed, one problem with viewing biology as the most powerful cause of teenage troubles is that it ignores the profound impact of our stressful culture and increasingly hectic family life.

Family and social dynamics also have a great deal to do with how teenagers learn to manage one of the central dynamics of teenage life: the urge—some would even call it a need—to take risks. Lynn E. Ponton, M.D., a professor of child and adolescent psychiatry at the University of California, San Francisco, has spent twenty-five years counseling teenagers and has raised two of her own. She says that risk-taking behavior is an inherent and essential part of adolescence. "I actually believe that risk taking is the primary tool in adolescence [that allows teens] to develop their identities," Dr. Ponton says. "It's really key. It's through risk taking that men become who they are." But all risks, she points out, are not the same.

"Our culture has come to believe that adolescence is naturally a tumultuous time, and this has blurred the lines between normal, exploratory behavior and behavior that is dangerous," Dr. Ponton wrote in her 1998 book *The Romance of Risk: Why Teenagers Do the Things They Do*. "When we assume that all risk taking is bad, we fail to recognize both the very real dangers some risks pose, and the tremendous benefits that others can yield."

Learning to face challenges and take acceptable risks is a key part of growing up, Ponton says, and is crucial to an adolescent's healthy development. Instead of seeing how fast he can drive or how a drug makes him feel, a teenager can take a healthy risk by conquering cliffs on his mountain bike, trying his hand at painting or acting, or traveling to a place he's never been. He can run for office on the student council or write articles for his high school paper. He can spend time volunteering at a homeless shelter or trying to save endangered wildlife. The teenaged sons of Bennett L. Leventhal, M.D., a child and adolescent psychiatrist at the University of Chicago, got their thrills by learning to scuba dive. "They were able to tell their friends they played with an octopus, which is pretty safe but feels and sounds thrilling and risky," Dr. Leventhal says.

The bottom line: When kids have an outlet for taking healthy risks, they're much less likely to take unhealthy ones.

One problem with assuming nearly all adolescents are going to take stupid or dangerous risks is that parents may throw up their hands and figure there's nothing they can do. Then they may reassure themselves that it's okay, because their kid will "grow out of" these behaviors once his hormones stop raging. That's a dangerous assumption, according to the authors of the Institute of Medicine report: "When adults overlook these problems, assuming they are an inevitable risk of adolescence and will be outgrown, they may be placing young people at risk."

THE YEARS OF LIVING DANGEROUSLY

One of the biggest transitions your child will face comes with the move from the protected cocoon of elementary school to the early-teen world of middle or junior high school. Suddenly, your child is in a big school with bigger kids who are tougher and more sophisticated. There are a lot more teachers, too, but no single one charged with looking out for each child.

"A lot of kids, particularly boys, were on a good track in elementary school and they get to middle school and they begin to fail," says Joy G. Dryfoos, a researcher and author of the book *Safe Passage: Making It Through Adolescence in a Risky Society.* "Some of it has to do with the nature of the institution. They start changing classes, they become much more autonomous, they don't get as much attention."

This jarring change in environment is often accompanied by big changes in behavior. For many kids it's a time when risky behaviors start to take hold. For example, 19 percent of ninth graders and 27 percent of twelfth graders report current marijuana use, according to the YRBS data.

Another survey, by CASA, documented the rising use of alcohol, cigarettes, and marijuana during these early teen years, from twelve to sixteen. The survey found that:

- Ninety-five percent of teens who smoke cigarettes start by the age of fifteen. The average starting age: twelve years, three months.
- Ninety-three percent of teens who drink alcohol start by fifteen. Average starting age: twelve and a half.
- Eighty-six percent of teens who smoke pot start by fifteen. Average starting age: thirteen and a half.

These numbers illustrate a sad fact: Much as you'd like to have that discussion about drugs or drinking when your son is a bit older, you really can't. If you wait until a child is fifteen, for instance, he may already have developed a drug or alcohol habit that's going to be difficult to break.

THE RISKS BOYS TAKE

Boys and girls tend to take risks in different ways, says Dr. Ponton. "Girls' risk taking turns inward," she says. "It's directed in towards themselves—cutting or disordered eating. Boys' risk taking turns outward toward the world. And I think that reflects the differences in boys' and girls' characters."

The difference in risk-taking style between girls and boys makes adolescence a more dangerous time for boys. Teenage boys are nearly three times as likely as girls to die, and the main causes are rarely natural and almost always preventable—a result of behavior not disease. In 2000, for example, 9,697 boys (and "just" 3,866 girls) between fifteen and nineteen died, and 75 percent of these boys died from just three causes: unintentional injuries, homicide, and suicide.

Teenage males are more likely than people of any other age group to be the victims of violent crime. Males are also more likely than females to be the perpetrators of crimes and to carry weapons. At schools across the country, according to the Mid Atlantic Equity Consortium, an education advocacy group, three times as many boys as girls carry weapons, twice as many boys have been threatened or injured with weapons, and twice as many boys have engaged in physical fights. Fortunately, there is some good news. Violent crime rates have fallen steadily since the mid-1990s, although the United States has the highest crime rate of any industrialized country in the world.

Drugs, alcohol, and violence are not the only risks that young people face, or even the biggest. The most common kind of unintended injury—and the biggest killer—by far, is automobile accidents.

IF YOU WORRY ABOUT ONE THING, MAKE IT BOYS IN CARS

There is good news and bad news when it comes to teenage drivers. The good news is the number of teenagers who die in cars has dropped substantially in recent years, by 36 percent since 1975. Males especially seem to be driving more safely. Deaths among teenage boys have dropped by 43 percent during this period.

The bad news is that teenagers remain the most dangerous drivers on the road, by far. Auto accidents are the leading cause of death among teenagers, accounting for nearly 40 percent of all teenage deaths. Mile for mile, teen drivers are four times more likely to crash than drivers of any other age group. Males are at especially high risk. In 2001, 5,582 teenagers died in automobile accidents and two thirds were boys, according to the Insurance Institute for Highway Safety.

Why are teenagers at such high risk when they climb into a car? There are a number of reasons:

- Teens are inexperienced drivers, and they're not always good at recognizing dangers or dealing with problems.

- Teens are more likely to drive when under the influence of alcohol or drugs, or to get in a car with a drunk or stoned driver. And teens that have been drinking are far more likely than older drivers to crash.

- Teenagers—especially males—have the lowest rate of seat belt use among all age groups. In 2001, 14 percent of high school students (18 percent of males) said they rarely or never wear seat belts. The trend is changing for the better, though: In 1993, 19 percent of high school kids said they never buckled up.

- Teens tend to be less careful. They're more likely to run red lights, make illegal turns, and speed. And some teens do things that are so dangerous—and dumb—it is hard to believe. In 1998, *Reader's Digest* surveyed 400 kids, ages fifteen to nineteen, about their experiences with teen drivers who had not been drinking or taking drugs. The results were frightening:

HAVE YOU EVER BEEN WITH A TEEN DRIVER WHO	PERCENTAGE ANSWERING YES
Packed in so many passengers that there weren't enough seat belts	57%
Drove 20 miles per hour or more over the speed limit	53%
Jerked the steering wheel to make the car swerve back and forth	35%
Had a passenger grab the wheel while the car was moving	21%
Tailgated, cut off, or tried to bump another car	14%
Let a passenger car-surf—ride on the outside of the moving car	12%
Did at least one of these types of activities	82%

Source: Bruskin/Goldring Research, 1998. Reprinted with permission from the June 1998 Reader's Digest. *Copyright © 1998 by The Reader's Digest Assn., Inc.*

More Is Not Merrier

Sometimes, even levelheaded kids who don't normally take silly risks slip, especially if a group of buddies piles in the car with them. When a teenager is driving, just having passengers in a car increases the risk of a crash. And the more passengers, the greater the risk:

- One passenger doubles the fatal crash risk.
- Two or more passengers ups the fatal crash risk to five time as likely.

Interestingly, passengers have no effect on the likelihood that an older driver will have a fatal crash. Teenagers, it seems, are more likely to turn around to talk to someone in the back, let a passenger take the steering wheel, or go along with a passenger who urges them to go faster. All of these things make an accident more likely.

Don't Let Your Son Become a Statistic

Now you know: The biggest risk that teenage boys face is a two-ton piece of rolling steel piloted by them or another teenager. So what can you do to protect him? Arm him with good sense. And good sense doesn't come from your lectures, but from what you do when you drive. Don't take risks behind the wheel. Don't laugh or show encouragement when you see other people drive recklessly. "Make your own driving as excellent as possible," says Dr. Ponton. "And admit your own mistakes so that they can really learn from that."

Encouraging safe driving starts long before a teenager gets behind the wheel, says Ponton. It should begin when your boy is learning to ride a skateboard or a bike. Teach him the rules of the road. Watch him closely to see how careful he is and how he follows your directions. Once he's a competent bike rider, be prepared to impose consequences if he violates safety rules by suspending his bike-riding privileges. When he starts driving, do the same with his driving privileges. In this way, he'll get the idea that he needs to take safety seriously.

Make Sure He "Graduates"

Teen drivers are dangerous, but sixteen-year-olds are in a risk class of their own. They are twice as likely to crash as seventeen-year-olds and nearly three times as likely to crash as eighteen- and nineteen-year-olds. Between 1976 and 1996, while the death rate among drivers older than seventeen was declining, the death rate among sixteen-year-olds was rising. In an effort to reduce the number of accidents and casualties caused by teen drivers, especially the youngest teens, many states converted to a system of graduated drivers' licenses in recent years. In this system, new drivers can get behind the wheel only with certain restrictions, and earn driving privileges in stages.

In the first stage, usually at age fifteen, a new driver gets a learner's permit and can drive only under the supervision of a licensed adult. The new driver is not permitted to drink any alcohol, must comply with seat belt laws, and must make sure all passengers wear their belts. After six months of safe driving, and after passing both a driver-education course and a road test, the learner can apply for an intermediate license.

During the intermediate phase, drivers can drive on their own during the day but must be supervised by a licensed adult after 10 P.M. They must continue to comply with the zero alcohol and seat belt policies. After six months of continued safe driving with no moving violations, they can apply for a regular driver's license.

These programs have been a success. Two recent studies looked at the impact of graduated license laws passed in Michigan and North Carolina in 1997 by comparing accident rates in 1996, the last year under the old system, and 1999. In Michigan, nighttime crashes involving sixteen-year-old drivers dropped 57 percent, and all crashes declined 25 percent. In North Carolina, fatal crashes involving sixteen-year-old drivers dropped 57 percent and nighttime crashes dropped 43 percent.

"In North Carolina, during 1999 alone, the result was dozens of lives preserved, thousands of injuries prevented, and millions of dollars saved," wrote Robert Foss, Ph.D., and his colleagues from the University of North Carolina, who authored one of the studies.

At least thirty-four states have now adopted some version of a graduated license system. If the state you live in hasn't gone to this system, you can impose one in your own family. The truth is that even if your state does have a graduated license law, you and your husband will still be the main enforcers. So pass a new license law at your house and impose similar restrictions on your teen's access to the car. Then drive with your teenager as often as possible and under as many conditions as possible.

Here are a few other suggestions to help get your son (and his passengers) home in one piece, drawn from the American Academy of Pediatrics and other sources:

RULES OF THE ROAD

- Require your teen to maintain good grades before he or she can drive. Check with your auto insurance company to see if "good student" discounts are available.
- Set a good example by not speeding or using alcohol or other drugs when driving, and by making sure that everyone wears a safety belt, including you and your husband.

- Remind your teen that it's important to stay focused on driving, without distractions from loud music or conversations on the phone or in the car.
- Let your teen know that driving after drinking or using other drugs will not be tolerated.
- Implement a no-questions-asked policy, too. If your kid has had a drink and has the good sense to call home for a ride, don't punish him or interrogate him about it. Talk it over later when everyone is thinking rationally. The important thing is to get him home alive.
- You can formalize these kinds of agreements in a contract. The group SADD (formerly Students Against Driving Drunk but now known as Students Against Destructive Decisions) has a copy of its "Contract for Life" on its website at *http://www.saddonline.com*.

SMOKING

For many years, the number of Americans smoking cigarettes declined among people of every age group but one—teenagers. Between 1993 and 1997, the percentage of high school students who said they were current smokers rose from 31 percent to 36 percent. The good news is that the trend finally seems to have reversed. In the CDC's 2001 Youth Risk Behavior Survey, the number of admitted current smokers was back down to 29 percent, while the number who said they smoked frequently dropped from 17 percent in 1997 to 14 percent in 2001.

But if the numbers are headed in the right direction, they are still unacceptably high. Every day, according to the American Lung Association (ALA), about 4,800 teenagers will smoke their first cigarette, and just under half of them will become regular smokers. About 4.5 million adolescents and teenagers ages eleven to seventeen are smokers. If they continue, one third will die younger than they should from heart, lung, and other problems caused by smoking. And one more sobering fact: According to the ALA, most adolescents who have smoked at least one hundred cigarettes—just five packs—in their lifetime say they would like to quit but are unable to do so. It doesn't take long to get hooked.

"The earlier adolescents start smoking, the more likely they are to remain addicted as adults," says Laurie Chassin, Ph.D., a professor of psychology at Arizona State University. "Even teens who reported 'experimenting' with smoking were more likely to become regular smokers five or six years later."

One recent study published in the journal *Tobacco Control* in 2000 found that children can become addicted to smoking in a matter of days and after smoking only a handful of cigarettes. A team of researchers led by Joseph DiFranza, M.D., of the University of Massachusetts Medical School, followed almost seven hundred twelve- and thirteen-year-olds for one year and found that nearly one hundred started smoking that year. Of the kids that started smoking, one in five began feeling withdrawal symptoms such as nervousness, anxiety, and irritability within four weeks. Sixteen students developed symptoms within two weeks, and several said their symptoms started within days.

This may seem surprisingly quick, but the researchers point out that after just two puffs on a cigarette—or two doses of nicotine—the number of nicotine receptors in the brain increases. The adolescent brain may be especially vulnerable to addiction because it is still developing. The researchers identified three types of smokers, depending on how quickly they get hooked:

- The "love at first sight" smokers got addicted almost immediately and seemed to sense right away "that nicotine had a powerful influence on them."
- The gradual addicts were a bit slower in developing symptoms of nicotine dependence, needing to smoke for months or years before they felt symptoms of dependence.
- The third group, dubbed "chippers," could smoke up to five cigarettes a day without becoming addicted.

What Can a Parent Do?

How can we make sure our sons don't become smokers? Do we have any influence over what they do? These are important questions to ask, especially when you consider that if a person makes it to twenty-one without becoming a smoker, there's only about a 10 percent chance he or she will smoke later.

We parents have more influence than we realize. The first and most powerful form of influence is our actions. Mothers who smoke during pregnancy seem to increase the chances that their child will become a smoker. And when parents are smokers who light up at home, their children are far more likely to become smokers. In one recent study, Arthur Farkas, Ph.D., and his colleagues at the Cancer Prevention and Control Program at the University of California San Diego looked at the influence of parents' smoking on their children. They found that adolescents who lived with smokers (usually their parents) were three times as likely to be smokers as those whose parents never smoked.

If you are a smoker, you should quit—for everyone's sake. It makes a difference. In his study, Dr. Farkas also found that kids who lived with ex-smokers are about half as likely to smoke as those whose parents still light up. And the earlier you quit, Farkas has found, the better the chance your children will never start.

If you can't quit, at least stop smoking in the house. Make your home a smoke-free zone and you'll reduce the chances your child will smoke. At least you can say you're doing something to try to help him. "Adoption of a smoke-free home policy sends a message to family members that smoking is not condoned, while the lack of such a policy may send the opposite message," wrote Dr. Farkas and his colleagues. The earlier you start this policy, of course, the better it will be for your child.

The Farkas study also found that teenagers who worked were less likely to smoke if they worked in a smoke-free workplace. So that's something to think about when your son (or daughter) is looking for a job (see page 208). You might want to insist that your teenager not work in a place that allows smoking.

The attitude you convey to your children about their smoking is also important. A recent study in *Pediatrics* by researchers at Dartmouth Medical School found that when kids think that their parents strongly disapprove of them smoking, they are less likely to start, particularly if both parents take the same antismoking stance. Most children really do care what their parents think (even if they don't want to admit it).

I was surprised to learn from the Dartmouth study that simply taking a strong position against your children smoking may be more important than whether you smoke yourself. There is some conflicting data on this point, but I would say this: Whatever you can do to let your son know how dangerous smoking is, and how much you want him not to smoke, the better. If you smoke, quit. If you can't quit, ban smoking in your house.

Here's another thing to think about. Kids who watch a lot of TV are more likely to smoke. A study recently published in the journal *Pediatrics* found that the more time kids watch TV, the more likely they are to smoke. Kids who logged an average of five hours of tube time a day were six times as likely to start smoking as kids who watched less than two hours. The kids in this study were surprisingly young; the average age was twelve and a half.

What lies behind these numbers? It's hard to say, but researchers point out that kids who watch a lot of TV see a lot of people smoking cigarettes. One quarter of all videos shown on MTV depict people smoking, often in glamorous, sexualized settings. In a review of eighty-one G-rated films, many of which end up on TV, thirty-five of them (43 percent) showed tobacco use for an average of two minutes per film. And even though cigarette ads are banned on TV, cigarette billboards, logos, and banners make their way on the tube through televised sporting events. "Television, with its frequent positive portrayals of smoking, may be an effective indirect method of tobacco promotion," wrote the authors of the *Pediatrics* study. Cut down TV time and you may reduce the chances your kids will start smoking.

Helping Your Son Kick the Habit

What can you do if your teenager does take up smoking? If you're a smoker your-self, the most effective thing would be to make a pact that you will both quit. Then you could both enroll in smoking-cessation programs. There are a number aimed at help-ing teenagers quit, but the results of these programs have been mixed. One that has demonstrated some success is the American Lung Association's NOT (No On Tobacco) program. Designed for use by high schools and community-based organi-zations, the NOT program provides training to teachers, school nurses, counselors, and other staff and volunteers who then facilitate a series of ten sessions for teenagers. The program separates boys and girls so each group can relax and deal with issues key to them. The goal is to help teens who want to quit or cut back by offering support and training in stress management and other skills.

A recent evaluation of the NOT program found that after six months, 22 percent of teens taking part had quit smoking. Of those who continued to smoke 65 percent had cut the number of cigarettes smoked during the week, and 75 percent reduced the number of cigarettes they smoked during the weekend. If your community group or high school is interested in setting up a NOT program, contact the local chapter of the American Lung Association (1–800-LUNG-USA) to find out if training is available in your area.

Smokeless Tobacco

As many as 20 percent of high school boys used smokeless tobacco, according to the Centers for Disease Control and Prevention. Of the 12 million to 14 million chewers, one third are under the age of twenty-one, and half develop the habit before they are thirteen! Imitating sports figures (it's big with baseball players) and adopting a macho pose are two main reasons boys start chewing. The problem is that smoke-less tobacco comes with serious risks (though many kids believe it is less dangerous than smoked tobacco), including mouth sores, cracked bleeding lips, receding gums that may lead to tooth loss, and ultimately throat and mouth cancer. The CDC's web-site has more information aimed at kids who use smokeless tobacco and suggestions for quitting (*http://www.cdc.gov/tobacco/sgr/sgr4kids/smokless.htm*). See Resources for a website that discusses how the National Spit Tobacco Education Program is working to get professional ballplayers to quit chewing.

ALCOHOL AND DRUGS

If you follow news reports about American teenagers' use of drugs and alcohol, you may feel a bit confused. One day, former Secretary of Health, Education and Wel-fare Joseph Califano is worrying at a press conference about an "epidemic of underage drinking" starting in junior high school. The program he now runs, the National Center on Addiction and Substance Abuse (CASA) at Columbia University, was releasing a report that found that almost one fourth of all the alcohol purchased in the United States is consumed by underage drinkers.

A few months later, current Secretary of Health and Human Services Tommy Thompson held another press conference to announce that "the youth in our high schools are increasingly acting like responsible young men and women" by reducing their use of alcohol and drugs. Two major national surveys in the past year have found that the number of teens drinking alcohol and using drugs is declining—modestly, to be sure, but declining nonetheless.

Whatever the exact numbers, it is clear that the consumption of alcohol and drugs remains a big problem for American teenagers. Surveys estimate that almost one half of high school students drink alcohol at least once a month and that 30 percent of students have consumed five or more alcoholic drinks in a row sometime in the previous thirty days, meeting the criteria for binge drinking.

Califano's group, CASA, reports that children are drinking at earlier ages than ever before. Since 1975, Califano says, "The population of children who begin drinking in the eighth grade or earlier has jumped by almost a third, from 27 [percent] to 36 percent." By the time young people get to college, almost half of them—44 percent—engage in binge drinking.

Califano also points out that the alcohol industry, especially beer makers, benefit hugely from the sale of alcoholic beverages to the young. "Without underage drinkers," he says, "the alcohol industry . . . would suffer economic declines and dramatic loss of profits." The dangers of alcohol consumption by teenagers are clear: Drinking plays a major role in fatal auto accidents and drownings, and contributes to a host of other risky behaviors. Teenagers who drink are twice as likely to have sex with multiple partners, increasing the risk of HIV and other sexually transmitted diseases (STDs).

Drugs are not quite as widely used by teenagers as alcohol. Still, almost half of all high school students have tried marijuana, and one in four report that they are current users. Anyone who thinks that drug use among teenagers is mostly a problem among poor kids in the inner city could not be more wrong. Surveys in recent years have found that affluent suburban kids are more likely to use drugs than kids from urban areas.

In one study, researchers from Columbia University surveyed almost five hundred tenth-grade students in the Northeast, half from well-to-do suburbs and the other half from the low-income inner cities. They found that 59 percent of suburban boys admitted to having used an illegal drug at least once in the past year, compared to 33 percent of inner-city boys. Among girls, 46 percent of the suburbanites and 26 percent of the urban kids reported that they had used a drug.

Marijuana is still the most commonly used drug, and it's usually one of the first drugs that teenagers try. That hasn't changed much since I was a kid, but in other ways, the drug scene has gotten more complicated. Back then, a lot of kids were using marijuana, and a few kids were trying LSD and harder drugs such as cocaine and heroin. All those drugs are still around, of course, but there are also a seemingly endless number of new designer drugs popping up all the time, drugs like Ecstasy, GHB, crystal methamphetamine, ketamine (a.k.a. Special K), and Rohypnol (a.k.a. Roofies), to name a few.

Teens try alcohol and drugs for similar reasons: because their friends—or older, "cool" kids—are using them; because they want to feel more grown-up, more powerful, and more confident; because they want to escape from painful feelings of anxiety and depression. They may also see alcohol, drugs, and cigarettes as glamorous, and think that the girls or boys they'd like to "hook up" with will think that they're cool if they use them. Finally, they also use them—and there's no point denying this—because they're fun, at least at first. Kids usually drink or take drugs together, so there's a big social aspect. Parties and raves where drugs are used are exciting—there's music, dancing, camaraderie, sex.

The problem, of course, is the unintended consequences many young people underestimate: the dangerous side effects, the dependency or addiction, and the stupid things that people do when stoned or drunk. We need to let our children know about these risks and to help them think through ways to avoid them.

Helping Your Son Avoid the Drug and Alcohol Trap

"Could my son be drinking or using drugs?" This is the big question most parents of teenagers are forever trying to answer. It's a reasonable and appropriate question to ask, but if you haven't thought about this issue—and been talking about it with your kids—long before they started high school, you've waited too long. This is an issue that you simply can't ignore in the hope that it won't come up.

"From the start, from day one, communication is the key," says Joy Dryfoos. "You can't start early enough. You can't wait until they're thirteen or fourteen and think that the message is going to get across. You have to start talking to kids earlier."

A lot of parents never have these conversations because they don't know what to say. Others don't bring up the issue because they think their thoughts and opinions don't matter to their children. If that's what you think, you're probably wrong. The 2000 CASA study found that teens whose parents talk to them frequently about the dangers of using drugs are, in fact, less likely to use them—even when drugs are easily available at school. In the study, half of the teens who did not smoke marijuana credit their parents' influence as the main reason.

Don't spend a lot of time agonizing about saying the right thing or bringing the issue up in the right way. When your kids are young, around nine or ten, talk about drugs and alcohol can come up naturally. If you're watching a sporting event with your son, and the umpteenth beer commercial comes on, take the opportunity to mention that the goal of all these beer commercials is to get people, including young people, to drink, and that's really bad. If you know of, or hear about, someone who dies or gets hurt or encounters legal trouble as a result of drinking or taking drugs, bring it up in conversation.

As your son gets older, ask him his thoughts and feelings about drugs. Find out whether he knows other kids who are drinking or using drugs. Use any opportunity, any moment you can find to teach and express your feelings about the great risks people expose themselves to by drinking or using drugs. Before he enters those tricky early teen years, he should know what you think and where you stand. Many experts recommend you have a zero-tolerance policy for any use of drugs or alcohol other than, say, minimal drinking at family celebrations or holidays. If this policy feels right to you, announce it to your children and tell them what the consequences are if they violate this rule.

A Matter of Time

One of the biggest factors in how your child fares during his teen years will be how he—and you—spend time. Studies show very clearly that the biggest predictors of whether teens drink or do drugs is quality parental relationships and parental involvement, including supervising your son's time and activities. If your kid has little or nothing to do, especially in the hours after school, he's far more likely to spend it doing things that you'd rather he didn't. If, like most parents, you're working when he gets home from school, make sure that he has interesting and useful things to do, and that a caring, responsible adult is supervising his activities.

It's not only a question of how he spends his time, it's also a matter of how much time you and your partner spend with him. Finding a way to spend time with your children is one of the most basic—and important—things you can do. "It has to do with creating a sense of family and creating family opportunities to spend time together," says Joy Dryfoos. "Sometimes parents have to give up some of their free time to be with their children. They have to shape their lives around their children to protect them from a lot of evil influences—advertising, stuff on the Internet, peer influences, all those things in kids' lives that are hard to counteract."

But even parents with the best of intentions may not be able to do this whole job themselves. Some parents simply won't be able to spend the time they'd like to spend with their children. Others may feel at different points that they're not communicating or interacting with their kids in the way they think they should. Single mothers who are raising boys alone, and even some married mothers whose husbands are preoccupied with their jobs, may really benefit from recruiting an interested and responsible male for their boy to spend some time with.

"I think it's the most important intervention parents can make," says Dryfoos. "A lot of parents just feel very incompetent, especially as their kids hit those middle or later years. If the parent is having trouble communicating, then it's terribly important to find another [adult] that the kid can relate to." What can this person do? To Dryfoos, it's pretty simple: "Listen. Care. Do creative activities. Help them with their homework. Follow their interests. Take them to concerts. Enrich their lives in whatever ways are possible. But listening is as important as anything."

If you think your son might benefit from having another man in his life, give some thought as to who might fill that role. Maybe you have a brother or other family member who'd be interested, a trustworthy neighbor your son likes, a college student that you're friendly with. If you can't identify someone from your own constellation of friends and family, check out groups such as Big Brothers that train and supervise people to fill this role.

A MOTHER'S TOUCH

Boys surely benefit from having a responsible, caring man in their lives. But Dr. Lynn Ponton also argues that women—moms—can play a key role in helping teenage boys learn healthy ways of channeling and managing their need to take risks. One way is to participate with their sons in fun, challenging activities—healthy risks.

Many fathers do this: They go whitewater rafting, canoeing, rock climbing, or backpacking with their kids. In the process, they not only have fun with their children, they also stay involved in their lives in a way that allows them to have some influence over how their kids approach and evaluate risks. Too many mothers shy away from these activities, ceding the territory to their husbands and undercutting their own ability to influence the way their children approach challenges and risks.

Moms can also play a role in helping their sons reflect on and broaden the kinds of risks they take. "This is a culture that encourages risk taking, not risk assessment, particularly for boys," Dr. Ponton says. "And it does not encourage emotional or social risk for boys. So a lot of males don't take social and emotional risks and they're left dwarfed in that area, even though their physical development is quite extensive. We can encourage them to get involved in social activities, to do volunteer work. And we can say that doing this does not make our sons either gay or female-identified. It makes our sons full people."

When a mother spends time with her son and plays a big role in his life, it also helps to counter other negative influences such as tendencies toward violence or negative attitudes toward women. "I think mothers have an unbelievably important role in this area," Dr. Ponton says. "Moms who do this don't get a lot of support, but it's absolutely mandatory. If you don't do that, you raise really one-sided human beings." She adds, "The key to healthy risk taking is good communication. The great thing about teens is that they'll really listen if they don't think you're lecturing."

RESISTING THE NEGATIVE INFLUENCE OF PEER CULTURE

Parents help their sons deal with and avoid dangerous risk taking by recognizing the power of peer pressure and helping them develop strategies for dealing with it. Help them think ahead about how they would respond to a challenge to do something dumb. Have them rehearse a snappy comeback or answer so they're ready the next time another kid suggests they do something silly, violent, or dangerous.

Parents also should not be afraid to express their disapproval and to intervene if they think their son is engaging in dangerous or inappropriate activities. This may seem obvious, but many parents try to look the other way, hoping their child will work his way out of a situation on his own. "When you see them engage in risky behavior, you have to implement consequences," Dr. Ponton says. "You don't cut them off—no 'tough love' here where you cut them off entirely. But parents have to show their disapproval."

It's also important not to give up on kids or to assume that you can't help them through a tough patch because you have no influence until their hormones calm down. "I think a lot of parents don't understand that if a teen is engaged in dangerous risk taking it's not hormones and his brain that are making him do it," says Dr. Ponton. "It means that your child has poor risk-assessment skills and you have to work hard to help him learn. Teens are not as bad as we think, but we have to take the risks seriously."

Baruch Fischhoff, Ph.D., a psychologist at Carnegie Mellon University, agrees. "By the time kids get to middle adolescence, they really are pretty capable," Dr. Fischhoff says. "Kids have all these big decisions thrown at them. Intimacy and sexuality. Who you are going to hang with? What are you going to do about drugs and alcohol? How are you going to drive? Their error rate may not be any worse than ours, but they are making so many decisions that there are just more things that are going to go wrong. Don't give up. They are capable of making good choices."

BOYS, DEPRESSION, AND SUICIDE

In early 2001, then Surgeon General David Satcher issued a report on the mental health of America's children. According to the report: "The nation is facing a crisis in mental health for children and adolescents." Two years later, the signs of kids in trouble are everywhere.

- In New York City, the number of children admitted to the emergency room of Children's Hospital of New York–Presbyterian for psychiatric emergencies has increased dramatically in the last decade. "Psychiatric emergencies in children have reached epidemic proportions," says Meredith Sonnett, M.D., the hospital's associate director of pediatric emergency medicine.

- At Yale–New Haven Children's Hospital in Connecticut, the number of children in need of emergency mental health care jumped 60 percent from 1995 to 2001.

- Since 1980, the suicide rate among children aged ten to fourteen has doubled, while the rate among kids from fifteen to nineteen increased 14 percent. In 2001, 19 percent of high school students said they seriously considered taking their own life. And while girls are more likely to attempt suicide, boys are three to four times more likely to succeed in their suicide attempts. Gay and lesbian teenagers are more likely than straight kids to attempt suicide.

- Prescriptions of psychiatric medication for children and adolescents have exploded, even among preschool-aged children. Most of these medications are prescribed not by psychiatrists but by pediatricians, many of whom lack significant training in the diagnosis and management of childhood depression and other disorders. An even bigger problem is that many children never receive proper treatment mainly because their psychological problems go undiagnosed.

- Juvenile detention facilities are overflowing with children with mental health disorders. A recent study of Chicago detention centers found that about three quarters of the girls and two thirds of the boys had at least one psychiatric disorder.

What lies behind these grim statistics? Much of it has to do with the unrelenting pressure that today's generation of teenagers—dubbed Generation Stress by some observers—live with.

Some low-income and inner-city children cope with the stress of violence, crime, and poverty, not to mention disintegrating schools. Many live in neighborhoods and walk on streets where the drug trade is brisk, police presence heavy, and shootings routine. Many have fathers, cousins, or friends killed by violence or locked up in prison. For these kids, high levels of danger and stress are the background music of daily life.

Middle-class teenagers are under a different kind of stress: the pressure to perform and prove themselves to parents, college admissions directors, athletic coaches, and peers. Too many are "obsessed with an almost unattainable vision of perfection: the best school, the hottest clothes, the coolest music, the nicest body, the greatest friends," wrote reporter Andrew Julien in the introduction of his series on adolescent mental health problems published in the *Hartford Courant.*

Teenagers of all classes and races face this heightened pressure at a time when many parents find it all but impossible to provide the support and guidance children need. They're divorced. They're juggling two or three jobs, or working all day and into the night. The result is a generation of adolescents left increasingly to their own devices, of kids who face greater pressures with less support than any generation in modern American history. In many ways, boys are especially ill equipped to deal with all this stress because they have such a hard time admitting problems and asking for help. Instead, many take what has become a classic male path for dealing with anxiety and depression: They drink, take drugs, or they express the only emotion that's acceptable for a male—rage. "They lash out with behavior that can run the spectrum from increased irritability all the way up to physical violence," says Terrence Real, a Boston area family therapist specializing in male depression (see chapter 19 for a full interview with Real).

Real fought his own battle with depression, as he struggled for years with the legacy of his violent, abusive father (an experience he recounts in his book *I Don't Want to Talk About It: Overcoming the Secret Legacy of Male Depression*). He believes that although adolescent girls and women are two to four times as likely to be diagnosed with depression as their male peers, the disease may actually be just as common in teenage boys and adult men. The difference, he argues, is that boys and men are less frequently diagnosed and so go uncounted. Unfortunately, parents, teachers, and mental health professionals frequently miss depression in males because the symptoms are different than in women. Real calls it "the holy triad of covert depression"—self-medication, social isolation, and violence. "When men have pain, we try to fend it off and move into action," Real explains. "But we also move into forms of escape that fuel many of the problems we think of as typically male."

In recent years, Real and other like-minded psychologists who work with boys and men—such as Harvard's William Pollack, Ph.D., and Dan Kindlon, Ph.D., and school psychologist Michael Thompson, Ph.D.—have been making the case that men's emotional lives, and their ability to connect to others, are stunted early in life by their need to adhere to a strict male code of conduct. Dr. Pollack calls this the "Boy Code," Real calls it the "Stoic Code," but it all boils down to the same thing.

"Human beings are wired to be social and to be connected," Real says, yet the stoic code pushes boys to cut off from being close to others. "When we quote-unquote turn boys into men, we enforce disconnection. Boys are taught to disconnect from their mothers and from their own feelings. They're taught not to reveal themselves too much to other boys and girls. They're taught not to care that much about what other boys and girls are feeling. We call that learning to be independent.

"This is what the stoic code means. The very phrase 'suck it up' means 'don't feel it' and 'keep going,' and there's a lot of merit to that. The [police and firefighters] on 9/11 who were faithful to that traditional code gave their lives and very heroically. There are aspects of this that are great, but there are aspects that aren't—the equating of masculinity with numbness, with not feeling or caring, with ultra-toughness. For some boys, these traditional qualities are a fit and they slip very naturally into them. But for many, many boys, it's injurious. We basically toughen up our kids and beat the sensitivity out of them. And it hurts.

"The Catch-22 for boys is this: If they comply with this code, then they have to squelch vital aspects of who they are, and that's traumatic. On the other hand, if they don't comply, then they're going to be punished for it often. These things may be changing in your living room, but it ain't changing on the playground. There's a strong line between boyland and girlland, and woe unto the boy who crosses that line. The enforcing of this code through humiliation and ostracism and even physical abuse can be ferocious."

Most boys don't take the chance. They go underground with their feelings, retreating into what Drs. Thompson and Kindlon call their "fortress of solitude." For most adolescent boys, they point out in *Raising Cain*, "emotional isolation has become virtually a reflex." Indeed, this kind of silent withdrawal is a common sign of emotional distress in boys, and can start in the early teens. It's a sign that should not be ignored, since it may often signal future drug or alcohol use or risky sex.

Another disturbing part of the American experience may also shape the personalities and attitudes of some boys: A surprising number are sexually or physically abused. Three years before releasing its study on men's health (see page 10), the Commonwealth Fund conducted a national survey of boys and found that one in eight had been abused by the time they were in high school. For a boy (as well as, of course, for a girl), physical and sexual abuse is linked to many problems. Four in ten boys who were abused suffered from symptoms of depression; a shocking 15 percent said they wanted to kill themselves, and more than half said they had thought about it. Abused boys were twice as likely as boys who weren't to smoke, drink frequently, or use drugs.

These unhealthy habits aren't the only negative results of abuse. Nearly half of abused boys don't tell anyone about it, and only 7 percent told their doctors. These boys went underground with their feelings and withheld from both parents and doctors key information about their health. Thus begins a dangerous and potentially lifelong pattern of not dealing with or talking about their health.

Looking for the Signs

So how do you spot the signs of depression in boys? It's not easy. "Symptoms of depression in boys may be hard to read or be missed because the boys often don't look sad or depressed," Drs. Thompson and Kindlon write. "They look edgy or angry, hostile or defiant." Since males are almost expected to act in these ways, adults may not pay much attention to these kinds of actions or attitudes.

Still, there are some signs to look out for: persistent dark moods, falling grades, and withdrawal from friends. But these red flags aren't always there, or at least can't always be seen. With some boys, Drs. Thompson and Kindlon say, withdrawal "comes in the guise of anger, sarcasm, or hostility" as verbally adept but insecure boys deflect their own feelings of inferiority or isolation by putting down others.

"Boys use shields of various forms to keep others away: irritability, sarcasm, nonchalance, stoicism, and others," Drs. Thompson and Kindlon write. "Whether they use offensive intellectualism and humor or muscle and meanness, boys . . . seek to camouflage their fears with an exaggerated image of strength."

Depression in boys often looks different than it does in girls or adults. For that reason, Dr. Pollack, the Harvard psychologist who codirects the Center for Men at McLean Hospital and wrote the book *Real Boys,* put together a new list of the warning signs of depression in boys. Some match items included in standard lists of diagnostic symptoms, but many are different.

WARNING SIGNS OF DEPRESSION

- Increased withdrawal from relationships and problems in friendships.
- Depleted mood or increased impulsiveness.
- Irritability or an increase in intensity or frequency of angry outbursts.
- Increased risk taking, bravado, or acting out.
- New or renewed interest in alcohol or drugs.
- Discussion of death, dying, or suicide.
- Increased aggression.
- Concentration, sleep, or weight changes, or other unusual physical changes or symptoms.
- Low self-esteem, harsh self-criticism, or perfectionism.
- School or academic difficulties.
- Denial of pain, denying others' help, or inability to cry.
- Shift in sexual activity or interest level.
- Inappropriate silliness or "clowning."
- Obsessive overworking in school or in sports.

If you see one of more of these signs in your child, talk to your pediatrician and consider getting a referral to a mental health professional.

Suicide

Suicide is the third leading cause of death among those aged fifteen to twenty-four, after car accidents and homicide. In 2000, suicide took the lives of 29,350 Americans; people under the age of twenty-five accounted for 15 percent of those deaths, the vast majority—75 percent—of which are boys. Though suicide rates among teenagers have declined slightly in the last few years, the trend over the past twenty years has been straight up. Why do so many more boys commit suicide? It seems strange, especially when you consider that girls are at least as likely to be depressed, and are, according to most estimates, about twice as likely to attempt suicide as boys. And yet boys are far more "successful."

Part of the reason is that boys tend to act more impulsively and they're more likely to use guns. Girls tend to attempt suicide by swallowing pills, and that allows time for someone to find them and get them to a hospital. Most boys use quicker, more lethal methods such as shooting or hanging themselves.

A Mother's Ounce of Prevention

Terrence Real has a prescription to help prevent the painful emotional disconnection that so many boys experience, and it's aimed largely at the mothers of boys and teenagers.

"Mothers, do not think that you have to let go of connection and nurture to your boys or they're going to become sissies. Do not buy into this myth, which you'll hear all the time, including from mental health professionals, that only men can raise men. This is a dreadful myth that disempowers perhaps millions of single mothers, and it's absolute nonsense. This idea has led a lot of women to abandon their sons emotionally, often against their own instincts. Yes, it's nice for boys to have a positive male role model, but they'll live without it. The job of parenting remains and women *can* parent their sons. It's about nurture and guidance and limit setting. So hold on to these boys and hold on to their wholeness. Explicitly value these qualities that our society holds in contempt for men. And surround your boys as much as you can with other families who are like-minded."

Stay connected with your son and make sure you listen to him closely. Pay attention to what's going on in his life. Use your common sense. "A lot of times being a parent is not knowing and just taking your best shot," says Real. "This is not rocket science, these are not subtle processes. If your kid is in trouble, you'll begin to see it. He'll look like he's in trouble, or he'll feel like he's in trouble."

Could My Child Commit Suicide?

Who would ever expect that your child would take his own life? Predicting a child's suicide is very difficult, though in most cases, young people who take their own lives have offered clues or let someone else know that they were having suicidal thoughts before actually taking action.

As hard as it is to know your son's intentions and to prevent him from taking his life, there are signs you can watch out for. Here are some of them, according to the American Academy of Child and Adolescent Psychiatry:

Signs that adolescents may try to kill themselves:

- changes in eating and sleeping habits
- withdrawal from friends, family, and regular activities
- violent actions, rebellious behavior, or running away
- drug and alcohol use
- unusual neglect of personal appearance
- marked personality change
- persistent boredom, difficulty concentrating, or a decline in the quality of schoolwork
- frequent complaints about physical symptoms, often related to emotions, such as stomachaches, headaches, fatigue, etc.
- loss of interest in pleasurable activities
- not tolerating praise or rewards

A teenager who is planning to commit suicide may also:

- complain of being a bad person or feeling "rotten inside"
- give verbal hints with statements such as: "I won't be a problem for you much longer," "Nothing matters," "It's no use," and "I won't see you again"
- put his or her affairs in order, for example, give away favorite possessions, clean his or her room, throw away important belongings, etc.
- become suddenly cheerful after a period of depression
- have signs of psychosis (hallucinations or bizarre thoughts)

If you see some of these signs, DON'T IGNORE THEM. You've heard this before and it's true: Suicidal behavior is a cry for help. If you intervene in an effective way, you may be able to keep your child from taking such a drastic step. Here are some things you can do:

1. **Listen.** Give your son the chance to talk about his troubles and his feelings. You don't need to say much; the point is to show your love and concern and to help

him feel a little less alone with his pain. Be patient, sympathetic, accepting. Don't argue, express disbelief, or give advice.

2. **Ask directly:** "Are you thinking about suicide?" Don't worry that you might suggest the idea; the idea is already out there. Asking this question can show your son that you really care and take his feelings seriously. If he is having suicidal thoughts, find out how far his ideas have progressed: "How were you thinking about doing this?"

3. **Don't leave him alone.** If you think he really is suicidal, make sure you or another responsible person stays with him.

4. **Get help.** If your son tells you that he is actually thinking about suicide, or gives you the impression that he is by his words and actions, call your pediatrician or seek help from a mental health counselor. If you don't know whom to call, or feel the situation poses an immediate crisis, call your local suicide hotline. If you can't find the number quickly, call 1-800-999-9999 to get a number for a hotline or crisis center in your area.

5. **Stay engaged.** Even if the immediate crisis fades, stay tuned in to what's happening with your son and make sure he gets the help he needs. That means checking in with him regularly and finding a counselor or someone else he trusts with whom he can talk and share his feelings.

Source: Reprinted from AACAP Fact Sheet No. 10, "Teen Suicide." Reprinted with permission from American Academy of Child & Adolescent Psychiatry.

The Boot Camp Bandwagon: Too Much Tough Love?

Melanie Hudson had reached the breaking point with her fourteen-year-old son, Tony Haynes. The teen had rebelled against both his parents and stepparents, and had been caught shoplifting. When he learned of her plans to send him to a boot camp for troubled teens, he slashed the tires of his mother's car. Hudson sent him anyway—to a five-week program in the Arizona desert run by a Phoenix-based group called the America's Buffalo Soldiers Re-enactors Association.

Hudson thought the program was the answer to her son's troubles. The literature for the camp promised to take problem kids—those who use drugs, defy their parents, or get in trouble with school officials or the law—and subject them to a military-style program of physical endurance and discipline, returning them home well-adjusted and happy. Instead, Melanie Hudson's son was returned dead.

Boot camps and "wilderness therapy" programs have grown in popularity since the late 1980s and early 1990s. By some estimates, there are more than one hundred such programs across the country, with thousands of kids enrolled. Many, like the camp where Tony Haynes died, are privately run, but others are operated by state juvenile justice programs, with children committed by juvenile courts. Unfortunately, many camps are poorly regulated, dangerous, and staffed by counselors with little training. Nationwide, complaints abound of boot camp counselors physically abusing children, denying them food and water, and pushing kids beyond their physical limits, in rare instances, to the point of death.

According to media reports, Tony Haynes was forced to stand in 114-degree heat for some five hours without access to water as punishment for saying he wanted to go home. When he began to hallucinate, counselors left him alone in a bathtub, in an unsuccessful attempt to revive him. When emergency medical assistance was finally summoned more than two hours later, it was too late. Haynes died, according to the coroner's report, from "complications of near drowning and dehydration due to heat exposure." Charles F. Long III, the camp's director, has been charged with second-degree murder.

Haynes's story is only one of thirty deaths at boot and wilderness therapy camps over the past decade, says Representative George Miller of California, whose congressional committee investigated boot camps in 2001.

In some states—especially those where teens have died or otherwise been abused—officials have cracked down, requiring the programs to get licenses and follow specific health and safety standards. Enforcement is difficult to carry out, however, and many states still have no regulation at all.

Clearly, however, all boot camps are not the same, and most have not been connected to children's deaths. Some juveniles seem to benefit from such programs, especially if the camps have highly trained medical and psychological personnel on staff. The best programs strive to involve the parents and other family members in numerous sessions before, during, and after their child's therapy. They also allow children to communicate with their parents frequently.

Still, there is little evidence that boot camps are any more effective at reforming teenage behavior than traditional approaches. Most studies of state-sponsored boot camps have found that 64 percent to 75 percent of juveniles reoffend in the year or two following release. Researchers at the Koch Crime Institute, a Kansas criminal justice think tank, did an effectiveness study on court-affiliated boot camps in 1998 and found that "the recidivism rates for boot camps are not that much different from the recidivism rates of traditional juvenile settings."

The controversial nature of these camps, their lack of proven effectiveness, and, above all, the many documented cases of abuse and even death should make parents extremely wary of shipping kids off to these programs. If a camp's philosophy seems to be centered around "behavior modification" or "breaking down" your child's rebellious spirit, it's a red flag. Ask yourself if you trust these people to tear down your son and build him back up again. Youth advocates encourage parents to explore all other avenues before sending their kids off to one of these programs. If you decide to use a camp, says Deborah Vargas, of the Center on Juvenile and Criminal Justice, investigate it thoroughly. Ask lots of questions: Your child's life may be at stake.

Most of all, be wary of claims that sound too good to be true. "These programs promise parents who are at their wits' end a quick fix, but there is no quick fix," Vargas says. "If you think that a four-month program in the desert is the solution, you're fooling yourself."

HOW TO INVESTIGATE A BOOT/WILDERNESS CAMP

- Find out if the camp is licensed through a state agency. If so, call the agency and ask about the program's reputation. Find out if any complaints have been filed against it and, if so, what they involve.
- Ask what kind of medical professionals are on staff and if they're available twenty-four hours a day. Make sure the camp counselors who will be hiking and camping with your son have medical and first-aid training.
- Ask what kind of mental health professionals are on staff and what their degrees and licenses are. (Check with any institutions named to make sure degrees and licenses are valid.) How many hours a day are they available?
- Find out what the ratio of children to camp counselors is (three-to-one is considered good).
- Ask about the backgrounds of the counselors, if you can you see their résumés, and if the camp has done criminal background checks on them.
- Find out the average age of the children in the program and how most children end up there. Are they sent by the courts or by their parents? What kinds of children will your child be with?
- Get detailed accounts of what types of activities your son will participate in, where he'll sleep, and what he'll eat. Make sure adequate, healthy food and water are not withheld as punishment.

Red Flags
Do not send your child to a camp in which any of the following is true:

- Use of force and/or restraints is permitted.
- The camp is not licensed through a state agency.
- Children's letters home are censored.
- Children are not allowed to phone their parents, or their parents aren't allowed to phone them, at least once a week.
- Parents aren't allowed to visit the facility unannounced.

BOYS AT WORK

Your fifteen-year-old son comes to you and tells you the exciting news. He's been offered an after-school job at a local burger joint, a nearby convenience store, or perhaps at a full-service gas station. He's feeling proud, and he's already counting his money, figuring out how he's going to spend it. All he needs now is for you to agree and sign his work permit.

Few things give teenagers a greater sense of independence than a paying job. All of a sudden, they earn their own money, buy what they want, or save for a down payment on a car. Desires like these drive millions of teenagers to enter the work force: Two million teens work jobs during the school year, and three million find jobs during the summer, according to the U.S. Department of Labor.

For parents, this may be a moment of great pride. Your son is showing initiative and maturity—qualities we all want to see in our kids. But that doesn't mean you should agree. There are important things for you both to think about before he starts flipping burgers or selling Slurpees at the 7-Eleven: safety, school performance, and his exposure to alcohol and drugs.

The kinds of injuries that teen workers get vary greatly, from back injuries sustained loading trucks to being shot while working at a convenience store. Teenage workers are twice as likely as adults to be injured on the job. It happens each year to about 230,000 teenagers, according to the National Institute for Occupational Safety and Health (NIOSH), and some 77,000 teenagers are injured seriously enough that they need hospital emergency room treatment. At least seventy teenage workers are killed in workplace injuries each year, a number the Institute of Medicine described as a likely underestimate. Nearly 90 percent of those killed on the job are boys, according to government studies.

Why do so many teenagers get injured? Because they're young and inexperienced. Because they don't get enough training. Because they don't know their rights as employees. In too many workplaces, little attention is paid to health and safety issues. A 1996 study of 122 teenagers working in retail establishments in North Carolina found that only half had been trained to avoid injury and only 40 percent had been taught how to deal with a robbery. Yet one in seven teens works alone after dark.

Another big issue to consider is how a job will affect your son's education. Some studies have found that working a limited number of hours helps kids later in life, both in going to college and in future employment. But balancing homework, job, activities, and friends isn't easy. Neither is figuring out the right number of hours to work. Some studies have found that working more than twenty hours per week hurts academic performance, but many teachers feel that even twenty hours of work won't leave enough time for homework and other important activities.

In 1998, the blue-ribbon committee convened by the Institute of Medicine urged

Congress to empower the Labor Department to limit the hours that teens under eighteen can work to twenty hours per week. The report noted that kids who work long hours during the school year are more likely to do poorly academically and are less likely to go to college. They're also more likely to drink, smoke cigarettes, and use drugs, to get too little sleep, to get involved in delinquent behavior, and to drop out of school. Some kids may use work as an escape from school where they are not performing well.

If your son applies for or gets a job, find out exactly what he'll do. Make sure it's safe and that he's old enough to do it by checking with your state's department of labor. Get to know his supervisors and find out with whom he'll be working. Even after the paychecks roll in, keep tabs on how the job progresses.

FIVE JOBS TO AVOID

Every year, the National Consumers League lists the five worst jobs for teens. These are the jobs your teen should avoid. This can be found at *www.nclnet.org/childlabor/2003pr.html.*

1. Delivery and other driving including operating or riding on forklifts and other motorized equipment.
2. Working alone in cash-based businesses such as convenience stores, gasoline stations, and fast-food establishments.
3. Construction including work at heights and contact with electrical power.
4. Work at heights: on ladders or scaffolds.
5. Traveling youth crews: selling candy, magazine subscriptions, and other consumer goods on street corners, in strange neighborhoods, in distant cities, and across state lines.

Source: Reprinted from www.nclnet.org/childlabor/2003pr.html.

8

Boys and Sex

When my son was only three years old, he uttered the words that have become famous in my family. "I yike that yady," he said, as he stared at a suggestive photograph of Catherine Zeta-Jones in the fashion magazine I was browsing. That would not be the last time my toddler noticed a pretty woman. Another day, as our family walked on a Manhattan street, an attractive woman swished by. My son's eyes nearly popped out of his head. "Wow," he murmured, from his perch on my husband's shoulders.

Until recently I harbored some of the classic double-standard notions about boys and sex. Somehow I had it in my head that my husband would handle the "sex talk" with our son. I, on the other hand, would talk exclusively with our daughters, who were, after all, more in need of sex information since they need to be "protected" from randy boys. But my assumptions about boys and sex were wrong. The single most important thing you will do to ensure that your son has a healthy, well-adjusted attitude toward women and sex is to keep the lines of communication open and be prepared to discuss topics you may find uncomfortable. If you don't do this, you leave it up to him to sort through the pervasive and confusing messages he will receive about men and sex through the media.

Kids today are exposed to more sexual images and discussion than ever—on TV, over the Internet, in movies, on billboards, in magazines, and, yes, in my lingerie catalogue. Even animated movies aimed at the kiddie set (such as *The Little Mermaid* and *The Emperor's New Groove*) feature scantily clad princesses and mermaids with impossible hourglass figures and deep cleavage. According to a recent report by the American Academy of Pediatrics, U.S. teenagers view nearly 14,000 sexual scenes or references on television each year during the seventeen hours of TV they watch each week.

Small wonder that kids today have a knowing air and use sexual language at an age when many of us were clueless naifs. They talk of "sexing," dress like Britney Spears, and sing or rap along with lyrics that boast of sexual conquests. But for all their seeming sophistication and all the sexuality in our culture, many know little about sex and the risks, dangers, and heartaches that go along with it. In fact, the apparent precocity of kids today is deceiving. We may think they're more informed than they are. We may say to ourselves: "Why should I bother to sit down with my kid for a chat about sex? He probably knows more than I do."

The truth is that in this, the age of HIV/AIDS and other sexually transmitted diseases, kids have more need than ever for useful, accurate information about sex. Eighty percent to 90 percent of parents polled favor comprehensive sex education in schools, yet most kids are not getting a whole lot of information about sex at school. The problem is that school-based sex education programs, which have never been especially strong, are increasingly constrained by politics.

In recent years, the federal government awarded substantial amounts of funding for abstinence-only education. Schools that accept this federal money are required to teach children that "sexual activity outside of marriage is likely to have harmful psychological and physical effects." A number of states and school districts chose to advocate abstinence—teaching children to refrain from sex until they are married—and that may be the *only* thing your son learns about sex. Today, according to researchers at the Alan Guttmacher Institute, a think tank that studies reproductive health issues, 35 percent of schools teach abstinence as the sole acceptable way of preventing pregnancy and STDs. The use of condoms and other contraceptive methods to avoid pregnancy and disease are not discussed.

As a doctor trained in the science of medicine, I find this new strain of political correctness appalling and destructive. American children have sex, and they do it by the millions. By the time they finish high school, 61 percent of American high school students report having had sexual intercourse. Sexually transmitted diseases are epidemic here, at rates higher than in any other industrialized country in the world. How can we *not* teach children how to protect themselves?

Teenagers in Europe and Canada are no less likely than American teenagers to have sex, yet the rate of STDs is far lower, as is the rate of premarital pregnancy. Compare U.S. teenagers to teens in Sweden. Both have sex around the same time, on average, yet the pregnancy rate among American teens is more than three times that of Swedish teens. More young people (aged fifteen to twenty-four) are living with HIV/AIDS in the Americas (6 percent) than young people in Europe (2 percent). Why the gap? There may be other factors but one is clearly this: In those countries, teens get comprehensive sex education from the early grades onward.

Okay, I've said my piece. Fortunately, other men and women in medicine and science see how misguided these policies are. In 2000, the Institute for Medicine, a research and advisory body chartered by the federal government, reported that abstinence-only programs had "no evidence of effectiveness" and criticized the government's investment in them as "poor fiscal and public health policy." The Institute called on Congress to stop spending public funds on abstinence-only sex education.

In 2001, then–Surgeon General David Satcher released a report on sexual health. In it, he made this commonsense point: "Given that one half of adolescents in the United States are already sexually active—and at risk of unintended pregnancy and STD/HIV infection—it also seems clear that adolescents need accurate information about contraceptive methods so that they can reduce those risks."

Since schools are doing an increasingly poor job of meeting that challenge, it means that parents have their work cut out for them. We need to do a better job sharing our ideas and values about sex with our children starting from an early age. This is a job we as women may take the lead on, but it's also an issue both mothers and fathers should think about, talk about, and do something about. It should not be a subject that gets discussed only between mothers and their daughters or between fathers and sons, as is often the case.

Lynn Ponton, M.D., author of *The Romance of Risk: Why Teenagers Do the Things They Do,* writes, "It is still remarkable to me, even after fifteen years of practice working with teens and their parents discussing sex, how different the sexual standards for girls and boys continue to be. The idea that 'boys will be boys' and that they need sexual experience, sometimes characterized as 'good, clean fun,' is pervasive. If parents are not able to teach sons about responsible sexual behavior, then who is?"

One striking bit of evidence that teenagers strongly internalize this double standard can be seen in a recent study published in the journal *Pediatrics.* It found that girls between twelve and fourteen with high self-esteem were much more likely to remain virgins than those who ranked low on the self-esteem scale. Just the opposite was true with boys. Those with high self-esteem were more than twice as likely to have sex over the next two years. "Early sexual initiation in boys may be seen as a badge of honor that is celebrated within the peer culture," wrote the study's authors, a group of researchers from the University of Indiana.

The double standard operates on many levels and has far-reaching consequences. Adolescent males are given little information about sexuality and reproduction, and as adults, they are not expected to play much of a role in birth control and other reproductive issues. One third of both men and women say men feel "left out" of the decision-making process around birth control, and roughly two thirds believe men should "play more of a role" in the process of contraception, according to a survey by the Kaiser Family Foundation.

It is important for your son to understand that young men aged eighteen and older are legally required to take responsibility for their biological children, thanks to strengthened child support and paternity legislation. Depending on the circumstances, genetic tests may be conducted to identify biological fathers of children born out of wedlock, and a young man can be required to cooperate.

On a policy level, too, men are the neglected half of the sexual health equation.

There are few reproductive health programs designed to reach out and educate men. Agencies such as Planned Parenthood, so successful in providing women with low-cost, quality reproductive health information and services, have virtually no male staff members and almost no male clients. Federal funding through the Title X Program pays for 4.5 million visits a year to reproductive health service providers; only 2 percent of these visits are by men. Even researchers ignore men: In 2002, when the Alan Guttmacher Institute published its report *In Their Own Right,* it was the first comprehensive analysis of data on the sexual and reproductive health behavior of American men of all ages ever published.

In the long run, this double standard hurts everyone. It's bad for women because it forces them to do the thinking about birth control and to bear the expense. She's the one who could get pregnant, of course, and if she does, she'll be faced with a huge decision. But men pay a price, too: They can end up as unwitting fathers, whether or not they're ready to fulfill the role and responsibilities. If they choose not to be involved, they can live with the guilt and pain of that decision for the rest of their lives. Ignorance and passivity can also put both men and women at greater risk of contracting and passing STDs, including HIV.

So how do we change this double standard? How can we as mothers most comfortably talk with our boys about sex? And if we have husbands or partners, how should we work with them in the process? The most basic answer is we must create, in our homes and in relationships with our children, an atmosphere that allows them to ask questions and feel comfortable talking about sexual issues. As parents, we also need to communicate with each other, to discuss honestly any differences we may have. And we need to start creating this open environment early in our children's lives, educating and providing boys with information that has historically been elusive.

Will boys, adolescents, and young men be receptive? The Planned Parenthood affiliate in northern New England launched an effort in 2001 to reach out to young men from eighteen to twenty-four and help them get information and services. They held focus groups with men to figure out what kinds of information and services men need, and how best to couch their messages. They produced and ran public service ads on radio and TV. They set up a telephone hot line called the Man Phone to provide information and counseling to men and received fifty calls a month during the ad campaign.

The Planned Parenthood focus groups brought young men together to talk about sexual health issues in a way that most men never do. At the end of one two-hour session, recalls Planned Parenthood's Nancy Mosher, one young man asked if they could please get together again. "None of the men in the group had ever had the opportunity to discuss these issues in a safe environment before," she recalled. "And they were hungry for more."

TEACH YOUR CHILDREN WELL—AND START EARLY

"Mommy, where's your penis?" "Where did I come from?" "Why don't boys have vaginas?" These and dozens of other questions about sex can start coming from kids as young as three. And they will probably continue and intensify until your child is a teenager, and too embarrassed to talk to you about sex—at least if anyone else can hear.

Start early. Send your young children healthy messages about sex by answering their questions simply, matter-of-factly, and in a way that is age- and developmentally appropriate. Let them know that it's fine for them to ask and be curious. Do your best to avoid turning red in the face when your little angel asks you some question about penises and vaginas. Kids are very perceptive. If they sense you are awkward or uncomfortable talking about sex, they may conclude that sex is shameful or a bad thing they shouldn't talk about. Studies show kids who feel they can talk freely about sex with their parents are less likely to engage in risky sexual behavior in their teens.

Even before they start asking questions, you can do a little teaching by naming their genitals right along with other body parts. "This is your nose, these are your toes, this is your penis . . ." Be sure you use the correct names, although you might also want to tell him some of the popular slang words ("Some kids call it a wiener"). Some kids, of course, may make up their own words for fun.

One of the first questions young kids are likely to ask is "Where do babies come from?" You can give young children a simple answer about babies growing inside their mommy's bodies in a special place called the uterus. As they get older and ask for more details, describe how Mommy has eggs inside her body and Daddy has something called sperm inside his, and the sperm and the egg together can turn into a baby. In follow-up questions, you can describe a bit about the mechanics of intercourse. A general rule of thumb for young children is to answer only the question they ask but leave the door open for further queries.

There are some great books you can read and show to your children that help answer some of these questions. *Where Did I Come From?* by Peter Mayle, Arthur Robins, and Paul Walter has been a classic for the past twenty-five years, thanks to its straightforward text and amusing illustrations. *What's the Big Secret?* by Laurie Krasny and Marc Brown (he is the creator of Arthur) is another useful book, providing answers to all those questions that tend to leave parents blushing and stammering. I read Dr. Ruth Westheimer's book *Who Am I? Where Did I Come From?* to my kids, and they laughed hysterically! (See Resource section for more.)

Young boys are quite fond of their penises and since they sometimes walk around in their birthday suits, their penises are readily accessible. They will fondle them and stroke them—often absentmindedly—and even point them at you like a gun. Don't let this bother you. For little boys, and little girls, touching and manipulating their genitals is completely natural and normal. They are very curious, and they really make use of the scientific method. They touch, pull, and otherwise experiment in order to find out what will happen. If your son senses that you don't like this or are uncomfortable about it, or worse yet, if you embarrass or humiliate him for touching himself, he'll learn that his natural interest in his own body is shameful.

Reverend Debra Haffner, a sexuality educator and director of the Religious Institute on Sexual Morality, Justice and Healing, points out that many parents are uncomfortable when their children fondle their genitals because they equate this with adult masturbation. As she writes in her excellent book *From Diapers to Dating*, "Understand that infants are not 'masturbating' in the adult sense of the word; they are simply learning that it feels good to touch all the parts of their bodies." That goes for young children as well.

It is perfectly appropriate, however, to let your boy know that if he wants to touch, fondle, or display his penis, he should do it in his room or in another private place.

SEX PLAY

Kids of both sexes are not only interested in their own genitals, they are also curious about each other's. Haffner says it's very common for young kids to strip off their clothes and engage in sex play with each other. For the most part, she says, there's no need to worry about it. What do you do if you walk into your son's room and he and the girl next door are lying down together, naked, or examining each other's genitals?

"First take a breath; try to calm down," she writes. "Try hard, really hard, not to look at this through adult lenses. Your three-year-old is not having sex with the [child] next door! She is most likely curious about how his body is different than hers and vice versa. Start by saying, in as composed a voice as you can muster, 'Tell me what game you are playing.'"

Tell the kids that it's normal for them to be curious about each other's bodies. Then redirect them to some other play, being careful not to shame them. When you see the parent of the other child, let him or her know what happened and be clear that you don't think it's a big deal.

It's also completely natural for young kids to dress up in girls' clothes or try on makeup, so if your little boy starts putting on dresses or skirts, or asking you to apply some makeup, don't worry. Your child is experimenting, but it doesn't mean he's confused about his gender (see chapter 1).

NUDITY AROUND CHILDREN: WHEN TO STOP

When should moms stop appearing naked in front of their sons? I don't believe there's a right or wrong answer to this question; it's really a matter of personal comfort. But know this: You're not going to damage your son by letting him see your naked body. As Elyse Zorn Karlin noted in her book *Sons: A Mother's Manual*, "We should remember that human beings did not always wear clothes and that in many societies today, nudity is still acceptable. Any discomfort we may feel stems solely from our cultural upbringing."

I like the approach to nudity outlined by Australian authors Ronald and Juliette Goldman in their book on children's sexuality, *Show Me Yours*. They urge parents to relax and not worry about nakedness within the family during children's early years, especially at bath time or at the beach. This will help reinforce the idea that genitals and breasts are normal, functional parts of the body and nothing to be ashamed of. At some point, though, you'll need to socialize them to the fact that even children are expected to behave differently when they're in public or with people not in their immediate family. Explain to them that some people are uneasy with nakedness and that it's important to respect their feelings and desires for privacy.

SEX ED FOR PREADOLESCENTS

Kids in their preteen years tend to be curious and to have lots of questions about sex. As awkward as it may be for you to have these conversations, you really do want your son to be asking you these sorts of questions. For one thing, it means you have the kind of relationship that lets your children feel comfortable asking you questions—about sexual and other issues. You want them to know that you're available and open to their questions and concerns and that you respect their privacy and feelings. And believe me, it's better that they get information about sex from you than from their peers or from older teens.

Educate Before Puberty

There are some specific things that kids of this age should learn about. Boys should know what to expect before they enter puberty. If he knows what's coming, he won't be shocked or worried when he wakes up one morning with wet, sticky sheets. Boys should also learn about what's going on with girls' bodies—why they're sprouting breasts and starting to menstruate. You could engage in a little covert operation by going to the library or bookstore and picking out a good, attractive, illustrated book on sex. Leave it in your son's room, or somewhere else he'll find it. In a few days, you can ask him what he thinks or bring up something engaging from the book. If he hasn't read it yet, some interesting comments from you may pique his interest. (See Resources for a selection of books.)

Get Ready, the Bar Gets Higher

Of course, some of their questions may render you momentarily speechless. Don't be shocked when, sometime during grade school, your child asks you what a blowjob is or simply uses the term. Stay calm and be ready to give a simple, matter-of-fact description of oral sex. You can thank the media and Ken Starr, along with Bill Clinton, of course, for the fact that every kid in America was hearing these words a few years ago. You don't have to answer every question. My friend Susie's young son caught her off guard one day when he asked her what it felt like to come. Susie held it together long enough to tell her son to ask his father. It's completely appropriate to defer a question to a partner. It's also okay to admit your discomfort with questions and to say you don't have an answer right now but will revisit the issue when you do. However, you should not answer deeply personal questions about your own sexual practices.

Keep Dad in the Loop and on the Same Page

Ideally, moms and dads will both be involved in thinking about their children's sexuality and in talking about it with them. There's no reason for moms to avoid talking about sex with their sons. The key thing is that you and your husband work from the same page. Before you have any big talks with your children, I would encourage you to do some reading about sexuality education and to sit down with your partner and discuss your attitudes and approaches on the subject. "There are certain issues that I think are better for men to talk about with boys and for women to talk about with girls," says Reverend Haffner. "A dad's gonna have a hard time explaining menstrual cramps or how to insert a tampon. I think a mom's going to have a hard time having a discussion about what you do if you have an erection in class and how to handle that."

Avoid Mixed Messages

Without realizing it, many parents give children mixed messages. They save the big talks about sexual responsibility for their daughters but say little to their sons. Be an equal-opportunity parent, says Reverend Haffner, who also wrote *Beyond the Big Talk*, a book that belongs on your reading list. "I have a bias here. I think it is important to give boys and girls similar messages. But that does not happen very often. I can't tell you how many times I have had a father say to me, 'I worry much more about my girls than I do about my boys.' " Reverend Haffner points to one study that found that mother-son conversations about sex made the boys more likely to abstain from intercourse, while father-son conversations had the opposite effect. The researchers didn't ask the mothers and fathers about the content of these talks, Haffner says, but she suspects there was a "go-for-it, do-me-proud, son" message from many of the fathers.

There are plenty of other reasons for you to engage with your son about his developing sexuality, even if your partner is taking the lead in talking about sexual issues with him. A recent study by researchers at the University of Minnesota found that teenage boys who felt close to their mothers were less likely to have sex.

According to the researchers, parents' attitudes and opinions about sex matter a lot more to children than most people realize, but only if they know how their parents really feel. When teens felt that their mothers didn't want them to have sex, they were less likely to do so, the study found. Trouble is, a lot of kids don't get that message from their moms, even though most mothers think they send it. "Kids will pay attention to their parents' values and beliefs about sex," says Robert Blum, M.D., one of the authors of the study and director of the University of Minnesota's Center for Adolescent Health and Development. "But talk alone does not get the message through."

Adolescence into Teens

As puberty hits and hormones rage, boys transform dramatically. Almost overnight, muscles harden, voices thicken, and genitals mature and enlarge. For most boys, this time of chaotic change also causes another big shift: They start thinking about sex almost constantly, fantasizing, visualizing, obsessing. They hide out in their room. They stare at themselves in the mirror. They masturbate—a lot. For many boys these changes make them feel more awkward and nervous then ever.

Boys (and girls) at this stage become increasingly less likely to answer questions that parents have about their sex lives or to listen to your unsolicited opinions. At least that's how they act. Don't push your son to talk, but do keep letting him know that you (and, we hope, your partner) will talk with him anytime. With luck, this will sink in, and when you least expect it, he may bring up something. This often happens in the car, a place where people talk casually without making eye contact.

Dr. Lynn Ponton, a psychiatrist and adolescent specialist, says a lot of parents are deterred by their teenager's negative reaction when the topic of sex comes up. "Many parents don't know that adolescents want to have such conversations and are put off by the teens' initial protest . . . and, often, by their own embarrassment," Dr. Ponton writes. "Acknowledging this embarrassment is a good place to start the conversation. Most teens, relieved to hear that their parents aren't experts, will benefit from casual, nonjudgmental conversations on [a wide range of] subjects."

The little ruse I mentioned earlier about buying a good book on sex and leaving it in your child's room can work with teenagers too, even if you've done it before. Teenagers, of course, are ready for more sophisticated books now, and some books are more detailed than others. Picking one that is right for your son will depend on age and level of sophistication. (See Resources for a selection of books.)

For you I include the column below by sex educators and mothers Charlene Giametti and Margaret Sargarese, reprinted from the iVillage website.

TEN BASES TO COVER WHEN YOU TALK TO YOUR ADOLESCENT ABOUT SEX

1. Admit that sexuality is positive (perhaps the hardest thing to admit to a child on the brink of lust and love). If you cast sex as negative, as in "Don't do it!" then your child will simply tune you out.

2. Don't give boys short shrift. Broaching sexuality is easier with girls, because you can start with menstruation. With boys, talking about wet dreams and ejaculation is far more disquieting. It's hardly surprising, then, that surveys show girls get far more information about their bodies and sexual urges than boys.

3. Define sexual behavior as a romantic progression. Explain that sexual attraction begins with a smile and proceeds along a path from kissing to touching and on to intercourse. Remember first base (kissing), second base (petting above the waist), third base (petting below the waist)? Ask if kids still use this home-run lingo. A step-by-step approach ensures that a child can stop at any time. Make that point.

4. Girls and boys require different instructions. Take the issue of consent, for example. Girls need to learn to say no firmly looking a boy straight in the face. Sometimes girls look away or say nothing; this can be misinterpreted by a boy who continues making sexual advances. Boys need to be warned of the danger of assuming consent. He may be liable for charges of date rape or sexual abuse.

5. Listen carefully to your child's comments. Each generation has different sexual expressions and values. Think back to the '60s or '70s. Remember your parents' take on free love? Begin to learn today's lingo and norms. Then you know where to start.

6. Clarify the danger of oral sex. In today's culture, oral sex is considered casual and convenient. Raised in the shadow of AIDS, our children seize upon oral sex, thinking it's safe sex and, technically, doesn't undo virginity. Explain that any exchange of bodily fluid can result in STDs or HIV. Define abstinence.

7. Offer a checklist for sexual decision making. How does someone decide it's right to have sexual intercourse? Discuss typical reasons. Love. Boyfriend or girlfriend pressure. Pressure from peers. Lower inhibitions after drinking or using drugs. Here is where you inject your values—when and why one would take this step.

8. Link sex to emotional consequences. Sex is a physical drive but with emotional connections. Put sex in a loving context. Explain how it bonds people deeply. Once sex happens, people are more vulnerable. Broken hearts hurt more. Reputations get juicier. Regrets happen.

9. No parent gets off the hook. Mothers and fathers each bring important perspectives to sex talks. Boys need to hear from their fathers about what is appropriate and what's not. Only mothers can demystify women to their sons; only dads can explain men to their daughters.

10. Take advantage of all the help you can get. TV, movies, magazine articles, newspaper stories—all provide teachable moments. Use everyday opportunities to comment and listen to opinions from your young adolescent. The sex talk is an ongoing educational conversation.

Finally, remember, having sex is not a punishable offense.

Source: Rollercoaster Moms. Courtesy of iVillage.

MASTURBATION

With the coming of adolescence, your boy is going to discover the pleasures of masturbation. At the peak of puberty, testosterone is surging through the bloodstream of an adolescent boy many times a day, leaving him in an almost constant state of excitement with frequent erections. Under these circumstances, masturbating is completely natural and nothing to worry about. And it's certainly a much better form of sexual release than getting a girl pregnant.

Still, this can raise issues that are awkward to discuss, especially for mothers who feel uncomfortable and are uninformed about wet dreams and ejaculation. For that reason, this is an excellent topic for Dad or another important male in your son's life. If that's not practical or possible, or if you simply want to have the conversation yourself, by all means go ahead. One question that may come up if your son's a bit of a late bloomer is why he's *not* having wet dreams yet when all his friends are. Just let him know that everybody's different and assure him that he'll start ejaculating soon enough.

One place to start may be a matter-of-fact discussion of hygiene. Ask him to put any stained bedding he might have directly into the laundry; that way, there's no need for conversation about it or for him to feel embarrassed. (This is something many boys do feel embarrassed about—enough to hide their stained sheets and pillows in the closet or under the bed.)

In his book *Speaking of Boys,* Michael Thompson, Ph.D., offered an excellent suggestion that came from a mother he knew. She noticed her son was covertly changing his sheets all the time and putting the dirty ones in the laundry. That was fine, but she didn't want all that extra laundry. Her solution, according to Thompson, was "handing him a bundle of new tube socks with the advice that 'a man once told me that clean tube socks work great, and you just toss them in the wash. That way, you won't have to explain yourself to anyone, and it makes life easier for both of us.' "

Probably the only time that masturbation might be a problem is if a boy is spending inordinate amounts of time in his room or the bathroom alone. To Dr. Thompson, that could be a sign that a boy is depressed, anxious, or lonely. "Perhaps they masturbate 'too much,' " he writes, "but their problem is really that they are disconnected from people and the relationship they have with themselves is the only gratifying one in their lives."

Thompson also worries about boys and pornography—not about boys who sometimes look at pornographic images, as almost every boy does, but about socially isolated boys who become addicted. His definition of addiction: "when the consumption of pornography takes on a compulsive quality and crowds out other activities in life." If your son is spending a great deal of time online looking at pornography, or is spending money on phone sex lines, or buying access to Internet porn sites, that's a sign of loneliness and compulsive behavior. You need to set some limits. You may also need to get him some help.

HEALTH, SEX, THE INTERNET, AND YOUR TEENAGE SON

A surprising number of teenagers and young adults—68 percent—use the Internet to get health information, according to a survey of teenagers and young adults aged fifteen to twenty-four conducted in 2001 by the Kaiser Family Foundation. Four in ten of the online users look for health information once a month, and 44 percent have searched for information on sexual health, including pregnancy, birth control, AIDS, and STDs. Because today's youth are so wired into the Internet, it can be a great way for them to get health and sexual information they might otherwise be too embarrassed to ask for. That's the good news. The bad news is there's lots of bad information on the net, as well as lots of inappropriate sexual material, including of course, pornography.

The Kaiser survey found that while they're on the Internet, 70 percent of teenagers from fifteen to seventeen say they have accidentally come across pornography, and nearly half professed to be upset by it. We all know, of course, that many teenagers go to the Internet looking for pornographic sites. Is this something to worry about? Well, I don't think it's the greatest thing in the world, and when my kids are old enough to be scouring the Internet by themselves, I'll probably make use of filtering devices to keep them from accidentally or deliberately looking at violent or inappropriate material. But let's be honest: Teenage boys didn't start looking at pictures of naked women with the Internet. Boys have been obtaining—and hiding under their beds—copies of *Playboy* and other magazines for as long as they have been published.

If you catch your son looking at pornography on the Internet or in any other form, my advice is don't freak out. Take a deep breath, calm down, and think things through. Talk it over with your partner or your son's father and perhaps your pediatrician or another professional you trust. One key question to consider is the same one posed by Michael Thompson about masturbation: Is a teenage boy's use of pornography becoming obsessive or crowding out social interactions? An occasional peek is one thing; spending hours on porn sites and downloading or printing or creating porn is another. If these things happen, take the situation seriously and get some professional advice.

There are a number of things you can do to keep your kids from inappropriate sites on the Internet. Keep the computer in a family room and use filtering software. A good article that outlines some of the possibilities can be found—where else?—online. The article, "Kids and Teens on the Internet: What Parents Should Know," can be found on the website of the Family Education network at *www.familyeducation.com*.

THE CONDOM CONUNDRUM

Once your son is sexually mature, you're going to wonder whether he's sexually active, and you're probably not going to know the answer. So do you talk with him about condoms and how he can protect himself from getting HIV or other STDs? Or are you afraid that doing so will send a message that you approve of sex at such a young age?

This is a tough question, and your answer is driven by your own values and attitudes. You may feel strongly that your son should abstain from having sex until he's out of high school and married or is at least in a committed relationship. You may feel this way, but the odds are that's *not* the way it's going to happen. Remember this: In 2001, 41 percent of tenth graders had sex, as had at least 60 percent of high school seniors, according to surveys of young people conducted for the CDC.

There is some good news in the recent patterns of teenage sexual engagement. The number of teen pregnancies has declined since the early 1990s. In fact, the 2001 birthrate for U.S. teenagers was at the lowest level reported in two decades, down 26 percent from its peak in 1991. As a result, the number of babies born to teen mothers, and the number of abortions, has declined. Why is this happening?

Advocates of abstinence-only sex education programs like to take credit, attributing the lower rate to their newfound influence and prominence in schools. But a 1999 study by the Alan Guttmacher Institute shows that about 80 percent of the decline in teen pregnancies is because sexually experienced teens were taking precautions and using contraceptives more effectively; only 20 percent of the drop in the pregnancy rate was a result of a drop in the number of teens having sex.

Despite the conventional wisdom about the inherent irresponsibility of teenage boys, they are part of the changing landscape of teenage sexuality. "It used to be that we thought we couldn't do a thing with these young men. Boys would be boys," says Freya Sonenstein, Ph.D., director of the Population Studies Center of the Urban Institute, a Washington think tank. "And so the focus was totally on the young women. What the data has shown us is that actually over time, young men's behavior has changed quite radically."

From 1991 to 2001, the number of teenage males reporting that they'd had sex dropped from 57 percent to 49 percent. The boys having sex are also more likely to be wearing condoms. In 2001, according to the CDC, 65 percent of sexually active high school–aged males used condoms the last time they had sex, up from 61 percent in 1995.

STATISTICS TO THINK ABOUT

- Worldwide, 42 million people are living with HIV/AIDS, and each year 5 million people are infected with HIV—58 percent of the new infections worldwide are among people under the age of twenty-five. Though improvements in treatment have greatly reduced the U.S. death rate in recent years, AIDS is now the leading cause of death worldwide. And while the number of new cases is declining for most age groups, it is holding steady among the young. At least half of all new HIV infections in the United States are now among people under twenty-five, and most contract the disease through sex. Additionally, young men of color, as well as young men who have sex with men, continue to be disproportionately affected by HIV/AIDS.
- The United States has the highest rate of sexually transmitted disease among all industrialized countries. Each year, there are nearly 10 million new STD cases among people aged fifteen to twenty-four. By twenty-four, at least one in three sexually active people will have contracted an STD.
- Each year, approximately 1 million teenage girls in the United States become pregnant—10 percent of all females between fifteen and nineteen. Nearly 80 percent of these pregnancies are unplanned, yet about half of them lead to births. Most teen pregnancies—six in ten—occur among eighteen- to nineteen-year-olds.

HOOKING UP, RISKY BUSINESS

As encouraging as these gains are, some of the apparent progress may be deceiving. Some teenagers try to remain technical virgins by engaging in sexual activity that they don't have to call "sex." Lots of teens have oral sex—usually without protection—as if that's going to keep them from contracting HIV or other STDs. In fact, researchers say that oral sex has become a lot more popular among teenagers. In studies of teen attitudes about sex, anywhere from 40 percent to 60 percent of all teens and young adults say they don't consider oral sex to be sex, and between 20 percent and 25 percent say that anal sex isn't technically sex either.

"It's like an added base," was the way one teenage girl described oral sex to a reporter for *U.S. News and World Report.* "Like shortstop or something," added another girl, who said she talked to her housekeeper about sex because her parents wouldn't answer her questions. The girls, of course, use the "sex as baseball" analogy where a home run means vaginal intercourse.

Nearly one in ten boys had sex before age thirteen, according to the CDC, and those kids have a much greater risk of contracting an STD. And nearly one quarter of male high school seniors has already had four or more sexual partners.

Millions of teenagers also mix sex with alcohol or drugs, part of what young people today call "hooking up"—meeting somebody for a drink and then having casual sex. Nearly one quarter of sexually active teenagers and young adults under twenty-five—5.6 million in all—report they had unprotected sex because they were drinking or using drugs, according to a survey by the Kaiser Family Foundation. Nearly one third of the young people surveyed say they went further sexually than they planned because they'd been using alcohol or drugs. The survey also found that teens and young adults who use substances, especially teens who use multiple substances, are less likely to use condoms, and that people who use drugs and drink a lot are more likely to have multiple sex partners.

SEX AND MASCULINITY

One factor that can lead boys toward risky behavior is the attitude they develop about what it means "to be a man." Joe Pleck, Ph.D., a social psychologist at the University of Illinois, has studied young men's attitudes about masculinity. He says that some young men hold very traditional views. They admire physical toughness and absolute confidence, think that men should always get respect, are "bothered" by guys who act like girls, and think that men are always ready for sex. Young men who hold those views most strongly are much more likely to have sex at an early age, have many sex partners, and not use condoms. They're also more likely to admit they've tricked or forced women to have sex.

"If we raise our children to endorse beliefs about being tough and getting respect—which is traditionally the core of what it means to become a man—it leads young men to engage in behaviors that endanger their health, their future, and their partners and their children," says Dr. Sonenstein. "If we could change their [beliefs] we might be able to curb some of these risky behaviors."

For parents, dads especially, this means acting in the ways you want your son to act, letting him know that men don't always have to be tough, that it's okay to make mistakes and admit it, that being considerate toward others is as important as getting respect from them. It also means challenging these backward ideas in the culture and the media when they arise. If you're watching TV and see examples of men behaving badly, take the opportunity to challenge the notion that this is "the way men are."

STAND BY YOUR TEEN

As difficult as your son may be, and as much as he may sometimes irritate you, the teen years are a time when you need to put yourself in your son's shoes and understand how he feels. If you can, remember this period in your own life and how intense, awkward, and confused *you* felt at times. Let your son know you remember those feelings, and that you understand what he's going through. Also remember that most kids do great during the teen years and that many experts believe we have "overpathologized" this time of life.

Keep reminding him how much you love and respect him, and that you will continue to—even if he makes mistakes. Dealing with peer culture during these years can definitely be a challenge. Your son will be around other boys who will boast of their exploits, of whom they had sex with, and how great it was (or more likely, how great *they* were). Most of these stories aren't true, of course, but your son probably won't know that. Boys feel pressure to have sex and may get teased for being a virgin. A 2003 survey by the Kaiser Family Foundation backs this up. They found that boys face particular pressure to have sex, often from male friends. One in three boys age fifteen to seventeen said they felt pressure to have sex; only 23 percent of girls said the same. This is intense and painful stuff for a young man in the midst of great change.

Boys who are either early bloomers or late bloomers can have an especially tough time. It's easy to sympathize with the late-blooming boys, who often feel very insecure as they look up at full-breasted girls who tower over them or boys with pubic and facial hair who are already sexually mature. But boys who mature way early can also be quite vulnerable, and are more likely to have sexual experiences before they're psychologically ready. Dr. Lynn Ponton, author of *The Romance of Risk: Why Teenagers Do the Things They Do,* worked with a fourteen-year-old boy who was six feet three inches and looked like he was in his twenties. He often got come-ons from older teenage girls and even young women. He and other boys like him need help realizing that it's okay to admit they're not ready for sex and that they don't have to be ashamed about it. "We need to teach our boys that they can say no," says Debra Haffner. "That boys . . . and men are not ready for sex all the time."

You can bolster your son's self-confidence and help him rehearse what he might do if friends start goading him to take a girl in the other room at a party. But you should also make sure that he knows where to buy a condom and how to use one. If you think he's having sex, or that he might start, you might even want to buy him some yourself, letting him know that you're not advocating that he have sex. And, please, don't forget to remind him of his responsibilities if his sexual partner gets pregnant. If this should happen, you have a role to play, too: to help your son and his partner talk about the situation and try to deal with it logically. Show respect for the fact that the decision is going to be made by your son and his girlfriend. Then try to help them think through all the different issues they're going to have to face if they go ahead with the pregnancy—finances, health insurance, the young couple's education, and so on.

Can I Tell If My Son Will Grow Up to Be Gay?

Suppose your son likes to play with dolls and put on Mommy's high heels. Does that mean he is going to be gay? No doubt this very question has crossed the mind of just about every parent of a young boy. Almost as soon as kids play, parents subconsciously—and consciously in many cases—monitor *how* they play. Play is often about mimicking adult behavior, and what adults do is, to some extent, gender driven. Mommies do nurturing things like bake cakes and take care of babies; daddies do things like drive cars and work. That's the broad concept for the gender script that kids are supposed to stick to, give or take a little. It's true that girls are given more leeway to be tomboys and experiment with more types of play than little boys. When boys deviate from this they stick out like sore thumbs. We would all laugh at a little boy in high heels and a dress but take little notice of a girl wearing a police hat and carrying a toy billy club.

The rigidity of gender roles, especially for boys, is part of what is known as the "Boy Code" (see chapter 1). Boys who don't follow the code are in for it. Part of the definition of the "Boy Code" is to avoid acting feminine. At some point a boy who acts "girly" is likely to be criticized, ridiculed, teased, even physically abused or beaten up. Fathers, especially, can be pretty hard on boys who demonstrate feminine traits. "You throw like a girl!" How many times have you heard that? Young boys learn quickly that doing something "like a girl" is one of the worst insults. There is some tolerance when boys are very young, but as they get older, tolerance wanes. By the age of six or so, most boys adhere pretty rigidly to gender stereotypes, probably because they have learned to avoid behaviors that bring negative reactions from peers or adults.

Not long ago a family friend became deeply concerned about how her young son was playing. Dresses, dolls, and even wearing a ribbon in his hair like his older sister became the major focus of play. Sure, he had lots of "normal" boy interests—he even had a terrarium with a live frog. But nothing could beat the reaction he got when he pulled the girl routine. He would dress up, tell his mother he was a girl, and then laugh hysterically as if playing a joke. It would have been funny to his parents if he hadn't continued to wear the dress long after the joke was over. Soon his parents really began to worry. They spent a lot of time discussing it, trying to figure out what to do. They even sought counseling for the boy. His mother was convinced he was gay or a cross-dresser and that this was an early manifestation. Eventually her son confounded everyone when one day he simply dropped all interest in dresses and announced he was bored with being a girl.

The confusion and upset this boy's behavior caused mirrors perfectly how per-plexing the topic of sexual orientation and gender identity is for all of us. It also exposes the prevailing prejudices and phobias about homosexuality. Was my friend's boy just going through a phase? Would he grow up to be gay, a cross-dresser, or a transsexual? Frankly, I had no idea. It's a confusing world with lots of pressure to con-form to expected behaviors, even at a young age, and prejudice against those who don't is still very much a part of our cultural landscape. One thing is for sure: My friend's son understood completely that wearing girls' clothes was distressing to the adults around him.

Does young child's play really predict anything? If a three-year-old boy's preferred toy is a doll, can you draw broad conclusions about his future identity or sexual ori-entation? The short answer is no. Most boys—and girls, for that matter—experiment with different sorts of play, both feminine and masculine play. Parents should not assume that boys who show interest in dolls or dress up are going to turn out to be gay. Lots of boys will show interest in "girly" activities, such as painting their toenails (my son Harry liked this at one point) but will also show interest in other more tradi-tional boy activities. I, for one, am all for boys having a range of interests and partici-pating in play that involves nurturing or caring. I have heard the criticism that "feminists" want to turn boys into girls by encouraging them to play with dolls. Frankly, these worries are ridiculous. The vast majority of men I know get as a much satisfaction and gratification out of caring for those they love as do women. Teaching boys that they are as entitled to the good feelings of love and connection that come from nurturing is as much a right for them as it is for girls. My own sweet son is just as likely as one of my daughters to admire a cute baby or care for a "sick" toy, and I am happy he is comfortable with that. Do I think we should try to create a perfect gender-neutral environment in which to raise our children, trucks for girls, dolls for boys? Well, you can certainly try, but it will never work!

Ma Vie en Rose

Ludovic, a seven-year-old boy, is the subject of the film *Ma Vie en Rose (My Life in Pink)*, set in France. Ludovic's desire to be a girl and wear girls' clothes exposes the prejudices and phobias of the adults around him in a humorous, touching way. Is a child like Ludovic more likely to be gay? This is a good place to make distinctions. The first thing to understand is that there is a difference between sexual orientation and gender orientation/identity. Sexual orientation is defined as which sex a person is attracted to romantically or erotically. Homosexuals prefer the same sex and hetero-sexuals prefer mates of the opposite sex. Bisexuals are attracted to both.

Gender orientation or identity is different. Gender identity is how a person sees himself. One may see oneself as a female or a male regardless of genitalia. By the age of three, most kids can identify themselves as boys or girls. A few years later, they achieve what is known as gender constancy. In other words, they know their gender is fixed and will never change. In most cases children behave pretty much as we would expect; boys act like boys and express no doubt about their sex. Girls act like girls. But in some rare cases, a child may become uncomfortable with his sex and even with his genitals and wish he were the other sex. *Transgender* is the term used when a person dresses or behaves opposite to his or her biological sex. It is a general term used to describe all people who do not feel their anatomical sex matches their gender identity, and whose appearance and behaviors do not conform to the societal roles expected of their sex. This includes male-to-female transsexuals, female-to-male transsexuals, as well as cross-dressers, drag kings, and drag queens.

Transsexuals are people who feel they were born into the wrong body and experi-ence a great disturbance or disconnection with their given sex, a condition known as *gender dysphoria*. A transsexual sees the world from the perspective of the other sex. Thus, an anatomically male transsexual feels that she is a woman trapped in a man's body. Feelings of resentment for her own male sexual characteristics may develop. A transsexual wants to have the sexual organs of the opposite sex and may opt for sex-reassignment surgery or hormone treatment to alter genitalia and secondary sexual characteristics. According to Carole R. Beal, author of *Boys and Girls: The Develop-ment of Gender Roles,* this is rare, occurring in 1 out of 25,000 people.

What happens to effeminate boys when they grow up? Some research suggests boys who are more comfortable with feminine gender roles and exhibit effeminate behavior are more likely to grow up to be homosexual or even transsexual. But this is hardly a certainty. Many adult homosexual men report they knew very early they were gay and preferred feminine activities from the time they were toddlers. Others say they did not have feminine interests as children. Predicting from these early experiences is almost impossible. The most important thing for a boy who acts in ways deemed effeminate is to help him feel as comfortable and happy with himself as is possible. If a boy shows a strong preference for exclusively feminine play *and* either he or the family is distressed or uncomfortable about it, then it is good idea to seek professional help.

Nature or Nurture?

Between 2 percent and 10 percent of the male population is thought to be homosexual. Despite years of debate and many studies, nobody can really say for sure exactly why. Is it in the genes? Does it happen in utero? Is it caused by certain parenting styles? Nature—meaning that a person is born with it—or nurture—meaning caused by the environment—is the age-old question. While there is certainly no resolution to the nature-versus-nurture debate, there are a few new twists. Some even question whether we should be asking why at all. Edward Stein, law professor at the Benjamin N. Cardozo School of Law in New York, believes it shouldn't matter why people are homosexual and that seeking a cause will ultimately hurt gay people. In his book *The Mismeasure of Desire: The Science, Theory, and Ethics of Sexual Orientation*, he argues that genetic and biological research could lead to attempts to "cure" homosexuality or abort fetuses that are at risk for becoming homosexual. What's more, he says, most of the research that points to one cause or another is deeply flawed. Sexual orientation may be too complex to ever be successfully studied, and society should accept how people are, regardless of cause. On the other hand, some advocates say that identifying a biological basis for sexual orientation will be helpful for gays, since it may prove once and for all that homosexuality is not a choice people make but a biological imperative they cannot change. The debate is charged because there still exists a deep homophobia within society. Not until 1973 did the American Psychological Association declare homosexuality to be neither a mental disorder nor disease. Yet many continue to believe it is. For this reason almost any exploration into the causes of homosexuality is charged with controversy.

Nevertheless, some scientists continue looking for a biological basis for sexual orientation. To Simon LeVay, Ph.D., the former Harvard and Salk Institute neurobiologist who first measured the difference in the hypothalamuses of gay and straight men, this is one piece of evidence that homosexuality is a product of nature more than nurture. Dr. LeVay notes in an article that measurable differences have been found between the fingerprint patterns of gay and straight men, a trait clearly set during pregnancy and thought to be controlled by exposure to male hormones. Other studies have found that homosexuality runs in families. "If you are a man and you have a gay brother, your own chances of being gay are increased about fivefold," says Dr. LeVay. Still other studies have linked index finger length and left-handedness to homosexuality. Ten years ago researchers even claimed to have discovered a gay gene, a claim that other researchers have so far been unable to confirm.

Does that mean being gay is strictly genetic? Probably not. One piece of evidence is that among identical twin brothers, if one is gay, there is roughly a 50 percent chance the other will be too, according to one study. But that means that half the time, a gay twin will have a straight brother. This could be a result of "environmental" influences: The boys were somehow treated differently by their parents or had other different life experiences that shaped their preference in sex partners. Or it could be that they were exposed to different levels of testosterone in utero, even though they both shared the same uterine home. Pregnancies are full of random events, and there has been some very early research that seems to indicate that the womb environment is much more important than previously realized.

Female fetuses exposed to higher than normal levels of testosterone (a condition called *congenital adrenal hyperplasia*) tend to have enlarged clitorises and engage in a more rambunctious, physical style of play. So it's possible that male fetuses that get less testosterone in their embryonic bath may be more likely to be gay. Obviously, the whole question of what causes "male" and "female" behavior, or gay and straight sexual orientation, is complicated and controversial. To me, the most reasonable explanation is that all these factors—genes and hormones (nature), and direct, personal experiences in the world (nurture)—interact. Scientists will be arguing about these questions for a long time to come. Focusing on the "cause," however, is not what is important if we want to help our gay sons.

Sorting It All Out

One of the main tasks of adolescence and puberty is to understand and accept one's sexuality, including one's sexual orientation. Sorting out all the intricacies of romance, sex, attraction, crushes, and so on may take time for teens. It is not uncommon for many boys to go through a stage where they question their sexual orientation. Because all boys are constantly confronted with negative messages about gays, this can be a time of great distress for those truly on the fence about their sexuality. Many boys pass through a stage where they have a crush on another teen or on a rock star or some other popular figure of the same sex. It is perfectly normal for boys and girls to have crushes or feel attracted to or aroused by members of the same sex. Sometimes these feelings persist and sometimes they fade.

Some teens act on their feelings of attraction to the same sex, but that does not mean they will ultimately identify themselves as gay. By the age of nineteen, 17 percent of boys say they have had one homosexual experience. Though many of these boys later say they are homosexual or bisexual, half later identify themselves as heterosexuals, according to *Adolescent Medicine,* edited by Hoffman and Greydanus.

By the later teen years homosexual boys have probably spent much time ruminating about their sexual identity and have concluded they are gay. According to the American Academy of Child and Adolescent Psychiatry, research has shown that the development of a homosexual identity goes through several stages.

Stage 1: Feeling Different

Having social experiences in the middle teen years that made them feel different from other adolescents, such as a boy's sharing few interests with other boys.

Stage 2: Identity Confusion

Reaching physical maturity and realizing that they are attracted to members of the same sex, causing emotional turmoil and a questioning of their heterosexuality.

Stage 3: Identity Assumption

Moving from private acknowledgment of sexual preference to admitting it openly, if only to other homosexuals.

Stage 4: Identity Integration

Adopting homosexuality as a way of life, both emotionally and sexually.

Source: Adapted from Your Adolescent: Emotional, Behavioral, and Cognitive Development from Early Adolescence Through the Teen Years *by the American Academy of Child & Adolescent Psychiatry.*

Coming Out

Muskogee, Oklahoma, population 37,000, a typical American small town—religious and conservative—is home to Joyce and Calvin Rock. Their son Jimmy is anybody's idea of the perfect son: student council president and Presidential Scholar from the state of Oklahoma during high school, active in the local Baptist church, even voted most likely to succeed. "The all-American boy," says his mother. When Jimmy was nineteen years old, he came out to her. "I was shocked. He had hid it very well," she reflects now. "At first when your son tells you he's gay and you've grown up in the Bible Belt, you think, 'Oh my god, he's going to move to San Francisco and get AIDS.'"

For Joyce that reaction was momentary. She loved her son and wasn't about to abandon him, but she worried about her husband's reaction. When she finally told him, it was a turning point for the family. "It was a great moment for me because I never would have believed that men could love their children as much as women do. His first words were 'I have got to find Jimmy. I have said things that hurt him.'" The reaction from the community was not as smooth. "You really learn who your friends are," she says. The family left the Baptist church they had been so active in and no longer socialize with people who could not accept her son's sexual orientation. The upside, she says, is that the family is happier and more closely knit than ever before. Since that time in 1997 when her son first came out, Joyce has become a spokesperson for Parents, Families and Friends of Lesbians and Gays (PFLAG), heading up a chapter in Oklahoma helping other families with gay children.

Jimmy was lucky. Despite years of anguish, worrying about how those around him would act (he knew he was gay in middle school but did everything he could to hide it), when he finally came out, his family embraced him. Many boys get the opposite reaction. Families disown them, abandon them, or distance themselves from them. David Tseng, executive director of PFLAG and a former White House senior policy adviser, says when kids come out of the closet, many parents go in. "They are embarrassed. They don't want the stigma." To me this is one of the saddest things for a parent to do to a child. All kids need the acceptance and love of their parents. Gay children, because of the prejudice they will face from much of society, need it more. There are no statistics on the percentage of gay children turned away by their families because they are gay. But if it happens once, it is certainly too often.

Fathers often have a harder time acknowledging or admitting their son is gay. They are, therefore, unable to support and reach out to their gay sons. One of the best things a mother can do is help the boy's father understand that being angry or trying to change the son will not work and will only lead to isolation and loss for both father and son. Gay teens need acceptance and love from their parents at the critical time they begin to acknowledge they are gay. When they lose the support of the family, they are at a much higher risk for problems in school, substance abuse, running away from home, or suicide. When the family holds religious beliefs that say homosexuality is a sin or fundamentally wrong, it can be much harder for them to accept their gay child. If a parent is having internal conflicts that get in the way of communicating positively with his or her teen, I recommend he or she read *Always My Child: A Parents' Guide to Understanding Your Gay, Lesbian, Bisexual, Transgendered, or Questioning Son or Daughter*, by Kevin Jennings and Pat Shapiro. This excellent book helps parents to recognize their own feelings and provides psychological insights into teens going through the process of understanding their sexual orientation.

As a boy goes through the process of understanding his sexual identity, it can provoke extreme anxiety. Effeminate or openly gay teens face verbal and even physical abuse from their peers. One of the worst insults one kid can hurl at another is calling him a "fag." Homophobia makes it extremely difficult for a gay teen to become comfortable with his sexual orientation.

This is probably a good time to talk about the role every parent has in combating homophobia. For all our sons, gay and straight, we need to foster a strong sense of acceptance and tolerance for homosexual friends and peers. Boys often inflict great injury—emotional and physical—on other boys who appear to be or are gay. As mothers of sons we have a responsibility to help stop this terrible injustice by teaching our own sons it is wrong. Teasing, taunting, or physically harming another boy because he is effeminate or gay is unacceptable. There is some hope that the tide is turning toward tolerance. Media images of gays have done a lot to soften intolerance. In many large cities and in certain industries, people are far less uptight about sexual orientation than in the past. Greater acceptance may be one reason that the average age that teens come out has dropped from twenty years old in 1970 to thirteen in 1998, according to a study by Richard Savin-Williams from Cornell University.

If you suspect your son is gay or he has come out, you may be in denial and shock. Many parents say they went through a grieving period when they first learned that their son was gay, feeling loss for the daughter-in-law or the grandchild they would likely never have. Some parents are angry or feel guilty that somehow they did something to cause their son to be gay. Given the social stigma within our society these feelings are hardly surprising. Not only does the child feel devalued by stigma, the family does as well. But while parents work through their feelings, they must not forget to show love and support for their child. It takes courage to come out, and parents need to acknowledge that courage and help their child be as comfortable as possible with his or her identity.

Helping Your Gay Child Stay Healthy

Staying healthy and happy is the goal for gay teens. The first step, according to David Tseng, is to become educated about gay issues. PFLAG has a website, *www.pflag.org,* that tells you how to find chapters throughout the country that assist parents in dealing with and understanding the sexual orientation of their gay sons and daughters. Reading about gay issues and talking to other families and gay advocates can help you learn about the important issues in your child's life. Parents should understand the unique risks gay teens face and focus their efforts on their children's health.

One way to stay on top of how your child is doing is to be familiar with his peers and learn about the school environment, says Tseng. If he faces verbal or physical abuse, parents need to work to make the school environment as safe as possible. According to PFLAG, the average high school student hears twenty-five antigay slurs a day and 97 percent of high school students regularly hear homophobic remarks. This takes a serious toll on gay kids, making them more likely to skip classes, engage in high-risk behaviors (alcohol, drugs, unsafe sex), drop out of school, suffer from depression, or even commit suicide.

"Parents need to stay actively involved to prevent abuse of the child when they are not at home. Be active in the school and help educate teachers, other parents, and counselors," Tseng advises. PFLAG's safe school initiative, launched with their From Our House to the Schoolhouse program, was started in 2000 and is now supported in over 350 cities and towns nationwide. This initiative helps to sensitize school administrators, educators, and policy makers about issues affecting gay teens in the school systems. Parents should also help their gay teens identify straight allies who can have a role in creating a safe environment for their child.

Some gay teens may need counseling. They may benefit from a support group and the opportunity to clarify their feelings. Therapy may also help the teen adjust to personal, family, and school-related issues or conflicts. But stay away from therapy aimed at changing homosexual orientation. This can be harmful for a teen who is unwilling. It will no doubt add to his sense of confusion and anxiety by reinforcing negative thoughts and emotions the child may already be struggling with.

Help gay teens stay physically healthy by first recognizing what risks they face and making sure they have an open and honest relationship with a doctor sensitive to their needs. Regular comprehensive checkups with attention to sexually transmitted diseases including HIV are important. Half of the estimated 40,000 new HIV infections in the United States each year are among people under twenty-five—and young males who have sex with males are at particularly high risk for infection. In addition, depression, substance abuse, and suicide are all more likely to occur in gay teens. Parents of gay teens need to take any sign of depression (see chapter 7) very seriously. In one survey, about 30 percent of gay and bisexual high school students had attempted suicide in the last year. Why? Societal stigma, hatred, and isolation lead to very high stress levels. Finally, many gay male teens become preoccupied with their body image to the point that it becomes pathological, working out obsessively or taking steroids. To learn more about body image issues in males, check out chapter 6.

9

Boys and Sports

Few things are more important to many boys and have more influence over their attitudes and behaviors than sports and the culture that surrounds them. Sports give boys a healthy way to channel their intense physicality and feel strong in their bodies. Sports help boys develop a sense of confidence and the satisfaction of working as a team. But the main reason that kids like sports is much simpler: They're fun.

"I think that physical activity—being able to run and move and leap and hurl your body through time and space—is tremendously important for boys," says Don Sabo, Ph.D., a sports sociologist at D'Youville College in Buffalo and a former college football player. "Kids need to move. They need that release."

Kids also like the challenge of learning new skills and of engaging in competition. But the big thing is the fun, and when sports stop being fun for a lot of kids, they stop playing them. That's something parents need to keep in mind as they think about their child's future involvement in sports.

Sports are good for kids in many ways. They keep them active and fit and help them avoid the obesity trap. As teenagers, kids involved in sports are less likely to smoke cigarettes or use illegal drugs, and less likely to commit suicide. High school students who play sports also tend to get better grades and to do better on standardized tests. Today, more children than ever—nearly 40 million—are playing organized sports.

But as healthy and fun as sports are for many kids, there are plenty of problems. Today's kids are being pressed at absurdly young ages to get serious and specialize in one sport, instead of taking part in and enjoying many on a more casual basis. Because so many kids now play a single sport all year long, overuse injuries from performing the same movement repeatedly are rising dramatically. From every quarter, the pressure to compete, to be the best, gets more intense. For many boys, the macho risk-taking culture that surrounds competitive sports in high school and college leads them to ignore pain, to drink and binge on alcohol, and to act in sexist, disrespectful, and sometimes violent ways toward women and others.

These days, different trends in the world of athletics butt up against each other. At the same time that more young children are playing organized team sports, school-based recreation programs and physical education classes are being slashed, making it harder for kids to play for fun without seriously committing to a sport. As the pressure to compete and perform moves down the age ladder, increasing numbers of kids are dropping out of sports activities and complaining that it's just not fun. At a time when growing numbers of children are overweight and sedentary, that is truly unfortunate.

So how do parents—and especially us moms—help our boys to be involved in sports and have a good time doing it? How do we know they're ready to play a certain sport or to move into the realm of competition? And how do we help them stay healthy and happy doing it? For me, these are not easy questions. I love sports and always have. Growing up, I loved skiing, running, tennis, and swimming, and I still do these things when I get a chance. But I've never gotten into the competitive team sports that boys and men seem to love. Now, thanks to my son Harry, all that must change. Harry loves sports of all sorts, and I can already see how important they are going to be in his life. For his sake, I will learn about RBIs and what, exactly, clipping is. I'm learning about youth soccer and T-ball, trying to figure out how my husband and I can both stay involved in this process, and, most important, thinking about ways that our whole family can engage in physical activities that can help keep all of us fit.

Start 'em Young Having Fun

Kids have enormous physical energy. When they're young, we have a vested interest in helping them find good ways to use that energy without wrecking the house. Family hikes, bicycle rides, rock climbing, even jogging or running races down the street—doing these things together lets us get needed exercise and introduces kids at an early age to the pleasures of physical activity. It also does something else that experts say is important: It models for them our own love of being active.

It doesn't matter if your child has natural athletic talent or if you do. In fact, it's probably even more important for parents who *don't* consider themselves athletes to find activities to engage in with their children. Eric Small, M.D., a pediatric sports medicine specialist in New York, devoted one chapter in his book *Kids & Sports* to "the non-athlete." He points out that these kids, who often have unathletic parents, frequently have low self-esteem. They feel clumsy and uncoordinated, get teased for their shortcomings by other kids, and often get excluded or chosen last in pickup games.

No parent can protect a child from these sorts of put-downs and problems. But they can show kids that you don't have to be a great natural athlete to enjoy sports, physical activity, and the outdoors.

Sports for Preschoolers

The early years, from around two to five, should be a time for kids to experiment and explore different sports activities. They can kick soccer balls, shoot or dunk basketballs into low baskets, and start playing with bats and whiffle balls. Low-key gymnastics classes, where they can tumble and bounce and leap, are great for many kids. Swimming classes in which parents take part can help kids feel comfortable in the water. Don't get competitive. The goal in these years is to introduce different things, let them have fun, and see where their interests lie.

If you can, do these activities with your son. Don't worry if you're not very good at a sport. What matters is that you do it together and that your boy is having fun. If you enroll him in classes or organized sports activities, look for classes that are developmentally appropriate for a preschool-aged child. That means, according to a report on kids and sports from the American Academy of Pediatrics (AAP), "exercise sessions should be short and emphasize playfulness, experimentation and exploration of a wide variety of movement experiences." A reasonable format, the AAP says, combines fifteen to twenty minutes of structured activity with thirty minutes of free play.

Remember that kids in this age range have short attention spans, limited eye-hand coordination, and a hard time tracking moving objects such as balls or judging their speed.

Sports for School Kids

The early school years, from ages six to nine, bring big leaps in children's skill levels. Eye-hand coordination, motor skills, and balance all improve a lot, and kids get better at tracking objects and judging speeds. Kids can now get the satisfaction of whacking baseballs, sinking basketball shots, and dribbling the soccer ball down the field.

Kids of this age still don't have great attention spans and are often more interested in playing with their pals than focusing on the details and rules of a game. They tend to do best with flexible rules and lots of time for free play. As a parent, remember to keep your eyes on the real prize: You want your child to have fun and feel good about his body so he'll want sports and physical activity to be part of his life for years to come.

"For children and preadolescents . . . fun, success, variety, freedom, family participation, peer support, and enthusiastic leadership encourage and maintain participation," says the AAP report. "Failure, embarrassment, competition, boredom, regimentation, and injuries discourage subsequent participation."

Sports for Preteens and Teens

When kids hit their preadolescent years, around ten to twelve, their motor skills, vision, and tracking ability improve to near-adult levels. They now have a much greater ability to concentrate and focus. They can plan and remember strategies, so they can play complicated sports such as football and basketball.

At this age, team sports become a bit more competitive as kids' skills improve and coaches get more serious. Do your best to make sure kids still enjoy themselves. As you enroll them in classes or organized teams, look for teachers and coaches who know how to keep things fun and relatively noncompetitive. This is also an age when many kids begin to drop out of team sports and cut back on physical activity. That's a big reason why the Centers for Disease Control recently launched a national media campaign aimed at showing "tweens"—kids between nine and thirteen—that it's hip to be physically active.

When it comes to athletic activities, kids today have more options than ever, but they're also more limited in their ability to engage in the kind of after-school free play that many of us took for granted as kids. These days, parents don't want their children playing outside without supervision, and many kids don't want the main alternative—organized, competitive team sports.

The result, says Dr. Small, is that "today there are two populations, the kids who are heavily involved in sports and those who do nothing. Thirty years ago you played in your yard, pickup games, a seasonal sport. Now both parents work, and kids are not allowed to play in their backyard or on the street because it's not safe. So you have one segment of the population training year-round in a sport—basketball, baseball, soccer, et cetera. And then there are kids who do nothing in terms of sports or activity, they just watch TV or play computer games or [log on to] the Internet for five hours a day."

The traditional team sports that we grew up with still attract plenty of kids, especially young ones. These include baseball, basketball, football, and hockey, with soccer now added to the mix and surpassing many of the others. But while millions of children still play these sports, especially in their younger years, participation in most team sports is actually declining. Instead, kids are gravitating to in-line skating, skateboarding, snowboarding, and off-road mountain biking—the so-called extreme sports that have exploded in popularity in the past decade.

According to a survey conducted for the Sporting Goods Manufacturers Association, basketball and bike riding are the two most popular sports activities, enjoyed by around 11 million youth (aged six to seventeen) each. In-line skating, with nearly 8 million young participants, follows. Between 1990 and 1999, the popularity of in-line skating, or Rollerblading, grew by 600 percent.

As for team sports, another survey by Sportstime.com found that basketball and soccer were the most popular team sports among seven- to eleven-year-olds and they attracted more kids than in 1990. But as kids get older, many drop out of team sports. Among kids between twelve and seventeen, participation in every team sport declined between 1990 and 1999.

Experts say it's not only the growth of extreme sports that's causing a decline in team sports; it's also that kids are alienated by the pressure and emphasis on competition creeping into sports earlier than ever before. The result, says Dr. Small, is that 75 percent of kids quit organized sports by the time they're twelve. "The more you push at kids (in sports), the more they burn out and quit," he says.

Sadly, the middle school years, when the greatest number of kids drop out of organized sports, are "the most critical time in a child's life" for them to be physically active, says Marty Ewing, Ph.D., a sports psychologist at Michigan State University. This is the time, she says, when kids need the physical and psychological benefits of being physically active and involved with others as part of a team. Instead, it's a time when lots of kids quit sports and devote their time to armchair activities like watching TV, playing computer games, or surfing the Internet.

THE SPORTS PRESSURE COOKER

The increasing pressure on kids to play competitive sports comes from a number of sources. But some of the biggest culprits are parents. They enroll their two- and three-year-olds in private tennis and golf lessons. They schedule daily practice sessions for children of six and seven. They start their three-year-olds in soccer classes.

I don't think there's anything inherently wrong with young kids taking soccer lessons, depending on how the lessons are taught and how much the kids are pushed to participate. When Josh, the son of my cowriter, Rob Waters, was four, his parents signed him up for a soccer class with some of his pals at a neighborhood park. Josh would generally kick the ball when it was his turn, and he paid attention some of the time. But he spent a lot of time practicing his fantasy "battle moves" or strolling with his arm around a friend. Josh seemed to enjoy the class, but when it was time to sign up for the next one, his parents gave him the choice, and he decided not to go back. Last spring, he took a baseball class and then, in the winter, a basketball class at the local Y. Just before his seventh birthday, he started playing on his first Little League baseball team. For the most part, he's enjoyed them all, because there's little pressure and he gets to have fun while he learns the basic skills and rules.

The problem is that for many kids, the pressure and competition build, especially if parents believe their child has real talent and they fantasize about his or her athletic future. "I think a lot of parents project future success onto whatever athletic activity their kid is currently involved in," says Don Sabo. "If a kid becomes captain of his middle-school basketball team, they see this as an indicator that he's a future CEO. There's enough pressure on kids already without attaching all these adult expectations and baggage."

The kids with athletic talent, and whose parents have big aspirations for them, are often the ones who get pushed to practice the same sport every day. The trouble, Small says, is that "making kids concentrate [on one sport] often takes the fun out of it. How many kids are going to be professional athletes? Less than one tenth of one percent. There's one Tiger Woods for every generation. If you push them at a young age, they end up quitting."

Former child tennis star Andrea Jaeger was winning tournaments at fourteen and was ranked second in the world at fifteen in 1981. But she worries that young children may be pushed to specialize in sports too early. "How do you know a child at age two wants to play tennis?" she said recently to an Associated Press reporter. "It might be bringing out an enormous talent, but how do you know there isn't another one in there?" Jaeger quit professional tennis at twenty-one after a shoulder injury.

The pressure on kids only intensifies as they get older and join competitive teams. Many parents push hard on their kids, perhaps in the hope that their child's athletic skills will earn him or her an athletic scholarship to college. This pressure often comes from overinvolved dads, who prowl the sidelines at games, screaming at their children to run faster or berating the coach for not playing their child enough. Since my son, Harry, started at a youth soccer league, I've been shocked by how intense and serious some of these dads are. I can easily see how there might be a problem with "sideline rage," and I'm glad to hear that the National Youth Sports Safety Foundation has developed a "parent code of conduct" aimed at getting parents to act appropriately around their children's participation in sports. You can check out this code of conduct at the group's website, *www.nyssf.org*.

Fathers are much more likely to get carried away and criticize their sons in insulting, even cruel ways, says Harvard's Roberto Olivardia, Ph.D., coauthor of *The Adonis Complex*. "I think a lot of fathers are threatened that if their sons aren't doing well, it's somehow a poor reflection on them. They'll say, 'Don't be a wimp.' 'Hit the ball.' Or— and I've heard fathers say this many times at baseball games—'You throw like a girl.' And that is the most shaming thing that a boy can be told."

The pressure may also come from coaches who fall into the win-at-all-costs mentality, humiliating players who makes mistakes, benching players who aren't as skilled, and pushing their players to be tough and play through their pain and injury. Some high school coaches these days recruit star athletes from junior high schools and even entice them to move or transfer from other schools. Some parents and coaches agree to hold children back an extra year in junior high school so they'll be older and bigger when they join the high school team the next year, a controversial process called "redshirting."

"A coach can exert a tremendous amount of influence," says Sabo. "If a coach is a despot, it can turn positive potential into negative consequences. Some coaches will use gay-bashing or girl-bashing to motivate boys and I think that's really dangerous. A coach will tell a boy, 'Do you want to trade in your shoulder pads for a training bra?'"

Many kids internalize all this pressure and turn it on themselves. They push themselves to practice harder, lose more weight, add more muscle, run even faster. They spend hours at the gym, stare at themselves in every reflection, and take strength-boosting steroids and supplements. They'll show that coach who needs a training bra.

A Parent's Role: Not Just Cheerleader or Chauffeur

So how can you help your boy navigate this perilous terrain? First of all, stay as involved as you can with your boy's sporting life and do it in a positive and support-ive way. Encourage him to be active and physical doing healthy things he enjoys, and keep bike riding, hiking, skating, or doing other active things with him for as long as he's willing to do them with you. But be sure to follow his lead about the sports he wants to play and how much he wants to play them. Nagging and hectoring won't get kids to enjoy sports, even if it gets them to play.

"Let the kids dictate how much they want to play," says Dr. Small. "Some kids will always walk around with a baseball glove or a basketball. Those are the kids who love it. But if you're saying, 'Oh, did you practice your baseball today? Did you do your bas-ketball?' then you know they're not into it. You can't preprogram these kids."

This means that if your husband is pushing too hard on your son, you need to find a way to get him to ease up. It's important to be aware of the dreams and aspirations that you (and your husband) have for your boy—and to be sure you don't impose them on him. It's his life, not yours, and the dreams he chases should be his own.

If your son plays on a team, go to his games and cheer him on. But don't limit your role to being a cheerleader or chauffeur. Your son's physical education demands more active involvement than that.

"People tend to think about sport as a magic pill," says Don Sabo. "All you have to do is expose your kid to the magic pill and suddenly good things happen. Most par-ents understand that if they send their kids to school, they have to pay a lot of atten-tion to what's going on in the classroom and their relationships with teachers. Parents should follow the same kinds of guidelines when it comes to their kid's involvement with sports. It takes effective coaching to draw out the positive lessons in sports, to teach boys when they're endangering their bodies. Parents need to monitor that in order to ensure not just the physical safety of their kids but their healthy development."

Check Out That Coach

When you sign your son up for sports classes or team play, talk to the coaches about their philosophy and make sure that the emphasis is on having fun and devel-oping skills, rather than winning at all costs. Look for coaches who want to get all players into the games, rather than favoring the stars and letting the less-skilled players warm the bench. Make it your business to know something about the coach and to have a relationship with him.

"You ask questions, you find out what's going on, you go to practice, you try to observe," Dr. Sabo advises. "You don't have to show up at every practice and stand on the sideline and interrogate the coach. But you can listen to what kids say about coaches. You can pay attention to how coaches respond to injured players on the field."

Be prepared to intervene if the coach is putting too much pressure on your boy, or is creating an environment you consider to be physically or emotionally unhealthy.

SPORTS INJURIES

With more kids playing sports—and playing at younger and younger ages—it's no surprise that sports injuries among children are rising. Each year, according to the United States Consumer Product Safety Commission, more than 3.5 million children under fifteen are injured playing sports badly enough to require medical treatment. Many of the sports injuries that doctors see today were rarely seen in the past. According to the CDC, there are 775,000 children under age fifteen treated in hospital emergency rooms for sports injuries each year.

"Ten years ago, three quarters of the injuries in boys were acute injuries, an ankle injury, a knee injury, a shoulder dislocation," says Dr. Small. "Now, three quarters are what we call 'overuse injuries' caused by too much, too soon, too fast."

Overuse injuries damage the body muscles, ligaments, tendons, and bones—by stressing them beyond their capacity with repeated or prolonged movements. Children whose bodies are not fully grown are particularly vulnerable, especially if they practice intensively, play the same sport throughout the year, or suddenly increase their training regimen.

For example, many kids play baseball in the spring, summer, and fall for as many as seven or eight months a year. A pitcher who throws one game a week in the spring and two or three games a week in the summer can develop shoulder tendinitis as a result, Small says. A kid on the track team who runs ten miles a week for most of the year, then logs thirty to forty miles during one week at a running camp, could be headed for trouble. "These super specialty camps

SPORT	ANNUAL NUMBER OF INJURIES REQUIRING MEDICAL TREATMENT
Basketball	574,000
Football	448,200
Baseball	252,665
Soccer	227,100
Hockey	80,700
Gymnastics	75,000
Volleyball	50,100
Total	1,707,765

Source: Figures reprinted from the National Electronic Injury Surveillance System of the United States Consumer Product Safety Commission.

and training year-round have caused an epidemic of overuse injuries," says Dr. Small. One of his recent patients went to five one-week intense soccer camps and wound up with foot and shin stress fractures.

Of course, more traditional sports injuries—the concussions, fractures, joint dislocations, and contusions that have always been a part of sports—continue to plague thousands of kids as well. The risks in high-contact team sports such as football, hockey, and basketball are well known. But the new and fast-growing extreme sports are also major sources of injuries. Here's a rundown on the most popular youth sports, the types of injuries that tend to go with them, and what you can do to help protect your boys.

BASKETBALL

Of all the team sports, basketball ranks first in injury to children, according to the CPSC. Players most often sprain or strain their ankles, knees, lower back, hands, and wrists. Eye injuries, usually from being poked by a finger, are also common. Some players get hurt playing outdoors when they collide with the backboard post or trip on poor playing surfaces.

One key to avoiding injuries in basketball or any sport is warming up properly. Cold muscles are more prone to injury. Players should warm up for three to five minutes with something mildly active, such as jumping jacks or running, then gently stretch their muscles. The right shoes are also important. Basketball shoes should fit snugly, provide support, and have good nonskid soles. High-top shoes provide more ankle support. Knee and elbow pads can protect kids from cuts and bruises, and mouth guards can protect teeth, lips, cheeks, and tongue. Make sure that backboard supports and walls are padded and the playing surface is free of holes, rocks, or other hazards, and has good traction.

FOOTBALL

Many experts consider football the most dangerous of the popular team sports because it carries the greatest risk of serious injury. In 1999, six high school football players died from brain injuries suffered on the playing field, according to a study from the University of North Carolina. And from 1977 to 1992, according to *Epidemiology of Sports Injuries*, 127 high school football players suffered spinal injuries that left them with permanent damage. Another 25,200 high school football players suffer concussions every year, according to the American Association of Orthopedic Surgeons. Overall, according to the CDC, 170,000 children under fifteen and 139,000 fifteen- to nineteen-year-olds were treated in emergency rooms for football-related injuries between July 2000 and June 2001. Football players can get injured in any part of their body, but the joints of the knee, ankle, and shoulder are especially vulnerable.

Preventing football injuries is difficult, to be sure—unless you forbid your boy to play. Many parents do just that while their child is young, figuring they're not yet big and strong enough to play safely. Ironically, football is a much safer sport for younger kids, those under fourteen, because kids are not yet all that big and strong. But in high school, when kids gain size and strength, and begin to hit more aggressively, football becomes much more risky.

Don Sabo, who played Division 1 college football for the State University of New York at Buffalo, hoped his own teenage son wouldn't play high school football because of the risk for long-term orthopedic problems. "I highly dissuaded him," says Sabo, "but I didn't forbid him." Making a sport off-limits is liable to backfire and make him want to play it all the more, Sabo says.

If your son does play football, make sure he wears the proper protective equipment and learns how to tackle properly. The biggest no-no when tackling is "spearing"— leading with the head or neck—which can lead to concussions and serious head and neck injuries. Kids should also be trained to drink plenty of water and take frequent breaks, especially during hot weather, to avoid heat exhaustion. See page 249 for more on heat exhaustion.

Realistically, if your son plays football, injuries may go with the territory. If he does get hurt, your goal is to prevent a reinjury, and that means helping your son resist the macho push to get back on the field before he's completely healed. Concussions are particularly worrisome. People who sustain one are prone to further concussions for weeks afterward, and people who suffer repeated concussions have a high risk of neurological problems.

BASEBALL

People think of baseball as a safe, noncontact sport, and by and large it is. Still, there are many ways kids get hurt playing America's pastime. They get hit by a ball (or bat), get hurt sliding into a base, colliding with another player, or jamming a finger. Injuries are more common early in the season, when players are not yet in their best condition.

Probably the most dangerous part of the game is getting hit with the ball. The traditional hard baseball—the kind used by the pros and still used by most Little League teams—can cause serious injury, even death, when it strikes the head or chest traveling even at relatively slow speeds of 40 to 60 miles per hour. Fixed bases can injure players when they slide or trip over them. Fortunately, there are ways to reduce the number of injuries.

In a 2000 study, researchers from the University of North Carolina compared injury rates on Little League teams that use a new kind of safety baseball and those that use the traditional baseball. Though it looks and plays much like a regular baseball, the safety ball, known as a reduced-impact ball, has a core of polyurethane instead of cork. Teams that used the safety ball had a 29 percent lower rate of ball-related injuries. And the teams that used face guards to protect players when they were batting and running bases cut the risk of facial injuries by 35 percent.

Previous studies found that breakaway bases, which give way on impact, can also prevent injuries. And the Consumer Product Safety Commission estimates that as many as one third of the injuries to young baseball players requiring emergency room treatment could be avoided if safety balls, face guards, and safety bases were used in all youth leagues.

A different kind of injury common to youth baseball is sometimes called "Little League elbow," and it's one of the most common overuse injuries in youth sports. It happens when children, especially pitchers, stress their arms by throwing too many pitches or using poor throwing technique. "The elbow is particularly vulnerable to overuse injuries, which result from throwing too hard, too fast, too early," says Mary Lloyd Ireland, M.D., an orthopedist at Shriners' Hospital for Children in Lexington, Kentucky, and team physician for Eastern Kentucky University.

Young pitchers risk damaging their growth plates, areas at the end of a bone, near the joint, where growth occurs. This area of developing bone is not very strong, and stresses on the arm from pitching can chip off pieces of bone around the growth plate. This chipping can prevent the arm from growing normally and could end a young pitcher's career.

A 2002 study by researchers from the American Sports Medicine Institute found that Little League pitchers aged nine to fourteen sustained more shoulder and elbow injuries when they threw a lot of pitches in a game or when they threw curveballs or sliders. The authors recommend that pitchers under fourteen not throw curves or sliders, and that they operate with a strict pitch limit—no more than seventy-five per game and six hundred over the course of a season. To avoid needing to precisely count pitches, young pitchers could also be limited to fifteen batters in a game and one hundred twenty in a season, the authors suggest.

Little League Baseball has no formal policy on pitch counts, but it does limit pitchers to six innings per week. I think that's not good enough, and that the recommendations in the Institute's paper make good sense. Keep your boy from throwing too much, and keep in mind that if he's a pitcher, he probably shouldn't play catcher or shortstop on the days he's not on the mound. Those positions also require lots of throwing and can add to the strain on his arm. Be sure, too, that he doesn't throw breaking balls until he's around fourteen, when those growth plates usually close. How do you know when it's okay? If a boy has facial hair, he can probably handle throwing a curveball, says Glenn Fleisig, a biomedical researcher at the University of Alabama who coauthored the Institute study. Remember this, and try to get it across to your boy: The glory of mastering a curveball early cannot compensate for going through life with an injured elbow. Kids need their joints, brains, and bodies to work well for the rest of their years.

In addition to monitoring the pitch counts of young pitchers, coaches or parents should encourage them to condition and strengthen their rotator cuffs and other shoulder-stabilizing muscles. Pitchers should gradually increase the amount and intensity of their throws to give their arms a chance to adapt to the stresses of throwing. Have a physical therapist or athletic trainer show a specific program to the young pitcher. If a pitcher feels pain in his arm or shoulder, he should leave the game immediately and avoid pitching altogether when the arm is sore.

IN-LINE SKATING

In the thirty years since it burst on the scene, in-line skating, or Rollerblading, has become enormously popular among children, teenagers, and young adults. Even some middle-aged types do it, often with their kids. It's exciting, fast-paced, fun, and relatively safe. Around 7.5 million children under seventeen go in-line skating at least twenty-five times a year, according to the Sporting Goods Manufacturers Association. Because most people skate on hard surfaces—usually streets and sidewalks—there are plenty of sprains and fractures. Despite potentially treacherous conditions such as potholes, many injuries are preventable. In one recent study, nearly half of all in-line skating injuries happened to skaters who were novices or skated infrequently. Nearly half the injured skaters wore no protective equipment at all. When asked why they don't wear pads and other protection, many people said they found them uncomfortable and unnecessary, plus they didn't like the way they looked.

In the study, about 40 percent of all injuries were fractures, and most were to the wrist, elbow, and forearm. And note this: thirty-two skaters fractured an arm, and only three were wearing a wrist guard. The wrist is the most commonly injured site, and two thirds of wrist injuries are fractures, according to the *New England Journal of Medicine*. According to an American Academy of Pediatrics statement in 1998, wearing wrist guards can reduce the number of wrist injuries by 87 percent, and wearing elbow pads can cut elbow injures by 82 percent.

To protect your kids, make sure they wear a helmet, wrist guard, and knee and elbow pads. The type of skate should be appropriate for a child's level of skill and experience. Three- or four-wheeled skates should be used by new, less experienced skaters; the high-performance, five-wheeled variety should be used only by skaters with plenty of experience.

SKATEBOARD AND SCOOTER INJURIES

As kids move away from team sports, they spend more time doing their own thing—and lots of it on skateboards and scooters. Around 4.5 million kids under seventeen ride scooters, and more than 3 million cruise on skateboards at least once a week, according to the Sporting Goods Manufacturers Association. These fast-paced action rides are pretty safe, with an injury rate less than half that of football or basketball. Still, the rate of injury to young skateboarders, at least, seems to be rising, especially among males, who make up about 76 percent of skateboard riders and 87 percent of those who get injured.

In 1999, according to the Consumer Product Safety Commission, 51,000 skateboarders under twenty were injured. During the first eight months of 2000, when lightweight scooters suddenly rocketed onto the scene, 10,000 scooter riders were injured, the CPSC says.

The thing that's troubling about skateboard injuries is that they are rising much faster than the number of kids who ride them. Between 1993 and 1998, the injury rate more than doubled. And as with in-line skating, many of the injuries could be prevented, if riders wore protective gear.

The American Academy of Pediatrics recommends a few safety rules for scooter and skateboard riders. Here are the most important:

- Kids under eight should not ride scooters without adult supervision, and kids under ten shouldn't ride skateboards unsupervised.

- Scooter and skateboard riders should both wear helmets, wrist guards, elbow pads, and knee pads.

- Parents should not allow kids to ride them on streets, in traffic, or at night.

SOCCER

Everyone who has kids has noticed the trend: Soccer has become the fastest-growing team sport in America, played by millions of boys and girls—some 3 million on organized teams, not to mention unofficial leagues.

Soccer is a great sport. It gives kids an aerobic workout, builds strength and endurance, and is safer than many team sports. But it also can cause injuries, including the usual variety of sprains, strains, bruises, and fractures. There's a fair amount of contact between players, who can get injured bumping or tripping each other as they vie for control of the ball.

Another danger is concussion, a problem that has drawn a lot of attention from sports medicine researchers in recent years. A concussion is a brain injury caused by a blow to the head. At the moment of impact, the concussion causes a huge increase in pressure within the skull, lasting for a few thousandths of a second. It may or may not cause a loss of consciousness, but by definition it always causes some alteration of mental function. Concussions are usually rated on a scale of I to III, with a grade I concussion producing dizziness and headache, and a grade III concussion causing loss of memory (amnesia) and a brief loss of consciousness. There's little likelihood of long-term brain damage from a single concussion, but repeated concussions, from activities such as boxing or football, can cause lasting mental problems. Newer research suggests that amnesia—not loss of consciousness—may be the main indicator of concussion severity and the best predictor of future cognitive problems.

There are a number of ways soccer players get concussions: hard contact with another player, with the ground, or with the goalpost. A series of reports in recent years has also raised concerns that the technique known as heading—in which players steer a kicked soccer ball by allowing it to hit their heads—may also cause concussions.

Studies of professional soccer players have found that many, if not most, suffered concussions during their careers. As a group, the studies have found, soccer players are more likely than others to suffer from headaches, neck pain, and neurological problems. One study found mild to severe deficits in attention, concentration, and memory in 81 percent of a group of former Norwegian soccer players.

However, a University of North Carolina researcher says there's really nothing to worry about. Donald Kirkendall, Ph.D., research assistant professor of orthopedics, reviewed over fifty studies dating back to 1943 on heading, head injury, and cognitive function. He concludes that heading poses little risk because players spread the impact of the ball over their whole body by tensing their neck muscles. "Purposeful heading of a ball is not something parents should be concerned about," he says.

To be safe, though, the American Youth Soccer Organization advises parents and coaches to keep children under ten from heading the ball and not to teach the technique to older children until they are ready and interested. When heading is taught, the group suggests using a soft Nerf ball or beach ball to prevent injuries. To limit the extent of cumulative impact, AYSO also recommends that heading drills with older children be infrequent.

OTHER CAUSES OF CONCUSSIONS

Soccer is not the only sport where players risk a concussion. In fact, kids who box, play football, or wrestle are far more likely to have a concussion, and perhaps more than one. According to the American Academy of Orthopedic Surgeons, nearly one third of all concussions that occur each year in the United States are suffered while playing football, and 20 percent of those happen to high school players.

Boxing is even more dangerous, but fortunately, far fewer young people engage in this sport. My advice to any parent whose child wants to box is simple: Don't let him. Boxing is simply too dangerous, and your child and his brain are simply too precious.

If your child plays other contact sports such as football, hockey, basketball, soccer, or rugby, he runs the risk of a concussion. The most important thing to understand about concussions is that there are big risks of further injury. The most extreme risk, known as second-impact syndrome, is quite rare but is believed to have caused the deaths of boxers and hockey players. It happens when a person returns to play before the symptoms of an earlier concussion have passed, then sustains another head impact, causing massive brain swelling.

Even after a person has recovered from a concussion, he or she has a risk of further concussions that may be as much as four times greater than someone who's never had one. Repeated concussion may cause cumulative neurological damage, eroding a person's cognitive capacity.

After years of discussing the threat posed by concussions, a group of sports medicine experts from medical groups including the American Orthopaedic Society for Sports Medicine and the American Academy of Pediatrics came up with a series of recommendations on how to deal with players who have suffered a concussion. Their suggestions, published in the *American Journal of Sports Medicine*, included these:

- Every athlete who sustains a concussion should be evaluated by a doctor.
- A player who loses consciousness should not return to play that day.
- A player should not return to play if he or she has any symptoms that last longer than fifteen minutes or that come on after a period of delay.
- If a player's mental or physical status takes a turn for the worse after the initial trauma of concussion, he should be taken promptly to the nearest emergency room that can provide neurological services.

IT'S TOO DARN HOT

Playing sports for many hours in high temperatures can suck the moisture out of a body, causing dehydration and a number of other problems. The biggest concern is heatstroke, which occurs when the body is unable to cool down and regulate temperature. Heatstroke can send body temperature shooting up to 106F or higher in the course of ten or fifteen minutes.

Unfortunately, deaths and injuries due to heat-related problems are not uncommon among professional, college, and high school football players practicing in heat while wearing heavy pads and equipment. In fact, until the mid-1980s, deaths occurred at a rate of four to five a year. Active efforts to keep players supplied with water improved the situation, according to a recent report by Julian Bailes, M.D., chair of neurosurgery at West Virginia University and a consultant to the National Football League Players Association. But in recent years, the number of deaths has climbed again. Largely, Dr. Bailes suggests, because of increasing use by athletes of nutritional supplements such as ephedra and creatine, which can cause body temperatures to spike. According to Dr. Bailes, four football players died from heatstroke each year in 1995, 1998, 2000, and 2001.

High heat causes other problems as well. An overheated body cramps and suffers muscle spasms in the stomach, arms, and legs, especially in people who sweat a lot, depleting the body of salt. High heat can also cause players to become confused and clumsy, leading to strains and fractures. And before a person ever gets to the severe stage of heatstroke, he usually passes through a phase known as heat exhaustion, which can produce a fast but weak pulse rate and fast, shallow breathing.

Children and, to a lesser degree, adolescents, are especially vulnerable to the stress of high heat. Compared to adults, children's skin makes up a greater proportion of their body mass, making them more vulnerable to rapid heat gain and loss. They also sweat less than adults, which makes it harder for them to rid their body of extra heat.

To protect young athletes from the dangers of heat-related problems, a few precautions can go a long way.

- On hot, humid days, young athletes should not exercise strenuously for more than about fifteen minutes without taking a break.

- Take it easy and get used to the heat. In warm weather, children's bodies need time to acclimatize to the heat, especially if it's also humid. Recent guidelines from the AAP suggest that when a person starts an exercise program (including sports practice) or moves to a warm climate, he should start off slowly and gradually increase the amount of workout time over a period of ten to fourteen days.

- All athletes, and especially young ones, need to have plenty to drink. Children frequently don't remember to drink enough, and they may not realize that they need to drink even more when they exercise in the heat. They should drink before starting to exercise, then drink periodically during the course of the game or exercise session. A good benchmark is five ounces of water or a sports drink like Gatorade every twenty minutes for a child weighing 88 pounds and nine ounces for an adolescent weighing 132 pounds. Sports drinks are better than water for kids who are running and exercising intensely for long periods for two reasons: They taste good, so kids want to drink them, and they contain important electrolytes—potassium, magnesium, calcium, and sodium—which help provide energy.

ORTHOPEDIC PROBLEMS
Slipped Capital Femoral Epiphysis

Few people can pronounce this disorder, much less know what it is, but it's a common hip problem among kids from eleven to sixteen, especially those who play sports or are overweight. It can cause serious problems if it isn't dealt with quickly.

It happens when the end of the thigh bone—the *epiphysis*—slips out of place, usually during an adolescent growth spurt. Boys are more likely to get this than girls, and African-Americans are more likely to get it than Caucasians.

The pain can be sudden, or build over time, usually in the knee or thigh. It may feel like stiffness in the hip and may get better with rest. But after a while, it usually turns into a limp that makes it too painful to play sports or even to stand. It may also cause problems such as the child being unable to turn the hip inward, having a foot that turns outward, and/or one leg noticeably shorter.

Most children with SCFE will be able to walk, although they may need crutches. Those with a form called unstable SCFE can't walk even with crutches and are in very intense pain.

If your son develops these symptoms, get him checked promptly. He may need surgery. Usually pins are inserted into the hips to stabilize the joint and help the growth plate close properly. The sooner the problem is treated, the better the chances for a full recovery. If you delay treatment, arthritis and even permanent deformity may result.

Osgood-Schlatter Disease

More boys than girls get this problem, which causes pain, swelling, and tenderness just below the knee bone. Despite its name, it's really not a disease at all but an overuse injury that strikes kids who do a lot of running, dancing, or jumping. The repetitive stress of all this activity causes inflammation and pain where the tendon meets the knee.

Osgood-Schlatter is most likely to hit boys during those adolescent growth spurts, between ten and fifteen. In many kids, the pain comes and goes, triggered by athletic activity.

If your child has these pains, see a doctor. He probably won't need to stop playing sports altogether, but he may have to slow down for a while until the pain eases. A doctor may advise taking a break from sports and running for a few weeks or months.

If your son is in pain, use the RICE approach to ease it:

> **R**est the knee from the painful activity.
> **I**ce the affected area three times a day for twenty minutes.
> **C**ompress the painful area with an elastic bandage.
> **E**levate the leg.

Usually, time and home treatment, along with pain relievers, take care of the problem. In some cases, your child may need to wear braces to reduce the pressure on the tendons and quadricep muscles around the knee. The pain rarely lasts beyond puberty—when a child stops growing, so does the pain.

GET A PHYSICAL

Before a child starts taking part in any team sport, especially one that involves contact, he or she should have a complete sports physical, which should be repeated each year (see chapter 5 for more on sports physicals).

PROTECT THE FAMILY JEWELS

Boys who play a contact sport should wear an athletic supporter and a cup. Cups and supporters both need to fit right, and the hard cup is a lot more protective than the soft kind. Unfortunately, getting your boy to wear this protection may not be easy, and you may be quite embarrassed to even have this conversation. Do it anyway (or get your son's father to). If you think talking about this with your son is embarrassing, wait until you go to buy them. To get you in the mood, here's a fun story that was posted on an Internet site:

A mother was complaining about having to go to the store to buy an athletic cup for her seven-year-old son, who was just starting in a soccer league. At the store, the salesman asked her what size of an athletic cup she needed. She shrugged and held her thumb and index finger about an inch apart. "He's about this big," she said. "No, ma'am," said the man behind the counter. "What is his *waist* size?"

Most young men are woefully unaware about why wearing a cup is a good idea. A study in the late 1990s of about five thousand football players from Ohio high schools found that only 21 percent wore them regularly and 55 percent never wore them at all. Yet one third of the athletes surveyed had experienced at least one testicular injury.

Why do so few male athletes wear a cup? There is no shortage of reasons, of course. They're uncomfortable, they irritate the groin, and they interfere with running, boys will say. If your son makes these arguments, says that wearing a cup is for sissies, or claims they're too uncomfortable, remind him of how uncomfortable he'd be if he took a cleat or a baseball to the groin. And tell him that, according to urologists, one of the big causes of infertility in adult men is a genital injury in their youth. Perhaps this will help do the trick.

Finally, if your son is playing a noncontact sport such as tennis or track, a cup and supporter aren't necessary, but it would really be wise if he wore briefs instead of boxers. I know how much teenage boys these days like to "sag" their pants so that their boxers show. But he should remember this too: Briefs don't offer a whole lot of support or protection, but boxers offer none. Hanging loose is not always a good thing.

THE RIGHT GEAR FOR THE RIGHT SPORT

Experts estimate that half of all sports injuries are preventable. One of the best ways to prevent them is by making sure your boy is wearing the right gear for the right sport. The following is an excellent rundown on sports gear that we've reprinted from *Pediatrics for Parents* magazine. Other sports tips for parents are available at the website of the American Academy of Pediatrics at *www.aap.org*. Just type "sports shorts" into the site's search engine and you'll see a list of articles on sports safety and preparedness.

In-Line Skating

Gear Helmet, elbow pads and kneepads, wrist guards.

Safety Stop Kids should skate only in designated areas and only on smooth terrain. Since 1992, at least thirty-seven children aged fourteen and under have died from in-line skating injuries. The majority of injuries and deaths were from collisions with motor vehicles.

Bicycling

Gear A snug-fitting helmet, the right size bike, a light, and reflective tape if they must bike at night. To size a bike, have the child sit on the seat with his hands on the handlebars. The balls of his feet should touch the ground.

Safety Stop Kids should ride in bike lanes and paths free from potholes and debris. Insist children under ten stick to sidewalks and paths, since the skills for judging speed and distance in the street are not yet developed.

Soccer

Gear Shin guards, rubber cleats.

Safety Stop Scan the field for holes and debris. Secure goalposts. Try a synthetic nonabsorbent ball. The regular type can become waterlogged in wet grass and make heading the ball dangerous.

Baseball/Softball

Gear Batting helmets with face mask, rubber cleats, full protective gear for catchers, an athletic cup for boys.

Equipment Check Inspect the diamond and outfield for debris. Encourage your league to use breakaway bases. These bases, which detach when a player slides into them, can prevent many ankle and knee injuries.

Basketball

Gear Shoes with ankle support, shatterproof eye protection for children who wear eyeglasses (this is true for any sport, not just basketball), elbow pads, mouth guard.

Equipment Check Anchor the goalpost securely to the ground, and make sure the netting won't disengage from the hoop. Check that the rim is out of reach—dental injuries can occur when a player's teeth snag on the net while hanging from the rim.

Football

Gear Helmet with face mask, mouth guard with keeper strap, full upper and lower body pads, athletic cup for boys, rubber cleats.

Equipment Check Make sure helmets meet requirements of the National Operating Committee on Standards for Athletic Equipment (NOCSAE). Kids must be matched in leagues by similar skill level, weight, and physical maturity.

What Else Can Parents Do?

- Make sure kids are properly supervised.
- Stress the importance of protective gear during practice.
- Encourage rest breaks.
- Offer lots of fluids.
- Discourage kids from "playing through an injury."
- Be sure the coach has an emergency plan that includes parents' numbers and doctor and hospital preferences.

Source: Jennifer Nelson. Reprinted with permission.

FINAL THOUGHTS

Mother to Son: Ten Tips for Talking to Your Boy About His Health

Mothers play a huge role in helping shape boys' attitudes towards their bodies and their health. They do it through the examples they set and the way they talk to their boys about health care issues. Richard Heyman, Ed.D, is the author of the new book *How to Say It to Boys*. He says moms can help their sons learn to listen to and respect their bodies by encouraging them to talk about what bothers them. Here are his suggestions for ways of talking to boys of all ages about matters of health.

1. **Know your son—his temperament and his reactions.** Then use your knowledge to adjust the way you talk about health. How does he react to illnesses or injuries? Is he timid or aggressive? Keep these things in mind as you talk to him. If he's very timid, be calm and take care not to alarm him. If he downplays things or doesn't want to talk about problems, be aware of that and don't let him off the hook.

2. **Encourage him to talk about health and hurts.** "Young boys under the age of five are quite open to talking about what's wrong with them and eager to show where they got hurt," Heyman says. But sometime after that, things often start to shift, as boys pick up the male pattern of not talking about health or hurts. "Boys, like men, don't like to talk about their injuries or their illnesses," he says. "And when they do, they claim they're not afraid. But I think they are. I think boys probably need more comforting about illness or injury than girls and women do, even though they won't admit it."

3. **Be there for your son—physically and emotionally.** At the age of two-and-a-half, Heyman had a cancer that required his left eye to be removed. "I remember being separated from my parents," he says. "And I remember being terrified. Boys need their parents there all the time—in the hospital or any kind of doctor's visit. And I think this goes right through adolescence."

4. **Make health care routine. And be a good role model.** Going to the doctor should be a regular occasion, not something that's done only in a crisis. One way to do that is by fostering your son's relationship with his doctor. "Start with the very first visit, making sure there's a good relationship between the physician and the child," Heyman says. The best way to be a role model, he says, is to "give that child all the good examples I can of the way I look after my own health. I'd want my boy to know that I go to the doctor for regular checkups."

5. **When problems arise, explain them clearly and without alarm.** "Talk to him in a positive way: 'This is what's going to happen.' But don't explain what's going to happen in a way that's going to frighten them. I would lie to a young child rather than tell them the truth if it was really something serious. I don't think children

at a young age can handle that. Your job as a mother is to give care, comfort and security so that the child knows you're always for them."

6. **Use positive, not negative examples.** The idea is not to scare your child into paying attention to his health. "Avoid saying things like, 'If you don't do this, this is what's going to happen.'" Instead, use positive examples that show the value of taking care of oneself and that encourage healthy behaviors.

7. **Don't make dramas.** "Kids really pick up on your moods. They pick up on how you say things, your tone of voice, your facial expressions, your body language. And the younger they are, the better they are at picking up on that. Don't overreact and make things bigger than they are. If they tell you about an injury and you go off the deep end and say, 'Oh my God, let's go to the hospital right away,' I think that's going to put them off telling you about a problem in the future."

   In other words, if you get excited or upset when a boy comes to you with a problem or an injury, he will stop coming to you with problems. If you overreact, he learns not to tell you anything.

8. **Don't be overprotective.** "Many parents are afraid their boys are going to hurt themselves. Well, boys do hurt themselves. They're going to get into situations that are relatively dangerous. You just want to make sure that the risk of injury is not extreme. With young boys, you've just got to let them do (adventurous) things."

9. **Get him to talk by being indirect.** Draw your son out with a story. "If you suspect that your boy is having anxieties or something like that, you might just make up a story and say, 'Hey, you know, when I was your age, I had da-da, da-da, da-da.'" Heyman suggests. "And you talk about something that may or may not be true. And then you say, 'Do you ever feel like that?'" What you *don't* want to do, says Heyman, is "to go straight ahead and say, 'All right, tell me. There's something wrong with you and I want to know what it is.'" That strategy simply doesn't work.

10. **Don't deny substance abuse or mental health problems in the family.** If your husband or another member of your family has a drinking or drug problem, or suffers from depression or another form of mental illness, you need to acknowledge that Daddy or Uncle Joe has a problem. "Kids always learn what men are like from watching other men," Heyman says. "If their father sets a bad example, if he smokes, if he drinks too much, if he's popping pills all the time, if he has anxiety attacks, I think the mother's job is to try to explain these things to the child. Don't deny them. Don't ignore them. Put it into a context the boy can understand. And counteract the example by providing a good example yourself. And point to other male role models who are doing the right thing."

PART TWO

Husbands, Partners, Lovers

10

Husbands, Partners, Lovers

INTRODUCTION

I'm a doctor, so when I got married and had kids, I naturally expected that I'd be pretty involved in important health decisions for our family. And what that meant, I figured, is that I'd take the kids to the pediatrician, make sure they got their shots at the right times, and be ready to diagnose them and take care of them when they got sick. What I didn't realize is that I'd end up in the role of first medical officer in charge of family health, and that the position includes managing the health care of my husband as well as my children. It's a position with a pretty broad job description and lots of responsibilities.

In our family, it means I think about what's healthy not only for me and the kids, but for my husband as well. I encourage him to see the doctor regularly (I even make the appointments myself sometimes). I remind him to follow up on the doctor's advice. I fill out all the paperwork for the family's medical insurance.

Do I do all this because I'm a doctor? No, I do it because I'm a woman and my husband doesn't always take very good care of his health. If you're a woman and you have a man in your life, you naturally care about his health and well-being. You love him. You want him to be happy. And you'd like to see him live long and prosper. For all these reasons, you're involved in looking out for his health. And this is likely true whether you've been married for fifty years or two. (By the way, when I use the term "husband" or "wife" in this chapter, I'm referring to all couples who share their lives and worry about each other's health, married or not.)

In many families, the woman monitors the health of everyone, including her partner. If he seems to be hurting or moving more slowly than usual, she sees it. If he hasn't seen a doctor in a long time, she notices that, too, and pushes him to go or simply makes the appointment. She buys the family's food and manages the family diet. And in many families, she also selects and deals with the family's health insurance. Having medical training is not the number-one qualification for this job, being a woman is. Dr. Mom doesn't have to be an M.D.

Most women don't even realize the influence they have over their family's health, and how much time and effort they put into it. Unfortunately, this work—like many things we do—is often quite invisible, unnoticed by our children, our husbands, and often even ourselves. This must change. Managing a family's health care is a profoundly important job that needs to be seen and acknowledged. And, yes, we ought to get some credit for doing it.

In the long run, we'd like to work our way out of this job, or at least hand off more of the responsibility. In the short run, we want our husbands to be healthier. One of the ways of making progress toward both of these goals is to shine more light on this issue, and to help men learn to pay more attention to their bodies and their health. We need to help them realize they're really not invulnerable. We need to remind them that healthwise, they're the weaker sex (even if we don't use that term). We must help them see that being strong and responsible means taking care of their health instead of ignoring it. And that part of being a good father is setting a good example for our sons.

After all, one of the main ways our boys learn to be men is by watching and emulating their fathers. So ask your husband a question. First, explain to him that right now men die, on average, six years younger than women and from a whole range of preventable illnesses. Is this a status quo that he's willing to accept, not only for himself but for his son? Is it okay with him if his son grows up to be as unaware of his health as he is?

If we want to help him take better care of himself and set a better example for our sons, we need to know more ourselves. When we become more familiar with men's health needs and with the major threats that they face, we do two things.

First, we may literally save our partner's life. "Wives saves lives," as the saying goes. Ask physicians who work with men and they will tell you about the men they've treated who came in only because they were pushed to do so by a woman. You may see or notice something before he does. You may urge him to get help for a nagging problem that turns out to be a big deal. You may even save him with your own hands by giving him CPR if his heart stops beating. (Rescues like this happen more often than you might think.)

Second, we can pass on our knowledge. We can talk to him about the things we learn. We can leave articles around for him to read about issues he needs to be aware of. The more you know, the more you can teach—and the more he can do for himself.

This is a story with two characters. It's a story of the average man and the issues he is likely to face—from love handles to sports injuries, high blood pressure to road rage. And it's a story about how these health issues affect you, the loving partner of that typical guy.

In this section, we'll talk about the major health issues, risks, and conditions that affect adult men. We're going to talk about his health as a process, something that happens in the context of your relationship. We'll look at the dynamics between partners that can either help or hurt the pursuit of good health. We'll give you some ideas about ways that you can help the person you love to make changes before problems strike. We'll talk about preventive care and the huge role that healthy eating and regular exercise can play in maintaining a man's health. And we'll look at how bad habits such as smoking and road rage can affect the entire family. Of course, we'll also cover the major conditions and illnesses men are most likely to face, and offer some advice on ways you can help.

PARTNERS IN HEALTH—FOR BETTER OR WORSE

There are lots of different ways in which husbands and wives deal with each other in the health-care arena. Some men are terrific at taking care of themselves and maybe you could learn from them. Others, well, let's just say they are less skilled. You'll see examples of both of these styles in the following sections, as we look at how some real-life couples dealt with major health issues in their lives with very different results.

THE HIGH PRICE OF DENIAL

Several years ago a close friend of my family—we'll call him Vinny*—complained to his wife of intense stomach pains. She urged him to go to the hospital, and he did. His father had died in his early fifties of a massive heart attack, a fact Vinny took lightly, though he was in his late forties himself. Because of his history and his frighteningly high cholesterol and blood pressure levels, he was admitted to the hospital, even though initial cardiac tests suggested his heart was not causing his pain.

The coronary care doctors told him he was lucky. He did not have a heart attack this time—it was probably his gallbladder—but they said he should immediately follow up with a series of tests after he left the hospital. They gave him an appointment for the stress test a week after he was discharged. He missed it. Time went by, and now and again I would ask him whether he had made a new appointment. These conversations almost always took place over dinner, which for him meant a large bowl of pasta followed by tiramisu.

"I don't need these tests I'm fine," he would say. "Besides, when my time comes, there is nothing I can do about it." Then he would laugh, raise his glass in toast, and point out that he had cheated the devil thus far and would continue to do so.

I was stymied by his denial. Seriously concerned, I told my husband again and again that our friend was "a massive heart attack waiting to happen." And unfortunately, I was right. One morning, several years after the stomach pain episode, I received a call that our friend had died suddenly of a massive heart attack after an hour of vigorous exercise, something he usually avoided. Later his wife told me that his failure to follow up with the doctors and to take the medicines that were prescribed, along with his foolish and boastful denial, were a frequent source of conflict between them. Eventually she gave up trying to convince him to take care of himself. He was forty-eight years old when he died.

NAGGED, DRAGGED—AND SAVED

Robert Smith* almost suffered the same fate. A few years ago, Smith, a forty-nine-year-old resident of south Florida, took up a vigorous new exercise routine that included lifting heavy weights at the gym. Bob began to feel pain in his left shoulder and neck. People at the gym told him he was lifting too much and not doing it correctly, so he assumed his pain was muscular. At home he complained about the pain, but went round and round with his wife July about seeing a doctor. She suggested, he declined. She pleaded, he refused. Finally she got fed up—and took him to the hospital. Larry Alexander, M.D., the emergency room director, performed an EKG, the standard test to look for signs of a heart attack. It was normal, but Dr. Alexander felt something wasn't right.

"The man continued to downplay everything," said Dr. Alexander. "But I listened to the wife's verbalizations about how and when the symptoms occurred. And I became concerned." So Dr. Alexander ordered a complete physical and lab workup. When the results came back, they showed that Bob's heart enzymes were elevated. He'd had a heart attack.

Bob was whisked to the cardiac lab where doctors found a complete obstruction of one coronary blood vessel and near-complete obstruction of another. The next day he had quadruple bypass surgery. Had July not nagged and then dragged her husband to the hospital, he would almost certainly have suffered a major—possibly fatal—heart attack.

THE COLLABORATORS

When New York Yankees manager Joe Torre learned just before the start of spring training in 1999 that he had prostate cancer, his wife Ali immediately became his medical partner—gathering information, considering options, and helping him make treatment decisions. "It was a very difficult experience to go through," said Ali Torre. "But when I learned that Joe had prostate cancer, there was no question that I'd be there for him. Although prostate cancer was first and foremost about my husband's life, it would be the two of us who would fight this disease, both on our own and together as a couple."

Torre had surgery and survived the disease, coming back in the middle of the 1999 season to lead the Yankees to victory in the World Series. Since then, Joe and Ali have been active with the American Foundation for Urologic Disease in urging couples facing prostate cancer to fight the disease together. "One of the reasons we want to talk about the 'couple effect' of prostate cancer is to encourage men to work with their spouses in fighting this disease, not shut them out," Joe says. "After the diagnosis, there is a lot of information to absorb. I knew if I missed something, Ali would get it."

I'd like to think that most couples work together in the model of the Torres, but I know that's not so. There are lots of families in which husbands don't easily accept their wives' assistance or counsel.

My goal here is not to turn wives or lovers into doctors or health cops. You are not your husband's doctor—and even if you are a doctor, you shouldn't be one to your husband. (Believe me, I should know!) No one is helped when women assume the role of health police or overbearing mother to their husbands. Admittedly, this is a fine line, and how it is drawn depends a lot on your and your husband's attitudes—just ask Bob and July Smith.

What we should strive for, in my view, is something quite different: to be caring companions who can help the men we love take better care of themselves. We want them to pay attention, to be more aware of their own health needs and better at managing their medical care. We're happy to help them, we already do—but we want to see them take more responsibility. When they do this, it helps them—and it also relieves us of a big burden and a lot of stress. But you have to start somewhere.

"Excuse Me, Madame, Do You Recognize Any of These Men?"

There are many different types and personalities among men. And when it comes to their health attitudes and practices, there are—well, not quite so many. Let's see, there are men who rarely think about their health. And men who never go to the doctor. And then there are a few athletes who are paid lots of money to take care of their bodies and stay in good health so they *have* to go the doctor. And that's about it, right?

All right, let me stop picking on men. There are, in fact, quite a few who think about their health and go to the doctor voluntarily. Actually, one of my closest friends from medical school takes exquisite care of himself. He simply eats well and exercises regularly. As a result, he looks not a day older than he did fifteen years ago, and his health is superb. His wife says it's all vanity, but the rewards for him go well beyond that. You probably aren't married to someone like my friend or you wouldn't be reading this book.

I think we can help men take better care of themselves if we pay a little attention to who they are, and how the attitudes and habits they've developed influence the way they deal with their bodies and their health care. Here, then, is our modest effort to describe some of the different kinds of men (in terms of their health attitudes and practice). But before we do, let's be clear that there really *are* lots of men who do a good job of looking after themselves. They see doctors when they ought to, get tests when they should, and follow up on problems when needed. These men, by and large, don't need our help, and they're not the men we're describing below. But, sadly, far too many men do fit into some of the categories below.

Indestructo Man

You know these men. There are probably more of them than any other category. Like most men, they were healthy as kids, healthy as teenagers, and healthy as twenty-somethings. So they never paid much attention to their health and now they never go to the doctor. Why should they? They're healthy and tough—almost indestructible. If something does bother them, they figure it will go away soon enough. Just like it always did before.

But the psychology of Indestructo Man is more complex than that. Since a good part of his ego is built on the idea that he is tough and invincible, he is deathly afraid of anything that will show that he is not. "I think there are a lot of men who have a fear of getting diagnosed," says Ken Goldberg, M.D., a Dallas urologist and men's health activist who has written several books on men's health. "But I think there's also a fear of a chink in their masculinity and a threat to their masculinity."

The Family Man

This guy is great at looking out for his family and works very hard to do so. He helps around the house, is supportive of his wife, and spends plenty of time with his kids. If anybody in the family's got a health issue or problem, he makes sure they get attention and help—anybody, that is, but himself. These are men like Gary Small, the man we met in the overview who was so busy working and looking after his kids that he just ignored the pain he was feeling, the pain that was telling him he was having a fatal heart attack.

The Tunnel Visionary

These men pay some attention to parts and problems, but they never really look at the big picture. If they have a sore shoulder, they might get it checked out. If they get sick, they might take some cold medicine. But they don't pay attention to prevention, so they don't think about getting screened for diseases. And they're probably not aware of their family's health history. The Tunnel Visionary's shortcomings are magnified by the way many overworked doctors operate. If a guy doesn't ask to have his cholesterol checked, or for a PSA test, the doctor doesn't offer it either. "If a man doesn't get his rectal exam, I don't know very many men who ask, 'Aren't you going to do it?'" says Dr. Goldberg. At least a Tunnel Visionary will call the doctor if a problem hits him in the face.

Risky Business Man

This fellow is a cousin of Indestructo Man. He loves to live on the edge. He drives fast, works hard, drinks heavily, and plays tough. If he's athletic, he'll probably keep wanting to play tackle football (without pads or practice) when he's in his thirties and forties. He never wears a seat belt, thinks bike helmets are for kids, and likes to drive his motorcycle full throttle. And watch out: If Risky Business Man cheats on you, he probably won't use a condom.

The Great Procrastinator

He's more or less aware of his health needs and problems, but he never has time to take care of them. He'll make that appointment with the doctor—tomorrow. He'll start an exercise plan—next week. He'll fill the prescription—when he has a chance to get to the pharmacy. And sooner or later, he may discover he has a disease that could have been treated if he had gotten medical care—yesterday.

GI Jim

This guy learned to follow orders, to do his morning calisthenics, and to see a doctor whenever he was told. For those men who got into the habit and still do their push-ups and jumping jacks, army life left a healthy exercise legacy. But their reliance on others to tell them when to get health care is more problematic.

"In the military we had regular, required, unavoidable physical exams that were very comprehensive," says David H. Gremillion, M.D., a former Air Force internist who now teaches at the University of North Carolina School of Medicine. "But it has the disadvantage of creating a passiveness on the part of the individual." Dr. Gremillion, who is also active with the Men's Health Network, believes that one result of this passivity is that former military men are less likely to see doctors and to get tests and checkups than they should.

Hank Hardbody

Hank goes to the gym, he pumps lots of iron, and he reads men's health magazines religiously. He likes the idea of high-protein diets, and Zone diets, and diets that pledge to "boost your testosterone" and give you "rock-hard muscle." Indeed, the idea of "rock hard" has a special resonance to him. He's a prime candidate for a condition that two researchers have dubbed the "Adonis complex" and others refer to as "bigorexia nervosa"—the obsession of many teenagers and men with the appearance of their body in a way that rivals what many women have been going through for years.

Trouble is that being obsessed with how his body looks on the outside doesn't mean he takes care of his insides. He's tempted to take steroids, which may do long-term damage, and he risks injury when he pushes too hard. And because he's so focused on his body being perfect he, like Indestructo Man, is likely to deny any flaws, imperfections, or problems.

THE STAGES OF A MAN'S LIFE

Whatever "type" your man is, he will go through various stages in his life that influence how he deals with his health. Authors Gail Sheehy (*Understanding Men's Passages*) and Daniel Levinson (*The Seasons of a Man's Life*) have each written about these stages. With a big nod of gratitude to them, here's a rundown of the stages we see, and the challenges and opportunities they pose for dealing with men's health issues.

Obviously, these stages don't begin and end on some magic day when a man suddenly morphs into a wiser or more mature man. In his detailed map of men's "adult development" stages, Levinson includes a lengthy transition period bridging each stage to the next. For our purposes, we're dividing things a bit more neatly, recognizing that every man is unique and that no one follows this like an appointment book.

Young and Invincible: Twenty- and Thirty-Somethings

Men in their twenties and thirties are, generally, in the prime of health. They rarely have health problems that make them *need* to see a doctor, and so they rarely go. And even when they do need to see a doctor, they put it off as long as possible. The Commonwealth study, *Out of Touch*, found that 30 percent of young men between eighteen and thirty would put off getting medical care as long as possible if they were sick or in pain. Another 20 percent would wait at least a week, and 38 percent would wait a few days. Only 10 percent said they would seek care as soon as possible. Men on the other side of thirty weren't much better: Only 14 percent of them would get help ASAP.

Before they have families, many twenty- to thirty-somethings tend to drink hard, play hard, and engage in riskier behaviors. And since many adults these days put off having families into their late twenties or thirties, that period lasts longer for many men than it used to.

The biggest risk to men's lives in these years are auto accidents, which are often linked to alcohol and/or drug abuse, followed by homicide and suicide. The chances of being a victim of violence, whether fatal or not, are much greater for men in this age group than for any other. That being said, it's important to note that despite all the attention given to school shootings and to violence among young men, the homicide rate among young men has dropped sharply since its peak in the mid-1990s.

Suicide has followed a similar pattern. Among young men, the suicide rate has dipped slightly in recent years, after rising for many years. The vast majority of these suicides are of young men. Indeed, fifteen- to nineteen-year-old boys are five times as likely and twenty- to twenty-four-year-old males seven times as likely to take their own lives as women in those age groups.

Though death and illness from other causes are quite rare, the health habits that men get into during their twenties and thirties are important. These are the years when people establish health habits—good and bad. If they don't see a doctor or exercise during these years, they can fall into a pattern of neglect, one they may pay for in the years ahead.

The Middle Years: Feeling Their Power, Sensing Their Vulnerability

For many men, the forties are a confusing time. Their families and careers are usually well established, leaving many men feeling good. They've got a nice house, they're making money, they're watching their kids grow up. But along with this sense of accomplishment comes a nagging awareness that they can't do all the things they used to do. They push too hard playing sports and end up with sprains and strains, or worse. Erections may be less automatic. They can't keep up with their sons in a race, and they watch with alarm as that spare tire grows around their bellies. And if they stay up late working or playing, it takes them longer to recover than it used to. This is the time when men start to feel their sense of invulnerability slipping away.

The forties can also be a time of great stress for many men. If their careers are going well, they may be under great pressure to keep it up or to do more. Or maybe their careers haven't flourished, and it seems as if everyone else's has. Maybe they're not getting along with their wives and they feel trapped in a dead-end relationship. It's a time when a lot of men take inventory of their life and wonder, "Is that all there is?"

During these years, the health risks men face start to change as the combination of stress, unresolved or developing emotional issues, and, for many men, poor health habits begin to take a toll. By the time men hit forty-five, heart disease has become enemy number one, a status it will maintain for the rest of their lives. Other related problems may be showing up, too: high blood pressure, diabetes, mounting cholesterol levels.

Ironically, for many men this new awareness of their own mortality can make it more likely that they will try to avoid seeing the doctor or doing anything that further exposes their vulnerability. On the other hand, many men who experience a health setback *will* resolve to do something about it. It's too bad, though, that it takes a scare to get him there.

Sixty and Beyond

With good luck and good habits, people can stay healthy longer than ever these days. We know now just how important good nutrition and routine exercise really are. If people eat well, move their bodies regularly, and get good medical care, they can, with a little luck, be working, playing, and enjoying their bodies into their eighties and beyond. The longevity gap that we've talked about so much may mean that the average man will die at age seventy-one, six years earlier than the average woman, but the truth is that there's no such thing as an "average" man or woman. The longevity gap is not a law of nature, it's a statistical average. It's based on the total population of men—including those who die early in car crashes after drinking too much, or those, like my friend Vinny, who suffer heart attacks too young after years of neglectful eating and poor exercise. Sadly, so much of what kills men early is largely or entirely preventable.

In the post-sixty years, men (and women as well, for that matter) really reap the benefits or pay the price for the health habits they established back in their thirties and forties. The biggest force that's operating here is not the law of averages but the laws of karma. What goes around comes around, to put it in a more American way. People who took care of themselves and their bodies are likely to be rewarded with longer and healthier lives.

People in their sixties, seventies, and even eighties can be extremely healthy and fit. Obviously, with advancing age, there are more things that can and will go wrong, which means that men in this age group need to have good doctors whom they see regularly. They need to pay close attention to their bodies' complaints and not delay getting care for problems or symptoms that pop up. And they need to work extra hard to be sure they're working their bodies in ways that strengthen and sustain them.

A WOMAN'S PLACE

Chances are that if you're reading this book, you're concerned about your partner's health and would really like to see him make some changes. You're convinced he won't change—hell, he won't even *try*—and your resentment builds and builds. You nag, you needle, you cajole, and after a while you get tired of it. Pretty soon, you're saying to yourself, "Well, damn him. If he wants to be an idiot and kill himself, then he can just go ahead." The only good thing I can say about this is you have lots of company—millions of other women. What can you do about it?

Well, first of all, here's some surprising news: As annoyed and powerless as you feel, you may have more influence over your partner than you think. Odds are, if your mate talks to anyone about a health problem, it's probably you. Hard to believe perhaps, but that's what studies suggest. In one survey reported in the *Journal of Family Practice,* family physicians agreed that men tend not to seek help or support for their health problems. But when they do, the report said, they usually turn to their female partners, not their male friends. And what prompts them to go to the doctor on those rare occasions when they make the trip? Usually, a woman is pushing them.

One doctor who participated in the survey said, "I can't recall ever being told by a patient that they have talked to a friend who said, 'Go to the doctor for that,' as opposed to hundreds of men who talked to their wife or female friend."

David Bell, M.D., sees this firsthand. He is the medical director of the Young Men's Clinic at Columbia University in New York City, one of a handful of clinics around the country that specialize in taking care of men. "We see anywhere from twenty-five to fifty-two guys in a four-hour session," says Dr. Bell. "And they do care about their health [but] sixty percent of the men we see are there because their partners tell them to go."

"Dr. Mom," an Unpaid Position

The changes in the roles played by men and women in America over the past forty years have been little short of breathtaking. Women have entered the work force in huge numbers. More than half of all college students are now women, as are nearly half of all newly admitted medical students. Fourteen women now serve in the United State Senate; sixty women sit in the House of Representatives.

On the home front, today's fathers are more involved with their children than ever. Men do more housework (though, of course, not enough), they help more with child care, and they do more cooking and shopping. Many of today's fathers are working hard at the balancing act that we women have been trying to pull off forever, trying, as one dad told author Suzanne Braun Levine, to hit the "Triple Crown" and successfully juggle family, work, and friends.

Unfortunately, one of the last areas to change seems to be the realm of managing the family's health care. Many young fathers change diapers like a pro but they still let their wives play Dr. Mom for the kids and Dad. Indeed, when a woman works more than forty hours a week, her husband's chance of being in good health declines by more than 25 percent. The reverse, though, isn't true. When hubby keeps late hours at the office it has no effect on his wife's health, according to a University of Chicago study in 2000.

For women, playing this role carries a price: extra responsibilities, extra worry, and a lot of extra stress. So why do we take it on? "We've been raised to expect ourselves to be Dr. Mom," says Braun Levine, a founding editor of Ms. magazine and author of Father Courage, a look at the struggles of today's new dads. "We want to be able to soothe anything that hurts and fix anything that's broken. It's a matter of pride that we can do it right. It's a big part of my self-image, there's no doubt about it."

Some feminists, like Barbara Risman, Ph.D., the University of North Carolina sociologist and author of Gender Vertigo, think Dr. Mom should go on strike and force men to change their ways. The thesis of *Gender Vertigo* is that the gender roles we all play perpetuate continuing gender inequality; in it, Risman advocates violating gender rules to the point of sparking chaos or vertigo. Only then, she says, can we create a more equal society.

"I think that women would be better off if they took the burden of caring for others off themselves," Dr. Risman told me in an interview. "When you love someone you want to take care of them. On the other hand, as a social pattern I think that until women tell men to behave like adults and take care of their own health they won't do so. I see it very much as analogous to 'Should we still scrub their shirts and pick up their socks off the floor?' Well, it's good for them, but it's not good for us. As long as women do it for them, they'll never do it."

I see things a bit differently. I agree that men must become more aware and more responsible for their own health. They need to change and we need to encourage that process. But that, clearly, is going to take some time. In the meantime, we simply are not going on strike as medical managers because to do so would hurt the very people we love most—our husbands and our children. In my view, one of the best ways to change men's attitudes and behavior about matters of health is to try to teach our sons a new way. The goal is generational change. We teach our sons and help them become more aware of these issues, and they'll adopt new attitudes and transmit them to *their* children.

To succeed in this effort, we'll need to get our husbands to join us. We can and should talk to our boys and work to educate them, but we should also realize the limits of our influence. In what they say and especially in what they do, dads may have more influence over boys as they develop their own attitudes and practices toward health. We need to encourage our partners to talk the talk—and to walk it, too.

If we're going to play the Dr. Mom role, we should do it consciously and find good ways to take care of ourselves so we don't become overwhelmed and resentful about the unfair burden we bear. This means we need to get some credit and appreciation from our partners. But it also requires us to adopt a nuanced and sophisticated attitude about our role in the family, an attitude, I think, along these lines: We're willing to be our family's health-care leaders and to manage this department for our kids. And we're willing to help our husband in his effort to stay healthy and on track. But that doesn't mean that our husband's health is our responsibility. If he's unhealthy, it's not our fault. If he doesn't take care of himself, it's not our failure.

In Sickness and in Health

The conventional wisdom about modern marriage and health used to boil down to something like this: It's good for men's health and bad for women's. University of

Washington psychologist Neil S. Jacobson, Ph.D., narrowed the idea a bit when he told *USA Today* a few years ago that marriage "protects men from depression and makes women more vulnerable." But more recent research challenges these assumptions. A more accurate statement might be this: Good marriages are good for people's health and mental health, especially men's; bad marriages are bad for people's health and mental health, especially women's.

Social relationships are enormously important to the health and well-being of men and women alike, so it's worth looking at how this plays out in the most important relationship in most people's lives—their marriage or long-term partnership. We'll do that in the discussion that follows. Don't be surprised, by the way, that the focus here won't just be on how marriage affects men. There are two people involved in your marriage, and the happiness and health of each of you has a profound impact on the happiness and health of the other.

A couple of years ago, researchers in Australia posed the following question: Does marriage improve the mental health of men at the expense of women? Their study followed more than ten thousand Australian adults and found that about 16 percent of both women and men suffered from some kind of mental disorder (women tended to be depressed and anxious, while men had more substance-abuse problems). But among men and women who were married, only about 13 percent had mental disorders.

Loneliness, on the other hand, is unhealthy, especially for the heart. According to John Cacioppo, Ph.D., a psychologist at the University of Chicago, social isolation causes as much risk to a person's heart as being obese, physically inactive, or a smoker.

Linda Waite, Ph.D., and Maggie Gallagher, authors of *The Case for Marriage*, argue that marriage is healthy for both men and women, especially men. They cite studies that have found that 90 percent of both women and men who are married at forty-eight are still alive at age sixty-five, compared to 60 percent of single men and 80 percent of single women.

One of the main reasons that being married can be healthy is simple: It's a built-in source of social support, and social support is increasingly recognized as a key to good health. "People in relationships use the health-care system more than people not in relationships," says Tamara Sher, Ph.D., an associate professor of psychology at the Illinois Institute of Technology. "They follow doctor's orders more—everything from taking medicine to starting an exercise program to stopping smoking."

At its best, having a partner can be like having a physician's assistant in your own home, someone to remind you to get that mole checked out or to go to the gym. With a multiyear grant from the National Institutes of Health, Sher is now studying ways to harness the power of relationship to help people facing a serious illness.

Bad marriages, though, can have a very different effect. Studies have found that people who describe their marriages as unhappy have more gum disease and cavities.

They may be more prone to ulcers and may have a harder time recovering from a heart attack. For one recent study, psychiatry professor James Coyne, Ph.D., and his colleagues at the University of Pennsylvania videotaped the arguments of couples in which one partner had congestive heart failure. In the couples who snarled and argued the most, the heart patient was almost twice as likely to die over the next four years, compared to patients who got along better. Another study, in the *Journal of the American Medical Association,* found that women who'd had a heart attack were nearly three times more likely to have another one if they were in a stressful relationship.

So what is it about a bad relationship that can make people—especially women—sick? Researchers know a few things. When couples get into arguments, blood pressure rises more rapidly for women than for men. A study published in the *Annals of the New York Academy of Medicine* found that wives were more likely to experience an increase in stress hormones and a weakening of the immune system during a big fight with their husbands.

Conflict in a relationship can weaken the immune systems of both partners and produce stress reactions in women. Researchers at Ohio State University took blood samples from thirty-one couples aged fifty-five to seventy-five before they talked about thorny issues and then several more times during the discussion. Couples whose test results showed they had weaker immune systems expressed more negativity toward each other during their talk. When the discussion got heated and negative, stress hormone levels in the women jumped but did not change in the men. "We believe that women show more response in hormone levels because they are more attuned to negative behaviors in their relationships and are more sensitive to them," said lead author Janice Kiecolt-Glaser, Ph.D.

Researchers at the University of Toronto found that when people who'd been in a bad marriage for three years were in the presence of their spouse, their blood pressure rose, and when they avoided their partner, it went down. Over the course of three years, the left ventricle of the heart also thickened among the people in bad marriages. For people in happy relationships, the reverse was true: When they spent time together, their blood pressure dropped.

Psychologist John Gottman, Ph.D., the well-known marriage researcher and author of *Seven Principles for Making Marriage Work,* points out that unhappy marriages can increase the risk of illness by up to 35 percent, while happy relationships can strengthen the immune system. What qualities allow partners to be happy? Dr. Gottman says that happy partners know how to pay attention to each other, even when it comes to little things. She'll notice his long face when he comes in the door and she'll ask about it. He'll pick up his socks after only one request and he'll accept her invitation to take a walk.

Dr. Gottman calls these everyday interactions "emotional bids," and he has found that men who are headed for divorce ignore them 80 percent of the time. Those in stable marriages turn this number around—they *honor* the request 80 percent of the time. Wives headed for divorce ignore their husband half the time, while women in good marriages ignore them only 14 percent of the time.

Happy couples manage to retain their sense of humor even during an argument and are openly affectionate to each other. Friendship, in other words, is at the root of their relationship. But other traits are deadly to a marriage, especially the ones Dr. Gottman calls the Four Horsemen of the Apocalypse—criticism, contempt, defensiveness, and stonewalling.

One stereotype about marriage and health is still true. When women become seriously ill, their husbands often leave them. Women, on the other hand, rarely abandon sick husbands. A few years ago, Michael Glantz, M.D., a neuro-oncologist at the University of Massachusetts, noticed that many of his female patients with brain tumors were having trouble in their marriages. He and colleagues followed 214 couples coping with brain cancer and found that 23 of the couples went through a divorce—and 18 of them involved a female patient. In another study of patients with multiple sclerosis, twenty-two of twenty-three divorces involved female patients. "The number of failed marriages among women with brain tumors is very alarming and suggests that male partners were not as supportive as one would hope," Dr. Glanz commented.

When Rich Stock, M.D., began his career as a radiation oncologist at Mt. Sinai Medical Center in New York City, most of his patients were women with gynecological cancer. "When I think about those women, I can't place the face of any of their husbands," he says. "They just were not in the picture." Now he treats mostly men with prostate cancer "and it's totally the reverse. When I come into the room, I see a man and a woman. Women are so much more supportive and so much more involved."

This certainly does not mean that *all* men are inconsiderate louts who run at the first sign of trouble. There are many wonderful men who provide great support and love to women who become sick. Of course, when men take on this nurturing role, they're often seen as heroes, while women are just doing what's expected, and with little credit. Scott Coltrane, Ph.D., a sociologist and researcher from the University of California at Riverside and author of *Family Man: Fatherhood, Housework, and Gender Equity,* thinks this is because expectations of men as fathers and spouses are exceedingly low. "This is changing, but my research on television imagery of family and gender shows that we still expect very little from men, and when they do anything, they expect praise and appreciation. Men feel entitled to be waited on and cared for by their wives and women feel obligated to provide care and domestic services to husbands and kids." The solution is to raise expectations.

When Bernie Smith's wife became ill with breast cancer, he and his son took loving care of her and made sure she was comfortable to the end. After she died, he started Men's Crusade Against Breast Cancer to help give a voice and a roadmap to the thousands of men every year whose wives are diagnosed with breast cancer. I've spoken to Bernie several times, and his devotion and love for his now deceased wife is inspiring. His Crusade is now four hundred members strong.

Personally, one of the most touching memories of my years as a medical student was of a couple where the roles were "reversed." A woman with terminal breast cancer was admitted to the hospital for pain control. Though her body was ravaged, she still wanted to be "presentable," but she could no longer manage to put on her make-up or do her hair. So her husband carefully applied her lipstick and eyeliner, and teased her thin hair until she was content. His love for her was evident in everything he did. He stood by her like a fierce lion, fighting to get her more pain medication when she needed it, making sure her last days were as comfortable as possible. I spent several hours listening to them recount the story of their marriage and travels. She could barely speak but would nod and smile as he talked about a trip they had taken many years before.

When she died, I was called to the room to pronounce her dead and fill out the paperwork. She was slumped over in the bed awkwardly. He went to her body, combed her hair into place, and adjusted her dentures. "I loved her no matter what she looked like," he said, "but I know Betty would never want to be seen this way." This man, so gentle, so superb at caring for his wife, was in no way feminine. I remember him as one of the most "masculine" men I've known, for qualities far different from those usually ascribed to that word.

HELPING SOMEONE YOU LOVE MAKE CHANGES

How do you help the man you love to make the changes that will help him stay healthy? How do you encourage your Great Procrastinator to get with the program? You hope that time will mellow Indestructo Man and moderate Hank Hardbody, but that's not always the case. In any event, you don't want to wait until he's fifty to finally agree to see the doctor. Your approach will depend partly on your husband's personality.

As a former Air Force doctor, Dr. David Gremillion is quite familiar with macho behavior. With men who display a lot of it—like Indestructo Man, Risky Business Man, and GI Jim—he suggests appealing to their sense of manliness by equating it with good health. One way to do that, he says, is to point out the weakness of a man you both know who didn't get medical attention for a health problem. "He was never strong enough to admit he had a problem, and follow through on it so he could stay healthy," you might say.

Another suggestion: Pick your shots. Don't ride him about every health issue that concerns you. Figure out the ones you think are really important, then choose the right moment to discuss them. (Obviously, I'm not talking here about emergencies. If one of these happens, you have to get help or call 911 immediately and ignore any objections he might make.) Milestone moments like birthdays or Father's Day can often present a good opening. "This is a grace period where men's egos don't get in the way as much as usual," Dr. Gremillion says. "It's a time in their life when they might be reflective about their own health." That's one reason, by the way, that the Men's Health Network worked to have the week before Father's Day declared as National Men's Health Week.

Another strategy you can use, especially with the Family Man, is to appeal to your husband's concern for your children, especially your sons. Remind him that he's a role model and that your sons really do watch his behavior carefully. Dr. Gremillion suggests delivering a message like this: "When you deny your pain or symptoms, it sends a message to our son and to all the young men in your life. Wouldn't it be great if they received the message from you that it's okay to have a pain here or there and tell someone about it?"

In the same way that boys may be more likely to listen to their fathers, and follow their leads, adult men may find it easier to hear messages about men's health issues from another guy. But that's only going to happen if your husband has a close male friend he can talk to. Since some men have trouble making social connections, or don't make it a priority to spend time with friends, Dr. Ken Goldberg urges women to help their men form these connections, and to encourage men to make time for their friendships. Try to develop or strengthen friendships with couples that include a man your husband connects with.

"There's no question in my mind that men will talk about their problems," Dr. Goldberg says. "They're not going to sit around the lunch table and talk about their problems getting erections. But they'll talk one-on-one with another man."

CAN YOUR PARTNER CHANGE?

Right about now, you may be thinking: You can't make someone else change. No one can change unless they really want to. We've heard these sayings a million times, and there's little doubt that they're true. A person *does* have to want to change. But that doesn't mean his or her desire must come solely from within. And it certainly doesn't mean that you have no role, or that you can't support or help inspire your partner to make changes.

Few things in life are harder than change. Whether it's giving up smoking or losing weight, learning to be optimistic or stepping back from a tendency to be bossy, making big changes requires a big effort and more than a little planning. Change often comes after a crisis such as being diagnosed with a disease or losing a job. In fact, most people wait for the bottom to fall out before they really get it together. When the Alliance for Aging Research, a nonprofit group based in Washington, D.C., surveyed baby boomers (thirty-eight- to fifty-six-year-olds), most admitted they would not change their lifestyle until they received an unwelcome diagnosis. They *know* they ought to change even before that, but until they know something is wrong they're willing only to take baby steps. Indeed, 43 percent of those surveyed said they would rather eat what they want and only live another ten years! This makes it especially complicated if you are trying to help someone else change.

But love is the most powerful motivator there is. If you offer someone your love and support to help him start down this road, that's a big source of strength he can draw on. Of course, you can't do it *for* him. But if you're in his court, and he's ready and determined, change is indeed possible.

Joel Kotin, M.D., proudly flouts the conventional wisdom that we can't really help someone else change. "That's absolutely incorrect," says Kotin, a psychiatrist and author of *How to Change Your Spouse and Save Your Marriage.* "When you're in an intimate relationship with someone, you have more power to change them. People can and do change each other, and it's really wonderful when it happens. I would not recommend that anybody give up on a member of the family who is not taking care of his health."

After all, Dr. Kotin adds, "If you care about someone, can you let them self-destruct? If you ignore a life-threatening situation, such as obesity, smoking, alcoholism, or workaholism, what kind of partner are you?"

Dr. Kotin argues that people change through their interactions with others. The more you are around a person, the more influence you have. The biggest reason you have this power is that your spouse loves you and wants to please you. "Even years after the glow of the new romance has worn off, people have a general tendency to want to please and to be accepted, valued, and loved," Dr. Kotin writes in his book. "This can work to your advantage in attempting to bring about change in your relationship."

But just because change is possible doesn't mean people will achieve it. In fact, many people who try to make big changes fail. For them, and for those who were pushing them or helping them to change, every failure is bitter proof of how fundamentally impossible change is. But perhaps the real reason that they failed is not because change is impossible or even because they were incapable of changing, but because they weren't ready or used the wrong technique at the wrong time.

THE STAGES OF CHANGE

James Prochaska, Ph.D., spent years watching his own father battle depression and alcohol. As he thought about his father's experience, and the way his family tried to help, he realized that the ways people often go about trying to make change are wrong. He recognized that change is a process with definable stages, much like the stages of grief that people go through after a loved one dies.

Today Dr. Prochaska, a psychology professor at the University of Rhode Island, is the reigning guru of behavior change. Along with researcher Carlos Diclemente, Ph.D., he studied the ways people change and how those around them can facilitate the process. The result of this research is a theoretical model, now widely accepted, called the Stages of Change. In Prochaska's view, people progress through the six stages one step at a time, completing one phase before moving on to the next. That's not to say that it is always a straight ahead process. People get stuck at one phase or another, they backslide, then backslide again. Some never get past the first two phases, which are the most common places to get stuck. But like Dr. Joel Kotin, Dr. Prochaska urges us not to give up on the people who keep getting stuck. Keep supporting them if you can, he says, and your support may eventually pay off.

According to Dr. Prochaska, one big mistake many people make—especially action-oriented Americans—is to start a change process before they're really ready. And the mistake many spouses often make is pushing their partners to take steps they're not ready to take. When the inevitable happens and the changes don't occur, people leap to the wrong conclusions, like "I told you to change and you didn't do it, therefore I can't help you change." To Dr. Prochaska, this expectation that people should change because we demand it is both wrong and potentially disabling. And it is not just spouses who make this mistake.

"Two thirds of American physicians have come to believe that their patients either cannot or will not change their behavior," Dr. Prochaska says. "They just become demoralized, they give up. [Their attitude is] 'Why waste my precious time if they're not going to change?'"

Think for a minute about a guy who has just been diagnosed with type 2 diabetes. Suddenly his doctor, his wife, and perhaps his own children are telling him he has to change his life—to change what he eats, to do frequent blood testing, to begin a complicated medication regimen. Odds are, the newly diagnosed patient is going to feel overwhelmed and may rebel against the whole thing. The result, Dr. Prochaska says, is an alienated and resistant patient and a demoralized doctor and spouse. But it doesn't have to be that way, he says. "When you match to the stage"—meaning you tailor the process to where a person is at—"you don't drive them away, you don't shut them down. They can do it."

Here's a rundown on Dr. Prochaska's six stages:

Stage 1: Precontemplation

This is where everyone begins and where many stay. People at this stage are not in the process of changing, and change isn't in their immediate plans. Some think they don't need to change, they don't believe they have a problem at all. Others don't want to confront their problem because they think the situation is hopeless. And still others recognize that there's a problem, but it's everybody else's, not theirs. Whatever the reason, precontemplators aren't ready to start changing. What this means for you as a spouse is that you need to tread very carefully. People in this phase are not likely to take kindly to directives like "You have to stop smoking" or "You must go the doctor." Try to push a precontemplator and he may withdraw into denial or cling stubbornly to his unwillingness to change. Worse yet, he might decide to get back at you by smoking, drinking, eating even more.

"You can't get them to take immediate action when they're not ready," Dr. Prochaska says. "And the majority of men won't be prepared. So when the wife tries to pressure, encourage, influence, or coerce them into taking action they're going to get more defensive and resistant. Then the person trying to help comes to the conclusion, 'You see? You can't get somebody else to change.'"

Your task at this stage is to provide information in a nonjudgmental, nonaccusatory, and nonthreatening way. Your goal is to get him thinking about the pros and cons of giving up cigarettes, altering his diet, or whatever change he ought to be making. Think of it as planting seeds that you hope will take root in your loved one's mind. So provide information and leave out the commands. But be prepared: No matter how you present the information, your partner may not be ready to receive it and may resent you for bringing it up.

One thing you can do for a little extra motivation is appeal to his sense of responsibility and love for someone else, in this case your children. As Dean Ornish, M.D., says, "People will often do things for someone else that they wouldn't do for themselves—but only if they feel like they're freely choosing to do so."

Even when your messages go unheeded, don't give up. Apathy can look like approval, especially to a precontemplator. Don't avoid the topic because you're afraid it could cause a rift. You don't want to fall into "enabling" behavior, such as covering for him or minimizing the impact of his actions.

One more thing about information. You can try to "scare him straight" and it may work in the short term, but it probably won't over the long haul. Lots of people know all the gruesome ways cigarettes can affect their bodies, but they continue to smoke. If there is new information about the dangers of a certain habit, then by all means pass it on. But don't expect action based only on fear.

According to Dr. Prochaska, about half of the people who enroll in smoking-cessation or weight-loss programs drop out, usually because they're not ready. Many of them started, Prochaska says, under pressure from a spouse or doctor. The message here is clear: Unless there's a life-threatening situation, don't apply the full-court press.

The use of directives as a way to get someone to change has a long and unsuccessful history, says Dr. Ornish, another expert in helping people change their health behaviors. "It goes back to the very first dietary modification intervention—which also didn't work—when God said, 'Don't eat the apple.'"

The bottom line is that in order to change, people need to feel they're in control. If you take that away they will never fully invest in change.

TIPS FOR DEALING WITH PRECONTEMPLATORS

- Clip newspaper articles and leave them or other health information around where he can see it.
- Tell him about somebody you know who overcame a similar problem.
- If you pass by a health booth at the mall, express interest. Then stop by and bring your partner along.
- The language you use is very important. Talk about yourself or use "we" a lot. Leave out "you" and by all means the "you should."

Here are a few examples:

"Did you know that Bob next door got screened for colon cancer and they found a tumor? Thank God they were able to remove it and he's going to be fine. But the doctor told him if he had waited any longer for the test, it almost certainly would have spread. Why don't we go see the doctor and get checked ourselves?"

"I love you so much I would never want anything to happen to you. Remember the doctor told us we were supposed to follow up with him about that high cholesterol level? Let's make an appointment."

"I feel so much better since I started walking to work and, look, I've lost three pounds. It's amazing what a difference exercise makes to your mood and overall health."

"I really think we need to set a better example for the children—and I really don't want our kids to be without their parents. I'm joining a stop-smoking program at work. If you want, I'll find out if spouses can come, too."

Stage 2: Contemplation

The person in this stage has begun to realize there might be a problem. He may still use excuses or denial—like "I'm okay" or "I feel fine" or "I'm too busy right now."

Despite the bluster, he knows there's a problem, and may even know the solution. But he's not yet ready to change.

People may spend years in this phase. They're ready for the next one only when they begin to focus more on the solution to the problem than the problem itself. Little by little they begin to acknowledge that the way they are doing things isn't so great, that they could get lung cancer or emphysema. They may notice how tough it is to walk a few blocks. But they still might not be ready to move on. Smokers in one study spent two years in the contemplation phase.

Contemplators are usually more receptive to messages and information than they were back in stage 1. You can help a contemplator by giving him every opportunity to express himself, his fears and doubts. Try to find out what he thinks will happen if he makes a change and correct any obvious misconceptions. This is also a good time to talk about the rewards of changing. Ask him what he would be comfortable doing if he were to make a change, but be sure to add "when you're ready." The most important thing you can do is to provide empathy and warm support.

Hopefully, one more thing will happen at the end of the contemplation stage: He'll make a decision to move ahead. He'll make this decision when he comes to the conclusion that the benefits of change outweigh the pluses of the way he's now living.

Stage 3: Preparation

A person in this stage plans to make a change within a month or so, and is usually quite happy to talk to you about it. He may tell you, for instance, that on such and such a date he'll see the doctor or will quit smoking for good. Ironically, your job may be to slow him down. Rushing through the preparation phase too quickly may hurt his chances for success. Far better to spend some time mulling over ways to confront looming temptations and how to cope with inevitable setbacks.

If your loved one tells you he's getting ready to make a change, resist the urge to push him. Let him come to it on his own terms but be sure to remind him how proud you are that he's thinking about making a change. And be sure to ask him specifically how he'd like you to help: What should you say—or not say—as his planned date for starting comes near? How can you best lend your support?

Some people may want you to leave them alone, while others may need daily stroking. Whatever the case, be sure you know his preferences. You may want to help him visualize what his daily routine will be like after he makes the change. If you know his goals, you may also help him avoid one of the biggest mistakes people make—trying to do too much too soon. If his plans seem too ambitious or optimistic, try to let him know that, delicately. Remind him that small steps are often more successful because big steps are so hard to maintain.

Stage 4: Action

People in the action stage actually begin to live the change. They stop smoking, see the doctor, or put the résumé in the mail. It's a busy and stressful time, and your role as a helper is crucial. Naturally, you'll cheer him on and offer lots of verbal support. But there are also other ways you can help. One is to sign a contract with your partner that puts both of your commitments into writing. For instance, he'll work to stop his angry outbursts at the kids and you'll give him praise for controlling his temper.

If he needs to make lifestyle changes, you can offer to do it together. If he's trying to quit smoking or drinking or wants to change his TV-viewing habits, Prochaska suggests rearranging the furniture or changing your daily routine so that the usual cues for the old behavior are removed. Keep up the support and remember to remain positive!

One more point: Look out for yourself, too. People who are trying to quit smoking or to make other difficult changes can be really grumpy, and that grumpiness can be aimed straight at you. It helps to have a thick skin, but it might be more helpful to spend some time doing things that take care of you—dinner with friends, a good massage, anything that helps you deal with the stress.

Stage 5: Maintenance

When someone changes his behavior, and keeps it up for six months, he moves on to what Dr. Prochaska calls the maintenance phase. This doesn't mean the battle is over. The challenge now is to continue on the newer, healthier path.

Getting to this stage is definitely cause for celebration. Be generous with praise and consider planning a special trip or event to mark the occasion. You might set it for a point when he reaches a certain goal, like the first anniversary of giving up smoking. You could also suggest saving up the money that would have been spent on cigarettes and buying something special. If he's lost—and kept off—a lot of weight, suggest splurging on new clothes.

Bear in mind that many people will relapse during this stage. Indeed, relapse is so common it should be considered a normal, expected part of the process. Yet for many people slipping up makes them feel as if they have failed and sends them back to earlier stages. Prochaska says that people can fall back many times, even going all the way back to precontemplation.

If your partner starts to slip back, be sure not to jump on him. Resist the urge to scold or finger wag. It's also important to remind him that relapse is normal; it doesn't mean he has failed. Let him know that you will help and support him even when he's had a slipup. One way to reassure him is to remind him that in the process of making this attempt, he's learned about what works for him and what doesn't, and he'll be able to put the experience to use during future attempts.

Stage 6: Termination

This is the promised land. The old problem is no longer a temptation or threat. A new life pattern has been established, and the old way is a thing of the past. People become comfortable with their redefined self. They are comfortable saying "I'm a nonsmoker" rather than "I'm trying to quit." You should keep patting your partner (and yourself) on the back so he knows you still care and are aware of all the effort that went into his change. Be aware that for many people, the termination phase may never be reached, and effort will be required to stay in the maintenance phase.

WHAT ELSE CAN YOU DO TO HELP SOMEONE CHANGE?
BECOME A MODEL

Writing instructors and film directors are fond of a simple slogan: "Show, don't tell." It applies to the field of behavior change as well. Sometimes the strongest statement you can make to a loved one is not what you say but what you do. If you're trying to help someone change, you might ask yourself if your own health habits are in line with what you're asking him to do. In other words, are you practicing what you preach? After all, if an overweight doctor counseled us to lose weight, how seriously would we take his advice?

Modeling can be a powerful influence on those around you, a convincing advertisement for a healthier way of life. It is the act of demonstrating to someone else how to do a task or make a change. It has one big advantage. When you start doing some of the things you're asking your husband to do—cutting out fat and salt, exercising several times a week, eating more fruits and vegetables—you'll be doing much more than setting a good example. You'll be doing great things for your own body.

AND NOW, A WORD ABOUT NAGGING!

Nagging has a bad reputation. Can you think of a worse insult (without using cuss words) that is hurled so often at women? A nag is almost always an unreasonably demanding woman or wife. Men are rarely tagged as nags.

But even though nagging has a bad rep, the truth is it's not all bad. (Even some men would agree with this.) There are lots of cases where a man, nagged by his wife, finally gets attention—just in time—for something that could have killed him. Nagging might just be one reason why married men tend to be healthier and live longer than their single friends. So I say *Viva la nag!* But I must also admit that there probably are more constructive ways to communicate.

Andrew Christensen, Ph.D., and Neil S. Jacobson, Ph.D., authors of *Reconcilable Differences,* have actually studied nagging. They say it sets up a dynamic in which one member of a couple tries to talk about a problem and the other wants to flee—as quickly as possible. Researchers call this the demand-withdrawal response, and not surprisingly, husbands are usually the withdrawers, and wives are most often the demanders.

Needless to say, this is not an especially pleasant or healthy pattern. If it happens a lot, it can be a sign of deep polarization and dissatisfaction within a relationship. Every couple does this at times, but the more frequent or extreme it is, the less happy they're going to be.

At its root, nagging is a battle for control. "I need you to hear me," the nagger is saying. From the nagger's point of view the "naggee" isn't listening. But from the naggee's standpoint, the nagger is trying to control his or her life. And that, as Dr. Ornish points out, is intolerable for many people.

"People will do things that they know are bad for them, that might even kill them," Ornish says, "to preserve something that's even more important than their life, which is the feeling of autonomy and control, of being a grown-up."

Your task, as the loving partner of someone who needs to make changes, is to search for ways to be encouraging and supportive as you make suggestions and to refrain from criticizing or badgering. It's one thing to make an offer to accompany your partner to the doctor or to offer to remind him of appointments, says Dr. Christensen. It's very different to get on his case and tell him, "You always forget about this," or "You don't care anything about your health."

Knowing your partner can help you tailor your message. Is he the type of guy who would be insulted if you made a doctor's appointment for him? If so, find some other way to suggest a checkup. Some men may not mind—they know if you don't do it, they'll never make the appointment. In the end, the best way to help your partner may be just to let him know that you are ready and willing to help in whatever way he'd like.

IF YOU'RE STUCK, CHANGE YOUR TACTICS

Sometimes trying to get someone else to do something can seem like running on a hamster wheel. You keep spinning the wheel, but nothing really changes. If what you're doing isn't working, you need to change your approach. For instance, if you and your spouse are at each other's throats, Kotin's advice is to take a break from pushing your partner. Give yourself and your spouse a six-week vacation from criticism. This doesn't mean you stop communicating; it simply means you can't use criticism as a way to deliver your message. If you can break this cycle, Kotin says, you may both open up and be more receptive to gentle messages.

In his book, *How to Change Your Spouse and Save Your Marriage,* Dr. Kotin outlines nine strategies for creating change including increasing communication (always the path to greater intimacy and understanding between couples), negotiation (I scratch yours, you scratch mine), mediation (an impartial third party to hear both sides and help resolve conflict), behavioral conditioning (change through overt and subtle rewards and punishments), manipulation (just what it sounds like), personal growth (enhance self-esteem and personal qualities as a way to influence a partner), ultimatum (a last resort), and getting professional help. If you find you and your partner are stuck, pick up a copy of this book and read more about how you can help change your marriage for the better.

11

An Ounce—or Two—of Prevention

For most of us, the way we live from day to day—what we eat, what we don't, how we use or abuse our bodies—has the biggest influence on our health and our likelihood of becoming ill. It's sad but true that men tend to have more unhealthy habits than women—but, hey, most of us women have plenty of room for improvement, too. Which means that we have every reason to work *with* our partners in an effort to help us all live healthier lives.

Later I'll discuss the major things that most often go wrong for men: high blood pressure, heart disease, cancer, stroke, and diabetes among them. These are the most common killers of adult men. The good news is that many of these problems are preventable.

If you really want to help the man you love, if you really want to promote his chance for a long, healthy life, the best thing you can do is to start being healthier yourself and invite him to join you in the effort. And that means, as you well know, doing two things above all others: Eating a healthy diet and getting regular exercise. Study after study shows that if you really want to cut down on bad cholesterol, reduce the risk of heart disease and stroke, avoid high blood pressure, and manage diabetes, you have to combine exercise with a sensible diet. Let's start by talking about exercise.

EXERCISE

If your partner is like a lot of men, his idea of a good "leisure time" activity is to turn on a sports game with a beer, a bag of chips, and a remote control unit at his side. According to the Centers for Disease Control and Prevention, 25 percent of men get no leisure time physical activity at all.

I've always had the feeling, though, that the tendency to be either a couch potato or to be active is catching within a family. When one family member gets on the ball—or gets out the ball—it can encourage others to get in the game. I know when I've been more diligent about my exercise routine it often motivates my husband to do the same.

The Couple That Works Out Together . . .

Studies show that people who work out with others are much more likely to stick to it than those who work out alone. Janet Wallace, Ph.D., of Indiana University found that married couples who enrolled together in the university's adult fitness program and also attended nutrition counseling sessions together were much less likely to drop out of the program than married people who came in alone. Married people who left their mate at home had a 43 percent dropout rate compared to a 6 percent dropout rate for the couples who came in together.

An added benefit of working out together is that you get to spend more time with your spouse. For busy two-career couples, that alone can be a real plus. But can it lead to too much togetherness or spur unhealthy competitiveness? That depends, says psychologist Thomas Plante, Ph.D., a professor at Santa Clara University who has studied the psychology of exercise.

"In general, exercising with people is a good thing," says Dr. Plante. "People are more likely to do it. And they are more likely to find it pleasurable, so it's less boring." Plante also found that when people work out together, the experience tends to leave them feeling more energetic, less tense, and less tired—even if they don't talk to each other during the workout.

But working out with a spouse is certainly not for everyone. Men and women often have different workout goals, and they may have very different skills and interests. So there's a danger of getting into conflicts that may mirror problems in the relationship in general. On the other hand, there's no rule that says you have to do your workouts side by side just because you go to the gym together. You could go together, do your own things, and then meet up to brag over lunch or coffee afterward.

My good friend Susan and her husband are an excellent example of how a couple can turn their lives around together, though not necessarily at the same time. After John received a less than glowing review from his doctor he got motivated and began biking, swimming, and lifting weights. Susan was reluctant to get active at first, and she held out for a year. But she began to miss her husband during his workouts so she decided to join him at the gym. At first he tried to instruct her on the equipment, but that left both of them frustrated. Eventually they sorted things out and both now have their own trainers. John got his health issues under control, and they say their relationship is stronger than ever because they both feel better and are sharing an activity they've both come to love.

PLANNED PARTNERHOOD

Here are a few things to consider before embarking on an exercise plan together.

- Try to pick a sport in which neither of you has a competitive investment or vastly superior skills. (Try to imagine Barry Bonds playing baseball with his wife—not a good idea.)
- Avoid the coach-player dynamic. If one partner is new to an activity but the other is accomplished, get a third party to teach it to that person. You can then avoid the "You're doing it wrong!" "No, I'm not!" "Yes, you are!" "You're always criticizing me!" cycle.
- Set goals and talk ahead of time about what you'd each like to accomplish. Is this a time for togetherness? Or do differing workout goals mean you each need to go solo? If you're hiking, biking, or running, do you expect to always go at the same pace? Or is it okay if one zooms ahead? Make sure your goals, and your expectations of each other, are clear going in.
- Don't criticize your partner's abilities, especially in front of others. If you are concerned that your partner is doing something that could lead to an injury, say so in a nonjudgmental way. Have fun and keep it light!
- No matter what kind of exercise you and your partner decide on, it's important that you exercise safely. That means warming up and cooling down, wearing the proper protective gear, doing the exercise correctly (get lessons if you don't know how), drinking plenty of fluids, and wearing sun protection when needed. Your goal should be to do some form of aerobic exercise most days of the week.

Test Your Fitness Together

If your partner isn't overweight and has no obvious physical problems, it can be hard to convince him that a consistent exercise routine is a good idea. You can yell. Or you can cajole—even bribe. But we know those methods don't work, at least not over the long term. Besides, even if they did work, who wants to be the nag all the time?

One way to break through this denial might be to take a fitness test. You and your partner can do it together and see how you each stack up. The test below was developed for individuals by the Cooper Institute for Aerobic Research in Dallas. I asked Institute researchers if they could adapt it for this book. Fitness is defined in the categories of cardiovascular endurance, muscular strength and endurance, and flexibility. If you take this test, it can tell you how fit you are and where you need to be going. It can also be used to monitor progress as you go forward. If both of you take the test it can be a good way to support each other in a new lifestyle.

FITNESS TEST

Before You Begin

If you haven't consulted a doctor recently, it's a good idea to do so, either in person or over the phone. Talking to a doctor is an absolute *must* if you answer yes to any of the following questions:

- When doing mild exercise:
    - Do you sometimes become extremely short of breath?
    - Do you ever have dizzy spells?
    - Do you experience chest pain or pressure?
    - Do you ever experience blurred vision?
- Have you ever noticed that your heart has skipped a beat?
- Do you sometimes feel your pulse racing?
- Have you had medical problems such as high blood pressure, diabetes, high cholesterol, heart murmur, or heart attack?
- Do you have musculoskeletal problems such as arthritis, tendinitis, or chronic back pain that might get worse with exercise?
- Are you currently or were you recently pregnant?
- Are you recovering from surgery or a serious illness?
- Do you currently have an acute infectious illness with a fever?

Get Ready
1. Wait an hour or two after eating before you start.
2. Wear comfortable, loose-fitting clothing and well-padded athletic shoes.
3. Do some warm-up exercises and stretching before you start.
4. Choose a comfortable time of day—not too hot, not too cold.
5. Rest between each part for as long as you need to.
6. Help each other with preparation, timing, and scoring. It will be easier and more fun for both of you.
7. Practice taking your pulse before you begin the test.

Warning Signs

If you feel any unusual pain or discomfort during or right after the test, stop immediately and consult a doctor. And if you experience any of these warnings signs, call 911 right away:

- Abnormal heart activity, such as irregular beats, flutters, or palpitations in the chest or throat, sudden bursts of rapid heartbeats, or sudden slowing of a rapid heartbeat.
- Pain or pressure in the center of your chest or in your throat.
- Dizziness, lightheadedness, sudden lack of coordination, confusion, cold sweating, or fainting.

CARDIOVASCULAR ENDURANCE
ONE-MILE WALKING TEST

Warning: Don't do the test if you are taking any of these medications: alpha blockers, beta blockers, calcium channel blockers, nitrates, combined alpha and beta blockers, centrally acting adrenergic inhibitors, nonadrenergic peripheral vasodilators, peripheral acting adrenergic inhibitors, bronchodilators, cold medications, tricyclic antidepressants, major tranquilizers, diet medications, and thyroid medications. They could interfere with your heart rate.

Get Ready
1. You need a watch with a second hand.
2. Don't drink any caffeinated beverages for at least three hours before starting.

The Test
1. Find a smooth, level surface that can be measured easily. A high school track or shopping mall is perfect.
2. Warm up for several minutes by walking briskly and stretching.
3. Walk (*do not run*) one mile as quickly as you can without straining. Keep a constant pace.
4. Write down how long it took to walk the mile. Most people do it in ten to twenty minutes.
5. Continue walking slowly to give your heart rate and blood pressure a chance to come down.

Score It
Use the chart below to get a picture of your cardiovascular fitness, based on your age.

Men	Women
UNDER FORTY (MINUTES)	
13:00 or less (excellent)	13:30 or less (excellent)
10:01 to 15:20 (good)	13:31 to 16:00 (good)
15:31 to 18:00 (average)	16:01 to 18:30 (average)
18:01 to 19:30 (below average)	18:31 to 20:00 (below average)
19:31 or more (low)	20:01 or more (low)
OVER FORTY (MINUTES)	
14:00 or less (excellent)	14:30 or less (excellent)
14:01 to 16:30 (good)	14:31 to 17:00 (good)
16:31 to 19:00 (average)	17:01 to 19:30 (average)
19:01 to 21:30 (below average)	19:31 to 22:00 (below average)
21:21 (low)	22:01 (low)

MUSCULAR STRENGTH AND ENDURANCE
ONE-MINUTE PUSH-UP TEST
Tests strength and endurance of arms, shoulders, and chest.

Get Ready

You need a watch with a second hand. You may want to use an exercise mat or well-padded surface to protect your knees.

The Test

1. Place hands on the floor roughly shoulder width apart. From the "up" position, bend your arms and lower your body until your chest comes within three inches of the floor. (You can also touch a three-inch high sponge). Keep your back, buttocks, and legs in a straight line. Then return to the "up" position. This is one complete push-up.
2. Men should have only hands and toes touching the floor. Women can do a modified push-up by keeping their knees, toes, and hands on the floor.
3. Do as many complete push-ups as you can in one minute.
4. Write down the number of push-ups you complete.

Score It

Based on your age, here's how many push-ups you should be able to do to be considered generally fit.

Age	Men	Women
Under 30	35	30
30 to 39	30	25
40 to 49	25	20
50 to 59	20	15
Over 60	15	10

SIT AND REACH TEST

Tests flexibility of lower back and hamstring muscles.

Get Ready

1. Tape a piece of masking tape about twelve inches long to the floor. Place a yardstick on the floor perpendicular to the tape so that the fifteen-inch mark is flush with the edge of the tape. Place several pieces of tape over the yardstick to secure it into place.
2. Do a few stretches to warm up before you begin.

The Test

1. With your shoes off, sit on the floor with your legs straight and straddle the yardstick.
2. Keep your feet as close together as possible and your heels flush with the edge of the masking tape. The "0" end of the yardstick should be closest to your groin.
3. Place one hand on top of the other and lean forward slowly, extending your arms. Reach as far forward along the yardstick as you can, exhaling as you perform the stretch. Be sure you keep your legs straight and don't bend your knees.
4. Hold this position for at least one second. *Do not* bounce down rapidly. Your score is the farthest point you can reach with your fingertips. Perform this three times and use the best score of the three.

Score It

Based on your age, here's how many inches you should be able to reach to be considered generally fit in this area.

Age	Men	Women
Under 30	18	19
30 to 39	18	19
40 to 49	17	18
50 to 59	17	18
Over 60	17	18

ONE-MINUTE SIT-UP TEST

Tests strength and endurance of the abdominal muscles.

Get Ready

You'll need an exercise mat or well-padded surface and a watch with a second hand.

The Test

1. Lie flat on your back on a well-padded surface with your legs together, your feet flat on the floor, and your knees bent. Cross your arms over your chest and tuck your chin to your chest. Have someone hold your feet firmly to the floor or slip your feet under something heavy like an armchair. Your buttocks should stay on the floor at all times.
2. Keeping your hands in place, curl your upper body off the floor until your spine is vertical or your elbows touch your knees. Exhale as you move to the "up" position, then lower your upper body back down to the floor. This represents one complete sit-up.
3. Perform as many correct sit-ups as you can in one minute.

Score It

Based on your age, here's how many sit-ups you should be able to do to be considered generally fit in this area.

Age	Men	Women
Under 30	40	35
30 to 39	35	30
40 to 49	30	25
50 to 59	25	20
Over 60	20	15

Source: Adapted from The Physical Fitness Specialist Manual, *revised 2003, The Cooper Institute, Dallas, Texas. Used with permission.*

When you've completed all the parts of this test, sit down and take a look at the results. You and your husband can use them to judge how fit you each are and to decide what, if anything, you need to do about it. If you decide to embark on an exercise routine, it's a good idea to check in with a doctor and see if there are any precautions you ought to take, especially if you've been something of a couch potato. The goal of a new exercise program should be to start out slowly and gradually build up. I know many middle-aged men—like my friend "Vinny," who collapsed and died at the gym—who think that their years of playing high school basketball will keep them fit forever. They're in denial about just how out of shape they are. So they push too hard too fast—and sometimes pay the price.

GET REAL

In this age of men's magazine cover models with massive chests and abs of steel, of action figure toys for boys with bulging pecs and beefcake thighs, it's important for your husband—and you—to keep your eye on the real prize. Fitness is not about having twenty-inch biceps or six-pack abs. It's not about how you look or even how far you run. It is about strength, flexibility, endurance, and—most of all—keeping your insides healthy.

Exercise helps to increase HDL cholesterol levels— the good stuff—and lower levels of LDL—the bad stuff (see page 407). It helps keep weight off and lowers your heart rate and blood pressure, reducing the risk of stroke and heart disease. It can delay the vascular complications of diabetes and stave off the crippling effects of arthritis. It can even help prevent depression.

So how much exercise does he (and do you) really need? Most experts recommend that people aim to walk briskly (or do other vigorous exercise) for at least thirty minutes most days of the week. Unfortunately, less than a third of adults actually do this or anything comparable. An excellent goal for walkers is twenty to twenty-five miles a week, but if you want to push up your levels of good cholesterol, the more the merrier. Keep in mind that you don't necessarily have to spend thirty minutes each day at the gym sweating it out on the treadmill. Brisk walking, taking the stairs, and just generally being active for half an hour will do. Add in weight training and you'll get the added benefit of reduced LDL levels, along with stronger bones and muscles, which can help prevent arthritis and osteoporosis, which, it may surprise you to know, strikes men as well as women, particularly as they age (see page 484).

One reason so many people—especially men—fail to keep at an exercise routine is that they set their sights too high. They want abs of steel overnight or they just don't see the point. One way to help someone stick with a routine is to encourage him to set reasonable, attainable, and sustainable goals. And that means choosing a program that emphasizes exercise for overall weight loss and cardiovascular health—not just doing endless sit-ups in a vain attempt to look like a *Men's Health* cover boy.

Another thing to avoid is the weekend warrior syndrome—the men who sit at their computers all week and barely walk beyond the parking lot, then go out and play football or take a long run on the weekend without building up or training. Weekend warriors put themselves at great risk of injury as well as heart attack or stroke. The guy who drops dead suddenly of a heart attack is often the guy who joins a gym and on his first day decides to work out like a maniac.

One final point about exercise: Whether you do it alone or together, exercise can be good for your relationship in many ways. "Since exercise lowers anxiety, depression, and stress, it just might inoculate people from future stress," says Santa Clara University's Thomas Plante, Ph.D. The point is that people who exercise tend to be happier and calmer—and that can only be good for your relationship.

Diet for a Healthy Family

Food is the best preventive medicine known to humankind. Does that sound like an exaggeration? It's not. Foods from the garden contain a rich bounty of vitamins and minerals that can help us fend off illness and disease. Study after study has shown that making positive changes in what we eat can lead to profound improvements in our health. Studies also show that eating the wrong foods can increase the risk of getting everything from heart disease to cancer.

Like it or not, we women have tremendous influence over what the members of our families eat. We still do most of the thinking and planning about health and nutrition, along with most of the food shopping and cooking. In general, we're much more aware of nutritional needs and take greater care than our burger-and-fries-loving husbands to make sure that the family eats right. I'm not saying that all men are incompetents or no-shows in the kitchen. My cowriter Rob Waters is a good and frequent cook, and my good friend Janice never lifts a finger in the kitchen because her husband Alvaro is a gourmet chef. We should all be so lucky!

In general, men today are doing a bit more of the shopping and cooking. The bad news is that we still do the vast majority. Recently, some researchers conducted a survey for *Prevention* magazine and the Food Marketing Institute on this issue. "Interest in health and nutrition doesn't hit men until middle age or older," they concluded, "while women—in their role as family caregiver or simply due to worries about their weight and appearance—seem interested throughout their lives."

In her book *Feeding the Family: The Social Organization of Caring as Gendered Work*, sociologist Marjorie DeVault, Ph.D., uses interviews with women and men to catalogue the huge amount of work that goes into feeding a family, work that she argues is largely invisible and for which women get little credit. We often fail even to credit ourselves. But it is work, important work that affects the health of everyone in the family.

Even couples who start out with every intention of creating "50/50" marriages often find that they slip into old gender roles and patterns of behavior. Shortly after the vow, she's doing a pile of laundry and he's offering to change the oil. A short time later she's on the mommy track and he's working overtime, barely getting home to see the kids. Most women work outside the home, of course, but even then, the tendency is to slip into the familiar roles when we come home. We put in a full day at the office, then come home to manage the household chores and the kids—the "second shift" as sociologist Arlie Hochschild called it.

That's not to say that men haven't been stepping up to the plate more than they used to. Indeed, since the 1970s, men have roughly doubled their contributions to chores such as cooking, cleaning, and washing, according to Scott Coltrane, Ph.D., a University of California at Riverside sociologist. Still, the reality is that as wives and mothers, we spend a huge amount of time shopping for meals and preparing them, as well as making sure that the food on the table is healthy.

What this means, in my view, is that we need to do two things: One, learn effective ways of getting our mates to help out more and be more aware of the importance of healthy dining. And two, use our control over the family diet to make sure that everyone eats right. We may not like that we have this responsibility but we shouldn't make the mistake of slighting its importance. The decisions we make about the food that goes on our table has a huge effect on our family's health. Like it or not, we have enormous power in this area and we should put it to good use.

The Food Police

The problem with having as much control as we do over our family's dining practices is that it puts us in the uncomfortable position of being the food police—a job I hate but often find myself doing. I have literally pulled food from my husband's hands as it is headed toward his mouth more times than I'd like to admit. In the long run, I don't think this approach really works. After all, I'm not with him most of the day. And I have enough trouble monitoring what goes into my own mouth.

The trick is to come to accept that people are generally going to eat what they want to—you can't compel healthy eating. What you *can* do is watch what you eat and what you bring into the house. If your husband does some of the shopping, you'll need to get him on board in this effort, too.

The Nutrition Information Fog

One obstacle to making wise choices about what we eat is that we are inundated with dubious, often unfathomable, and frequently conflicting information about nutrition and healthy eating. If you've looked at a magazine rack or walked down the health and nutrition aisle of a bookstore, you know there's no shortage of advice on healthy diets. Some of these books are worthwhile, but others are fad-of-the-moment diets that have little real science behind them. It's easy to become overwhelmed and throw your hands up in despair. Even the U.S. government's recommended food pyramid—that classic chart of what we Americans should eat—has come under fire. And with good reason. The pyramid recommends that we limit how much fat we eat, that we increase our consumption of carbohydrates, and that we eat meat or other proteins as often as three times a day. Trouble is, it doesn't distinguish between the different kinds of carbohydrates, proteins, or fats. Most people probably know that Americans eat too much fat, but they don't know that some fats are actually good while others are extremely unhealthy. There is also mounting evidence that we're eating too many of the wrong carbohydrates, simple carbs such as potatoes and refined grains (white bread, white rice, and pasta).

Many experts believe the official food pyramid is giving out bad advice. One of its most prominent critics is Harvard University physician and public health researcher Walter Willett, M.D., the author of *Eat, Drink and Be Healthy: The Harvard Medical School Guide to Healthy Eating*. "The food pyramid is tremendously flawed," Dr. Willett said in an interview with Harvard's public health newsletter. "It says all fats are bad; all complex carbohydrates are good; all protein sources offer the same nutrition; and dairy should be eaten in high amounts. None of this is accurate." Thus, the official advice from the U.S. government may be worsening—instead of solving—a growing public health menace: the epidemic of overweight, unhealthy Americans.

Men and women are about equally likely to be obese, but men's diets seem to be a bit less healthy overall. Men are more likely to have heart attacks, strokes, and other problems at a young age, which may be linked to their weight and diet. Still, before we start feeling too superior, it's not like our diet is *that* much healthier than men's. As a group, women do eat a bit better than men do—but not much. According to the Centers for Disease Control, 81 percent of American men do not get enough fruits and veggies in their daily diets. For women, the number is 73 percent. So let's face it: We could all improve!

The Problem with Meat and Potatoes

Make no bones about it: Most men love meat and potatoes. If they had their druthers, many men would eat a big steak and a baked potato every night for dinner. And I am not talking only about older men. Steak and potatoes remain staples of the masculine diet for men in their twenties and thirties as well. But man can't live on meat and potatoes alone, not if he wants to keep living. The problem with meat is that it is high in saturated fat, the biggest contributor to heart disease. The problem with potatoes is that they contain a lot of rapidly absorbed starch that is quickly converted to glucose, a form of sugar. Over time, this excess of glucose in your system can increase the risk of diabetes, as we'll explain later.

Bottom line: The "masculine" diet of meat and potatoes promotes heart disease and diabetes (not to mention stroke, prostate cancer, and colon cancer) and should be abandoned if we want those we love to live long and healthy lives. I'm certainly not saying that you should never eat meat and potatoes. Rather, the goal should be to make them occasional treats rather than everyday staples.

To understand this better, let's take a closer look at the typical American diet and its two most controversial and problematic ingredients, fats and carbohydrates.

The Skinny on Fat

Most people—and most experts—would probably agree with this statement: High-fat diets are unhealthy. Over the past thirty years or so, that message has been so broadly repeated and so relentlessly drilled in that nearly everyone accepts it as gospel. During the 1980s and '90s, it sometimes seems, the whole country went on a low-fat frenzy. Fat became the Great Satan, and low fat became the Holy Grail. We had low-fat muffins, low-fat ice cream, and low-fat cheese. Drug companies made pills that tried to block fat absorption, and snack food companies made potato chips with a chemically altered "fake fat" said, bizarrely, to be "fat free."

What was the result of this focus on fat? Fat consumption fell across the land. And Americans got a lot fatter. Sixty percent of all Americans are now overweight. Rates of diabetes have soared, even among children and teenagers. From a nutritional perspective, Americans are less healthy than ever.

One problem with our tunnel-vision focus on fat was that it ignored an important reality: All fats are not the same. Some fats—especially the saturated kind found in meat—are truly unhealthy, especially in the quantities many Americans consume them. And other fats—the unsaturated kinds found in some oils, nuts, and some fish—are both healthy and necessary in a balanced diet.

Another problem with obsessively cutting fat is that it inevitably gets replaced by something else. For most Americans, that something else is carbohydrates, and with carbohydrates come calories. We've traded high-fat foods for high-calorie carbs, and it isn't a very good bargain.

Fats: The Good, the Bad, and the Ugly

There are three basic kinds of fats (also known as *lipids* or *fatty acids*) that we need to be concerned with: two that exist in nature and one that's the result of engineering by food processors. One of these fats is good, one is bad, and the other is so bad, it's ugly. Let's do a quick review of the chemistry. All fats of any kind are chains of carbon atoms with varying numbers of hydrogen atoms connected to them. What distinguishes one kind of fat from another is the number of hydrogen atoms it holds and the way the fat behaves as a result.

The Good Fats: Unsaturated

Unsaturated fats are those found in vegetable oils and many nuts. There are two kinds:

Monounsaturated Fats

The chain of carbon atoms that make up all fats are connected by single or sometimes double bonds. Monounsaturated fats have one (thus, the "mono") double bond, which causes a bend in the otherwise straight line of carbon atoms and reduces by two the number of hydrogen atoms held by the carbon chain. At room temperature, monounsaturated fats are always liquid. They are found in olives, olive oil, and canola oil, as well as most nuts, peanuts, peanut butter, and avocados. Monounsaturated fats raise HDL (high-density lipoprotein) cholesterol (the good kind) and lower LDL (low-density lipoprotein) cholesterol (the bad kind).

Polyunsaturated Fats

Polyunsaturated fats differ from monounsaturated fats in just one way. Instead of one double carbon bond, they have several, each one causing a bend in the carbon chain. Like monounsaturated fats, they are liquid at room temperature and will boost good cholesterol and lower the bad. One polyunsaturated fat that seems to do good things for the heart is omega-3 fatty acid, which is found in several kinds of fish, including salmon, sardines, mackerel, and herring.

The Bad Fat: Saturated

Saturated fats are the kind found in red meat; in dairy products such as whole milk, cheese, and butter; and in coconut and palm oil. In a saturated fat, each carbon atom in the chain holds as many hydrogen atoms as it can—they are "saturated" with them—and each carbon atom is connected to the next with a single bond in a straight chain. This makes them very stable and that's the reason they are solid at room temperature. Think of lard, butter, or the fat that congeals after it drops off a piece of meat and cools. The fact that they're more solid and stable is also the reason they're more likely to clog arteries. Saturated fats increase the levels of bad LDL cholesterol and raise the risk of heart disease. They are also associated with an increased risk of cancer of the colon, rectum, breast, endometrium, lung, and prostate. Indeed, prostate cancer is much more common in countries where people have high-fat diets. Go ahead and eat them occasionally, but you really should try to limit your intake.

The Ugly Fat: Trans Fats

In 1869, a French chemist named Hippolyte Mège-Mouriès rose to a challenge issued by Napoleon III: Anyone who could create "a suitable substance to replace butter for the navy and less prosperous classes" would receive a prize. Margarine was born. In Mège-Mouriès's formulation, it was a mixture of beef fat with milk, but that gave way to an oil-based version in the early 1900s, when a German scientist, Wilhelm Normann, discovered a way to "harden" unsaturated oil by adding an extra hydrogen molecule in a process known as hydrogenation.

Hydrogenation creates what food chemists call *trans fatty acids,* or *trans fats,* which are found today in most hard margarines, shortenings like Crisco, and endless varieties of commercial baked goods and fast foods. Any list of ingredients that includes "partially hydrogenated vegetable oil" or "vegetable shortening" contains trans fats. Most experts say that these synthetic fats are the least healthy fats of all since they lower HDL (good) cholesterol levels and raise LDL (bad) cholesterol levels, while also boosting two other bad substances—triglycerides and lipoprotein A, both of which are linked to heart disease. Bottom line: Avoid all trans fats whenever possible.

THE FAT CHART			
WORST *Trans Fats*	**BAD** *Saturated*	**BETTER** *Polyunsaturated*	**BEST** *Monounsaturated*
Most margarine, vegetable shortening.	Meat: beef, lamb, pork, poultry, and lard.	Oils: corn, cottonseed, sesame, soybean, safflower, sunflower, walnut.	Oils: olive, peanut, canola, and most oils made from nuts
Partially hydrogenated oil.	Brazil nuts, macadamia nuts, pistachios.	Margarine made with above oils (no trans fats).	Nuts: cashews, almonds, walnuts, pecans, filberts, peanuts, peanut butter.
Deep-fried food: chips, french fries.	Dairy: milk, butter, cheese, ice cream.	Seeds: sesame, sunflower, pumpkin, walnuts.	Avocado.
Commercial baked goods: cakes, cookies, donuts.	Chocolate. Coconuts, coconut oil, palm oil.	Fish.	Olives.

The Trouble with Carbs

If you follow health news, you've watched the pendulum swing back and forth on many nutrition subjects. But on few issues has it swung more wildly than on the value of carbohydrates. One day, carbs are great and we should all eat plenty of pasta (as long as it's topped with low-fat sauce). The next day, carbs are bad and we should purge them from our diet and eat protein instead.

The truth is that carbohydrates, like fat, come in many forms and lumping them all together as an undistinguished mass is neither useful nor healthy. They also affect people differently depending on how physically active they are. The conventional wisdom about carbs used to be that simple carbohydrates were bad and complex carbohydrates were good. But carbs, like life, aren't that simple. So let's start with some carbohydrate basics.

Simple carbohydrates include sugars such as glucose (the form sugar takes in our blood), fructose (the kind in fruits and vegetables), sucrose (table sugar), and lactose (milk sugar). Each provides the body's tissues and cells with needed energy. To ensure that cells have a consistent, available supply of energy, the body chemically regulates levels of glucose in the bloodstream so they stay within a narrow range.

Complex carbohydrates are simply chains of sugars linked together. Starch, the carb we eat most of, is a chain of linked glucose molecules. Some complex carbs are easily broken down by our digestive systems into their component sugars. Others, called fiber, can't be digested so easily and pass through our digestive tract largely unchanged.

Highly refined carbohydrates containing little or no fiber—white rice, pasta, white bread, or other things made with white flour—are rapidly absorbed and turned into glucose. When the glucose level in your bloodstream rises, it causes your pancreas to pump out a hormone called insulin to process the glucose. As the insulin level rises, it causes a crash in blood sugar and a subsequent craving for more food. If, on the other hand, the glucose level drops too much, the pancreas will stop making insulin, and the liver will start releasing some of its stored glucose. Over time, these spikes of glucose and insulin can tax your pancreas, increasing the risk of diabetes and heart disease and making it hard to control your weight.

For people who are already overweight, these refined, quickly digested carbohydrates may be especially problematic. "The low-fat, high-carbohydrate diet recommended by the National Cholesterol Education Program and the USDA Food Guide Pyramid may be among the worst eating strategies for someone who is overweight and not physically active," writes Dr. Willett in *Eat, Drink and Be Healthy.*

In contrast, when you eat whole-grain foods such as brown rice or oats, or fiber-rich food such as beans, fruits, or vegetables, you slow the roller coaster to a more leisurely pace. The body simply can't absorb and process these foods as quickly. Remember this: Fiber comes only from plants, and good sources of fiber include beans of all kinds, dried fruit, and a number of fresh fruits.

Carbohydrates and the Glycemic Index

A few years ago, nutrition researcher David Jenkins and his colleagues at the University of Toronto developed a scale called the glycemic index to rank these various kinds of carbs. Carbohydrates that are quickly broken down into glucose are said to have a high glycemic index. You don't need a degree in nutrition to know which carbohydrates are the bad ones: white bread, potatoes, donuts, and cookies, along with those ready-to-eat cereals with funny names that your kids probably clamor for.

Good carbs, the ones that contain more fiber and are absorbed more slowly, are said to have a low glycemic index. They don't send glucose and insulin levels soaring, and can help you feel fuller longer. Green veggies and whole grains top the list of good carbs, which also includes whole fruits and beans.

Simple enough, right? Actually, it's a little more complex than it first appears. Some foods, such as carrots, actually have a relatively high glycemic index. Does that mean we should avoid carrots? No, we should eat them like bunnies, and here's why: The glycemic index is based on a person consuming 50 grams of the carb in question. Since a carrot has only 4 grams of carbohydrate, you'd have to eat a pound and a half to get 50 grams, something no one is going to do! That's why many experts believe that a better measure of how a food affects blood sugar is the *glycemic load*, which factors in a food's glycemic index as well the amount of carbohydrate in a typical serving. Other factors can also affect the glycemic load: how a food is processed, how it is cooked, and the amount of fat and fiber in the food.

Glycemic index, glycemic load—all this can get rather complicated. If you are interested in learning more about the glycemic index and the individuals values for specific foods, check out *www.glycemicindex.com*, a website managed by the University of Sydney. The important thing to remember is actually quite simple: In shopping and in eating, go for fruits, vegetables, and whole grains. Stay away from processed foods, white breads, cakes, and cookies.

The Great Protein Debate

One of most common nutrition misconceptions among Americans is that they have to be vigilant to make sure they eat enough protein. The truth is that very few Americans are protein deficient. It's quite easy for most of us to get all the protein we need, and we don't need that much. The Recommended Daily Allowance (RDA) established by the National Academy of Sciences calculates that a healthy adult needs 0.36 grams of protein per pound of body weight. So a 160-pound man needs about 58 grams of protein a day and a 120-pound woman needs about 43. A six-ounce serving of chicken contains about 42 grams of protein. Most Americans get about twice that much. One reason it's so easy for us to get all the protein we need is because it's in so many foods: dairy products, meat, fish, poultry, nuts, and beans.

The American male's love of meat has helped make the Atkins Diet probably the most popular diet in the country. This so-called diet revolution calls for people to eliminate carbohydrates from their diet in favor of lots of protein. Most of this protein, of course, is animal protein—red meat—which means lots of saturated fat. I think the Atkins Diet is bad nutrition. It addresses one problem—overconsumption of carbohydrates—by creating another—overconsumption of saturated fat. The likely result: higher rates of heart disease and several types of cancer that have been linked to high intake of saturated fat. That's what I call a bad bargain.

PYRAMID SCHEMES

Critics have been pointing out the flaws of the official USDA pyramid and urging the government to revise it for at least eight years, but to no avail. Walter Willett argues that the U.S. Department of Agriculture, which created and updates the pyramid, is simply more interested in promoting U.S. agriculture than in protecting the public's health. The influence of the meat and dairy industries on the department is just too great, he says. In his book, Dr. Willett outlines his own "healthy eating pyramid" as an alternative to the official USDA pyramid. It recommends that people:

- Eat lots of whole grains, fruits, vegetables, nuts, and beans.
- Sharply limit red meat, potatoes, and refined grains such as white bread, white rice, and pasta.
- Consume dairy products (or calcium supplements) only once or twice a day.
- Replace unhealthy saturated fat with healthier unsaturated vegetable oils.
- Take a daily multivitamin (see page 317).
- Drink limited amounts of alcohol.
- Finally, at the base of the pyramid, Willet makes a suggestion that has nothing to do with food but everything to do with good health: Get daily exercise.

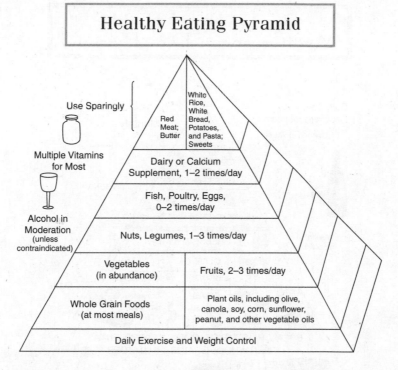

Source: Reprinted with the permission of Simon & Schuster Adult Publishing Group from Eat, Drink, and Be Healthy by Dr. Walter C. Willett. Copyright © 2001 by Presidents and Fellows of Harvard College.

Great Ideas from the Mediterranean

Another reasonable and achievable alternative to the standard American diet (and the official USDA food pyramid) is the popular Mediterranean diet. It calls for a relatively high fat intake (good fats, of course), about 35 percent of daily calories. But its emphasis on whole grains, fresh fruits and vegetables, fish, garlic, and olive oil, as well as moderate, daily intake of wine makes it rich in antioxidants, fiber, and heart-healthy nutrients, including omega-3 fatty acids. The Mediterraneans also tend to eat less meat and greater amounts of nuts, legumes, beans, and healthy carbohydrates than Americans. The value of this diet was shown in a study of Greek adults. Those who closely followed a Mediterranean diet had a reduced mortality rate overall and were less likely to develop heart disease and cancer. The study was published in June 2003 in the *New England Journal of Medicine.* In 1993, the nutrition research group Oldways Preservation and Exchange Trust created a food pyramid based on the Mediterranean diet. The group has since developed other pyramids based on healthy eating practices from different cultures.

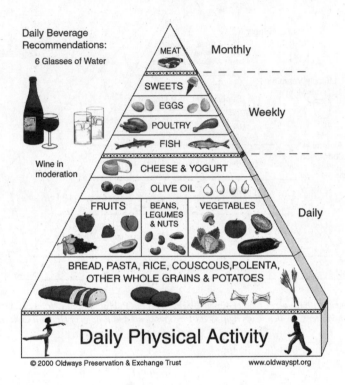

The Traditional Healthy
Mediterranean Diet Pyramid

Daily Beverage Recommendations:

6 Glasses of Water

MEAT — Monthly

SWEETS
EGGS — Weekly
POULTRY
FISH

Wine in moderation

CHEESE & YOGURT

OLIVE OIL

FRUITS   BEANS, LEGUMES & NUTS   VEGETABLES — Daily

BREAD, PASTA, RICE, COUSCOUS, POLENTA, OTHER WHOLE GRAINS & POTATOES

Daily Physical Activity

© 2000 Oldways Preservation & Exchange Trust   www.oldwayspt.org

Wisdom from the East

We can learn even more by traveling halfway around the world and visiting the people of Okinawa, a group of Japanese islands in the East China Sea. According to researchers, the Okinawans may just be the healthiest people on Earth. They have the longest life expectancy in the world—people there often live well past one hundred—as well as the lowest rates of heart disease, stroke, and cancer, the top three killers among people in the West. Breast and prostate cancer, for example, are almost unknown among Okinawans. How do they do it?

The people of Okinawa eat a largely plant-based diet high in unrefined carbohydrates and low in saturated fat: lots of whole grains, tofu and other soy products, fresh fruits and vegetables, and fish. They eat very little of the things we eat lots of, refined foods and animal fat. What's more, they also get lots of exercise, have close relationships with friends and neighbors, and strong and satisfying spiritual connections.

There is compelling evidence that their lifestyle—not their genes—is what allows the Okinawans to live such long, healthy lives. When they move away from their homes and adopt Western diets, they succumb to the same diseases we do.

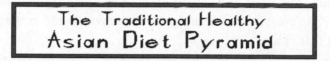

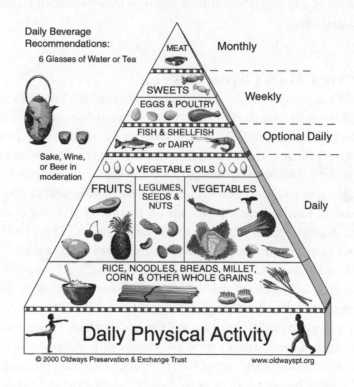

The Traditional Healthy Asian Diet Pyramid

Daily Beverage Recommendations:
6 Glasses of Water or Tea

Sake, Wine, or Beer in moderation

MEAT — Monthly

SWEETS
EGGS & POULTRY — Weekly

FISH & SHELLFISH or DAIRY — Optional Daily

VEGETABLE OILS

FRUITS | LEGUMES, SEEDS & NUTS | VEGETABLES — Daily

RICE, NOODLES, BREADS, MILLET, CORN & OTHER WHOLE GRAINS

Daily Physical Activity

© 2000 Oldways Preservation & Exchange Trust   www.oldwayspt.org

From Right Here at Home

Of course, you don't have to go to Okinawa to find people who advocate healthy eating and living. People like Dr. Walter Willett and Dr. Dean Ornish have been working for years to convince people—including those in Washington—that changing the way we eat is the cheapest way to improve the health of the nation. Dr. Ornish, the author of the best-selling book *Eat More, Weigh Less,* became famous for the ultra-low-fat vegetarian diet he created for people with severe heart disease. His plan is simple but radical: Eat no animal products at all except egg whites and nonfat dairy foods like yogurt.

Eat so little fat that it provides less than 10 percent of your calories. Then eat as much as you like of fruits, vegetables, and unrefined grains—there's no limit on calorie intake.

The Ornish diet has been studied not just for heart disease. Working with early-stage prostate cancer patients, he was able to show that a strict vegan diet and no alcohol consumption, combined with aerobic exercise and meditation, modestly reduced their levels of PSA (prostate specific antigen), an enzyme found in the blood that can be a marker of that cancer.

Clearly, this diet is not for everyone and you don't have to go to this extreme to have a healthy diet and life. If you simply begin to lean toward an Ornish-style diet, you will be doing better.

THE WAY TO A MAN'S STOMACH . . .

When Judy LaCour enrolled in a medical study called the Women's Health Initiative (WHI) in the early '90s, she hoped it might help her improve her diet. The study, funded by the National Institutes of Health and run by researchers at medical centers across the country, aims to track the health of some 160,000 postmenopausal women as they age, looking, among other things, at how women's diets affected their chances of getting various cancers and heart disease. A devout meat and potato family, Judy and her husband, Ray, had each grown up on fried food and had changed little as adults. "There was no organized system to our eating habits," says Judy. "We ate what was quick and easy. That of course included a lot of red meat and fat." To top it off, they both worked in sedentary jobs and got little exercise.

Ray was already feeling the effects of a lifetime of poor eating habits. He was twenty to thirty pounds overweight, and high blood pressure, high cholesterol, and diabetes were taking a toll on his health. Still, Ray was not exactly pleased when Judy announced she was enrolling in a health study that would require radical changes in her diet. Since she prepared the food and took care of the shopping, that would mean big changes for him as well. "If left to his own devices, he would just as well go to McDonald's," Judy says.

Women who enrolled in the study took classes on how to lower their fat intake so they were getting no more that 7 percent of their calories from saturated fat. Judy attended the classes and soon began cooking in a new way. She used more vegetables and less fat. She stopped using butter. She replaced regular salad dressing with low-fat versions and used less. The results were remarkable: She lost thirty pounds and has kept much of it off.

Ray was slow to buy into this new way of eating. But little by little he noticed a change. He lost weight and felt better, and his blood pressure dropped enough that he could stop taking his blood pressure medication. Now he's a full-fledged convert. "Anyone can do it," he says. "[You just have to] start with small steps."

Ray and Judy's experience is by no means unique. Though not a single man was enrolled in the WHI, the study had a clear—though unintended—effect on men's health. James Shikany, Ph.D., a preventive medicine researcher at the University of Alabama and WHI co-investigator, surveyed some of the women's husbands and found they had dropped their intake of fat from 37.4 percent to 35 percent, and their saturated fat from 12 percent to 11 percent of total calories.

These men had adopted their wives' healthier habits, not because they saw the light about the evils of dietary fat, but because they ate what their wives fed them. And while a drop of a couple percentage points might not sound like a lot, Shikany says, "even a relatively small decrease in fat intake could have a major public health impact if it were to occur over a population."

There are two big lessons here. The first is that, as daunting as it may seem, dietary change really is possible. Just ask Ray and Judy. The second inverts an old cliché: The best way to a man's stomach, it seems, is through his wife. If a family's diet is to improve, the person best able to spearhead that effort is usually the woman.

Clearly, this has good and bad sides. Many men have been socialized to have their food choices dictated to them by their mothers and then their wives, and they never learn for themselves how to choose, eat, or prepare healthy food. This is a domain where women have a great deal of influence—far more influence, in fact, than most of us would like! So, yes, we can be forces for change, but sooner or later men need to step up to their own plates. The trick for women, as we'll discuss in more detail later, is to do what we can to put healthier food on the table, while at the same time encouraging our men to learn more and do more for themselves. The goal is to model good behavior, not to enfeeble our loved ones. So here are some basic dietary principles that you should know and pass on to everyone in the family.

PRINCIPLES TO EAT BY
Cut the Bad Fat: Eat Less Red Meat

Limit saturated fats that come from meat and full-fat dairy products. Avoid those trans fats—found in commercially baked goods and processed snack foods—altogether if you can. Use healthy oils like olive or canola oil instead of butter or margarine. If you use margarine, choose the versions that are trans fat free. Peel the skin off chicken before you cook it. This does not mean that an occasional steak is verboten. It just means that it should be a rare treat, not a staple. When you do serve meat, try preparing it in small bits combined with vegetables, instead of big chunks.

But remember this too: The real key to a healthy diet is not to obsess about fat but to consume plenty of fruits, vegetables, and whole grains instead of processed foods that may be low in fat but are high in calories and loaded with carbohydrates.

Go Fishing

One delicious food you can use to replace some of that red meat on your family's dinner plates is fish. Fish is low in calories and high in the good omega-3 fatty acids that help protect against heart disease and stroke. Unfortunately, though, we've managed to foul our own nest sufficiently to make some kinds of fish dangerous to eat. The FDA and the EPA have found that levels of mercury and some other industrial chemicals in some species of fish now make it too risky to eat, especially for young children or pregnant mothers. They advise avoiding four types of ocean fish that have been found to contain high levels of mercury: shark, tilefish, swordfish, and mackerel. Be sure to keep up with the latest information on the mercury levels of fish in your area by contacting your local health department. The good news is that salmon, a favorite for many people, seems to be okay.

Join the Rainbow Coalition

"What color is your diet?" asks David Heber, M.D., director of the UCLA Center for Human Nutrition in his book by the same name. If your answer is brown or beige, he says, you're in a lot of trouble. Those are the colors of burgers and fries, steak and potatoes, pork and pasta.

Dr. Heber and other nutrition advocates suggest instead that you try to make your plates colorful. That means serving a variety of fruits and vegetables, not just green ones. Fruits and veggies are loaded with vitamins and phytochemicals (*phyto* means plant) that your body needs and loves. And different colored foods—I'm talking *natural* colors here—contain different valuable ingredients.

Tomatoes, for example, get their red hue from lycopene, which seems to protect against prostate cancer and heart disease. The blue in blueberries comes from anthocyanin, an antioxidant with powerful cancer-fighting properties. And the orange color in apricots, pumpkins, and carrots comes from beta-carotene; it and other substances found in these foods may slow the aging process and protect against cancer.

Fight Portion Distortion

Eaten at a restaurant lately and noticed how much food is put on your plate and poured into your glass? Supersizing has swept the country. Many researchers believe this trend, coupled with the fast food industry's huge advertising presence, has contributed to the obesity epidemic in a huge way. But do bigger portion sizes really mean that people eat more? It seems so.

A study by researchers at Pennsylvania State University used college students to see just what effect large portions have on eaters. When they gave men a 2-cup serving of macaroni and cheese and told them to eat as much as they wanted, the men ate 1.9 cups of it. But when they fed them a 5-cup serving of it they ate 2½ cups, felt equally full either way, and couldn't tell any difference in how much they actually consumed. By the way, women in the study did pretty much the same thing. Bottom line: The more on their plate, the more people eat! What we should do about it: Serve smaller portions at home. And make trips to fast food restaurants rarer than an undercooked burger.

What's really amazing is the huge and growing gap between the superportions that have become the norm in restaurants and the small portion sizes the government uses in defining servings in its recommended nutrition guidelines. The list below gives examples of what the U.S. Department of Agriculture considers a serving of food. Take a look.

WHAT COUNTS AS A SERVING?

Grain Products Group (Bread, Cereal, Rice, and Pasta)
- 1 slice of bread
- 1 ounce of ready-to-eat cereal
- ½ cup of cooked cereal, rice, or pasta

Vegetable Group
- 1 cup of raw leafy vegetables
- ½ cup of other vegetables—cooked or chopped raw
- ¾ cup of vegetable juice

Fruit Group
- 1 medium apple, banana, orange
- ½ cup of chopped, cooked, or canned fruit
- ¾ cup of fruit juice

Milk Group (Milk, Yogurt, and Cheese)
- 1 cup of milk or yogurt
- 1½ ounces of natural cheese
- 2 ounces of processed cheese

Meat and Beans Group (Meat, Poultry, Fish, Dry Beans, Eggs, and Nuts)
- 2 to 3 ounces of cooked lean meat, poultry, or fish
- ½ cup of cooked dry beans or 1 egg counts as 1 ounce of lean meat
- 2 tablespoons of peanut butter or ⅓ cup of nuts count as 1 ounce of meat

Source: U.S. Dept. of Agriculture, http://www.nal.usda.gov:80/fnic/dga/dga95/box02.html.

Don't Bring Junk Food into Your House!

As we all know, kids love snacks and junk food. (Grown-ups have been known to eat them as well.) But because they're so bad for our health, I try my hardest not to buy them—and especially not to bring them into the house. If you were to look in my cabinets, you would never find potato chips, and cookies are a rare treat. In fact, I don't buy anything that is overly processed.

I've also worked to train my husband. Now, after a few years of struggling with this issue, he no longer expects to find unhealthy foods in the house. Be warned, though: If you try to implement a policy like mine, you'll probably hear a chorus of complaints and anger. So it might be wise to start out slowly. Get rid of one kind of junk food at a time and keep eliminating until none are left.

This often leaves my husband wandering forlornly from cabinet to cabinet late at night. But I know that if the junk were there he would surely eat it. So what about those family members who *can* control themselves and eat only small portions of goodies? It probably is unfair to them, but they too can do without it.

Don't Scarf Down Your Meals

One of the practices that keeps the people of Okinawa so slim and healthy is that they practice a habit called *hara hachi bu;* roughly translated, it means stop eating when you are eight-tenths full. It takes some minutes for your stomach to signal your brain that you are full. So if you stop eating when you're only 80 percent full and wait twenty minutes, you'll find you are satisfied with what you've eaten. Cutting calories this way is easy—if you can handle the wait.

Don't Go on a Weight-Loss Diet (or Push Your Husband To)

Diets may work for a while, but study after study finds the same thing: They do not work in the long term. The only option we have if we want to be slim and healthy is to choose healthy food day in and day out, and to get plenty of exercise. Going on a diet not only won't work, it will set a bad example for your husband and children. Remember: The way you eat and deal with food exerts a powerful influence on your family.

Have a Cup of Tea

Heavy tea drinkers (black or green, hot or cold) are more likely to survive a heart attack, according to an article in the American Heart Association's journal *Circulation*. Tea drinking has also been linked to a reduced risk of a number of cancers, possibly because flavonoids found in tea act as powerful antioxidants.

And a Few More Tips

1. Aim to get less than 30 percent of your calories from fat.
2. Eat fried foods only when you've won the lottery.
3. Eat whole-grain cereal for breakfast with lots of fruit.
4. Eat beans—as side dishes or by putting them in salad.
5. Always remove the skin from chicken and turkey.
6. Use olive oil instead of butter.
7. Eat eggs occasionally. Really. The word from experts now is that up to one egg a day is just fine for most people.
8. Avoid weird diets. If it sounds weird or gimmicky, it is! As Dr. James Shikany says, "Don't go on any diet you wouldn't consider staying on for the rest of your life!"

CHANGES AT HOME
Learn the Basics About Nutrition and Then Pass Them On!

I hope some of the ideas and suggestions we've just gone over will pique your interest in learning more about healthy eating. If we women incorporate a few basic principles about nutrition and make a concerted effort to pass some of our knowledge to our husbands and children, it could make a big difference. Unfortunately, most men don't really pay any attention to nutrition until they start feeling vulnerable. And by then, they're often set in some awfully bad habits. If we can help our partners understand just how important healthy eating is today, and if we can get them to be better role models for our children, that might help the next generation avoid the bad habits that too many of us fell into.

Get Men to Shop and Cook

The closer people are to the source of their food, the more they know about it. So why not make your partner more responsible for buying food? It can ease the burden on you and help him learn more about good nutrition and healthy eating. And this really does set a good example for the kids, especially boys.

Here's one idea. Pack him and the kids off to the local farmer's market or fruit store and they can get some shopping done and learn a little about buying produce while you get some time to yourself!

If he needs some shopping lessons, go with him a couple times. My own husband will more than happily trot off to the store for food, but—forgive me, Avery—when I used to ask him to buy fresh fruits and veggies, he usually came home with spotted apples or mealy pears. I've found that going shopping together and showing him how to choose good fruit and vegetables has helped a lot.

If your partner already shops—or if you succeed in getting him to start—what about cooking? Many men are becoming more interested in cooking these days (at least compared to our parents' generation), thanks to the proliferation of star chefs like Bobby Flay made popular by the Food Network and CBS's *The Early Show*. Granted, this could be dangerous, but the truth is a lot of men can learn to cook if they're willing to try and you're patient and give lots of praise.

Strategies for the Chore Wars

Pushing men to do things around the house can lead your family into conflicts and minefields. We know how resistant some men can be. In her book *Halving It All, How Equally Shared Parenting Works,* Francine M. Deutsch catalogues some of the ways that men squirm out of chores. Why do they do this? In short because equality at home is an idea that mostly benefits women. And since most women I know are too busy to enforce or continually negotiate with their spouses, they often give up the fight. And even when men do pick up some slack they usually choose tasks that can be done at their leisure (change the oil) rather than jobs that have to be done routinely or on someone else's schedule (feed the kids).

If you decide that it's time for change in your family and you want your husband to take on more responsibilities, be aware that it could take some time. And you should probably start pushing for this before you're about to snap from frustration. From his research and interviews with women and men, Dr. Scott Coltrane has learned a couple of useful strategies from wives who have been successful in recruiting their husbands to do more child care or housework.

First, he says, define the work as a shared responsibility. Get men to buy in to the idea that the work is important, and that it's unfair to assume that the woman should automatically do it. What's more, if you can, get Dad to do chores with the kids. Boys who prepare meals, run errands, or do laundry with Dad are likely to be better behaved and have more friends, according to one study by Coltrane.

Second, give your husband responsibility for a clearly defined task and let him do it the way he wants to. "This is hard," Dr. Coltrane says, "but if you give up micro-managing, it allows him to assume more authority for the task and to 'own it' as his responsibility." This means you'll have to pick a few things that you can let go of controlling and live with them being done to standards different than your own.

"A lot of men are threatened by women and feel insecure when they think they're being judged," Dr. Coltrane says. "So they often avoid putting themselves in situations where they will be monitored by a woman with authority, including their wives. This sets up a double bind for women who want change but also feel responsible for protecting her husband's feelings and maintaining harmony in the family."

Many women say they want men to do more around the house, but then they get too frustrated or controlling to allow it. Instead, they find themselves saying, "I'll do it! You can't do anything right," and all that 50/50 stuff goes right out the window. Many women take a lot of pride in the work they do managing their home and family—and well they should. But some women's sense of identity is so connected to these jobs that they actually feel usurped or diminished if a man takes over some of them. If you start feeling this way, it's important to think and talk about it, and to look for other ways to feel good. If you want more sharing of chores around the house, you have to be prepared to be less than 100 percent satisfied with the job your loved one does. And if he does do something well, you need to praise him and allow yourself to enjoy it.

Make Changes Slowly

If I were to go home and announce to my husband that as of now we were total vegetarians, I probably wouldn't get much support. But I also know that over the years we have worked together to improve our eating habits. It's a slow process and it continues, but we no longer have desserts on a regular basis, I almost never cook red meat (though we occasionally order it), and breakfast is rarely anything more elaborate than an egg-white omelet. This has evolved over the years and has helped us keep to a reasonable weight (though, of course, we could both improve further).

Negotiate If You Must

If you're fighting an uphill battle with family members who just don't want to change what they eat, try to negotiate. Sit down and talk about healthy eating and try to come up with a plan you both can live with. Propose a swap: He agrees to eliminate one unhealthy item and you replace it with something healthier. The husband of a good friend of mine is a big meat eater; he insists on meat at nearly every meal. My friend has tried everything to get him to cut back. She finally broke through when she showed him the bill from the butcher and he saw what his meat habit was costing. After that he agreed to have one meat-free night per week, when my friend prepares a vegetarian casserole—not perfect, but a lot better.

Eat Dinner Together As a Family If You Can!

One of the most important things you can do for your family is to have dinner together as often as you can. I know it's not easy. Most people these days are working way too much, spending hours in horrible commutes, and ferrying kids to soccer practice and after-school events. But taking time to sit down and eat together not only keeps families talking and feeling connected, it also helps us all eat healthier meals.

When we eat at home, we're not grabbing greasy, high-fat fast food and eating it in the car. We are more likely to eat a balanced meal. Studies also show that when families dine together, kids eat better. One study of some sixteen thousand children conducted by researchers at Harvard found that the more often families ate dinner together, the more fruits and vegetables kids ate, and the less fried food and soda.

A TOAST TO GOOD HEALTH

Is a daily drink or two healthy? This is another area where the pendulum has swung back and forth. At this point, the preponderance of scientific research suggests moderate drinking is beneficial. A Harvard study published in the *New England Journal of Medicine* in 2003 followed 38,000 men for twelve years and found that those who drank alcohol every other day cut their risk of having a heart attack by one third. Slightly better results came from drinking every day, but it didn't take much alcohol to get those results. Men who had half a drink a day get about the same benefit as those who had three a day. Surprisingly, it didn't much matter whether people drank hard liquor, beer, or wine—all of them seemed to keep the heart healthier.

Moderate drinking also seems to reduce the risk of stroke, according to a recent review of thirty-five studies published in the journal of the AMA. The review, conducted by researches at Tulane University, found that moderate drinkers have roughly a 20 percent lowered risk of stroke, but that heavy drinkers may double their stroke risk, compared to nondrinkers.

Experts are quick to point out that heavy drinkers face many other health risks as well, including high blood pressure, cirrhosis of the liver, pancreatitis, cancers of the head and neck, and stroke. And then there are all the social problems, like drunk driving, family strife, and poor job performance, to name just a few.

So what constitutes moderate drinking? That depends on your age and sex. For women of any age, up to one drink per day is considered moderate. For a man under sixty-five, most experts consider up to two drinks per day to be moderate; for men older than that, moderation ends with the first drink. The threshold is lower for older men because the amount of muscle tissue decreases with age, while the amount of fat increases. As a result, the same dose of alcohol will produce a higher blood alcohol level in older men than it will among men who are younger.

So does this mean you should push a glass of wine on your teetotaling hubby? No. Nobody should be pushed to take up drinking. In fact, there are lots of people who should be encouraged to avoid it altogether. Those include people with a family history of alcoholism; those who have trouble restricting their consumption; and those on medications that might interact with alcohol. It is also important to know that men tend to get into more trouble with alcohol than women, which makes pushing your partner to drink a doubly bad idea. There is also some evidence that taking up alcohol late in life to reap health benefits may keep you from having a heart attack but increase your risk of death from other causes.

The American Heart Association does not make a specific recommendation about alcohol beyond saying that if you do drink, do so moderately. The group also points out a few other things to consider about alcohol:

- It has calories, an issue if you're counting them.
- Its protective effect is not evident in all populations, particularly African-Americans.
- If you drink heavily, cut back. It reduces your risk of stroke.

There's another thing worth thinking about. How much a person drinks seems to be less important than a person's pattern of drinking. Having one drink every day is more beneficial—and much less dangerous—than downing seven shots at one sitting and none for the rest of the week. Binge drinking, even occasionally, carries lots of risks. If your partner seems to have a problem with bingeing or regularly drinking too much, see chapter 16. Even moderate drinkers may want to review their alcohol consumption periodically with their doctor to make sure it continues to be a healthy habit.

Finally, any amount of alcohol can impair your ability to drive a car or operate machinery. Waiting a few hours before doing anything that requires skill or coordination is important—even for the moderate drinker!

To sum it all up, let me make use of one of the oldest scientific methods known to humankind—common sense. Common sense tells me that a little bit of alcohol is okay and too much is bad. And that if you don't drink at all, there's little reason to start. There are better ways to prevent heart disease. You should also bear this in mind: Alcohol affects different people differently and general pronouncements about alcohol are just that—general. They may or may not apply to you or to your loved one.

VITAMINS AND SUPPLEMENTS

Walk into any vitamin or health food store and you'll see bottles, jars, and tubs filled with pills, powders, and potions that promise to make a guy look like Arnold and make love like Marc Anthony. In 2002, *American Medical News* reported that 43 percent of Americans have used some form of vitamins or dietary supplements and are spending an estimated $40 billion a year on these products. But many of these products don't do much, except make your wallet lighter. Some may even be dangerous. Not long ago, I watched as a colleague lost twenty pounds using a supplement that suppressed his appetite. He looked great—for a while. Slowly the weight crept back on and now he's right back where he started. In fact, he's heavier. And since the product he was taking contained ephedra, a powerful stimulant that has been linked to heart problems and death, he put his health at risk for no reason.

The trouble with many of these supplements is that there is little or no scientific information to back up their frequently extravagant claims. In fact, the grander and more extreme the claims, the less likely there is to be any evidence to support them. This makes a foray into a health food store a real challenge, even for the savviest shopper. The first thing to realize is that no vitamin, mineral, or supplement can give a couch potato super energy, snap a depressed guy out of his funk, give a flabby guy washboard abs, or give a seventy-year-old the libido and stamina of a twenty-year-old. Not one.

If you're using vitamins and supplements, you need to be skeptical and use common sense, remembering that these products, unlike those sold by prescription, do not have to meet the rigorous standards for safety and effectiveness that the Food and Drug Administration requires of prescription and over-the-counter drugs.

Like so many areas of nutrition, this is one area where definitive answers are elusive. Disagreements among experts abound, and weak science leaves plenty of room for all sorts of claims from manufacturers and individuals looking to make a buck. Now, because so many Americans are taking such large quantities of these products, some health experts are concerned that many people are getting way too much and that this will ultimately backfire, making them sicker rather than healthier. Remember vitamin and mineral supplementation came about because people developed diseases related to deficiencies that simply don't exist today for most people in the United States.

For these reasons, I tend to be very cautious about using or recommending nutritional supplements. I acknowledge that many practicing doctors will have their own opinions and they may be different than mine. There is one thing, however, of which I am supremely confident: No vitamin, supplement, or pill will make up for a poor diet. You cannot eat junk food all day and then pop a multivitamin before bed and believe you've got it covered. You don't. A healthy diet such as those mentioned in this chapter and on page 421—the DASH diet—will do more for your health than any pill or potion you buy in the health food store.

Before taking any over-the-counter supplement, vitamin, or mineral I urge you to talk with a doctor or registered dietician. In some cases, seemingly benign products can have side effects in people with certain medical conditions. Discourage family members from taking megadoses of any vitamin, supplement, mineral, or herb. This is dangerous and can be deadly!

The Multivitamin: Good Insurance or Waste of Money?

Having said all that, let me also tell you that the daily multivitamin was recently endorsed in the *New England Journal of Medicine*—the most influential medical journal in Western medicine—by some highly respected medical experts, Walter Willett, M.D., and Meir Stampfer, M.D., of Harvard University. They wrote: "Given the greater likelihood of benefit than harm, and considering the low cost, we conclude that a daily multivitamin that does not exceed the RDA of its component vitamins makes sense for most adults."

Not everyone agrees with this position, of course. Benjamin Caballero, M.D., director of the Center for Human Nutrition at Johns Hopkins University, told *The New York Times* in 2003 there is no disease he knows of that is prevented by multivitamins, so he personally doesn't take one.

The problem—and the reason equally respectable experts disagree—is there are no definitive studies showing that a daily multivitamin will do anything for you. You or your partner may want to take one if your diet is not what it should be. But remember, taking a multivitamin does not make up for a poor diet. If it's a choice between a healthy diet and a multi, choose the healthy diet. If your partner (or you) eat a reasonable diet, then a multivitamin might not be necessary.

If your partner does decide to take a multi, the question is whether he should choose one with or without iron. There is some evidence that iron can contribute to heart disease by speeding the oxidation of cholesterol and increasing the chances that it will stick to artery walls. This is controversial and not everyone is convinced. However, studies have found that men who donated blood (thereby decreasing iron stores) have a lowered risk of heart attack than nondonors. Some experts also speculate that women's generally lower level of iron helps fend off heart disease until well after menopause when menstruation stops and iron levels rise. Bottom line: Nearly all experts agree that if a man is not anemic, iron is not necessary.

The best way to make a decision about a daily multivitamin is for your husband or you to speak to a doctor, preferably one with some nutrition knowledge, about your own health and risk factors. A registered dietitian may be able to help you sort it out if the physician seems unfamiliar with this area.

The Antioxidants

For a while, antioxidants were the rock stars of vitamins. Every day, it seems, we heard about their curative powers for everything from heart disease to cancer. More recently, though, the air has leaked out of this bubble. Antioxidants such as beta-carotene, vitamin A, vitamin E, selenium, and vitamin C are clearly powerful agents that can affect our health, but they are not the panacea we might hope for—at least not when taken as supplements.

Antioxidants help rid the body of potentially harmful substances that are created through normal cellular activity. They act as scavengers of particles known as oxygen-free radicals, the by-products of the body's normal chemical processes. Free radicals are the bad guys. They can damage genetic material or cell membranes, contributing to atherosclerosis, which may help trigger cancer. Free radicals are increased by smoking, environmental toxins, and stress.

Would most men benefit by taking antioxidants in supplement form, or can they get what they need by eating foods that contain them naturally? For most of these vitamins, there's probably no need to take supplements if you consume a healthy diet. In fact, it is possible to get too much of some of these vitamins, especially vitamin A, which can be toxic at high doses and may contribute to osteoporosis.

When it comes to vitamin overuse, vitamin C is the all-time standout. Many of my friends and colleagues take large doses of vitamin C, especially during cold season. The problem is that the body doesn't hold on to these large doses, and there is little evidence that taking so much will do anything for you besides give you expensive urine.

Vitamin E

Preventing or treating heart disease with vitamin E has been one of the great hopes of health researchers. Hopes were so high many cardiologists were taking it as a supplement long before it was proven it could help. Now it looks like it doesn't—and many of these cardiologists have stopped. The most recent knock on vitamin E comes from researchers at the Cleveland Clinic who analyzed numerous studies and concluded in a report in *The Lancet* that vitamin E had no effect on heart health and that people should give up on the idea that vitamin E in supplement form is the magic pill they have been waiting for. Investigators are also looking at whether vitamin E might help reduce the risk of prostate cancer, but it is way too soon to tell if it does.

There is mounting evidence that other antioxidants such as beta-carotene—a form of vitamin A—taken in supplement form may actually be bad for your health and may even increase the risk of cancer and cardiovascular disease. Trying to best Mother Nature by putting these nutrients in pill form has not worked so far, and I don't think it ever will. But that's okay. Mother Nature provides us with plenty of antioxidants in fresh fruits and vegetables, as well as some other healthy foods. Another reason that Mom was right about eating your vegetables!

The B Vitamins

While the antioxidants have lost luster in the past few years, the Bs have gained new status. The darling of the Bs is folate, also known as folic acid. The buzz about folate began when it was established that women of childbearing years who take folate supplements before and during pregnancy reduce the risk of neural tube birth defects (primarily spina bifida) in their babies. And some more recent research suggests that folate may also help men make healthier babies. A study in *Fertility and Sterility,* found that men with low levels of folate seem to have decreased sperm counts and sperm density.

There is also some evidence folate can help prevent heart disease by reducing levels of homocysteine, an amino acid normally found in the blood that seems to increase the risk of heart attack and stroke at higher levels. Homocysteine may damage coronary arteries or make it easier for blood-clotting cells called *platelets* to clump together and form a clot. Since homocysteine has also been linked to brain atrophy and vascular disease, it is also possible that folate could reduce the risk of both of these problems.

In 1998, the FDA recommended that all cereal-grain products be fortified with folic acid. As a result, most people are getting more folate than in the past, though it is probably still not enough, since many of us don't eat as well as we should. You can make sure you're getting enough by eating a healthy diet (include lots of dark leafy vegetables and wheat germ).

Other Bs that appear to be helpful are B_6 and B_{12}. A recent study found that these two, in combination with folate, decreased the risk that coronary arteries would get reblocked after angioplasty. B_{12} deficiency (documented through a blood test) may be a problem for some older men, and in those cases supplementation may be necessary. For most men, though, a well-balanced diet will supply enough folate, B_6, and B_{12} to maintain good health.

Vitamin D

One vitamin men should consider taking as a supplement is vitamin D. This is especially true for men living in northern states, where exposure to sunlight is limited. Vitamin D is found in food, but it can also be made in the body after exposure to ultraviolet sunlight. Supplementation is useful for those who do not drink milk. By law milk must be fortified with vitamin D. Also known as "the sunshine vitamin," vitamin D is necessary for the effective absorption of calcium. The goal is to get enough vitamin D to reach the RDA of 400 IU. If your family does not live in a sunny clime, and your husband does not get a few minutes of strong sunshine every day, then taking a supplement makes sense. Sunscreens with a sun protection factor of 8 or greater will block UV rays that produce vitamin D, but it is still important to routinely use sunscreen whenever sun exposure is longer than ten to fifteen minutes.

Minerals

Do men need calcium? At least one nutritional expert, Dr. Willett, thinks the calcium crisis for adult Americans has been overstated. He says guys will do just fine if they get no more than 1,200 mg a day and they can probably get by with much less. While women have a particularly high need for calcium to protect them for the risk of osteoporosis and hip fractures, men, too, are at increasing risk of developing osteoporosis as they age (see page 484). Older men should get at least 1,000 mg of calcium daily. If your husband's diet doesn't include enough dairy or other sources of calcium to meet or exceed that goal, dietary supplements are appropriate.

The use of selenium is being studied as a possible way to reduce the risk of prostate cancer. It acts like an antioxidant, but until studies now under way are complete, it's still too early to say whether men should take it in supplement form.

Finally, before buying any supplement, check for the logo of the USP (U.S. Pharmacopoeia is a nongovernmental organization that promotes the public health by establishing state-of-the-art standards to ensure the quality of medicines and other health-care technologies). This notation means that the manufacturer has followed standards set by the USP and will help you be sure that the ingredients listed on the package are actually in the supplements, in the listed amounts, and that they are potent.

Herbal Supplements

When it comes to herbal supplements for men, things get even more murky. I personally do not take herbal supplements because product analyses have frequently found they simply don't contain what they claim. How can we trust a product that does not contain what it promises on the label? Still, I know many people enthusiastically take herbal supplements and swear by them.

There are lots of books and hundred of websites that provide information on herbal remedies. A quick web search or a trip to the bookstore can help you, if you find a trustworthy source. Here are two that I think are reliable:

Consumer Lab (*www.consumerlab.com*) tests all kinds of supplements for purity and strength and maintains a large encyclopedia of information on vitamins, minerals, and herbs, including information on drug interactions. It is also indexed by medical condition. Some information is free; most is available for a small subscription.

Joe and Teresa Graedon, well-known experts on pharmaceuticals and medicinal herbal products, are the authors of many books, including *The People's Pharmacy*. Their website of the same name (*http://www.healthcentral.com/peoplespharmacy/peoplespharmacy.cfm*) includes articles, answers to questions about drugs and herbal products, and a library of medicinal herbs. In addition, the National Institutes of Health maintains a useful website (*http://www.cc.nih.gov/ccc/supplements*) on vitamins and supplements.

MEN AND DOCTORS

Rikers Island, New York, is one of the few places in America where men look forward to seeing their doctor regularly, and talking about their health worries freely and at length. That's because Rikers Island, located in the middle of the East River, a stone's throw from Manhattan, is the largest municipal jail in the nation. On any given day there are nearly fifteen thousand men (and a handful of women) incarcerated in the jail's ten facilities. It's more a way station than a penitentiary; most inmates are being held pending final sentencing or trial, but that can be a very long wait. In the meantime, they have to survive, and that's no mean feat in a place as rough as Rikers. To escape the jail's pervasive environment of fear, to get some relief from the constant state of vigilance they must live in, the men find all sorts of reasons to see the doctor. I know. I was one of their doctors for two years. What seems to the rest of us as one definition of purgatory—sitting for hours in a doctor's waiting room—is heaven for the men of Rikers Island. They can't wait for their next appointment and will more often than not fabricate an illness just to get out of their cells and down to the infirmary.

But for men elsewhere in America, a doctor's office is often threatening territory, a place of last resort. And the notion of actually seeking out the advice of a doctor, much less visiting one for routine checkups, is almost unthinkable. After all, to do so is to place one's fate in the hands of another, to lose control, to admit vulnerability. It also means paying attention to what's going on inside one's body, to notice the signs of potential problems, rather than to ignore them or to shrug them off. And let's face it: None of this comes naturally for most men. I am sure this is one important reason why men die, on average, five years earlier than women.

To be fair, there are some men who take great care of themselves, seek medical attention in a timely manner, and take the physician's advice to heart. I have several great friends, all doctors, who do just that. Their wives, I am sure, play almost no role in how they care for themselves. They have successfully applied their medical knowledge to their own lives without being nudged by anyone. However, even though the men I know who do this are all doctors, don't draw any broad conclusions about how most male doctors manage their health.

Many doctors, in fact, are partially negligent about having a source of regular health care. A recent Yale study of more than nine hundred doctors who had graduated from the prestigious Johns Hopkins University School of Medicine found that

34 percent of them had no regular doctor themselves. And these weren't fresh-out-of-med-school interns—their average age was sixty-one. Sixty of the doctors even said their primary care doctor was the one they saw in the mirror every morning! Kind of reminds you of that old adage about lawyers who represent themselves having a fool for a client.

Dealing with Avoidance

A colleague of mine, a famous newsman who will go unnamed, prides himself on not seeking help for a painful knee. Sure, it's not a fatal problem, but it clearly causes him discomfort and affects his quality of life. Every once in a while I point this out to him and remind him that the longer he waits to get it treated, the more serious and involved the treatment becomes (read: knee replacement—hello!). A dirty look and a growl is all I get for my trouble. Macho guys who love sports don't see doctors for little problems. He is not my husband, though, so I don't put on the full-court press. I figure one day he simply won't have a choice.

Even when health care is free, men don't take advantage. Wajdy Hailoo, M.D., head of Occupational and Environmental Medicine at State University of New York Stony Brook School of Medicine, found that out when he was hired by several companies to provide free health care to employees. Only 15 percent of the men who worked for these companies took advantage of the offer for free exams and services.

Sad to say, this kind of attitude toward getting medical care is typical of a lot of men, and it's one of the biggest reasons there's such a disparity in the health of men and women. A case in point: There are hundreds, perhaps thousands, of women's health clinics around the country, yet hardly any men's health clinics. They are so few that we could find no hard data on exactly how many exist. And even if they were built, there is no guarantee that men would come. Male resistance to going to the doctor runs deep and the reasons for resisting are many. "There probably is no more threatening an environment for men than the examination room," says Dr. Kenneth Goldberg, a Dallas urologist who, for eleven years, operated the Male Health Center, a men's clinic in Dallas. Goldberg closed his center for personal reasons in 2000, though he continues to operate a website (*www.malehealthcenter.com*) that provides a wide range of information about men's health.

Just how threatening to men are doctors' offices? In an annual survey conducted by the editors of *Men's Health* magazine and CNN, one third of all men said they would not go to the doctor even if they were experiencing severe chest pain or shortness of breath—two signs of a possible heart attack.

And remember that report that we discussed in the Overview, the one with the perfect name—*Out of Touch: American Men and the Health Care System?* It found that one third of men had no regular doctor, one quarter of men had not seen a doctor in the previous year, and one third of men over fifty had not been screened for prostate or colon cancer in the past five years.

What reasons do men give for shunning the doctor's office? The number one reason, according to the CNN/*Men's Health* survey, was that it's "too much trouble to get checked when nothing is bothering you." Being too busy was also a major excuse for avoiding the doctor. In the 2000 survey, 61 percent of men said they would go to the doctor if it only took ten minutes or it was free.

But if these are the reasons men admit to, there are others that go much deeper and may, in fact, be more telling. Men are raised in our culture to pride themselves on their toughness and self-reliance, to be active rather than passive, and to value independence over dependence. In other words, men like to be in control and they don't like to feel weak. Even with the most enlightened and progressive of doctors, being a patient means admitting to a degree of vulnerability and weakness. It means sitting, waiting, and letting someone else be the expert, the one in charge. It means giving up a degree of control and having to ask for help.

But there's another element that, on the surface, doesn't seem to fit with these macho characteristics: fear. I think a lot of men are scared to go to the doctor. They're scared of what they might learn, they're scared of the very vulnerability that they know they have but feel they can't admit, they're scared of pain and worried that they'll respond to it in ways that are "unacceptable." One result of all this avoidance is that by the time men go to the doctor for medical attention, their problems are often much more serious and difficult to treat.

One way many men deal with their reluctance to get the help they need is to seek it indirectly. They'll go to a doctor with a sports injury and hope the doctor will ask pointed questions that get to the real problem—his worries about his sexual function, for instance.

In the end, I think that these deeper psychological and cultural factors combine with the kinds of practical issues that turned up in the CNN/*Men's Health* survey to keep men out of the doctor's office. In a 1999 report in the *Journal of Family Practice,* a group of family doctors noted that men seem especially put off by long waiting periods before they can see a doctor. This may be more than just an issue of wasted time. Since some men tend to feel embarrassed by even going to the doctor, sitting for a long time in a public waiting room may be especially hard for them to tolerate.

Another point mentioned in the *Journal of Family Practice* report was that men may be reluctant to discuss their medical problems on the phone or in person with female receptionists and staff members or within earshot of other patients.

So How Can You Help?
Be Convincing

Tell your husband how much his health matters to you and to the rest of your family. Appeal to him as your loving man, reminding him how much you love and need him and want him to remain in your life (and your bed). Point out to him that if he isn't well, he won't be of much use to anyone, including the very people he wants most to help and take care of. If he's resistant and if you think it might help, include your kids in this conversation, assuming they're old enough.

There are national screening days or awareness weeks for a variety of diseases (see Resources). When one of these weeks comes up, and it's for a problem you think your husband might be at risk for, use the opportunity to start a conversation with him. Let him know that this is something you're concerned about and talk together about what he might be able to do to find out more about his health and level of risk for the disease.

Often one of the best ways to cajole a man to go is to tell the story of a friend who went to the doctor and was helped. You might also include a story where a man didn't go and had a bad outcome!

Be Clever

Look for sneaky, stealthy ways to get him "in" to the health-care system. Check out the newspaper or TV for listings about free health screenings that are coming up. Then just happen to show up together at the mall or state fairgrounds when the screenings are taking place. You could ask him to accompany you to your routine ob/gyn or prenatal appointment. Then, while you're there, ask the nurse to check his blood pressure.

Doctors from Washington University School of Medicine set up a study that did exactly that. At four obstetrical offices men who came in were offered a free blood pressure check and some two hundred accepted. Surprisingly, 20 percent of those tested had high blood pressure, though their average age was only thirty.

Be Assertive

Recruit backup if you need to. His mother might be a good candidate to help convince him to go to the doctor. So might his best friend or his boss. If you have to, make an appointment with the doctor yourself at a time when you know your husband will be free. When the day comes, get him in the car and take him there. You can decide for yourself when to tell him.

Obviously, since you know your husband, you'll have a good sense of which of these techniques might work best and which might blow up in your face. Whatever approach you choose—and you may have your own creative ideas—be sure that the underlying message comes through: You love him, are worried about him, and want him to get the care he needs.

One practical suggestion: If long waiting times really bug him, he—or you—may be able to minimize this by calling ahead before he goes and making sure the doctor is running on time.

Help Find the Right Doctor

My husband is the kind of man who just won't put up with superior attitudes or with people who lack a sense of humor, even a doctor. For that reason, we've looked around quite a bit to find someone who suits my husband's personality. By asking friends for recommendations and doing some footwork, we've been able to find someone my husband can relate to. And since he now likes his doctor, going to see him is less of a chore.

To my mind, finding the right doctor also means finding someone who believes that talking with patients and counseling them about health behaviors is time well spent. If you can find someone who incorporates this into his or her practice, it can make a difference. A study in the *Journal of the American Medical Association* showed that when doctors or other health-care workers provided just three hours of counseling over a two-year period, their sedentary male patients started getting more exercise. Unfortunately, most doctors don't do this very often or very well. Despite research that indicates physicians are successful in encouraging smokers to quit, a recent survey of Rhode Islanders found that physicians are doing so only about half the time. Investigators Michael G. Goldstein, M.D., and colleagues from the Brown University School of Medicine asked 3,037 adult smokers who had visited physicians within the last year whether they had received advice about quitting. Just 46 percent said they had.

It's true that HMOs and managed care make it difficult to find a doctor you can connect with and who has enough time to get to know you. But even in HMOs, you will have a choice of primary-care doctors, so don't settle for one you don't like. Before you choose a doctor, learn as much as you can about those on the list for your HMO. Credentials are important, for sure; they should be board-certified in their specialty. But word of mouth from friends or other patients about a particular doctor can be enormously revealing. If a doctor is always hurried or rude with a friend of yours, chances are you'll get the same treatment. There are several books that I think are worth reviewing if you are not savvy at getting the best out of an HMO. I really like *Don't Let Your HMO Kill You,* by Drs. Jason Theodosakis and David T. Feinberg. The title may seem a little dramatic, but this book gives excellent suggestions for working within a deeply flawed system to get the best care possible. Also check out *The Complete Idiot's Guide to Managed Health Care,* by Sophie M. Korczyk and Hazel A. Witte, and *The Castle Connolly Guide to the ABCs of HMOs: How to Get the Best from Managed Care.*

Does a Doctor's Gender Matter?

A generation ago, medicine was an overwhelmingly male field and the stereotype of a doctor was Marcus Welby. Today, one in four doctors are women and almost as many women as men are entering medical school. That means that gender dynamics, preferences, and politics are as much a part of the field of medicine as they are any other part of our society.

So how do men feel about the gender of their doctors? And how does the gender of doctors affect their relationship to male patients?

First of all, studies show that both men and women prefer doctors of their same sex for intimate health needs such as gynecology or urology. But here's the surprise: With the exception of these areas, women and men alike still overwhelmingly prefer male doctors. Among male patients, the preference for male doctors is a bit higher.

That said, men who reflexively choose male doctors may be missing out on some qualities they would actually appreciate, if they could get past their biases. A review of twenty-six studies published in the *Journal of the American Medical Association* suggests that women doctors spend more time with their patients, listen more attentively, ask more questions, and are less likely to dominate the conversation. They are also more likely to ask about emotional and social issues that may play a part in the medical issues at hand. Female physicians, studies suggest, are also more likely to recommend preventive tests and to discuss behavior change as a way to better health. Ironically, these kinds of concerns and sensitivities among women doctors could make them especially helpful to men, who in general have a stronger need to make changes in their diets, lifestyles, and habits than women. And indeed, one study of patients at an HMO in Northern California found that the most satisfied patients were males who had chosen female doctors. (Curiously, the least satisfied were female patients who chose female doctors—possibly because they had expectations of their female doctors that the docs couldn't meet in the context of a busy, time-pressured HMO practice.)

Another study of physicians found that a doctor's ability to motivate a patient to change and adopt healthy habits was enhanced when the doctor talked about his or her own health habits, something that female physicians are more likely to do. And another study, in *The Lancet*, finds that when doctors offer advice in a compassionate, understanding way, they are more likely to be listened to than those who take a more formal, informational approach devoid of reassuring words. And once again, the warmer style of interaction is more common among female doctors.

In all of this it's important to say that when we talk about the styles and tendencies of female and male doctors as a group we're talking about just that—tendencies. In these studies, patients are surveyed and doctors are observed interacting with their patients. But the fact that certain patterns are noticed in many members of a group tells you nothing about the bedside manner and approach of any individual doctor, male or female. I can think of plenty of female doctors that so lack warmth and personality I wouldn't let them examine my pet snake. And I have met many wonderful male doctors whose humor and humanity could win over anyone.

There are, of course, many other reasons men may have for preferring doctors of one gender over the other. Some men may prefer women because they are competitive by nature and don't want to discuss weaknesses with other men. Others avoid women doctors because they're afraid they will get an erection (it happens). And then there are men who don't want to be touched by other men because they are homophobic.

So what does all this mean for you and your partner if you're trying to help him develop an ongoing relationship with a doctor? Mostly this: If your partner is physician-phobic or resists seeing a doctor, one thing to try to discuss with him is what kind of qualities he would like to have in a doctor. Has he had negative experiences with a doctor that keep him from wanting to go back? The more involved he gets in thinking about these issues and in choosing a doctor, the more likely he'll be to want to return for regular visits.

Help Him Organize His Thoughts Before You Go

Have you had this experience? Your husband complains to you several times about headaches that he seems to keep getting. On other occasions he mentions that he's having trouble sleeping and that his knee feels unstable. You suggest that he make an appointment with the doctor, and he waves his hand at you like you've taken leave of your senses. "I'm not going to the doctor for this. This is nothing," he says. "Besides my physical's coming up in a few weeks. I'll talk to him then."

The weeks go by, and he finally has his physical. When he comes home, you ask him what the doctor said about his headaches, his insomnia, and his knee. He gives you a blank look. "We didn't talk about it," he tells you. "It didn't come up."

Or perhaps your husband has been found to have the early signs of coronary artery disease. He meets with a cardiologist who outlines the different steps he could take. Then he comes home and you ask him a million questions. "I don't know," your husband keeps saying. "He didn't talk about that."

Many men just aren't that used to going to the doctor. They tend to minimize the seriousness of their problems and are not accustomed to thinking deeply or strategically about medical issues. Plus, studies show that men approach doctors differently than women do. A lot of men won't come right out and tell the doctor what's bothering them—unless they have a sports-related or other injury. They'll make an appointment for a general health exam, hoping the doctor will ask pointed questions that get to the real problem. Most men could really use some assistance here, and there's a lot you can do to help.

Even highly educated men may need some help dealing with doctors and asking them questions. A few years ago, Maury Waters, a retired university professor and the father of my cowriter, Rob Waters, was told by his urologist that a recent rapid increase in his PSA scores was worrisome and might indicate prostate cancer. A biopsy was scheduled, and while they were waiting for that appointment, Maury and his wife, Elly, read lots about prostate cancer and various approaches to treatment.

Despite his years of education and teaching, Maury, like many men, is not good at asking questions of health-care providers. So Elly drew up a list of questions about the condition and the pros and cons of various treatments. At their next meeting, the doctor performed the biopsy and answered all the questions. In fact, he was so impressed by them that he asked for a copy to show his urology residents. At their next meeting, the couple got doubly good news: The biopsy was negative, and the residents had found the questions very useful in understanding the patient's point of view.

If your husband has an important medical appointment coming up, or even a routine one, spend a little time talking with him a few days before the visit. Ask him what he wants to bring up with the doctor. If he hasn't done so, suggest that he make a list of the things he wants to discuss with the doctor and the questions he wants to ask. Other questions will surely arise based on what the doctor says during the appointment, but if your husband's like mine (or like me), he'll forget an important question and then kick himself later for not asking.

Tell him that you'll be happy to go over the list with him. You should also suggest that he think about and write down the medical history of close family members, making some calls to fill in the gaps in his knowledge, if necessary.

In addition to his family history, he should think about his own health history and his current habits. If he thinks about this ahead of time, he will do less hemming and hawing and have less difficulty with recall. He should write down on a piece of paper all the significant things that have happened through the years: surgeries, abnormal test results, and bouts of serious illness. Don't forget to include a mental health history. If he's had past problems with depression or substance abuse, that's very important for a doctor to know.

It's also a good idea to have a list of medications. It should include prescriptions, over-the-counter medications, vitamins, and supplements taken regularly or even sporadically. The list should include the dosage, how often it is taken, and what it's taken for. This can be very helpful. especially when a patient sees more than one doctor or takes more than one medication regularly. A thorough list can save a lot of time and will help give you and your spouse a more complete understanding of his overall health.

A word about organizing your records. I am a big fan of *The Savard Health Record: A Six-Step System for Managing Your Healthcare,* by Marie Savard, M.D. This binder system of organizing your medical records is one of the best I have seen and can really help you pull everything together. You can buy it online at either Barnes & Noble (*www.bn.com*) or Amazon.com. Most of us don't have this thorough a record of our own health, and I believe this can be a huge help when you see a doctor or have an emergency.

How Healthy Is His Family Tree?

If you and your husband want to know more about his risk for different health problems, a good way to start is to find out the medical history of his close relatives. If several of his immediate relatives died young from heart disease or cancer, this is a big red flag. If, for example, there is a family history of diabetes, high blood pressure, or mental illness, this is helpful to know. If you're aware of the medical conditions hiding in the branches of his family tree, you, your husband, and your husband's doctor should develop a plan for prevention and early, aggressive testing. The trouble is that it's not always easy to get this vital information, especially for (or from) men.

In times past, people didn't like to talk about health problems, and intimate information was often cloaked in secrecy. In most families, people who fell ill were cared for by the women. As a result, the details of Aunt Millie's cancer or Uncle Joe's heart condition were probably known to the women and not much discussed outside their circles. For all these reasons, your husband might be unfamiliar with his family's medical history. However, it's really important that he learn as much as he can—even if it means that he or you have to ask some uncomfortable questions of his mother or other family members.

Carol Krause's quest to learn her family's history literally saved her life. She put the lessons she learned into her book *How Healthy Is Your Family Tree,* a step-by-step guide on how to uncloak family medical secrets by sleuthing for medical records and deciphering doctor-speak. If your husband is uncomfortable questioning his mother, father, or other relatives, you might offer to do it for him. It is important to learn as much as possible about both sides of his family and important to remember that some problems can resurface in different forms across genders. For example, having a mother with breast cancer puts a son at risk for prostate cancer. Your doctor will be able to make these connections and devise an appropriate follow-up plan.

Of course, good news can sometimes be squandered. A man may think that since many of his ancestors lived to one hundred, he's somehow super-protected and doesn't have to worry about diet or smoking or exercise. Big mistake. Knowing your family genes tend toward longevity is nice, but it is no guarantee. Plenty of people with long-lived relatives die young from heart disease or cancer brought on by unhealthy habits.

Should You Snitch on Your Husband to His Doctor?

Here's another scenario: After much cajoling from his wife, Bob has finally agreed to see a dermatologist about some moles. The doctor asks Sarah and Bob to come into his office so they can talk before he examines the moles. He asks Bob a series of questions, including how often he uses sunscreen and if he covers up when he goes outside. Bob replies that he is careful about the sun and wears a hat and sunscreen often. Sarah's eyes pop out of her head. In fact, Bob, who is balding, never protects his head from the sun and puts sunscreen on only when Sarah reminds him to. That past summer, Bob had a bad sunburn on top of his head. Should Sarah correct her husband in front of the doctor? Should she snitch?

I believe this scenario is played out in doctors' offices all the time. I've seen it happen with my own husband, and I'm sure many women reading this book have heard their partner give doctors a highly sanitized version of his own health habits. It usually falls to the wife to point out that no, he doesn't actually go to the gym three times a week and he smokes a pack a day, not just a few cigarettes.

The good news is that many physicians are familiar with this phenomenon and know that people—especially men—tend to shade the truth. An experienced doctor may ask patients, "Is there anything your wife would tell me if she were here today?" Or, better yet, he or she will turn to the wife and ask her directly.

"I often have a separate conversation with the wife and get a very different story than what I get from the man," says preventive cardiologist Lori Mosca, M.D., of Columbia University in New York City. "I think that the truth is usually somewhere in the middle. There doesn't necessarily have to be a single truth. There can be a perspective that the wife sees, but the wife isn't with the man all day long and she may not see what his competing priorities are."

The question becomes how far to go? It probably depends on the seriousness of the problem and how great the denial. Obviously this puts us women in an awkward position. After all, it's his health and his doctor, and most of us wish we did not have to monitor his health so closely. But we often feel that we do.

I snitched on my husband once when we met with a famous cholesterol doctor. The doctor asked about his eating history, how much he exercised, and what kind of stress he was under. My husband said his cholesterol problem was relatively new and that he ate a fairly healthy diet. My jaw dropped. The truth is he's had high cholesterol for years and has never met a Snickers bar he didn't want.

I was shocked by what my husband told the doctor and felt it was important he know the truth. So when Avery got up to go to the bathroom, I told him. "What my husband just told you is not entirely true," I said. "Duh," the doctor said. "They all lie, I know that." I probably did not to need to say a word, since my husband's cholesterol levels spoke for themselves.

Providing doctors with complete information is important, but so is picking your battles. Dr. Mosca's advice is to try to remain in a supportive, not controlling, role. "It's hard enough for men to open up," she says. "And when you get a woman in there trying to finish his sentences and tell him that he's not communicating reality to the physician—I've seen the man shut down completely. So not unlike marriage counseling, it may sometimes be a good idea for the woman to meet with the doctor separately, give her perspective, let me meet with the husband separately, and then do the educational intervention together."

One frustration for many women is that a doctor can tell a male patient the exact same thing his wife has told him numerous times—only then he'll listen because it's coming from a doctor. "I just sit there and watch [women] roll their eyes and say, 'How many times have I told him this and he didn't listen,' " says Dr. Mosca. What can I say? As a physician and a wife, I know this one from both sides. (See the Resources section for books that address patient-physician communication.)

TESTING, TESTING, 1, 2, 3 . . .
The Basics of Routine Health Care for Men

The following is a description of the basic evaluation men in generally good health need as a baseline and then as follow-up. This is an outline only. Many men may need more sophisticated or more frequent testing, and only a doctor can determine that. Some tests are offered to everyone in a certain group when they reach a certain age or if they have certain risk factors, such as their ethnicity or their family history. These tests are called *screening tests*. Other tests may be given to individuals because they have symptoms that may point to a particular condition and doctors want to get additional information. These are called *diagnostic tests*.

Whether or not these tests are covered by insurance will depend on your plan. For a brief discussion on dealing with managed care see page 325. The checklist below is a quick rundown of the tests men should consider having during each decade of life. I admit that this is an ideal—few men get all these tests. In addition, it is important to know that not everyone agrees on all points within this checklist. Using a variety of sources and my own experience, I have crafted a quick reference checklist for men's health. Because there are differing opinions, don't be surprised if other health professionals make different recommendations. You can also see a checklist by the U.S. Department of Health and Human Services Office of Women's Health (yes, they keep a checklist for men) by going to *www.4woman.gov/screeningcharts/mens.htm*.

Following my checklist is a more detailed discussion of some of these tests.

QUICK REFERENCE CHECKLIST FOR MEN'S HEALTH

Test/ Procedure	Ages 18–39	Ages 40–49	Ages 50–64	Ages 65 +
Routine Physical Exam				
Every 3–5 years	✔			
Every 1–2 years		✔		
Yearly			✔	✔
Weight/BMI				
At every visit or at least:				
Every 3–5 years	✔			
Every 1–2 years		✔	✔	✔
Blood Pressure				
At every visit or at least:				
Every 1–2 years	✔	✔	✔	✔
Cholesterol				
At least:				
Every 5 years	✔	✔	✔	✔
Diabetes Screening				
At least:				
Every 3–5 years	✔			
Every 3 years (high risk more frequent)		✔	✔	✔
Prostate Cancer Screening		✔ (high risk)	✔*	✔*
Colon Cancer Screening				
Fecal Occult Blood Test (every year)		✔	✔	
Colonoscopy (every 3–5 years)		✔ (high risk)	✔	

* See discussion, pages 334–46.

Test/ Procedure	Ages 18–39	Ages 40–49	Ages 50–64	Ages 65 +
CBC/Metabolic Panel As needed or at time of routine physical exam for baseline	✔	✔	✔	✔
Urinalysis Every 3 years Every 2 years Yearly	✔	✔	✔	✔
TB Skin Test Every 5 years	✔	✔	✔	✔
ECG Baseline Every 4 years Every 3 years	✔	✔	✔	✔
Cardiac Stress Test	If indicated*	If indicated*	If indicated*	If indicated*
Vision Every 2–4 years Every 1–2 years		✔	✔ ✔	
Teeth Every 6 months	✔	✔	✔	✔
Lung Cancer Screening	Controversial*	Controversial*	Controversial*	Controversial*
Vaccinations Flu shot Tetanus booster Pneumococcal Pneumonia Vaccine	Yearly (optional) Every 10 years	Yearly (optional) Every 10 years	Yearly Every 10 years	Yearly Every 10 years Once at age 65

See discussion, pages 334–46.

ROUTINE PHYSICAL EXAM

The physical exam is one of the most dreaded parts of routine health care for many men. One of the main reasons is the digital rectal exam (DRE). I can't tell you how many times I have heard men tell me they avoid the doctor like the plague because they don't want that "finger test." Make no mistake about it: Men hate the DRE.

It's hard for us to have much sympathy about this one. I mean, give me a break. We give birth, for crying out loud! But what can I say? Apparently, these big, brave men who can grin and bear horrible pain are almost traumatized by this test and the way it makes them feel invaded.

The good news is that most men can get a reprieve from this test until they turn forty. But after that, it should be part of the "regular" physical. Which brings me to my next point: I asked a few men around my office recently—all of them thirty-somethings—about the last time they had seen a doctor for a routine checkup. Not one had *ever* seen a doctor just to check in and see where they stood, though most had visited for the flu or an injury and had had their cholesterol and blood pressure checked for one reason or another.

By and large, these men are healthy so they don't think much about their health. But there's a good reason for even healthy young men to have at least one good checkup with a doctor. It gives the doctor a chance to take a thorough history and provide the man with some insight about health risks he may face down the road and what he can do to try to reduce them. This will happen only if the doctor questions the man thoroughly, gets a reasonably complete family history, and learns about the man's habits—exercise, diet, smoking, drinking, drug use.

The checkup should also include a physical of course, and—sorry, guys—that DRE, if he has hit forty. This exam is one way to look for cancer or other problems in the prostate as well as signs of colon or rectal cancer and even hemorrhoids. Another thing that ought to be part of any checkup—though it rarely is—is a thorough skin exam for signs of possible skin cancer. This test can literally mean the difference between life and death. Men who are at high risk for skin cancer—because they have fair skin and a history of the disease in their family, for example—may want to find a dermatologist to do this exam annually.

So how often should men get a physical? The Men's Health Network, a national advocacy group, recommends that they get a physical exam every three years before forty and then every two years until they reach fifty. After that, it should be an annual affair. The truth is that very few men will get all this done, and that's too bad. But whatever a man does to get prevention-oriented checkups will be a whole lot better than nothing.

BLOOD PRESSURE

High blood pressure, or hypertension, is a silent killer, yet many people don't take it seriously. Until the disease is advanced, there may be no symptoms at all. But make no mistake: This disease can have deadly consequences. If your partner is diagnosed with high blood pressure, take it seriously!

The American Medical Association recommends that men who are younger than thirty should have their blood pressure checked every two to two and a half years—unless they are at high risk. "High risk" means having a family history of any one of the following: high blood pressure, heart disease, kidney disease, or stroke. Men who smoke, are overweight, have diabetes, or consume more than two drinks a day are also considered high risk.

My own feeling is that high blood pressure is so common, yet is so simple to check, and is so easy to address when it's detected early that it ought to be tested once a year. What's the big deal? If nothing else, you can get a free screening at the shopping mall, or at many hospitals, clinics, or community service organizations. This disease is just too common and the consequences of not treating it too serious to let hypertension go undetected. Men's Health Network agrees with this. See chapter 15.

BODY MASS INDEX

This simple measurement of body size assesses a person's weight in relation to his height and is the way doctors define whether a person is overweight. It also serves as an indicator for a whole host of problems including increased blood pressure, heart disease, diabetes, and even cancer. The goal is to have a BMI of between 19 and 24. A BMI of 25 to 29 is considered overweight and a BMI of 30 or greater is obese. For more on how to calculate BMI and on weight issues, see chapter 15.

BLOOD FATS

Cholesterol Level

There's good news and bad news about cholesterol. The good news is that years after the long-running Framingham Heart Study first linked cholesterol to heart disease, just about *everyone* knows they ought to watch their cholesterol. Indeed, more than 70 percent of Americans have had their cholesterol checked in the past five years, according to the American Heart Association.

The bad news is that while Americans' knowledge of cholesterol is a mile wide, it's barely an inch deep. People approach me all the time with questions about cholesterol, but it's a rare thing for them to know anything more than that they have high cholesterol. They'll often have a number—one number—but to really understand your cholesterol, you need to know two or three numbers. So here's a quick rundown on cholesterol and what those numbers mean, along with a couple of other terms.

Cholesterol is a soft, waxy substance found among the fats, or lipids, in your bloodstream and in all your body's cells. Your body makes it on its own, but you also get it from eating meat and dairy products.

Total Cholesterol

This is the number most people know. It represents the total amount of cholesterol in your blood when you add the two kinds of cholesterol together. The goal is to have less than 200 mg/dl (milligrams per deciliter of blood). But the real goal is to have the right kinds of cholesterol, as indicated by the next two numbers.

LDL (Low-Density Lipoprotein) Cholesterol

The bad guy! This type of cholesterol loves to sit around in your arteries causing fatty buildup and eventually dangerous blockages. You want this number to be as low as possible, but 160 mg/dl is the highest acceptable level for people who don't have heart disease or other risk factors. People with two or more risk factors should aim to keep this number below 130. And people who have heart disease need to keep it even lower—below 100.

HDL (High-Density Lipoprotein) Cholesterol

The good guy! This type of cholesterol goes around and cleans things up, taking fatty deposits away from the arteries. Men should have as much of this as possible—above 60 if possible, but at least above 40.

Triglycerides

Another kind of fat found in the blood that is thought to increase the risk of heart disease. Triglycerides can jump after a meal so it's important to schedule blood tests after an overnight fast. The goal is to keep them below 150. Doctors used to think they were a concern only in people who also had high cholesterol levels, but the current thinking is that high triglycerides can increase the risk for cardiovascular problems even in people with normal cholesterol. High triglycerides have also been linked to type 2 diabetes and stroke.

Risk Ratio

Cholesterol numbers can be confusing, and they can also be deceptive. For instance, a person can have high total cholesterol but if it's mostly HDL, their risk is actually low. Because of this, doctors calculate a risk ratio, which is the total cholesterol divided by the HDL. A ratio of 4.5 is average, a higher ratio means a higher risk. For example, if a person has a total cholesterol level of 265 and an HDL of 65, their risk ratio is about 4.1, which is okay. On the other hand, if their total cholesterol is 265 and their HDL is 35, then their risk ratio is 7.6—very high. The ideal ratio is 3.5 or below.

Confused? It gets a bit worse. Government health officials in 2001 raised the bar on cholesterol, changing the numbers that are considered healthy. As a result, many men will need to adjust their goals. In the past, if your partner had an HDL level of 35, he would likely have been told he was okay. Today, however, that number's not going to cut it.

How often should you and your husband check your cholesterol levels? The government's new guidelines say that everybody twenty and older should have their cholesterol levels checked at least once every five years. People whose levels are high should be tested more frequently. The Men's Health Network recommends testing every three years before forty, every two years until fifty, and once a year after that.

DIABETES

High blood sugar is a sign of diabetes. Normally insulin, a hormone made in the pancreas, allows glucose to enter your body's cells and be used as fuel. Insulin lowers glucose levels in the bloodstream. People can have too little insulin—this is type 1 diabetes—or the cells of their body can be resistant to insulin—type 2 diabetes. Unused glucose builds up in the blood and this is what doctors test for.

Our big concern is type 2 diabetes, which is now reaching epidemic proportions in this country. That's primarily because so many people are overweight or obese, as more than 80 percent of people with diabetes are. Even minor weight gains can put people at risk for adult-onset, or type 2, diabetes. Still, being overweight or obese does not mean you will always become diabetic.

Knowing one's blood sugar, or glucose level, is the best way to find out about problems before symptoms set in. The American Diabetes Association recommends that all people over forty-five be screened for diabetes every three years if they don't have risk factors; earlier if they do.

Another group, the American College of Endocrinology, thinks people should start being screened even younger—at thirty—due to an explosion of diabetes among thirty-somethings. During the 1990s, diabetes increased by 33 percent, but grew a frightening 76 percent among people in their thirties. So just because a man is young doesn't mean he's not at risk.

There are a couple of ways to check for diabetes in people who don't have symptoms. One is to take a random blood glucose level without a person fasting beforehand. A glucose level of 200 milligrams per deciliter (mg/dl) or higher strongly suggests diabetes.

The better way is the fasting plasma glucose (FPG), in which blood is drawn after an eight-hour fast. A level of less than 110 mg/dl is normal; 126 mg/dl or more means diabetes.

Catch this one early and you may stave off serious problems like blindness and kidney disease. See chapter 15 for more on diabetes.

PROSTATE CANCER SCREENING AND THE PSA BROUHAHA

In addition to their fame, Rudolph Giuliani, Norman Schwarzkopf, Bob Dole, Harry Belafonte, and Joe Torre all have one thing in common: Like some 220,000 other American men each year, they developed prostate cancer. Because so many high-profile men have been speaking so openly about this disease, it has shed light on this increasingly common cancer and helped many other men cope. These celebrity cases have also increased the awareness of screening tools, especially the Prostate Specific Antigen (PSA) blood test. When celebrities endorse a test like the PSA, it can give the impression that such a test is without controversy. The value of the PSA test, however, is hotly debated among scientists, doctors, and researchers.

The PSA measures a protein produced by the prostate. It can be elevated as the result of cancer, inflammation, or enlargement. While an elevated level can signal that something is wrong, it doesn't necessarily mean cancer. In fact, as men get older, the prostate gland enlarges, which can raise the PSA level. If the PSA is above 4 ng/ml (nanograms per milliliter), doctors may want to do other tests or simply repeat the test over time.

The problem with the PSA test is that it's not all that accurate. Nearly three quarters of the time, men with an elevated PSA turn out not to have cancer; this is called a "false positive." And sometimes, men with a low PSA score still have cancer—a "false negative." The inaccuracy of the test leads to many men getting biopsies that end up finding no cancer. And since cancer in the prostate tends to grow very slowly, it's often not that dangerous for many older men. Without treatment, many of these older men *with* prostate cancer will die from some other disease such as heart disease, not *from* prostate cancer.

Critics of routine PSA screening argue that it sets in motion a chain of events that can take on a life of its own: An elevated PSA score leads to a biopsy. A biopsy may lead to surgery to remove a cancerous prostate that might never grow large enough to affect a man's health. The surgery often leads to impotence and sometimes causes incontinence. The concern is that the PSA test will be overused finding cancers that would not spread and would cause no harm, but because the cancer was detected, men will undergo treatment that may lead to complications. The problem is figuring out which tumors will cause trouble and which ones won't, and right now there is no good way to do that.

Other experts, however, are convinced that the PSA is saving lives. They argue that inaccurate though it may be, the test can tip men off that they may have prostate cancer in time to actually treat it and prolong lives. Cancer experts in favor of screening point out that prostate cancer death rates among American men have dropped decisively in the last decade, following the introduction of the PSA test. The National Cancer Institute last year documented a "dramatic decline" in the prostate cancer death rate per 100,000 men ages fifty and older since 1992; before 1992, the rate had been rising steadily. Others argue that it is not possible to know whether this decline is a result of the PSA screening itself or earlier and better treatment, or both.

Bottom line: There's little agreement among experts on the value of PSA testing. Two large clinical trials now under way will help determine whether routine testing saves lives. Unfortunately, results won't be in for several years. In the meantime, professional groups have interpreted these uncertainties in different ways, though all agree patients must talk to their doctors about their individual situation and make informed decisions. Here's what they say.

- The National Cancer Institute has no specific guidelines on PSA testing.
- The American College of Physicians, the American Society of Internal Medicine, and the U.S. Preventive Services Task Force (a panel of experts convened by the government) say doctors and their patients should discuss screening and make individual decisions.
- The American Cancer Society and the American Urological Association recommend that following an explanation of the benefits and limitations of testing, men be given the option of undergoing an annual PSA and DRE at age fifty or younger if family history warrants it.

Recently a large study called the Prostate, Lung, Colorectal, Ovarian Cancer Screening Trial sponsored by the National Cancer Institute suggested that men who have very low PSA values (below 2 ng/ml) be offered the test less frequently—every two to five years. Eventually data from this study may help shape clearer guidelines, but for now each man must discuss his own situation with his physician.

African-American men have a dramatically higher risk for prostate cancer, and this should be taken into account when decisions about screening are made. For this reason, many experts suggest that African-American men, and any man with a family history of prostate cancer, start getting the PSA test at forty.

If your husband, or any man you love, is considering taking the PSA test, encourage him to talk it over with his doctor and to read some of the literature. He might also ask his doctor about a new test called the free PSA. When performed after a regular PSA, this test may provide a more accurate picture and better help predict who needs additional testing. Personally, I think that some form of screening should be strongly considered and that eventually the data will show that finding and treating prostate cancer in the earliest stages can save lives. And remember, just because you have had a PSA, it doesn't mean you don't need a DRE!

SCREENING TESTS FOR COLON AND RECTAL CANCER

In 1998, the husband of *Today Show* co-anchor Katie Couric died from colon cancer. After mourning her husband, Couric launched a media blitz aimed at increasing awareness of the need for colon cancer screening. The blitz included a segment on the show where Couric herself underwent a colonoscopy. Millions of Americans saw the inside of Couric's colon, which turned out to be perfectly healthy. This was far from typical morning news fare and the results were amazing—an almost 20 percent increase in the number of people getting screened for colon cancer. Yet despite all the publicity, screening for colon cancer lags behind the tests for other cancers, such as breast and cervical cancer. Only about 44 percent of people over fifty had been screened appropriately when they were surveyed in 1999, according to the Centers for Disease Control.

Apparently, many people just don't realize that cancer of the colon and rectum (known together as colorectal cancer) is the third most common cancer in the United States. It affects women and men at equal rates until age fifty; after that it strikes women more often, mostly because we live longer. In 2002, the American Cancer Society estimates that 148,000 new cases were diagnosed.

When colorectal cancer is detected early, a patient's prospects are excellent, with a five-year survival rate of 90 percent. Unfortunately, many cancers are not found early enough, and the result is that some 48,000 men and women were expected to die from this cancer during 2002.

There are several ways to screen for colorectal cancer. We already talked about one of these tests, the infamous digital rectal exam. Here's a rundown of the others.

Fecal Occult Blood Test (FOBT)

This test can find microscopic traces of hidden, or "occult," blood in the stool, which can be a sign of colon cancer. If the results are positive, then a colonoscopy or other tests can be performed. To do this test, you have to provide a small stool sample to your doctor or lab technicians.

Sigmoidoscopy

A sigmoidoscope is a flexible lighted tube, two feet long, which is inserted into the rectum and extends about halfway into the colon. It allows doctors to look for polyps, precancerous lesions, and cancer. If any are seen, a biopsy can be done to evaluate the problem. If an abnormality is found, a colonoscopy is usually recommended.

Colonoscopy

A colonoscopy is similar to a sigmoidoscopy but with three key differences: The colonoscope's greater length allows doctors to visualize the entire colon. It is equipped with tiny instruments that will allow the doctor to immediately remove and biopsy any polyps that are found. And it extends all the way into the colon's full length, making it the most comprehensive and accurate screening method.

Double-Contrast Barium Enema

In this procedure, barium sulfate and air are pumped into the colon, expanding it in a way that allows high-definition X rays to be taken. This allows for a complete radiological examination of the entire colon. This technique was developed to allow patients to avoid the discomfort of a colonoscopy. But it is not as sensitive as a colonoscopy, and if polyps or lesions are detected, a colonoscopy will still have to be performed. For these reasons, double-contrast barium enemas are no longer widely used.

"Virtual" Colonoscopy

This high-tech method has been developed as a less-invasive alternative to colonoscopy. It uses a CT scanner and virtual-reality software to look inside the body. Unfortunately, there are lots of drawbacks. It requires that air be pumped into the colon to inflate it, which also causes some discomfort. It cannot visualize the smallest polyps, which can be seen with a traditional colonoscopy. And again, if polyps or lesions are found, a colonoscopy will still be needed to remove the polyps and test them for cancer.

Not everybody agrees on the best way to screen for colon cancer. Some doctors recommend that all men undergo colonoscopy beginning at age fifty whereas other doctors feel that fecal occult blood testing and/or sigmoidoscopy is a good alternative. What's really important, though, is that every adult should get screened one way or another, and on a regular basis. The best screening test, many experts say, is the one that actually gets done.

On the horizon, researchers hope, are tests that are less invasive and more sensitive than the virtual colonoscopy. One of the most promising is a test that can measure changes in genetic material found in the stool that can signal cancer. If this test lives up to its promise, it could improve and expand screening for colon cancer and save thousands of lives.

In the meantime, think about this: Being screened for colon cancer isn't much fun, but the alternative is far worse. So why not make this something you do together with your partner? You can each talk to your doctor and agree on a screening plan that makes sense. You can each get screened the same week or month. Then reward yourselves for your diligence with a celebratory dinner or other prize. The family that gets screened together stays healthy together.

BLOOD TESTS

The doctor will often order blood tests to have as a baseline. These tests can also be ordered if he or she suspects a particular problem such as anemia, infection, or kidney or liver problems, to name just a few. After a baseline, if there is nothing suspicious many doctors will not routinely order these tests on every visit.

Complete Blood Count (CBC)

This is one of the most common tests and is often done as part of a routine physical. It tells the doctor about the number and size of red cells (oxygen carriers), the number of white cells (infection fighters), and the amount of hemoglobin (a key protein in red blood cells). A low red count can signal anemia, among other things. A high white count can signal an infection. This test may also count platelets, which help the blood clot properly. Unless there's a reason to suspect a problem, a CBC is not needed every time you get a physical.

Blood Chemistry (Metabolic Panel)

This test can give the doctor an idea of how well your liver, kidneys, pancreas, and even bones are working. Blood salts such as sodium, potassium, and chloride are measured, and their numbers can tell the doctor things about your blood volume and whether or not your kidneys are working properly. It may also include your glucose level, which is discussed below. Like a CBC, a metabolic panel does not need to be done frequently. Most often these tests would be used as part of a diagnostic workup for a particular disease.

URINALYSIS

A urinalysis can reveal things such as diabetes, kidney disease, and even the potential for bladder cancer. The Men's Health Network says it should be done every three years before forty, every two years during the forties, and yearly after fifty.

TB SKIN TEST

This tests looks to see if a person has been exposed to tuberculosis. It should be done every five years, more frequently if a person works in high-risk occupations such as some health-care positions.

TESTS FOR THE HEART

Electrocardiogram (ECG; Also Called by Most People the EKG)

This test looks at electrical activity throughout the heart and can reveal if there are rhythm abnormalities, a history of heart attack, or other problems such as an enlarged heart. This test is useful because it allows doctors to track changes over time. According to the Men's Health Network, this test can be done as a baseline for men in their thirties who are at average risk for heart disease. Beginning at age forty, it should be repeated every four years. Men in their fifties should have it done every three years. If problems arise, doctors may suggest that it be repeated more frequently.

Cardiac Stress Test

To find out how your heart performs during exertion, and whether it has any blockages, you can take an EKG while running on a treadmill or pedaling a bicycle. You need to reach at least 85 percent of your target heart rate in order to have a true reading, which normally takes about ten or fifteen minutes. The doctor checks your heart for signs of distress and looks to see if any symptoms develop. For about 75 percent of people, the test will reveal whether they have coronary artery disease. In fact, a recent study in the *New England Journal of Medicine* found that a cardiac stress test can be the best single predictor of mortality, better than things like cholesterol level. If a problem is picked up, the doctor will probably want to do additional tests.

Your blood pressure should go up during exercise. If it doesn't, that could signal a serious blockage or weakness of the heart. This test will also show what kind of condition you are in, referred to as your "functional capacity." If your heart rate rose significantly before you worked very hard, you are not in good shape.

If you and/or your husband are about to embark on a program of vigorous exercise, it's important you take this test first, especially if there is a history of heart disease in your family, or you are older than forty and have other heart risks. While not routine, many physicians will recommend this test for patients who have coronary risks. If you've already had a heart attack, it may be done to evaluate the extent of damage to your heart.

VISION

People under forty who don't need glasses or have other vision problems don't really need regular eye exams unless they experience visual changes or pain in their eyes, or start seeing flashes of light, spots, ghostlike images, or wavy or distorted lines or edges. The American Academy of Ophthalmology recommends eye examinations every two to four years for people over forty who don't have vision problems, and every one to two years for people over sixty-five.

People who have a higher risk for eye-related problems such as glaucoma, cataracts, or macular degeneration should have their eyes checked more often. (Discuss a schedule for checkups with an ophthalmologist.) This would include anyone with a personal or family history of eye problems, people with diabetes, and African-Americans over forty.

TEETH

Here's a surprise—well, not really. According to the Academy of General Dentistry, men are less likely than women to get preventive dental care. In fact, men are inclined to neglect their dental health for years, preferring to wait for a problem to develop. Everyone should have their teeth cleaned and examined every six months, no matter how old they are. As Soupy Sales used to say, "Be true to your teeth and they'll never be false to you."

LUNG CANCER SCREENING

Chest X Ray

There's disagreement over whether to use chest X rays in the general population as a way to screen for lung cancer or other problems such as an enlarged heart. In smokers over forty-five there is probably good reason to do annual screenings for lung cancer, although it's far from clear whether this will save lives, given how hard it is to treat lung cancer. Individual doctors have their own ideas about this. It's important to discuss this with your physician if you have a history of smoking. Remember: Lung cancer is the leading cause of cancer death in both men and women, with over 160,000 new cases discovered every year.

Spiral CT Scan

This has become an increasingly common way to look for lung cancer in its earliest stages. The spiral CT scanner is faster, gives a clearer picture, and can find nodules that are much smaller than can be seen on a chest X ray. This test is growing in popularity though its value remains controversial among experts.

VACCINATIONS

Little boys aren't the only ones who need shots; sometimes big guys do, too. But usually they don't think about it until they step on a rusty nail or cut their finger on a tin can in the garbage. Then they wonder when they last had a tetanus shot. Often they do need a tetanus booster, but that's probably not the only immunization they need if they want to be sure to keep nasty diseases at bay. The other vaccines to think about include: influenza, hepatitis B, pneumonia, measles, mumps, and rubella, as well as chickenpox. Discuss each one of these with the doctor to see if you or your husband ought to get them.

Let's talk about tetanus first. Adults who received the routine childhood vaccination should get a booster every ten years, unless they've gotten some kind of wound that would be considered "dirty." Dirty wounds are not only rusty ones caused by stepping on rusty old nails. In fact, rust has nothing to do with tetanus; it's the dirt that can contain the tetanus bacteria.

If an adult has not had a tetanus booster within the past five years and he has a wound that could be considered dirty, he should go ahead and get a tetanus booster. It's usually given along with diphtheria and is called the "Td." If he never received the childhood series of tetanus shots, he should also talk to a doctor about the possibility of receiving the tetanus immune globulin (TIG), which can help prevent the onset of tetanus while the vaccination takes effect.

Another important shot to consider is the yearly flu shot. Many large corporations provide them every year free of charge or for a small fee. Not a bad idea for a man who doesn't like to miss work or has a lot of family obligations.

Men who were born after 1957 and did not have a measles, mumps, rubella (MMR) shot should receive at least one dose of the vaccine. If a man did not have chickenpox as a child, the varicella vaccine should be considered. Chickenpox is a much more unpleasant disease in adults than it is in kids.

Men who are sixty-five or older should have the pneumococcal vaccine that protects against pneumonia. Two other shots to be considered are the hepatitis A and hepatitis B shots. These are given to adults who fall into certain high-risk groups, including people who've had many sex partners in a short period of time, sexually active gay men, intravenous drug users, and people who traveled to certain countries with high rates of hepatitis.

To decide whether your husband or you need additional shots, check out the website of the Immunization Action Coalition (*http://www.immunize.org*). It includes a quick quiz that can help you decide which shots you may need.

12

Bad Habits

Doesn't it sometimes seem as if men collect bad habits like loose change? Now, to be fair, we probably have a few bad habits ourselves—I mean, nobody's perfect, right? But unfortunately, a lot of the bad habits men have are in the more serious vein, habits that can make them sick or kill them. Like cigarette smoking, risky driving, and alcohol and drug abuse. Here's a rundown—and some ammunition you might use to change things.

SMOKE GETS IN YOUR EYES—AND LUNGS

Everyone knows the dangers of smoking, so I won't bore you with a long list of all the ways it can hurt you. But if your loved one is a smoker, or if you are, there is one thing you should know that I think many people don't realize.

We tend to think of smoking as causing lung cancer, and indeed 157,000 people died of lung cancer in 2000, the overwhelming majority of them from smoking. But even more people will die from cardiovascular and chronic lung disease related to their smoking—about 250,000 people per year.

Here's why. Carbon monoxide makes up 1 percent to 5 percent of cigarette smoke and has a great affinity for *hemoglobin,* the protein in red blood cells that carries oxygen to the cells of your body. Inside the red blood cells, carbon monoxide competes with oxygen, pushing it out of the way, leaving the cells of the body—including your heart muscle—starved for oxygen. Smoke also raises your blood pressure, causes the heart to beat faster, and narrows and constricts blood vessels. For these reasons, many heavy smokers have a pale or blueish hue to their skin, especially around the mouth. Over time, all of this leads to stiffer, less elastic blood vessels. And when arteries become less elastic, they're more prone to blockages, which can lead to heart attacks and strokes.

CIGARS, PIPES, AND CANCER: THE PRICE OF LOOKING COOL

Cigars became cool in the go-go '90s, as a way for hot-shots to flaunt their wealth and as an alternative to cigarettes. Between 1993 and 1998, cigar sales soared by 57 percent, even in California. In 1996, for instance, almost 9 percent of California men were smoking stogies, nearly double the number from six years before. Cigar magazines have fueled the craze by putting celebrities on the cover, promoting the idea that cigars are sexy and suave. But there's a price to be paid for being this hip. Cigar smokers have much higher rates of cancers of the esophagus, larynx, and mouth than nonsmokers, and they're also more likely to have respiratory problems and heart disease.

Cigars pack way more tar and nicotine than cigarettes do—up to forty times more for big cigars. So even though people smoke fewer cigars, and don't tend to inhale the smoke, they can still do plenty of damage. Not inhaling won't prevent exposure of the mouth to the carcinogens; just holding an unlit cigar between the lips exposes the person to cancer-causing agents. And even though they don't inhale, cigar smokers who smoke more than five cigars a day still have three times the rate of lung cancer as nonsmokers.

Some people cultivate a different look—that professorial, intellectual pipe-smoking mystique. But pipe smokers are not as smart as they look: They're almost as likely to get lung cancer as cigarette smokers. And they have a high risk of developing cancer of the lips.

CHEW AND SPIT

"Just a pinch between cheek and gum." That old advertising pitch makes it sound harmless, but chewing tobacco is anything but. Men who chew tobacco—and 95 percent of chewers are men—increase their risk of cancer of the cheek, gum, and lips by a factor of 50. They pay a high price: Every year, some 30,000 people get diagnosed with some form of oral cancer, and 9,000 die. Nearly all of those people use tobacco in one form or another.

Chewing tobacco is alarmingly common, especially among young people. Around 6 percent of American men—and 14 percent of male high school students—were using chewing tobacco or snuff in 1999. Young men often start to chew tobacco in the baseball dugout. For years, baseball players have been big users of spit tobacco. The great Babe Ruth, for instance, chewed tobacco all the time—and died at age fifty-three of throat cancer.

Pitcher Curt Schilling, who helped lead the Arizona Diamondbacks to their World Series victory in 2001, started chewing tobacco when he was sixteen. It quickly became a habit that lasted fifteen years. During spring training in 1998, Schilling and one hundred forty other baseball players had their mouths checked for signs of cancer. More than half of the players checked, including Schilling, had tobacco-related mouth lesions, a precursor to cancer. For Schilling, this was a wake-up call, especially since his own father, a lifelong smoker, had died of lung cancer. Within a month, Schilling quit and has stayed away from chewing tobacco since.

In recent years, health advocates and former players like Joe Garagiola, the well-known broadcaster, have spearheaded a drive to raise awareness about the problem and to keep young players from getting hooked. Chewing tobacco is now banned in minor-league baseball, but incredibly it still is not banned in the majors. To its credit, though, Major League Baseball has participated in education and early detection efforts like the screening that led Curt Schilling to kick the habit.

> ### WARNING SIGNS OF ORAL CANCER
>
> - A mouth sore that fails to heal within two weeks.
> - A lump, thickening, or soreness in the mouth, throat, or tongue.
> - A white or red patch in the mouth that doesn't go away.
> - Difficulty in chewing, swallowing, or moving the tongue or jaw.

The one good thing about oral cancers is that they can often be detected at an early, curable stage, by looking for signs of sores in the mouth and by getting regular dental checkups.

WAYS TO HELP SOMEONE YOU LOVE QUIT

If you and your husband both smoke, the very act of smoking can become an important part of your relationship. Many couples do a lot of smoking together, and this ritual can become part of the glue of the marriage, an important way for them to spend time, relax, and connect with each other. At the University of Arizona researchers Michael Rohrbaugh, Ph.D., and Varda Shoham, Ph.D., have been looking at how relationships affect a person's or a couple's ability to quit and what sort of interventions will help them in that effort. Results of their study are not yet published, but Dr. Rohrbaugh says a few things have emerged. First, if you both smoke, it's a good idea for you to sit down together and take a hard look at the role smoking plays in your relationship. Once you've examined it and put it on the table, then you'll have a better shot at figuring out what to do about it. Instead of smoking together, maybe you'll agree to go for a walk or jump in the Jacuzzi.

If your husband smokes and you don't, you've probably been pushing him to kick the habit. And it's probably a big source of tension. One thing that is clear from their research, Dr. Rohrbaugh says, is that if one partner nags the other about quitting, it can backfire. In fact, he says, pushing too hard may lead someone to smoke even more. Earlier (see page 277), we talked about ways you could support your partner's effort to make big life changes by keeping in mind the stages of change. Here are a couple of additional points to consider if you want to get the smoke out of your lives.

The first thing to think about and talk to your husband about is the effect his smoking has on you and your children. If he smokes in your home or around members of your family, he is putting your health at risk. According to the Environmental Protection Agency, 3,000 nonsmokers die from lung cancer and 37,000 from heart disease every year as a result of being exposed to secondhand smoke. On top of that, as many as 300,000 infants and children suffer from respiratory tract infections, according to the EPA. Secondhand smoke can also make kids more susceptible to everything from pneumonia to ear infections to asthma.

And there's another big reason you and/or your partner should stop using tobacco: to set a good example for your children. No matter how often you tell them that they shouldn't smoke, what's really going to have an impact is what they see you doing. Children whose parents smoke are far more likely to pick up the habit than are the kids of nonsmokers.

Appealing to a smoker's concern for the children can be a powerful motivation. Another argument is financial. Smoking is an increasingly expensive habit. You could save a lot of money by quitting, money that could be used for a vacation or to buy a new treat or toy.

And here's an argument that might be the most seductive of all. Smoking is more than just a turnoff: After all, who wants to kiss a mouth with yellow teeth and nicotine breath? It also causes impotence. That's right, impotence. In California, health officials have used this as a centerpiece of a new antismoking campaign. Billboards there show a Marlboro Man–type with a limp cigarette hanging out of his mouth and the caption SMOKING CAUSES IMPOTENCE.

This is a powerful argument, says Dr. Dean Ornish, because it can give men an important and positive reason to want to give up the habit. "That means a lot more to guys than 'Smoking causes cancer, emphysema, heart disease.' All those things are so horrible that most people don't even want to think about them and so they don't. Whereas improved sexual function—people say, 'Well, gosh.'"

When smokers are polled, two thirds say they want to quit. So they are in the contemplation phase (see page 279). That is, they're *thinking about* quitting and they may even have a plan to quit at some future time. Supporting someone in this phase means helping him think through the different methods for quitting and maybe helping him find a buddy who has been through the drill and can serve as a guide. Your family doctor might also be a help. Studies show that when doctors take the time and encourage their patients to quit, they're more likely to do so. It is also a fact that when employers or health plans offer smoking-cessation counseling—even for free—very few people avail themselves of the service. Find out what is available at your partner's job or the local hospital and take advantage.

Probably the best thing you can do to help your partner to quit is to encourage him to join a program. While lots of men want to go it alone, their chances for success are very slim: Only 2.5 percent of people who try to quit cold turkey on their own actually succeed. Joining a group pushes the odds way up. Some 20 percent to 40 percent of people in smoking-cessation groups succeed.

Before they can quit for good, most people need to try more than once, and usually many, many attempts are made. So part of your job as a helper is to remind him that even if he's tried and failed before, that doesn't mean he won't succeed this time, or the next time. After all, each attempt is a learning experience.

The toughest part of helping someone else quit is when he first puts down his cigarettes. Withdrawal symptoms can make quitters irritable, anxious, stressed out, and hard to live with, so be prepared. Once he's gone six months without smoking, he's made it through the toughest period. Then your work will be to help him avoid a relapse.

> **TIPS FOR PARTNERS OF QUITTERS**
>
> - Avoid restaurants where smoking is allowed.
> - Reward progress with something special: a dinner, an outing, a trinket.
> - Offer praise frequently.
> - Remind him of the healthy life he'll enjoy without tobacco.
> - Keep a piggy bank for money saved by kicking the habit and break into it at the end of the year.

Whatever you do, try to keep in mind that you are in this together. Dr. Rohrbaugh says that a sense of "communal coping"—of being partners on a team that is tackling a tough problem—can be a big help. Remind him that you are there for him and that together you will kick the habit!

OPTIONS FOR SMOKING CESSATION

Finding the best method to assist a person with smoking cessation is sometimes difficult. Here are five options for quitting smoking:

Cold Turkey

This method requires that the smoker stop smoking cigarettes abruptly. This method has been very successful for some smokers. Other smokers require several attempts at quitting cold turkey before they are successful.

Factors to Consider

- This process can be managed alone.
- Quitting cold turkey is a one-step process.
- The cost is minimal.
- The smoker must be highly committed to the goal of quitting.
- The nicotine withdrawal symptoms (such as irritability, headache, or difficulty sleeping) may be severe for some, especially if the cigarettes smoked contain high levels of nicotine.

Nicotine Fading

The smoker is instructed to reduce the cigarettes smoked by 30 percent for one week, by 60 percent the second week, and by 90 percent the third week. During the fourth week, the smoker quits cold turkey. This method helps reduce the nicotine withdrawal symptoms.

Factors to Consider

- Easy to follow.
- Inexpensive.
- The smoker must have a high level of motivation.

Nicotine Gum

Nicotine gum provides a substitute source of nicotine to reduce the withdrawal symptoms during the quitting process. The smoker may need to chew ten to twelve pieces of gum each day over a three- to six-month period. The amount of gum chewed each day is slowly reduced during the last few weeks of the therapy.

Factors to Consider

- This process can be managed alone.
- The smoker must have a high level of motivation.

- The smoker must stop smoking completely when using the nicotine gum.
- Minor side effects may include lightheadedness, nausea, sore mouth, hiccups, and excess amount of saliva.
- The gum is not recommended during pregnancy, following a heart attack or other heart problems, or if there is joint disease of the jaw.
- Denture wearers may not be able to use the gum.
- Long-term smokers are more likely to become dependent on the gum.
- Cost of the gum for twelve weeks of therapy is approximately $250 to $500, depending on the dose.
- Most insurance does not cover the cost of the gum.
- Nicotine gum is available over-the-counter.

Nicotine Skin Patch

The nicotine patch provides a substitute source of nicotine to reduce the withdrawal symptoms during the quitting process. The patch is worn for eight to twelve weeks.

Factors to Consider

- One patch is applied every twenty-four hours.
- The smoker must have a high level of motivation.
- The smoker must *not* smoke when using the patch.
- Common side effects may include skin redness at the patch site when the patch is removed and restless sleep.
- The patch is not recommended during pregnancy or if there is a history of high blood pressure or other forms of heart disease.
- The cost of the nicotine patch is approximately $200 for twelve weeks.
- Most insurance does not cover the cost of the patch.
- The patch is available over-the-counter.

Zyban (bupropion HCl)

Zyban is the first nicotine-free pill that helps to reduce the urge to smoke. Zyban is thought to work on the biology of nicotine addiction by acting on the "reward" and/or "withdrawal" pathways in the brain associated with nicotine addiction. The smoker starts taking Zyban within one to two weeks before the quit date. Then on the quit date the smoker stops smoking and continues Zyban as recommended by the health-care provider. Zyban therapy may last from seven to twelve weeks.

Factors to Consider
- Zyban is not for everyone. There is a risk of seizure associated with Zyban.
- You should not take Zyban if you have a seizure disorder, are currently taking MAO inhibitors, Wellbutrin, Wellbutrin SR, or have an eating disorder.
- The cost is dose dependent and approximately $135 to $266 for three months of therapy.
- The most common side effects with Zyban are dry mouth and trouble sleeping.
- Zyban is available by prescription only.
- Health insurance may pay for Zyban.
- Zyban may be used in combination with the nicotine patch; however, blood pressure should be monitored during treatment.

COUNSELING SERVICES

All of these options are most successful when combined with modification of behaviors that were previously associated with smoking. Additional counseling may address stress management, weight control, and tips for preventing relapse.

Source: Copyright-protected material used with permission of the authors and the University of Iowa's Virtual Hospital, www.vh.org.

HE DRIVES ME CRAZY

Not much comes between many men and their beloved wheels. Whether they're tinkering or driving, these men love their cars and motorbikes. Too bad that something that gives them so much pleasure can also cause them—and us—so much pain. Whether it's road rage or drunk driving, men are far more likely than women to get into trouble behind the wheel.

Aggressive Driving and Road Rage

We all know the mild-mannered fellow who gets behind the wheel and suddenly transforms from Clark Kent into some sort of demon Superman. It's as if all of his bottled-up anger is unleashed and channeled into aggressive driving. He speeds, weaves, tailgates, runs red lights, and makes angry, obscene gestures to other drivers. The results can be grim: The National Highway Traffic Safety Administration (NHTSA) says that two thirds of all traffic fatalities are caused by aggressive driving—passing on the right, running red lights, speeding, and tailgating. A 1997 analysis by the American Automobile Association Foundation for Traffic Safety found that this kind of driving increased 51 percent between 1990 and 1996. Running red lights alone causes 1 million injuries a year, while some 6,000 Americans are killed each year because drivers run stop signs or speed through intersections, according to the U.S. Department of Transportation.

Even worse than aggressive or unsafe driving is road rage. This is more than just discourteous or unsafe driving, it is using the car as an actual weapon. Aggressive driving is a traffic offense, but road rage is a criminal offense. Surveys show that men are twice as likely as woman to be both aggressive drivers and to experience road rage. One reason, no doubt, that 22,000 men are killed on the nation's highways each year, compared to 10,000 women. Not surprisingly, the most likely candidates for road rage are young men; the older a man gets, the less likely he is to be a victim of his own anger on the road.

So what can you do if your partner is an aggressive driver or has bouts of road rage? Leon James, Ph.D., and Diane Nahl, Ph.D., authors of *Road Rage and Aggressive Driving: Steering Clear of Highway Warfare,* have some suggestions. First, they say, understand that for many men, road rage functions as a way to exercise control, to be the boss in a way they don't often get a chance to outside the car. "This is a role in our society where men use their given powers to lord it over women in the car," says Dr. James. "And many of them are actually terrorizing women. Children are very frightened by their behavior as well."

In this sense, car culture is about freedom, independence, and power. Being in a car allows a certain degree of anonymity as well, so people can feel removed from the consequences of their behavior. Even commercials and movies help to enhance the car's cultural significance as an instrument of power. The single car winding down a beautiful stretch of highway, driven by a solo male driver sends an appealing message: "You're in control, you're powerful." Unfortunately, says Dr. James, driving is not an individual activity but a social, community endeavor.

The good news is that you can help someone get a handle on his aggressive driving tendencies. James should know. He was an aggressive driver himself who came to recognize the problem only after his wife, Dr. Nahl, insisted he had to change. As a result, the couple launched their study of aggressive driving and became experts on the phenomenon.

There are many good reasons to change aggressive driving behavior, and not only because you may fear for your own life. When children witness a father (or mother) who drives in an angry or aggressive way, or hurls verbal insults at other drivers, they learn the same behavior. Another reason: You can actually save money on gas if you lighten up on the pedal.

The key to getting an aggressive driver to change is to make him understand that, as a passenger, he is actually violating your human rights. Sound extreme? Not according to James and Nahl. "We had to get that extreme [for them] to realize what they are doing in the car is really holding people captive," says James, "Because [passengers] can't leave if they're uncomfortable. There's no way to get out."

James and Nahl's strategy is to elevate the passenger to a partner and coparticipant who has rights and feelings that deserve to be heard. The goal is to make an agreement that the driver will listen to the passenger about what makes him or her comfortable and uncomfortable—and that the driver must do this without retaliating.

Using the car to vent anger can be a deadly exercise, not only because it may cause a crash, but because people who are this aggressive and hostile, over time, greatly increase their chances of getting heart disease or cancer. If your driver is out of control, you might want to check out James and Nahl's book. You can also try videotaping an aggressive driver in action. When you play it back to him, it may shock him into recognizing that he is over the line.

"DONORCYCLES"

"Donorcycles"—that's what ER docs all around the country call motorcycles. It's a grim joke, but you get the point: So many young men die riding motorcycles that they constitute a major source of organs for transplant. What's scary is that there's been a huge increase in deaths among older motorcycle riders in the last few years—forty-something men that you'd think would know better. In fact, the increase in deaths among boomers has been the chief cause of this trend: After reaching an all-time low in 1997, the number of people killed in motorcycle accidents has climbed more than 35 percent since. Here are a few other facts about motorcycles:

- In 2000, nearly 2,900 motorcyclists were killed and 58,000 were injured in crashes on America's highways.
- More than 90 percent of those killed in motorcycle crashes are men.
- A motorcyclist is about sixteen times more likely to die in a crash than is someone in a car.
- Head injury is the leading cause of death in motorcycle crashes. Wearing a helmet reduces the likelihood of death by 29 percent in a crash.

In states that have enacted mandatory helmet laws, motorcycle deaths have declined. Yet incredibly, only twenty states make helmet use mandatory for all riders and two states, Texas and Arkansas, recently repealed their mandatory laws. In both those states, helmet use declined and deaths increased immediately.

If your partner is a motorcycle rider who likes to ride without a helmet, show him these statistics and see if it changes his mind. Too bad more people don't get a tour of the morgue at the local ER. If that doesn't convince you, nothing will.

BASEBALL AND BEER AND THE RIDE
HOME FROM THE GAME

For many guys, beer goes with watching baseball (not to mention football, hockey, basketball, and wrestling) like ice cream goes with apple pie. Trouble is, when a game ends, a lot of male fans get behind the wheel and drive home, even if they've been drinking. One recent study published in the *Annals of Emergency Medicine* surveyed more than one thousand men at baseball games. Their blood alcohol level was tested, and they were asked how they'd get home. Here's what they found:

- Forty-one percent of all men tested positive for alcohol.
- Fifty percent of men between twenty and thirty-five tested positive, and 10 percent were legally intoxicated.
- Five percent of all men tested were intoxicated and said they would drive home.

So what can you do about this? Probably not a whole lot. You could urge him to take public transportation or suggest that the men split the cost of a taxi. You could also offer to pick them up at the stadium or the bus station. If nothing else, suggest your spouse and his buddies pick a designated driver.

13

Dealing with Emergencies

How worried should you be about your partner's health? When should you get on the phone and call 911, and when should you just push him to make an appointment with a doctor? The answer, of course, depends on what his symptoms are.

Whatever the state of his health today, the day may come when he, or someone else you love, requires immediate medical attention. If you learn to recognize important symptoms, you may literally save a loved one's life.

What follows is a brief guide to medical problems that often strike men and require action immediately, in some cases, and in the near future, in others. Hopefully, this guide will help you figure out when to act quickly, and when you can relax a bit and work on helping your partner make long-term changes.

CALL 911!

Knowing when to call 911 is important. Usually, it's obvious, there's been a car accident or a serious injury. At other times, people can be unsure and slow to react. Not knowing when to call 911 or waiting too long to do so causes thousands of deaths every year. When in doubt, err on the side of caution. Call 911 right away. Delay costs lives.

Get Help Fast!

The American College of Emergency Physicians says you should call 911 if any of the following warning signs are seen:

- Difficulty breathing, shortness of breath.
- Chest or upper abdominal pain that lasts two minutes or more.
- Fainting.
- Sudden dizziness, weakness, or change in vision.
- Change in mental status (such as unusual behavior, confusion, difficulty waking).
- Sudden, severe pain anywhere in the body.

- Bleeding that won't stop after ten minutes of direct pressure.

- Coughing up or vomiting blood.

- Suicidal or homicidal feelings.

If you're debating about whether to take someone to the hospital yourself or to call 911, check out the following questions. If you answer *yes* to any of them, call 911.

- Is the victim's condition life-threatening or could it become so on the way to the hospital?

- Can you safely move the victim yourself or does it require the skills or equipment of paramedics?

- Would distance or traffic conditions cause a delay in getting the victim to the hospital?

Be Prepared

Other tips to help you be ready in the event of an emergency:

- Keep a list of all emergency numbers by the phone, including the police and fire departments, local poison control center, local hospital, and numbers for the family's doctor(s).

- Keep a list of all the medications and dosages for each family member.

- Keep a list of drugs family members are allergic to.

- Keep a well-stocked first aid kit at home and in the car.

- Take a first-aid class.

- For a copy of the Home First Aid Kit recommended by the American College of Emergency Physicians, go to their website: *http://www.acep.org/* and enter "home first aid kit" in the search box.

PREPARE AN EMERGENCY PLAN

An emergency plan can help any family, but it's especially important if someone in the family has a heart condition or other serious health problem. You simply make a plan about what you would do if someone has a heart attack or other health emergency. Do some research and find out which hospitals in your area can most capably and readily treat a heart attack. Make sure other family members, friends, and coworkers know about this plan and understand the symptoms they need to watch

360 I FROM BOYS TO MEN

out for. Rehearse the plan. In addition, follow the suggestions from the American College of Emergency Physicians, above.

Emergency Preparedness: A Few Basic Tips

- Keep a list of all emergency numbers by the phone. This should include the police, fire department, poison control center, local hospital, ambulance service, and numbers for all family doctors.
- Keep a list of medications and dosages for each family member.
- Keep a list of all family members' allergies, especially to drugs.
- Keep a well-stocked first aid kit at home and in the car.
- Take a first-aid class.

DON'T LET HIM DIE OF DENIAL

Denial is a powerful force and one of the big reasons that people—especially men—die when they don't need to. It's the mechanism that allows a man with severe chest pain to declare "It's just indigestion, it'll pass."

Most of the time you see things more clearly than your partner does. And thankfully, that's why so many men are dragged into the doctor's office by their wives, and often just in the nick of time. But there are also times when a woman either doesn't want to challenge her husband or else colludes with him in failing to recognize what's really going on. Even doctors sometimes deny serious problems. A patient may call complaining of vague symptoms and the doctor advises taking it easy and calling back in a few days if the symptoms don't go away. Meanwhile, the patient is in the middle of a heart attack.

CARDIAC EMERGENCIES
Warning Signs of a Heart Attack

- **Chest Discomfort.** Uncomfortable pressure, squeezing, fullness, or pain in the center of the chest that lasts for more than a few minutes, or goes away and comes back.
- **Discomfort in Other Areas of the Upper Body.** Can include pain or discomfort in one or both arms, the back, neck, jaw, or stomach.
- **Shortness of Breath.** Often comes along with chest discomfort, but may happen before the chest discomfort.
- **Other Symptoms.** These may include breaking out in a cold sweat, nausea, lightheadedness, unexplained anxiety, weakness, or fatigue.

The symptoms on page 360 can signal a heart attack in progress. Notice that they are not all like the "Hollywood" version of a heart attack, i.e., chest-clutching pain. If you are with someone who has these symptoms call 911! Don't take no for an answer! Don't waste time negotiating! Don't wait more than five minutes! Don't let the person drive himself to the hospital or to the pharmacy to pick up some aspirin!

Going by ambulance is the safest way because paramedics can monitor and treat a patient on the way. They can even restart the person's heart if it becomes necessary. Also heart attack victims who arrive by ambulance get treated faster. If you have a choice of hospitals and you can persuade the ambulance driver, go to a hospital that has a twenty-four-hour emergency room and one with an intensive care unit or, even better, a coronary care unit.

If you are trained in CPR and the person becomes nonresponsive, perform it.

Many heart attack sufferers will deny that they are having a heart attack and try to resist calling 911, delaying the arrival of help. In fact, experts say you should expect a person with these symptoms to be in denial. It's so common that it's considered normal. Even some men who *know* they're having a heart attack will resist help! They may be embarrassed—they don't want neighbors to see the ambulance, or they don't want to create a fuss. Some even say they don't want to bother the doctors and nurses at the hospital!

A recent American Heart Association study of nearly 800,000 patients who had heart attacks found that only half of them called 911 for an ambulance. The other half drove themselves, or had someone else drive them to the hospital, thus delaying life-saving treatment. Younger patients, especially males, were more likely to drive themselves.

Because of this tendency toward denial, it's a good idea to discuss in advance with other family members how to deal with medical emergencies, including heart attacks. This is especially important if anyone in the family has heart disease. Develop an emergency plan and be sure everyone knows how to recognize the symptoms of a heart attack (see page 360).

Should You Give an Aspirin?

Aspirin can be a lifesaver when given to someone who's having a heart attack. But that doesn't mean you should delay calling 911 to *find* one! If you've got one, call 911 and dispense the aspirin. In that order. Emergency department personnel should give a person experiencing a heart attack an aspirin to chew as soon as they arrive. If the person is allergic to aspirin or has a bleeding problem, don't give aspirin and tell the ER people about this history.

Heart Attacks and Angina: Similar but Different

Angina is a recurring pain or discomfort in the chest that happens when some part of the heart is not receiving enough blood. An episode of angina is not a heart attack, though sometimes people with angina have a hard time telling the difference. Most people who suffer from angina use some form of nitroglycerine that they can take to relieve the pressure. But even in those cases, if the pain lasts longer than ten minutes, and is not relieved by nitroglycerine, they may be having a heart attack and need prompt attention. (For more on prevention of heart disease see chapter 11.)

STROKES

Time is also of the essence for people who suffer stroke. Unfortunately many people don't know that and will not seek immediate medical attention when they or a loved one has a stroke. New clot-busting drugs can prevent death and reduce the disability in some stroke patients if they are given in the first three hours after symptoms begin. After three hours, the drug may be ineffective and can even be dangerous. What this means is that waiting to seek help could deprive a stroke victim of the benefit of these drugs.

A stroke, or "brain attack," as they are sometimes called, is like a heart attack of the brain. Strokes occur when the blood supply to the brain is suddenly interrupted by a blockage in the arteries or bleeding into the brain.

Warning Signs of a Stroke

- Sudden numbness or weakness in the face, an arm, a leg, or one side of the body.
- Sudden confusion, trouble speaking or understanding speech.
- Sudden vision problems such as dimness or double vision in one or both eyes.
- Sudden trouble walking, dizziness, loss of balance, or problems with coordination.
- Sudden severe headache with no known cause.
- Fainting, convulsions, or coma.
- Sudden nausea and vomiting that comes on very rapidly.

In some cases the symptoms of a stroke last only a few minutes and then disappear. This is called a *transient ischemic attack* (TIA), also known as a ministroke. Since the symptoms of a TIA go away on their own, many people ignore them, never seek medical help, and indeed never even mention them to their doctor! This is a *huge* mistake. These TIAs are often warnings of worse to come, like a really big stroke that can disable or kill. According to the National Stroke Association, one in five stroke victims will have a secondary stroke within the next five years.

If you think someone is having a stroke, call 911 immediately! If he recovers quickly, make him see his doctor anyway, and soon. If he tells you about having strokelike symptoms when you weren't around, do the same thing. Make him go to the doctor ASAP. And don't take no for an answer. (See chapter 11 for more on prevention of strokes.)

SUICIDE

In 2000, more than 29,000 Americans took their own lives. The vast majority—80 percent—were men. Women attempt suicide three times as often as men, but men are far more likely—four times—to complete the act. Every day, sixty-four American men take their own lives. Men kill themselves for a wide range of reasons, but many share a common pattern. They are part of a culture of individualism that keeps many men from sharing their problems with others. They bottle up their problems and pain and medicate themselves with alcohol and drugs. Then, in a spontaneous fit of depression, they pull out their gun or steer their car into a freeway retaining wall.

If your partner, or anyone you know and love, begins talking about or threatening to commit suicide, or showing some of the warning signs below, take the person seriously and try to get him to see a counselor, clergy member, or another professional. Suggest that he call a suicide hotline. If you don't think the person will call, then phone a suicide hotline yourself and get some advice.

Call 1-800-SUICIDE and you can reach a trained telephone counselor twenty-four hours a day, seven days a week through the National Hopeline Network.

Signs Someone Is Thinking of Suicide

- He talks about suicide or death, even jokingly.
- He has great trouble eating or sleeping.
- His behavior and mood seem to change drastically.
- He has recently suffered great losses, of a loved one, a job, or money.
- He withdraws from friends or activities.
- He hoards pills or purchases a gun.
- He increases his use of alcohol or drugs.
- He gives away prized possessions.
- He has attempted suicide previously.
- He writes notes or poems about death.
- He changes his eating or sleeping habits.
- He neglects his personal appearance.

GET HELP SOON

Heart attacks and strokes are true medical emergencies. Every second counts if you are going to help your loved one. Other conditions may not require an ambulance, but they still call for prompt medical attention. Unfortunately many men may wait and hope that symptoms will pass. If your partner seems to have any of the problems below, you should do more than gently suggest an appointment with a doctor. You need to push him to get on the phone and make an appointment or pick up the phone yourself. Bear in mind that these symptoms can be vague and come on slowly over time. Vague complaints can be harbingers of problems to come, especially if they persist.

Warning Signs of Diabetes

People with undiagnosed diabetes often confuse their symptoms with aging or being overweight. As a result, they may ignore them—one reason that so many people with diabetes are untreated. The symptoms below may point to diabetes and are definitely reason to seek medical attention. (See chapter 15 for more on diabetes.)

- Frequent urination.
- Excessive thirst.
- Unexplained weight loss.
- Extreme hunger.
- Sudden vision changes.
- Tingling or numbness in hands or feet.
- Feeling very tired much of the time.
- Very dry skin.
- Sores that are slow to heal.
- More infections than usual.

Warning Signs of High Blood Pressure

People with high blood pressure may have it for years without experiencing any symptoms. Long-standing disease may cause these symptoms though many other diseases can be associated with these as well:

- headache
- blurred vision

In rare cases, a person's blood pressure can rise to dangerously high levels. That, of course, is a real medical emergency that requires immediate treatment. Symptoms may include drowsiness, confusion, headache, nausea, and loss of vision. People with a history of hypertension should call a physician immediately if these symptoms appear. (See chapter 15 for more on high blood pressure.)

Warning Signs of Sleep Apnea

- Bursts of snoring and snorting, sometimes quite loud, when sleeping on back.

- Morning headache.

- Person may appear to stop breathing briefly when sleeping, then inhale with a snort.

- Person is fatigued and drowsy during the day and may be quite irritable.

According to the American Lung Association, more than 18 million Americans—that's 6 percent to 7 percent of the U.S. population—suffer from sleep apnea, a sleep disorder that interferes with a person's ability to breathe while sleeping. It is most common in overweight men.

Most people with sleep apnea have an obstruction in their throat that blocks the flow of air through their mouth and keeps them from breathing easily. They typically snore, stop breathing for a short time as a result of the obstruction, and then are startled awake momentarily by their need for air. They then fell back asleep and the cycle continues.

People with sleep apnea tend to sleep poorly and to be very tired and irritable during the day. Because of their fatigue, they are prime candidates for falling asleep at the wheel. And since recent studies suggest that drowsy drivers are about as impaired as drunk ones, sleep apnea really can be a dangerous problem. Untreated, sleep apnea can lead to serious health problems, including heart disease.

If your partner snores at night, seems to start during his sleep, and is frequently tired, get him to make an appointment with a doctor or a sleep specialist. If he won't, do it yourself and drag him there. After all, you can tell him, all that snoring is keeping you awake, too. (See chapter 20 for more on sleep apnea.)

Warning Signs of Lung Cancer

In the early stages, lung cancer usually causes no symptoms. By the time a tumor has grown big enough to cause problems, it may be in an advanced stage. Then symptoms include:

- Persistent, hacking cough that may bring up blood or bloody mucus.

- Wheezing and hoarseness.

- Unexplained weight loss and loss of appetite.

- Shortness of breath.

- Unexplained fever.

- Repeated bouts of bronchitis or pneumonia.

- Chest or back pain.

As we all know, smoking is far and away the biggest cause of lung cancer. In fact, before cigarettes became popular, lung cancer was relatively rare. If your partner or someone you love still smokes, do everything you can to get them to stop. (See section on quitting smoking, beginning on page 349.) If he has any of the symptoms above—especially if he is a current or former smoker—get him to make an appointment with his doctor. While few lung cancer patients live for five years or longer, a person's chances of survival are much better if the cancer is detected early.

Warning Signs of Colon Cancer

Cancer of the colon or rectum often shows no signs or symptoms in the early stages. The first warning signs often include these:

- Changes in bowel habits including diarrhea or constipation that lasts for several days, "pencil" stools that appear narrower than usual or a feeling that the bowels are not completely empty after a bowel movement.
- Blood in the stool or red-streaked or black, tarry stools.
- Persistent gas pains, cramps, or tenderness in the lower abdomen.
- Unexplained weight loss or loss of appetite.
- Unexplained weakness or fatigue.

If your partner or other loved one experiences changes in their bowel movements like those listed above, call the doctor and ask for an appointment as soon as possible.

Warning Signs of Prostate Cancer

Prostate cancer normally causes no symptoms until the cancer has grown quite large. Eventually, if the tumor grows, it may cause the following symptoms:

- A weak or interrupted flow of urine.
- Difficulty in starting or stopping the flow of urine.
- Frequent urination that may be painful or bloody.
- Persistent pain in the lower back, upper thighs, or pelvis.

If your partner or another loved one experiences symptoms like those above, call his doctor and ask for an appointment as soon as possible. (See chapter 17 for more on cancer.)

Other Signs of Coming Trouble

The sad truth is that many men will only seek medical help after a brush with death, serious illness, or disability. By then, of course, it's often too late. One way to deal with this pattern is to use other, less serious problems as an opportunity to get him to seek attention before disaster strikes. Maybe he's had a sports injury, a really bad case of the flu, or heartburn that keeps him up at night. No matter how small the problem seems, it may be a way to get him to connect with a doctor.

One of the great by-products of Viagra was that many men made visits to the doctor for the first time in years. Doctors were then able to detect thousands of cases of high blood pressure, diabetes, high cholesterol, and even cancers that might otherwise have gone unnoticed for years.

Here are a few examples of relatively minor health problems that you can tell your husband need to be checked out by a doctor. *Carpe diem!*

- Heartburn, acid reflux, or burning pain in the stomach. (Long-standing heartburn has been linked to esophageal cancer!)
- An old injury that flares up.
- Frequent headaches or migraines.
- Rectal pain or itching. (Hemorrhoids can be a good reason to see a doctor.)
- Pain with urination or difficulty urinating.
- He is more than ten pounds overweight.
- He has high cholesterol, high blood pressure, or another chronic problem but has not had it checked out in a year or more.
- He seems depressed or especially moody.
- He stops taking a prescription medicine because of a side effect.
- He hasn't seen a doctor in many years or can't remember the last time he saw one.

14

"Houston, We've Had a Problem"

When the now-famous words "Houston we've had a problem" were transmitted back to Earth from 200,000 miles away, they did little to convey the seriousness of the situation the astronauts of *Apollo 13* were in. Seconds earlier, a loud explosion had rocked their ship, leaving the craft so damaged, the crew was unlikely to make it back to Earth. Then Jack Swigert uttered the famous words in a voice so low that Mission Control asked him to repeat it. Typical man—not a hint of panic in his voice despite the fact that his crew was facing near-certain death. Another famous phrase also came out of the rescue effort. "Failure is not an option!" shouted flight director Gene Kranz to other members of Mission Control. And failure indeed was averted.

In many ways, these astronauts and their ground crew epitomize the male character and approach to problems, including health. Most men give little thought to their health or vulnerability until a problem hits them in the face. When it does, they often roll up their sleeves and tackle it. Men are marvelous at responding and acting in a clinch. What they're not so good at is minimizing risks, preventing problems, and doing the little daily things that are hard to see or measure.

Those things often fall to us. Then when problems arise, we act like members of the ground control crew—we rally, gather information, and help get them out of the fix they've gotten themselves into. We're women—wives and girlfriends, mothers and sisters; it's what we do.

The section that follows will offer you some ways to coax your partner into being more active in his own behalf. It's not meant to be an exhaustive look at every health problem or disease. My intention is to point out the most common major diseases, to show how you and he can recognize these diseases, and most important, to make suggestions on how—together—you can keep manageable problems from becoming deadly threats.

At some point, nearly every man faces a "Houston, we've had a problem" moment. He won't be in a damaged space capsule, of course, but he may confront other dangers—a heart attack, cancer, or a stroke. Or it may just be the sudden realization after a lifetime of feeling invulnerable that he's not an iron man, he isn't immortal, and the way he's now living could kill him. That doesn't necessarily mean that he'll *do* anything about it, but often it takes a big problem to make a man wake up.

We women can help a great deal. We can win an Oscar for best supporting actress, but we're not in the starring role. Only your husband can do that. Only he can keep failure from becoming an option, and poor health from becoming a reality.

RULES OF THE ROLE

To help you keep your role straight, here are some useful rules to consider as you assist your husband in dealing with his health:

- You are not your husband's nurse or doctor.

- You are helping because the man you love is in need.

- Your goal is to help your partner become more in tune with his own health needs so he can take better care of himself.

- Helping and being in charge are two different things. If you take responsibility away from him, it will make him less connected to his own body and more dependent on you.

- It's not your fault if he becomes ill, so don't let yourself feel guilty.

- Patience is still a virtue. Recognize that change takes time.

PUBLIC ENEMY NUMBER ONE: HEART DISEASE

Every winter, thousands of men put on their coats, take shovels in hand, and venture out into a blizzard to lift and heave great mounds of wet snow. What could be more helpful or more manly? And for too many, what could be more deadly? Hundreds of men have heart attacks and many die this way every year. A middle-aged man, perhaps overweight, who hasn't exerted himself in months, suddenly starts throwing around heavy heaps of snow. His blood pressure and his heart rate jump at the very moment the cold causes his arteries to constrict. For many men's hearts, it's a perfect storm. And indeed, heart attacks go up 22 percent during a big snowstorm, according to a recent study in the *American Journal of Cardiology*.

My point here is not that you should leave your sidewalk buried under snow, but rather to show how ubiquitous heart disease is in the lives of our men. It is far and away the number one killer of men. It kills lots of women, too. We just tend to get it about ten years later in life, when our estrogen levels drop.

Death from heart disease has fallen dramatically in the last fifty years, yet it remains the top single killer of adults—not breast cancer, as many women fear, and not prostate cancer, as many men fear, but heart disease. In 2000, some 1.1 million Americans suffered new and recurrent heart attacks, and more than 520,000 died as a result. For some 250,000 of them, death came without warning; they did not reach a hospital in time to be revived. All told, cardiovascular disease kills more Americans than cancer, accidents, Alzheimer's disease, and AIDS combined.

More than 1 in 5 Americans—62 million people in all—have some form of cardiovascular disease, which includes high blood pressure, heart disease, and stroke. Consider this: Every year, 355,000 people undergo bypass surgery, 600,000 have coronary angioplasty performed, and a whopping 1.4 million get catheterizations.

> **PRECAUTIONS FOR SNOW SHOVELING**
>
> - Dress warmly and breathe through a scarf.
> - Don't eat a large meal before going out.
> - Use a small shovel and lift as little weight as possible.
> - Take your time.
> - Make sure you know if you are at risk for heart disease.
> - Make sure you are in good shape.

A Brief Primer on Heart Disease

So what is heart disease (also called coronary artery disease or ischemic heart disease) and how does it work? It's a disease that affects the vascular system—mainly the arteries that feed blood to the heart muscle. Fatty plaque builds up and narrows the arteries, reducing the flow of blood to the heart muscle. In some cases, this clump of plaque can rupture and lodge inside an artery, creating a blood clot that blocks the flow of blood. The heart becomes starved of blood and the oxygen it delivers. Since the heart needs the oxygen to keep going, a reduced supply can damage its ability to pump.

As the problem gets worse, several things can happen. The most dramatic is sudden cardiac arrest. The blockage is so severe, it cuts off blood to part of the heart. The heart's rhythm becomes too disturbed to pump efficiently. Without immediate care, the person dies.

In other cases, the blockage doesn't completely cut off the blood supply but reduces it enough to cause pain called *angina pectoris*. If it lasts long enough, the reduced blood supply can starve the heart muscle cells of oxygen and kill them. When cells die due to a lack of oxygen, it's called an *infarction*. When it happens in the heart, it's called a *myocardial infarction*—a heart attack.

Beginning in the 1960s, deaths from heart disease started to decline. Unfortunately, this decline began to slow in the 1990s, as the obesity rate among Americans exploded. The sad truth is that the best drugs and the greatest technology can do only so much. If Americans keep eating too much, smoking, and failing to exercise, heart disease—and a host of other related problems—will continue to kill people before their time.

Because men tend to suffer from heart problems earlier than women, many women are first exposed to cardiovascular health issues through their husbands. But couples that live together often share bad habits, such as being overweight, smoking, and eating an unhealthy diet. Many women whose husbands have heart problems today will experience the same problems a few years down the road.

The point: Don't let a good lesson go unlearned. Changes made for the gander can be just as good for the goose! Preventing heart disease should be a family affair.

Are You Looking a Heart Attack in the Face?

Gaze over at your sweetheart. You can tell a lot about his heart attack risk by looking at some of his physical traits.

Is Your Hubby Tubby?

Does your sweetheart have a roll around the middle? You know, love handles, a beer belly, a Buddha belly. Whatever you want to call it, weight that builds up around the middle is much more likely to lead to heart disease and diabetes than extra inches on the thighs or behind. In fact, weight around the middle has become such an important measure of risk that experts now urge doctors to measure their patient's waists to help them assess their risk.

"Hundreds of studies have led to the conclusion that any fat can be problematic, but it's much, much more dangerous when it's accumulated in the abdomen," says Jeffrey S. Flier, M.D., an endocrinologist at Beth Israel Deaconess Medical Center in Boston.

Why does belly fat cause so much trouble? There is no clear answer to that question, but there are some strong theories. Abdominal fat, it seems, acts very differently than fat stored in the hips, thighs, or other places. Fat in the hips, for instance, tends to stay where it is until you need it for fuel. It's like deep storage. But fat in the abdomen is much more available, metabolically speaking.

For various reasons, men are more likely than women to store fat in their bellies. We get big in our hips and butts; men get thick in the waist. But how thick is too thick? Rules of thumb can be dangerous, since everyone's body is different. But experts say a person's hip-to-waist ratio can be a good barometer of their health and fitness. To get this number, simply measure the waist (at the navel), then the hips. Now divide the waist size by the hip size.

$$\frac{\text{Waist (inches)}}{\text{Hip (inches)}} = \text{hip-to-waist ratio}$$

If this number is bigger than 1.0—meaning the waist is bigger than the hips—the risk of heart attack and stroke goes up. You can also estimate risk from a waist measurement alone. Men with a waistline greater than 40 inches have higher risk of various problems.

Thin on Top? Hair in Your Ear Canals? Finger or Leg Length?

Life's not fair. Men—at least white men—who are balding on top seem to have an increased risk of heart disease. A study in the *Archives of Internal Medicine* found that men with hair loss on top of their heads had a 34 percent increased risk for developing coronary artery disease compared to men with full heads of hair.

Hair in the ear canals and creased earlobes seem to mean higher risk as well, according to researchers who study these things. And then there's this one: British researcher Dr. John Manning says men whose index fingers are longer than their ring fingers—that's opposite the normal pattern—have a greater risk of heart problems that could begin in early adulthood. On the other hand, he's also found that professional soccer players have much longer ring fingers. One Brazilian soccer star—with a $12 million contract, no less—has a ring finger nearly 5 percent longer than his index finger. (Plenty of room for a nice fat diamond, I guess!) Men with longer ring fingers may also be candidates for depression later in life, Dr. Manning says.

But wait, it gets even wackier. Another British study has found that men with short legs are 10 percent more likely than long-legged men to suffer from diabetes and heart disease. Short men—under five feet three inches—are twice as likely to have a stroke as men over five feet seven inches, according to another English study.

Of course, none of these physical attributes can predict whether a particular man is going to have problems with his heart. Still, if your short-legged husband's head glints in the sun, he has extra weight around his waist, and he has hair growing out of his ears, he (and you) might want to pay attention to his health. And you know what that means—getting regular checkups and being sure to eat right, exercise, and not smoke.

Gums and Hearts

People with periodontal problems—gum disease—may have an increased risk of heart disease, according to some studies. If borne out in future research, this may help explain why some people who don't smoke and aren't overweight get heart disease at an early age. But what's the possible connection between these two health problems? Researchers at the University of North Carolina think that the release of bacteria from diseased gums may trigger the release of a *C-reactive protein*, which has been found to greatly increase heart disease risk. Periodontal disease may also be linked to stroke .

Assess the Risk

If you're worried about your husband's risk, you might suggest that he complete a cardiac risk assessment with his doctor. He can also get an online assessment of his chances of having a heart attack in the next ten years at *http://hin.nhlbi.nih.gov/atpiii/ calculator.asp*. If an assessment puts him in a high-risk group, it might motivate him to make some changes.

Know the Warning Signs

You never know when you may be called upon to help your husband or someone else who has suffered a heart attack or stroke. Even if your husband's already had a heart attack, and you think you know the symptoms, check out the list on page 360 because the symptoms may be completely different the second time around. Remember this too: Heart attacks don't always have that Hollywood presentation. They can be a lot more subtle. If you're in doubt, get help.

Learn CPR: Fight Sudden Death

Sudden cardiac arrest is the number-one cause of death in adults. More than 600 Americans die this way every day. That's over 4,000 a week, 220,000 a year. Three quarters of these deaths take place at home, which means that if your husband has one, you might be the only person who could help save his life. But you must take quick action and you must know CPR.

It's important to understand what happens in sudden cardiac arrest. In most cases, the heart goes from beating normally to a quivering rhythm known as *ventricular fibrillation*. In this state, the heart contracts in a rapid, chaotic rhythm that makes it unable to pump blood to the rest of the body and the brain. An electrical shock—defibrillation—can reverse this and restore a normal rhythm in most people if it is applied within a few minutes.

There's no time to waste. Brain death will start to occur in just four to six minutes after the heart stops. Tragically, more than 95 percent of cardiac arrest victims die before reaching the hospital. Two things can help improve this dismal statistic.

First, CPR, quickly performed, can act as a bridge until defibrillation can be provided by sending a trickle of oxygenated blood to the brain and heart to help keep these organs alive longer. Experts say that if CPR is started within four minutes of a heart stopping, and if defibrillation is provided within ten minutes, the person has a 40 percent chance of survival.

The sooner defibrillation is administered, the better the victim's chances of survival. In cities where defibrillation is available within five to seven minutes, the survival rate from cardiac arrest is as high as 49 percent. In recent years, defibrillators placed on airliners, and in airports, sports stadiums, and casinos have saved many lives. Now many experts and groups would like to see defibrillators placed in homes within communities, where neighbors trained in CPR and the use of a defibrillator could provide life-saving assistance until paramedics arrive. The American Heart Association estimates that 40,000 more lives could be saved each year if defibrillators were more widely available.

Saving Your Husband's Life

Learning CPR could allow you to save the life of your husband or someone else. Just ask Ann Miller of Stanwood, Michigan, or Cindy Reynolds of Indiana. Or better yet, ask their husbands Larry and Rick. Here's what they'd tell you.

In May 2000, Ann Miller took a CPR class offered to her and fellow employees of the city of Big Rapids. "I never thought I'd use it, but it was free, so why not?" Ann says. A few months later, she woke up to the sound of Larry making a strange noise. She turned on the light and found he had stopped breathing. She called 911 and told the operator she knew CPR. "She told me to start it up," Ann remembers. "And I did."

She pulled Larry onto the floor and began giving him chest compressions and rescue breathing, keeping it up for seven minutes until the ambulance arrived. "I was so calm during that whole time," Ann says. "I didn't break down until three months later."

When the paramedics arrived, they shocked him twice and put in a breathing tube, but he didn't regain consciousness for two days. Though the doctors originally gave him only a 1 in 10 chance of surviving, he's made a full recovery, with only minor memory loss. "I feel good now," he says. "But if it wasn't for Ann, I wouldn't be here."

The Reynolds' story is just as dramatic. The couple was out driving in the late afternoon on a hot summer day in August 2000. Rick began to feel sick in his stomach and told Cindy he needed to stop. They went to a restaurant and had just ordered dinner when Rick suddenly collapsed. With the help of a busboy, Cindy moved him onto the floor and began performing CPR, which she had learned only two months before. She continued for the rest of the fifteen minutes it took paramedics to arrive, restoring Rick's color but not his pulse. The paramedics zapped him nine times with a defibrillator and were able to get his heart beating. Still, he remained in a coma for three weeks.

Rick's condition today isn't as good as Larry's. He has a badly diseased heart and is kept alive by a pacemaker and medications he must take twice a week intravenously. But the couple recently celebrated their thirtieth wedding anniversary. "That's the ultimate gift," Rick says. "It's beyond what was in any of our wedding vows."

AFTER THE HEART ATTACK: THE POST-"EVENT" FAMILY

My heart racing, I park and run through the darkness toward the double doors marked emergency. Where is my husband? The ambulance he arrived in stands empty and there is no sign of him. Only an hour ago we were safely curled up in bed, watching TV and comparing notes on the details of our day. His sudden chest pain and an urgent call to 911 have led me to this door, where I stop, take a deep breath, and realize I don't know what to do.

—RACHAEL FREED

Source: From Heartmates: A Guide for the Spouse and Family of the Heart Patient, *3rd ed. Copyright © 2002 by Rachael Freed. Reprinted with permission of Fairview Press.*

Doctors refer to heart attacks and other medical occurrences as "events." It's a sterile, dispassionate word that conveys nothing about the impact and gravity of a human tragedy, one that not only affects a patient but often devastates a whole family.

Rachael Freed knows this world intimately. Her husband suffered a major heart attack in 1981 when he was forty-four. It sent the entire family into a tailspin and forever altered their lives. As her husband slowly recovered, Freed, a social worker, decided to write a book because she realized there were no resources available to families to help them cope with the experience.

"Heart disease is invisible and people do indeed recover from the event," Freed says. "And it looks like they are fine. People are supportive as long as you're giving an update of the patient's health. But once you say, 'He's back on the golf course' or 'He's back at work full-time' they stop calling. And rarely do they ask, 'Well, how are you and the kids doing?'"

Wives whose husbands suffer heart attacks are not patients, but the intensity of their experience is, in many ways, quite similar to that of people who have fallen ill. They grieve and mourn for a lost way of life. They struggle to get back to normal but find they rarely can. Freed counsels that the family's task is to learn to live with uncertainty, to discover a "new normal" that incorporates the realities of heart disease. Thanks to new medications and cardiac rehabilitation programs, heart attack survivors live, but they and their loved ones may live with uncertainty for years, even decades.

Some women become angry and resentful, feeling—if not actually saying—"Why didn't he take better care of himself?" Then they feel guilty for having such thoughts in the first place.

Others become overprotective, smothering their husband with lavish attention. "Did you take your medicines?" "Don't do that, you may have another heart attack." Many become so involved in their husband's health that it takes over their lives as well.

"My life is a twenty-four-hour worry over him," says Nancy Broom, the wife of a fifty-year-old heart attack survivor.

Many women whose husbands have suffered a heart attack take on a dizzying number of roles in an effort to keep him alive: like nurse, chef, appointment secretary, traffic cop, and de facto single parent. But by focusing so heavily on caring for their ill spouse, they often ignore their own needs. They blame themselves for their husband's condition, especially right after the heart attack.

"I didn't feed him a low-fat diet." "He was too stressed at work, and I didn't support him." "I didn't get him to the hospital on time." "I should have seen it coming." Thoughts like these often add to the guilt that many women feel simply because he's ill and she's not.

Women believing they're at fault fit right in with the attitudes of some men, who don't want to take responsibility for their own actions. Lori Mosca, M.D., a preventive cardiologist at Columbia University Health Sciences in New York, says she sees it all the time.

"The men say 'It's my wife's fault. She cooks too good. She gives me too much of this,'" Dr. Mosca says. "We see a lot of that, generally in older men. The younger men aren't so bad about that anymore.'"

In their determination to help the man they love, many women take on so much responsibility that their husband is left with none. In the years since she wrote her book, Freed has worked with many spouses and families who are grappling with the effects of a husband's heart disease. Many of them try but fail to control their husband's habits and grow frustrated, even bitter about it. "I can't tell you how many spouses I have worked with over the years who have said, 'He's going to die because he won't eat the diet I'm trying to make him eat,'" Freed says.

For Freed, one of the hardest lessons is learning that you can't control or save another human being. She learned this herself when her husband told her, "Let's not forget that when you make me an invalid, you invalidate me."

When our husbands are hurting and in need, it's natural that we want to be there to support and help them in any way we can. The problem is that a lot of women lose sight of the need to take care of themselves as well. "The best way we can help our spouses," says Freed, "is by taking good care of ourselves first so that we don't burn out and sabotage their recovery."

Depression is common among spouses of patients recovering from a heart attack. In fact, many wives experience substantial and persistent psychological problems up to eighteen months later. A study in the journal *Heart and Lung* looked at the wives of men undergoing cardiac rehabilitation to see how they were coping. It found that 66 percent of them felt distressed and tense and had trouble falling asleep. Distress was particularly common among the younger wives—those in their fifties—compared to older women.

The nature of a couple's relationship has a profound effect on how both partners cope with the stresses of heart disease. Just as the seemingly endless caregiving and worry can have dramatic effects on a woman's physical and emotional health, her ability to cope can also have a big effect on his health and recovery. Indeed, one fascinating study published in the *Journal of Health Psychology* found that when spouses (usually wives) of heart patients were optimistic and had good support systems of their own, their partners recovered better.

There's also lots of evidence that heart patients who get strong emotional support from family members have a much better chance of recovering than those who get little family support. The bottom line is that if your husband has suffered a heart attack and you find yourself looking after him, you need to find a way to take good care of yourself as well. It's critical—for your frame of mind and for his ability to recover.

Of course, some men have a lot of trouble coping with their brush with mortality. Some men who would never have thought about an extramarital affair before a heart attack wind up cheating on or leaving their wives as a way to affirm their masculinity. Interestingly, death during sex is more common during sex with a mistress than during sex with a spouse.

COPING WITH THE AFTERMATH

Whether your husband's had a major heart attack or been diagnosed with underlying heart disease, your family's life is going to change. The changes are far more sweeping than many people would imagine. Your husband is now, in many respects, a different man. He needs to eat differently, to monitor his habits and activities, and to exercise in ways he probably never did before. He'll probably be taking medications, perhaps several of them, and may be struggling with how to keep track of them all. On top of all this, he may feel very differently about himself and his abilities; he may feel vulnerable in a way he never has before.

Many women say their husband experienced a profound change in personality or a deep depression after a heart attack. And indeed, research has shown a strong link between heart disease and depression—a link with a tremendous effect on a patient's ability to recover.

Canadian researchers followed 200 acute heart attack patients and found that those who were depressed were four times more likely to die within the next six months than patients who were not. They concluded that depression is just as important a predictor of a heart patient's future prospects—his chances for life or death—as is his measured level of cardiac function.

Is this because depressed people are less likely to take their medicines? Because they don't follow a healthy lifestyle? Or is it due to hormonal or neuronal changes that weaken the body's ability to withstand the shocks it has experienced? In all likelihood, all of these may play a role. What is clear is that for heart patients who are depressed, treating the depression is as essential as treating the heart disease itself.

A Wake-up Call—for You

Women whose husbands have heart disease may not spend much time thinking about their own chances of having heart problems. But they should. Researchers at the University of Nebraska Medical Center in Omaha, Nebraska, looked at the wives of more than 170 men who had had a heart attack or undergone bypass surgery. When the researchers assessed the women's risk factors, they found that many of them were overweight, obese, smoked, or had high cholesterol levels. In other words, they were prime candidates for heart attacks themselves.

"In some cases," says Lynn Macken, R.N., coordinator of cardiac and pulmonary rehabilitation at the Regional West Medical Center, in Scottsbluff, and one of the authors of the study, "the women's risk factors were even higher than their husbands."

When you think about it, this should not be all that surprising. When people live together, they eat the same meals and often have similar habits. So if one partner smokes and rarely exercises, there's a good chance the other one does too. But because men tend to have heart attacks earlier, they get put on notice about the need to change their habits sooner. In fact, in the Nebraska study, almost 90 percent of the men who smoked quit after their heart attack (at least for a while), but half of the women kept right on puffing.

What this means is pretty clear: In many, many cases, it's not just your partner who needs to make changes in how he lives. You may need to make them, too.

The Changing World of Heart Treatment

The last thirty-five years have brought radical changes in both the understanding and treatment of heart disease. Every few years, it seems, a new procedure is developed or an old one refined. The rapid pace of change makes it hard not only for patients but for many doctors to keep up. The good news is that doctors are now able to treat heart problems less invasively than ever before. The other good news is that there is more awareness than ever that the way we live, eat, and exercise can help us avoid heart disease, or live with it if we get it. Here is a brief rundown on the most important ways of treating heart disease or preventing a second heart attack. It's important to remember that most people will need to combine two or more of these approaches.

CHANGE YOUR LIFESTYLE: EAT RIGHT, EXERCISE, STOP SMOKING

If we all did this, few people would ever get heart disease in the first place. But it's never too late to change. Even people with serious heart disease who make substantial changes in their diet and get on a regular exercise program can greatly improve their prospects. One key, of course, is controlling fat and cholesterol. Reducing your intake of the bad kinds and increasing your consumption of the good kinds can make a big difference in the state of your arteries and the condition of your heart. Regular moderate exercise is also important. Just remember to consult your doctor before starting and to build up slowly to more vigorous exercise. Finally, snuff out that butt and you'll reduce your risk of another heart attack by 50 percent after just one year.

Of course, all of these changes are much easier to talk about than to do. And for many people they're easier to start than to stick with. In one study published in the *Archives of Internal Medicine,* one third to one half of patients who survived a heart attack or stroke were unable to make changes in major risk factors like blood pressure and cholesterol. In other words, the same issues that got them into trouble in the first place keep them in trouble later.

This is an area where you can play a huge role in helping your husband adopt a more heart-healthy routine. And the good news is that as you make changes in your home to help your husband, you and the rest of your family will also benefit. "Whether we want to admit it or not, we are primary role models for our husbands and our children," says Dr. Lori Mosca. "If we change habits, then they change habits. Attitudes change. Physical activity levels change. And the children benefit because the cooking will change."

ASK ABOUT MEDICINE—THEN TAKE IT

If someone you love has suffered a heart attack or been diagnosed with a heart condition, the right medication can be critical. Surprisingly, many heart attack patients are not prescribed appropriate medications when they're discharged from the hospital. For example, beta-blockers have consistently been shown to reduce mortality rates when given shortly after a heart attack. Yet many patients are discharged from the hospital without a prescription for beta-blockers. Low-dose aspirin is also recommended for heart patients, yet many are not taking it. The sad truth is that many doctors simply fail to discuss these medications with their patients. That means your husband or you need to bring it up, to ask the doctor about what medications he or she recommends and why.

Taking lots of pills can be difficult for many people, so you may want to help your husband get organized. Still, if he is able, he should get and take his own medicines.

When women take over all responsibility for managing his disease, including medications, it disempowers the man. When that happens, says cardiologist Paul Kligfield, M.D., of Cornell University Medical College in New York, "the men think they are not responsible for their own medication. You say, 'What medications are you taking?' And they say, 'I don't know, ask my wife.'" Not a good plan. A man who has had a heart attack needs to learn as much as possible about his disease and to take responsibility for making the necessary changes in his life.

Here's a quick review of the various classes of heart medications you should ask your doctor about.

Aspirin

For more than one hundred years aspirin has been used to treat fever, pain, and inflammation. More recently, this jack-of-all-trades medicine has found a new career as a low-cost way to help fend off heart attacks and strokes. Here's how it works: In people with congested arteries, a blood clot can cause a complete blockage and trigger a heart attack. Aspirin inhibits the action of platelets, the tiny bits of blood cells that trigger the blood to clot. Experts now urge people to chew an aspirin at the first sign of a heart attack.

But it's not only heart attack patients who should be taking aspirin. Anyone who has as little as a 3 percent chance of having a heart attack over the next five years should consider taking aspirin, according to the U.S. Preventive Services Task Force, an independent group of experts sponsored by the government. In those people, the task force says, the benefits of taking aspirin outweigh the risks (bleeding in the stomach or brain). Bottom line: If you (or your husband) have just one risk factor for heart disease, talk to your doctor about whether aspirin makes sense. Do not begin taking aspirin without first talking to your doctor.

Risk factors include being a man over forty, being overweight, being a smoker, or having high cholesterol, high blood pressure, or diabetes. To figure your five-year risk, go to *http://www.med-decisions.com/cvtool/pati.html* and use the online calculator. (You'll need to know your total and HDL cholesterol levels, as well as your blood pressure.) Again, a risk of over 3 percent means you need to consider aspirin therapy. But always consult a doctor first!

Despite these recommendations, a lot of people who should be taking aspirin aren't. One recent study found that 20 percent of people with diagnosed heart disease weren't taking aspirin. That's too bad, especially when you consider how easy and cheap it is. You don't need a high dose to get the benefit—a baby aspirin will do. Just 81 mg a day or 325 mg every other day can reduce a man's risk of heart attack by as much as 25 percent to 40 percent. It can also prevent certain types of strokes and there is some preliminary evidence that it may reduce the risk of colon cancer and Alzheimer's disease.

Beta-Blockers

These drugs help the heart beat slower and less forcefully by countering the effects of adrenaline and other substances produced by the body. By lessening the stress on the heart, they reduce the heart's need for oxygen and ease angina (chest pain). They also help regulate irregular heartbeats and reduce high blood pressure. Because they improve the survival of heart attack patients, beta-blockers should be prescribed to nearly all heart attack patients. Brand names include Lopressor, Sectral, and Tenormin.

ACE Inhibitors

ACE inhibitors block the body from making *angiotensin,* a hormone that causes blood vessels to constrict. The medication thus lowers blood pressure, making it easier for the heart to pump blood. Given after a heart attack, ACE inhibitors may prevent continuing damage to the heart muscle and increase survival. Brand names include Capoten, Vasotec, and Prinivil.

Calcium Channel Blockers

These drugs keep arteries open by limiting the amount of calcium that can enter the smooth muscle cells that line the arteries. They can be helpful after a heart attack because they reduce blood pressure and ease the burden of pumping on the heart. They are often used by people who can't tolerate beta-blockers or have heart rhythm abnormalities. Brand names include Cardizem, Dilacor, and Tiazac.

Vasodilators

As the name suggests, these drugs relax the smooth muscles of the heart's blood vessels, widening them and allowing more blood—and oxygen—to reach the heart. This eases the heart's need to pump forcefully, lowers blood pressure, and relieves the pain of angina. Nitroglycerin, a vasodilator, is the most commonly used heart drug in the world. Men who take nitroglycerin or other nitrates should not take Viagra or Levitra.

Cholesterol-Lowering Drugs

These drugs don't directly treat the symptoms of heart disease but do address an underlying cause. Some boost HDL (good cholesterol) levels, others lower LDL (bad cholesterol) levels or triglycerides. They may be prescribed individually or in combination with other drugs. Some of the common kinds of cholesterol-lowering drugs are statins, nicotinic acid, bile acid sequestrants, and fibrates (see chapter 15).

HEART PROCEDURES

Angiogram

This outpatient procedure is used to diagnose the state of the arteries. Doctors insert a thin tube called a catheter into an artery in the groin or arm and guide it up to a coronary artery. Then they inject a dye and take an X ray that will provide an image of the arteries, including any blockages. The procedure takes about ninety minutes from preparation to removal of the catheter.

Angioplasty

Here doctors guide a catheter to the coronary artery. A thinner catheter is then inserted that has a balloon attached. The balloon is inflated at areas that are blocked, pushing back the plaque to make more room for blood to flow through. A thin wire-mesh tube called a stent is often placed into the artery to keep it from closing down again. The patient may spend the night in the hospital for observation before going home.

Coronary Artery Bypass Surgery

In this surgery, a blood vessel is taken from another part of the body, usually the leg or chest, and used to create a detour or bypass around the blocked part of a coronary artery. If more than one artery is blocked, doctors may perform more than one bypass—i.e., triple or quadruple bypass surgery. According to the American Heart Association, this is the most commonly performed of all surgeries, with more than 500,000 performed in 2000.

Bypass surgery is major surgery and will usually require a three- to five-day hospital stay plus more recovery time at home. Many patients who undergo it suffer from some decline in mental ability and memory after the surgery. It is important to look for signs of depression after the surgery and get help if you see symptoms. Many researchers believe this is a result of patients being placed on a heart-lung machine to keep blood circulating while doctors operate. In an effort to minimize the risk of cognitive decline, many surgeons are now performing bypass surgery on a so-called beating heart—that is, they don't stop the patient's heart or use a heart-lung machine.

RECOVERING FROM HEART ATTACKS OR SURGERY

Whatever treatment your partner gets, the immediate aftermath can be a challenging and stressful time. You and your family members have to suddenly learn to care for a man who used to be the co-captain of the family. He has to deal with the new reality of his dependence and inability to live the life he used to. It will help everyone to gather as much information as you can about recovery and ways of coping and helping once a patient gets home. Fortunately, this is easier than ever to do. There are literally hundreds of websites, organizations, and books. The local affiliates of the American Heart Association can help link you up with support groups in your area. Rachael Freed's book *Heartmates* is also an excellent resource for you and your family.

Some patients experience post-traumatic stress disorder (PTSD) as a result of a heart attack. In one study of 102 patients who had heart attacks, about 10 percent developed PTSD. Not surprisingly, this hampered their ability to deal with their recovery. The researchers found that people with the most severe cases often failed to take prescribed medications or follow their treatment plan.

How a man is treated emotionally as well as medically in the hospital can have a lot to do with how well he recovers. The total hospital experience—including doctor-patient communication, social and emotional support, and discharge planning—can have a big impact on recovery. A Harvard study published in the *Journal of General Internal Medicine* found that people who did not have good experiences as inpatients were sicker one year later than those who did.

Cardiac Rehabilitation

Cardiac rehabilitation is a multipronged approach to help a patient (and the whole family) recover from a heart attack and/or surgery. It involves physical therapy and exercise, education about dietary changes, and social support for patients and part-ners. Studies show that cardiac rehab can go a long way toward helping to prevent fur-ther heart disease. The problem is that many people who could benefit aren't getting it. In Western Europe, *everyone* who suffers a heart attack gets cardiac rehab; in the United States, perhaps 25 percent of patients do, at best. That's because rehab is not always reimbursed by Medicare and private insurance companies, because it's unavailable, or because the treating doctor fails to recommend it. Don't let this hap-pen to your spouse! Dr. Paul Kligfield, director of cardiac rehab at the New York Hospital–Cornell Medical Center, says: "If I had to make one recommendation for someone who's advocating for a spouse who has had a heart attack, it would be to try to find a good cardiac rehab program and fight like heck to get it."

Cardiac rehabilitation is about managing a chronic disease and teaching a patient how to control his or her risk factors. Studies show that a twelve-week cardiac rehab course can reduce mortality over a three-year period by 20 percent to 30 percent, a result, Dr. Kligfield says, that is "nothing short of spectacular." But beyond improved survival, the most important thing cardiac rehabilitation does for a heart attack sur-vivor is put him in charge of his own life again. Why is this important?

One reason is that it can help men avoid depression, which frequently follows a heart attack or heart surgery. Men who are depressed may neglect to take medicine or follow a healthy diet. They are much more likely to have further "events" and to die. If your spouse shows any signs of depression, it's important to get help and to treat it.

Good rehab programs treat the spouse as a key member of the patient's recovery team. In many rehab centers, programs welcome and cater to the spouse with everything from cooking lessons to stress-management sessions.

To enter a cardiac rehab program you must be referred by your doctor. If your doctor fails to discuss it with you and you want to find a cardiac rehab center in your area, the American Association of Cardiovascular and Pulmonary Rehabilitation (AACVPR) can help you find one. Check the website *http://www.aacvpr.org/* or call 312-321-5146.

Is There Sex After Heart Attack?

The question of whether and when they can have sex comes up for lots of couples in the aftermath of a heart attack or treatment for heart disease. But although many couples are worried about resuming a sex life, they are often too embarrassed to ask the doctor about it.

One common fear is that the sex act itself will bring on another heart attack. While this does happen, it is rare (the untimely death of a former vice president notwithstanding). The good news is that while each case is different, there is little reason for heart patients to be afraid of sex. A few years ago, researchers at Harvard actually studied this question by interviewing thousands of heart attack patients and their spouses. They concluded that having sex increased the risk of a heart attack, but only slightly. They also concluded that this increased risk was virtually wiped out if a patient exercised regularly. Experts say that sexual intercourse exerts about as much strain on the heart as walking quickly up a couple of flights of stairs.

A 1994 article in *Physician and Sportsmedicine* found that if a person can walk a mile in seventeen minutes without adverse symptoms, then he or she can safely engage in sexual activity. More recently, experts at an international conference came up with a plan to help doctors and patients assess the risk:

- **Low risk:** If your partner has gone six to eight weeks after a heart attack, angioplasty or bypass surgery, and if he has two risk factors or less, he should feel free to have sex. The same applies to men whose hypertension or angina is under control.

- **Moderate Risk:** Men who are two to six weeks out from a heart attack or heart procedure, who have three or more major risk cardiac risk factors, or have a history of heart failure, stroke, or peripheral vascular disease should have a detailed cardiac evaluation before resuming sexual activity.

- **High risk:** Men who've had a heart attack within two weeks, or who have severe angina, uncontrolled hypertension, severe heart failure, dangerous arrhythmias, or moderate to severe heart valve disease should hold off until their medical conditions have improved.

Viagra, by the way, is said to be safe for men with low to moderate risk unless they are taking nitrate medications—that is, all forms of nitroglycerin. If you're concerned about this issue, discuss your fears with your mate and get some guidance from his doctor. When you do resume activity, take it slowly at first. Wait several hours after a meal and take any scheduled medications prior to making love. At first, it makes sense to choose positions that are less strenuous, but most couples eventually resume normal relations over time.

Some of the medications used to treat heart disease can interfere with sexual function, as can cardiovascular disease itself. Some men have stopped taking their medicines for this reason and suffered heart attacks as a result. Not a good idea. If you and your partner are concerned about this issue, talk to the doctor about it, but don't stop taking a medicine on your own.

HEART FAILURE: A GROWING THREAT

Over time, heart attacks, coronary artery disease, high blood pressure, diabetes, heart valve disease, and even infections and alcoholism can cause the heart to weaken. When a heart becomes so weak that it can no longer pump blood throughout the body efficiently, doctors call this heart failure. Blood backs up into the veins, causing tissues in the legs or the lungs to swell.

Some 5 million Americans suffer from congestive heart failure and more than 500,000 new cases are diagnosed each year, according to the American Heart Association. More men than women get the disease, which kills 51,000 people each year and plays a role in the death of thousands more. These numbers have increased 148 percent since the late 1970s, according to the American Heart Association, a result of the aging population.

Symptoms of heart failure include fatigue, shortness of breath, difficulty breathing, wheezing, trouble lying flat, and swelling of the legs. Despite the increasing numbers, there is some good news for people with this condition. Nearly a third of heart failure patients will experience significant improvements by combining a pacemaker with medication, according to a recent study. This therapy, called *cardiac resynchronization,* helps the heart muscle beat more effectively and may help some patients avoid or delay getting a heart transplant.

WHAT ABOUT STROKE?

A few years ago, a good friend of my husband—I'll call him Jerry—spent a Saturday morning hitting golf balls at the driving range. Jerry was the picture of good health, a trim, athletic forty-year-old who'd never had an illness more serious than the flu and certainly no problems that would put him at risk for any major disease.

On Sunday night, when he went to bed, he started to get a headache. At first, he thought nothing of it, but when he woke up the next morning, it had gotten so painful, he could barely lift his head off the pillow. Strangely, his left eye also seemed to be drooping and tearing.

"I didn't know what to do because it didn't fit any illness I'd had before," he recalls. "My wife Karen kept pushing me to go the doctor." It was a good thing she did, even though it took a while for the mystery of his condition to be unraveled. When the headache did not go away he saw his regular doctor who diagnosed a sinus infection. But the X rays he ordered showed no infection. What followed was a round-robin of doctors and specialists. An eye doctor, a dentist, and an ear, nose, and throat specialist offered their opinions of the problem. The dentist even performed a root canal, unnecessarily, as it turned out. Finally, one of the doctors ordered an MRI. The result was almost as surprising to the doctors as to Jerry and Karen. Jerry had suffered a stroke.

Forty-year-old men are not supposed to have strokes, and for the most part, of course, they don't. In fact, when people think about likely stroke survivors, they tend to think of old people and of angry people who can't control their rage. Like many perceptions, both of these have a strong element of truth. Most strokes do happen to people over sixty-five, and people who vent their anger a lot have a bit of a higher risk of having a stroke. But sadly, most people are woefully ignorant about what a stroke actually looks like. A survey taken in 1998 found that most Americans could not identify even one symptom of stroke. Symptoms of stroke are on page 362.

Apparently, men and women may experience symptoms of a stroke quite differently. A study in *The Annals of Emergency Medicine* found that women are more likely to experience some of the less classic symptoms such as limb pain, disorientation, and fluctuations in consciousness. Nevertheless, if you notice any of these symptoms in your husband or anyone else, call 911 right away!

In the past, having a stroke was like being sentenced to death or severe long-term disability. But these days such a fate may be avoided, especially if the patient is a candidate for clot-busting drugs known as *tissue plasminogen activators (tPAs)* and *if* the patient gets quick treatment. If clot busters are given in the first three hours after the start of symptoms, the chance of suffering from a severe disability is significantly decreased in many patients.

In their cause, most strokes are quite similar to heart attacks. In fact, they're sometimes referred to as "brain attacks." In a stroke, the supply of blood to the brain is suddenly interrupted. The most common form is called an *ischemic stroke*. Usually, this happens when arteries become narrowed by deposits of fatty plaque. These plaques can rupture and form clots that block the artery. In other cases, a condition known as *atrial fibrillation* leads to strokes. Atrial fibrillation is a condition where the heart beats abnormally. This may create blood clots that can break off and travel to the brain, blocking blood flow. *Hemorrhagic strokes* occur when a blood vessel in or around the brain ruptures, causing bleeding into the brain and interrupting the normal blood supply. TPA is not used in these patients. In either case, if the proper flow of blood to the brain is cut off for more than a few minutes, brain cells begin to die.

In some cases the symptoms of a stroke last only a few minutes and then disappear. This is called a *transient ischemic attack* (TIA) or ministroke. Since the symptoms of a TIA go away on their own, many people ignore them, never seek medical help, and never even mention them to a doctor. The problem is that TIAs are often harbingers of worse things to come, namely, a really big stroke that can disable or kill. According to the National Stroke Association, one in five stroke survivors will have another stroke within the next five years. So if your husband or someone you love has symptoms like these that resolve quickly, be sure they get prompt medical attention.

WHO GETS STROKES?

Strokes are more common among older people. Seventy-two percent of strokes occur in people over the age of sixty-five. Men are more likely than women to have strokes at most ages. But in old age, when strokes happen in the greatest numbers, the rate of stroke among women shoots up. The result is that more than 60 percent of the people who die from stroke are women. In fact strokes kill twice as many women as breast cancer.

The good news about strokes is that treatment has improved so much that even though there are more strokes occurring than ever, the death rate is declining and people who have strokes are surviving longer and with less impairment than in the past.

Depression and Stroke

Depression and anxiety in men can lead to a higher risk of stroke. A study in *Stroke: Journal of the American Heart Association,* found that men who were depressed or anxious were more than three times as likely to die from a stroke as other men. Why? The researchers speculate that depressed people do not take care of themselves and neglect to take their medications.

Not Just a Disease of the Old

Many doctors fail to recognize stroke symptoms in young people because they don't think of them as being stroke candidates. But about 28 percent of strokes happen to people under sixty-five, a group not normally seen as "at risk." What causes strokes among the young? The traditional things, of course: high blood pressure and high cholesterol. But many strokes that hit the young have little to do with traditional risk factors.

Migraine headaches seem to increase the risk of stroke in both men and women, especially before the age of fifty. Many of the stroke-related migraines are so-called complicated migraines. These migraines are accompanied by neuro-logic changes such as paralysis of an eye or one side of the body. Compounding the risk for aging male baby boomers is the fact that they may ignore the pain and push on, says Patrick Lyden, M.D., chief of the Stroke Clinic at the Veteran's Affairs Medical Center in San Diego and director of the Stroke Center at University of California, San Diego Medical Center. "They have a serious migraine, yet they're inclined to go to work, ignore the pain, ignore the symptoms, and push through it," Dr. Lyden says. "And after a week, they have a stroke. Because they are boomers they feel a sense of omnipotence and invulnerability."

The use of cocaine, especially smoked crack cocaine, has also fueled an increase in strokes among the young. "Since 1985, the incidence of cocaine-related strokes has reached epidemic proportions," writes one researcher for the National Institute for Drug Abuse. The likely reason is that cocaine causes blood

> **STROKE**
>
> • It is the third leading killer in the United States. In 2000 more than 167,000 people died of stroke, according to the CDC.
> • It is a leading cause of serious, long-term disability in the United States.
> • Every year some 700,000 Americans have strokes. If ministrokes (transient ischemic attacks, or TIAs) are counted, the number rises to 1.2 million.
> • Fourteen percent of persons who survive a first stroke will have another stroke within one year.
> • The risk of stroke goes up with age. For people over fifty-five, it doubles with each successive decade.
> • Twenty-eight percent of strokes occur in people under sixty-five.
> • Only 1 percent of Americans think they are at risk for stroke, according to a survey by the American Stroke Association.

vessels to contract and pushes blood pressure up, problems that can also lead to heart attacks and seizures. The use of diet pills and herbal supplements containing ephedra can sometimes produce the same results, says Dr. Lyden.

A condition known as *carotid dissection* can also lead to stroke in younger people. A carotid dissection is a small tear in the carotid artery of the neck that sends blood directly to the brain. A similar but less common injury can occur to the other artery that feeds the brain, the *vertebral* artery. As a result of the injury, bleeding occurs inside the wall of the artery. Then a small clot forms, which can break off and travel to the brain, blocking blood flow. Carotid dissection can occur as the result of a trauma to the neck such as a fall or whiplash, from athletic activity like football, or even from manipulation by a chiropractor.

Though exact numbers are hard to come by, Dr. Lyden says this type of stroke is on the rise among baby boomers. "We see somebody here every week for possible dissection," he says. And since most people don't think stroke happens in the young, Dr. Lyden says, family members have a hard time understanding it: " 'How can my forty-five-year-old husband be having a stroke? It's impossible.' " But with newer diagnostic techniques like CT scans and MRIs, neurologists are finding that this form of stroke is more common in middle-aged people than previously thought.

"More people remain active longer," says Dr. Lyden. "We all used to give up basketball and soccer when we were in our late twenties. Now we are continuing to do this into our late forties. People are skiing and falling or surfing and falling. More people are going to chiropractors, and that can cause dissection. So we are seeing a lot more dissections." Even coughing or a violent jerk of the head can, in rare cases, trigger this problem. More common, though, are patients who have dissections and strokes from lifting weights, playing football, or even swinging a golf club.

After the MRI revealed that our friend Jerry had suffered a stroke, his wife Karen did a flurry of research and found a stroke specialist with a lot of experience with young stroke patients. He quickly figured out that Jerry's stroke was caused by a carotid dissection.

Jerry spent the next year on the blood-thinning medication warfarin, to try to prevent blood clots from forming. His carotid artery is completely blocked off and cannot be surgically repaired so all blood now flows to his brain through the vertebral artery. While he has made a complete recovery and has no neurological symptoms, he will have to be extremely careful for the rest of his life to avoid injuring his remaining functional artery. This new reality has forced a reluctant shift in his attitude.

"I was in denial," he says. " I kept thinking, 'What do you mean I can't work out anymore? I have to take medicine?' I wasn't grasping that I had a serious neurological problem. I finally realized I had to change so that this wouldn't happen again." Together, Jerry and Karen have found ways for him to exercise safely and avoid activities that could injure his neck.

Stroke Treatment

Treatment of stroke has improved tremendously in recent years. Studies have shown that specialized stroke units in hospitals can improve the odds of recovery from a stroke. Like specialized cardiac units, stroke units are equipped with the latest diagnostic and treatment equipment and have staff members who are specially trained in stroke treatment.

Experts and advocates would like to see more stroke centers established in cities around the country. Studies in Europe suggest that stroke units not only increase people's chances of surviving a stroke, they leave them functioning at higher levels five and ten years later and reduce the likelihood that stroke survivors would need to be placed in institutional care. A group called the Brain Attack Coalition is pushing for improved treatment and the development of stroke centers around the country. The American College of Emergency Physicians also has advocated for stroke centers, but at a time when many emergency departments are already overwhelmed and underfunded, the needed funding is hard to come by. More than one thousand emergency departments have closed in the past ten years, and the remaining emergency departments are treating an increasing number of patients—up to 108 million in 2000. Many hospitals are diverting ambulances to less crowded hospitals to avoid jeopardizing the care of patients already in the emergency room.

If your husband is at risk of having a stroke, do a little research and find out if there is a stroke treatment center in your area. If he has a stroke, insist on going there. "Of course, this may not be possible if the hospital emergency department is diverting ambulances to other hospitals," said George Molzen, M.D., president of the American College of Emergency Physicians. Steven Warach, M.D., the chief of the Stroke Diagnostics and Therapeutics Section of the National Institute of Neurological Disorders and Stroke, urges people to advocate for the creation of more stroke units. "It would be a good idea for people to lobby their own hospital and ask, 'Why don't you have a stroke team?'"

STROKE REHABILITATION

Some two thirds of stroke patients survive their initial stroke and then need help to relearn some of the basic skills they lost as a result of the damage to their brain. They may need help learning how to walk, eat, bathe, and dress again. These services usually begin in the hospital, often within a day or two of the stroke. Most stroke patients will regain some of these skills in the first thirty days through spontaneous recovery—meaning the effects of the stroke resolve on their own.

There are, of course, limits to what rehabilitation can do. It all depends on the nature and severity of the stroke. Some people are helped greatly by rehabilitation services; others are not helped much at all. In some cases, rehabilitation may not be recommended, and this can be very disappointing for a family. For this reason, it's important to get a good assessment, and perhaps more than one. This can be especially useful if you have to fight with a managed care company that's resisting paying for rehab.

THE POSTSTROKE FAMILY

Stroke is the number-one cause of major disability among Americans. Strokes affect not only individuals but whole families. According to the National Stroke Association, four out of five families will be touched directly or indirectly by strokes. In their aftermath, stroke survivors and their loved ones have to adjust to a new normal, a whole new way of life. Financially, logistically, emotionally, psychologically, stroke transforms the landscape of family life.

Let's examine for a moment the effect on you and your family if your husband were to have a stroke. First of all, there are all the worries. You may fear it will happen again. You may not want to be alone with your husband because you're afraid you won't know what to do. You may fear that friends and family will abandon you. And you may be afraid that your husband won't be able to adjust to disability or will have to be placed in a hospital or long-term care facility.

If your husband was the breadwinner, your family is now deprived of his income. If he is disabled, you must now arrange and pay for not only medical treatment but also care and support. You must now run the family's affairs, make more decisions, deal with fixing the roof or the toilet when they leak. Most difficult, you're deprived of the kind of companionship and support you once had. A study in the July 2001 issue of *Stroke* showed that spouses experience a sharp decline in their sense of well-being and a sharp rise in their psychological stress within the days after their mates had a stroke. This, they say, can affect the spouse's ability to support a stroke survivor, which is so important to the recovery and rehabilitation process. The message: Doctors and other members of the health team need to pay attention to and support spouses. If you are a spouse and you are having trouble dealing with the new challenges, don't be afraid to ask for help. If you don't take care of yourself you will not be able to take care of the person you love.

Depending on the severity of the stroke, the quality of a couple's sexual relationship is likely to change. Fears can interfere—the fear of being unable to perform, of having another stroke during sex, and of being rejected by a mate. Stroke survivors also must often adjust to a new body image.

Contending with such profound changes can be emotionally difficult. In addition, the needs of the caregiver are often overlooked in the effort to rehabilitate the patient. And while you might assume that the hardest part of being a caregiver to a stroke victim would be meeting his physical needs, many people find the psychological, emotional, and behavioral changes the most troubling. It is not uncommon for people who have suffered a stroke to experience mood swings, irritability, confusion, and memory loss.

No wonder then that depression, anger, resentment, blame, and guilt are commonly felt by not only the stroke survivor but also by the patient's spouse. Studies have found that as many as half of caregivers will become depressed or suffer other emotional problems. Not surprisingly, the greater the degree of impairment of the stroke victim, the greater the severity of the emotional upheaval felt by the spouse.

All of this, of course, can damage a spouse's ability to provide the support that is so crucial to rehabilitation and recovery.

The key to avoiding this scenario, according to experts, is for you, the spouse, to get your own support quickly. If you are the only caregiver, then the burden and potential for problems will be great. If you have a broad support network of family and friends, it will be less. The key is to ask for help. If family and friends step forward to help, try to get them to commit to particular times and tasks. This can help create much-needed routine, and it can also give you an opportunity to take a break and do something to renew your own energy levels.

Stroke support groups can also be helpful for stroke survivors, as well as spouses, children, friends, and caregivers. The Stroke Family Support Network at 1-888-4-STROKE (478-7653) is a free information and referral service offering information to stroke survivors, caregivers, family members, and health-care professionals. Many of the specialists responding to the calls are stroke survivors or caregivers themselves. The American Stroke Association, a division of the American Heart Association, operates the Stroke Family Warm Line (1-888-4-STROKE) designed to help family members through the emotionally trying times after a stroke. The ASA can also link you with more than two thousand stroke support groups around the country.

Caregivers are vital to the recovery process. But you can't be a good caregiver to someone else if you don't take care of yourself. Make some time for you, and your whole family will benefit.

FOR MORE HELP

If you are confronting the diagnosis of heart disease or a related condition for the first time, you are probably feeling a bit overwhelmed—whether it is your spouse who is suffering or you. As we pointed out, spouses are often more stressed than the person with the disease. There is certainly much to learn. A new tool, one I like very much, is the American Heart Association's Heart Profilers Program, which you can find at *www.americanheart.org*. This can help you and your spouse learn about heart disease and the role of various health and lifestyle risk factors. It may also help you decide, along with your doctor, on the best treatments for a particular disease. The program takes you through a series of questions and gives treatment information on a variety of heart related conditions including atrial fibrillation, coronary artery disease, and heart failure as well as high blood pressure and cholesterol. In addition it can connect you to the latest experimental clinical trials in your area as well as give you the latest information from the medical journals. It will even download specific questions you need to ask your doctor about your loved one's condition. And it's free!

15

The Usual Suspects

We've all heard about or know people who seem to be in perfect health, have no obvious risk factors, and then have heart attacks anyway. But before disaster strikes most people in the form of a heart attack or stroke, there are hints, little warnings that could help avert an "event" if only they were noticed and heeded.

The things that can cause big problems for most people are hardly mysteries. I like to call them the usual suspects: obesity, high blood pressure, high cholesterol, and high blood sugar (diabetes). These cause the damage that leads to heart attacks and strokes.

Recognizing and dealing with these problems can make all the difference in the world. That's why every year, public health experts seem to press harder to raise the public awareness of these issues. And every year researchers come up with new data and recommendations to more clearly define how much fat and cholesterol people can handle and be healthy, how much glucose in their blood poses a risk. For example, health experts say that if more people got their cholesterol treated, and kept it within a normal range, hundreds of thousands of lives could be saved every year.

As you read through this chapter, keep in mind that almost always a person will have not just one risk factor but two or more. The goal of this chapter is to give some helpful advice for each risk factor. Keep in mind that if you can get a handle on one risk factor, you are likely reducing all other risk factors.

So let's take a look at these usual suspects and look for ways we can begin to improve. We'll begin with the mother of all risk factors, the problem that is challenging cigarette smoking for the title of "public health enemy number one."

THE GIRTH OF A NATION

Americans are too fat. About this there can be no argument. The latest official word is that 61 percent of American adults qualify as overweight or obese, according to the U.S. Surgeon General. Every year since 1985 the number has risen, and now more than 100 million Americans are classified as overweight or obese. And there's no end to the problem in sight.

Another glimpse of the extent of obesity can be seen in two U.S. maps printed in the front of a report on obesity issued in 2001 by former Surgeon General David

Satcher. The states of the union are color coded to indicate the percentage of obese people living in each state in 1991 and 2000. Light blue and light green indicate lower levels of obesity (less than 10 percent and 10 percent to 14 percent of a state's population, respectively). Dark green and dark blue indicate higher levels (15 percent to 19 percent and more than 20 percent, respectively). The change in the map is truly striking. The 1991 map is all pale colors, with just four states shaded dark green. For 2000, the map is a solid sea of dark colors, nearly half of them dark blue, with only one state in the whole country still shaded a pale color. America truly is on a dangerous course.

How Fat Is Fat?

In 1998 the federal government released new guidelines to guide doctors and patients about body weight. Rather than looking at how many pounds a person may be over a so-called ideal weight, the guidelines were based instead on his or her Body Mass Index (BMI), waist circumference, and risk factors for other diseases and conditions.

Body Mass Index Table

The BMI is a measure of your weight relative to your height. Find your height and your weight on the table. Read up to the top of the column where the numbers intersect to find your BMI (see table on page 395). Or you could also calculate your BMI.

$$BMI = \frac{your\ weight\ in\ pounds}{(height\ in\ inches) \times (height\ in\ inches)} \times 703$$

Here's how to judge your BMI score:

Below 18.5	Underweight
18.5–24.9	Normal
25.0–29.9	Overweight
30 and above	Obese

Waist Circumference

Waist circumference is a good indicator of your abdominal fat and can help predict your risk for future problems such as heart disease or diabetes. Place a measuring tape snugly around your waist at your navel. If the measurement is over 40 inches in men and over 35 inches in women, your risk is high.

You can find more information about calculating and assessing your BMI score at this National Institutes of Health website: *http://www.nhlbi.nih.gov/health/public/heart/obesity/lose_wt/risk.htm.*

The site also includes a table that lets you look at your BMI and waist circumference together and helps you assess what it means. Or try the Centers for Disease Control website: *http://cdc.gov//nccdphp/dnpa/bmi/bmi-adult.htm.*

Other Risk Factors

To further gauge your risk of various health problems, take into account whether you have any of the following risk factors:

- high blood pressure (hypertension).
- high LDL cholesterol ("bad" cholesterol).
- low HDL cholesterol ("good" cholesterol).
- high triglycerides.
- high blood glucose (sugar).
- family history of premature heart disease.
- physical inactivity.
- cigarette smoking.

Body Mass Index Table

	Normal						Overweight					Obese										Extreme Obesity														
BMI	19	20	21	22	23	24	25	26	27	28	29	30	31	32	33	34	35	36	37	38	39	40	41	42	43	44	45	46	47	48	49	50	51	52	53	54
Height (inches)												Body Weight (pounds)																								
58	91	96	100	105	110	115	119	124	129	134	138	143	148	153	158	162	167	172	177	181	186	191	196	201	205	210	215	220	224	229	234	239	244	248	253	258
59	94	99	104	109	114	119	124	128	133	138	143	148	153	158	163	168	173	178	183	188	193	198	203	208	212	217	222	227	232	237	242	247	252	257	262	267
60	97	102	107	112	118	123	128	133	138	143	148	153	158	163	168	174	179	184	189	194	199	204	209	215	220	225	230	235	240	245	250	255	261	266	271	276
61	100	106	111	116	122	127	132	137	143	148	153	158	164	169	174	180	185	190	195	201	206	211	217	222	227	232	238	243	248	254	259	264	269	275	280	285
62	104	109	115	120	126	131	136	142	147	153	158	164	169	175	180	186	191	196	202	207	213	218	224	229	235	240	246	251	256	262	267	273	278	284	289	295
63	107	113	118	124	130	135	141	146	152	158	163	169	175	180	186	191	197	203	208	214	220	225	231	237	242	248	254	259	265	270	278	282	287	293	299	304
64	110	116	122	128	134	140	145	151	157	163	169	174	180	186	192	197	204	209	215	221	227	232	238	244	250	256	262	267	273	279	285	291	296	302	308	314
65	114	120	126	132	138	144	150	156	162	168	174	180	186	192	198	204	210	216	222	228	234	240	246	252	258	264	270	276	282	288	294	300	306	312	318	324
66	118	124	130	136	142	148	155	161	167	173	179	186	192	198	204	210	216	223	229	235	241	247	253	260	266	272	278	284	291	297	303	309	315	322	328	334
67	121	127	134	140	146	153	159	166	172	178	185	191	198	204	211	217	223	230	236	242	249	255	261	268	274	280	287	293	299	306	312	319	325	331	338	344
68	125	131	138	144	151	158	164	171	177	184	190	197	203	210	216	223	230	236	243	249	256	262	269	276	282	289	295	302	308	315	322	328	335	341	348	354
69	128	135	142	149	155	162	169	176	182	189	196	203	209	216	223	230	236	243	250	257	263	270	277	284	291	297	304	311	318	324	331	338	345	351	358	365
70	132	139	146	153	160	167	174	181	188	195	202	209	216	222	229	236	243	250	257	264	271	278	285	292	299	306	313	320	327	334	341	348	355	362	369	376
71	136	143	150	157	165	172	179	186	193	200	208	215	222	229	236	243	250	257	265	272	279	286	293	301	308	315	322	329	338	343	351	358	365	372	379	386
72	140	147	154	162	169	177	184	191	199	206	213	221	228	235	242	250	258	265	272	279	287	294	302	309	316	324	331	338	346	353	361	368	375	383	390	397
73	144	151	159	166	174	182	189	197	204	212	219	227	235	242	250	257	265	272	280	288	295	302	310	318	325	333	340	348	355	363	371	378	386	393	401	408
74	148	155	163	171	179	186	194	202	210	218	225	233	241	249	256	264	272	280	287	295	303	311	319	326	334	342	350	358	365	373	381	389	396	404	412	420
75	152	160	168	176	184	192	200	208	216	224	232	240	248	256	264	272	279	287	295	303	311	319	327	335	343	351	359	367	375	383	391	399	407	415	423	431
76	156	164	172	180	189	197	205	213	221	230	238	246	254	263	271	279	287	295	304	312	320	328	336	344	353	361	369	377	385	394	402	410	418	426	435	443

Source: Adapted from *Clinical Guidelines on the Identification, Evaluation, and Treatment of Overweight and Obesity in Adults: The Evidence Report.* National Heart, Lung and Blood Institute, National Institutes of Health.

CALCULATING YOUR RISK

So you've got all this information. You've figured out your BMI, measured your waist, and counted up any risk factors you or your husband might have. Now what do you do with this data? The government guidelines say you should try to lose weight if:

- You're obese: Your BMI is 30 or higher.
- You're overweight: Your BMI is 25 to 29.9 *and* you have two or more of the risk factors listed on page 394.

Even a small weight loss (10 percent of your current weight) will help to lower your risk of developing diseases associated with obesity. That means if you weigh 200 pounds, you need to get down to 180 pounds.

If you're overweight, but don't have a big waist, and you have fewer than two risk factors, you can probably focus on maintaining weight, rather than trying to shed pounds.

SO WHAT'S A FEW POUNDS?

It's easy to discount the risks of carrying around extra weight. After all, some people, though not most, can carry around extra pounds without it adversely affecting their health. For most people, however, obesity poses a heavy burden on their health. Researchers at RAND, a California-based think tank, say obesity presents a greater risk to health than smoking, heavy drinking, or being poor combined. They and others argue that obesity is now the nation's top public health threat. In a recent survey, RAND researchers found that nearly half of the people who were obese had two or more health problems such as heart disease, high blood pressure, or diabetes. The obese respondents had 30 percent to 50 percent more medical problems than smokers or heavy drinkers.

In January 2002 the *Journal of the American Medical Association* quantified just what those excess pounds can cost a person. A young black woman who is severely obese (a BMI of greater than 45) can expect to lose four to five years of life. A severely obese white woman can lose up to eight years. The biggest shocker of all, however, was what a young severely obese man loses—thirteen years for Caucasians and twenty years for African-Americans!

Obesity is expensive not only in years of life lost but also in dollars. A study in 2003 in the *American Journal of Health Promotion* looked at 178,000 employees of General Motors and found that overweight and obese individuals incur up to $1,500 more annual medical costs than people of healthy weight.

In his report, Dr. Satcher said that the obesity epidemic threatens to undo all the progress that has been made in the fight against heart disease, cancer, and other ailments. He estimates that over 300,000 lives could be saved every year if all Americans maintained a healthy weight. And he pegs the price tag for obesity-related diseases at over $100 billion annually.

For Satcher and other health guardians, the sheer scope of the obesity epidemic requires a major national response. They want to see a nationwide campaign on obesity similar to the one on smoking. Dr. Satcher's report, in fact, was called *A Call to Action.*

Here are a few of the reasons why public health experts feel the need to act so urgently:

- People who are obese have a 50 percent to 100 percent increased risk of dying compared to those whose weight is in the normal range. This higher death rate stems from many causes, but the biggest by far is heart disease.

- More often than not, obesity is a package deal that comes with high blood pressure (the most common obesity-related problem), high cholesterol, and diabetes. Some people have all four. Any of these problems alone can lead to heart attack and stroke.

- Obesity is often associated with cancer, especially esophageal, colon, and prostate cancer.

Even if being overweight doesn't kill you, it can make you pretty uncomfortable. When I was pregnant with twins I gained nearly ninety pounds! And wow, was that an experience. I understood firsthand just how tough all that extra weight made everyday living. After the babies were born, things didn't improve right away. It took me nearly a year and a half to lose the weight. During that time I had a litany of physical complaints from low back pain to knee pain to trouble breathing. So believe me, extra pounds can make life difficult—or worse! Here are a few examples.

- Obesity can cause or aggravate hernias, low back pain, arthritis, gout, carpal tunnel syndrome, and other problems involving nerves in the wrists and hands.

- Obese people have an increased risk of gum disease, cataracts, and gallstones.

- In men, obesity can lower testosterone levels, which can affect sexual function.

- Obesity is a strong risk factor for adult-onset asthma. Obese people need to work harder to breathe and tend to have inefficient respiratory muscles and diminished lung capacity. That puts them at risk for *hypoxia,* a state in which oxygen is insufficient to meet the body's needs. *Pickwickian syndrome,* named for an overweight character in a Charles Dickens novel, occurs when severely obese people experience a lack of oxygen that causes profound and chronic sleepiness and, eventually, heart failure. It is also called *obesity hypoventilation syndrome* (OHS).

- People with obesity and type 2 diabetes are at higher risk for a kind of hepatitis called *nonalcoholic steatohepatitis* (NASH) that produces liver damage similar to that caused by alcoholism. It can be very serious and require liver transplantation.
- People who are obese have a much higher risk of sleep apnea, which can lead to heart arrhythmias, stroke, right-sided heart failure, and car accidents.

Being overweight or obese can also lead to a whole set of social problems including discrimination. Studies have shown that obese people are less likely to be hired or promoted and are less likely to achieve higher educational status. Many obese people have trouble finding a mate. And society's attitude toward obese people can be harsh and punitive. They're often looked down upon and seen as inferior. Many people believe that being overweight is the fault of that person, a result of weakness or lack of will.

Because of this, groups like the National Association to Advance Fat Acceptance (*http://www.naafa.org/*) are fighting to change society's view of people who are fat. And while the exact causes of the obesity epidemic are not known, what is clear is that people who are overweight or obese should not be discriminated against because of their body size. Being obese will in time affect people's health, and it's critically important to seek out the causes of the epidemic and work to change it in a positive way. What we should not do is punish people who struggle with their weight.

So Why Are So Many of Us Overweight or Obese?

On one level, it's not that much of a mystery. For the vast majority of us, being overweight or obese comes from the discrepancy between the large number of calories we consume and the significantly lower number of calories that we expend: too much poor-quality food coupled with too little exercise. But it's not really that simple. There are a variety of genetic, cultural, and psychological factors at play, and researchers are exploring them all.

A few experts pin much of the blame on the low-fat craze that swept the nation a few years ago. Fat went out, and high-calorie, low-fat foods came in. Trouble was people started eating less fat but more calories, so we gained weight instead of losing it. Others say that the low-fat craze should not be blamed; Americans simply eat too much of everything, except healthy foods!

Another big—make that super-sized—factor is our increasing tendency to buy our meals from restaurants, especially fast-food joints, where serving up high-fat, high-calorie fare in ever larger portions has evolved into a fine art. Today fast-food purveyors encourage calorie gluttony with huge portions, and promote them with store banners and staff members adorned with pins urging customers to "super-size it." McDonald's 610-calorie super size french fries is three times greater than the single size the company offered when it opened in 1955. The 7-Eleven Double Gulp soda is a whopping 64 ounces—that's *half a gallon* of sugar and calories—designed to be consumed by one person. To be fair, some "big food" companies are getting the message. Kraft foods announced in July 2003 that it will reduce portion sizes and work to improve the nutritional content of its food products.

Fast-food marketing never lets up. Fast-food advertising is an overwhelming presence on television, especially during children's programs, helping to hook kids on junk food from an early age. Cash-strapped schools contract with fast-food purveyors to supply kids with fast-food lunches; the hallways outside many school cafeterias are lined with vending machines dispensing candy and chips.

But genetics plays a big part, too. Obesity tends to run in families, and not just because families tend to share dining habits. Identical twin studies have helped researchers isolate the effects of genes. In one famous study, researchers at Laval University in Canada overfed identical twins by 1,000 calories a day for fourteen weeks and didn't allow them to exercise. They all gained weight, but there were huge variations in the amount. Some sets of twins gained only 9 pounds, while others gained 29. Within each pair of twins, though, the weight gain was quite similar.

Lack of exercise is a big issue, too, as schools continue to gut sports programs and kids spend more time in front of TVs and computers. Depression or other mental health problems could also be a factor, causing people to eat more and exercise less than they should. All of these things combine to tip the scales against us.

Ironically, at the same moment that obesity has been identified as a public health problem, the cultural and social forces that help fuel it are as strong as ever. And there are also significant barriers keeping overweight or obese people from getting the medical and professional help they need. For instance, most health insurance companies and managed-care programs—even Medicare—will not pay for weight-loss treatment (though weight-loss programs are now tax deductible). Many physicians devote little time to obesity management because they believe that obese patients get that way from a lack of will and that there is little that they, as doctors, can do to influence their patients' behavior. Most doctors are not trained to counsel or treat people with weight problems, so many do not advise their obese patients to lose weight. Doctors and many experts disagree about whether obesity is or is not a disease. In my view, such an argument doesn't matter all that much. What is very clear is that obesity is a chronic condition that is difficult to treat and requires lifelong management.

DOES MARRIAGE MAKE MEN FAT?

In nearly all ways, marriage is good for men's health, as we discussed earlier in chapter 10. But there's one area where that may not be true. "Marriage," says Jeffrey Sobal, Ph.D., a sociologist at Cornell University, "seems to make men fatter." He says the weight gain from marriage can range from a couple pounds to double digits. Married women gain a few pounds, too, but that's because of aging and having children, Sobal says.

So why does wedded life make men fatter? Sobal suggests a few possibilities. One factor could be that many men stop smoking when they get married and that usually causes people to put on a few pounds. Another is that many men exercise less after marriage. Plus many men and women eat more when they're married because they're eating together. Instead of grabbing a sandwich alone, a man may eat an elaborate meal with a main dish, side dishes, and dessert. (The good news here is that although some men get tubbier after marriage, they're probably safer than their single friends who carouse all night drinking, smoking, and crashing their cars.)

Of course, when men put on a few pounds, they don't tend to become emotionally tortured about it, like we women do. Studies have shown that women and girls who are overweight tend to blame themselves, while men and boys blame outside factors.

IF YOUR HUBBY IS TUBBY

No matter how overweight your husband is and how much you worry about it, there's only one person who can get him to shed pounds, and that's him. You can help him, you can support him, you can modify your diet and even exercise with him. But the motivation to change must come from him. If it doesn't, your efforts won't work. And pushing and nagging will only drive you both crazy. So before you embark on a weight-loss program with or for your spouse there are some important differences between women and men that you need to understand. First, many men don't think they have a problem even if they have a belly that hangs over the belt. Surveys show that 25 percent to 29 percent of men and 40 percent to 44 percent of women are trying to lose weight at any given time. Karen Miller-Kovach, chief scientist at Weight Watchers, says there is not a lot of research on men and weight loss, but her experience tells her that men don't think of themselves as overweight or fat, they think of themselves as "big." Miller-Kovach says, "Women are constantly thinking about their weight, struggling with their weight, going on a diet, doing this, doing that. Men are very, very late to come to the realization that they even have a problem. It's very unusual to find a man who will say 'I am overweight.' Guys are big, they aren't overweight. They don't have weight problems."

But once they've decided they do want to lose a few pounds, they often tackle the problem head on; no sitting around wondering what the emotional reason was behind that extra piece of cake they ate for lunch. "They don't mess around. They don't play with diets the way women tend to by and large," Miller-Kovach observes. "They just decide they're gonna do it. And they do." They do it alone, too. Only 5 percent of Weight Watchers members are men because, hey, guys don't need backup. "The idea of being in a group support environment, of talking about weight as an issue, of trying to find solutions that will help is just antithetical to the way that men tend to approach weight loss," adds Miller-Kovach. "You don't sit down with your enemy and negotiate a settlement. You say, 'I hate you. I'm gonna conquer you.' And that's the end of it. They declare war!"

Men don't generally blame their extra pounds on emotional upheaval; they overeat because "it's there" or "it tastes good." In other words, asking your partner what he was feeling when he ate those four chocolate donuts won't get you very far. Miller-Kovach says: "If women try to help men lose weight their way, it will usually fail. There will be a lot of frustration on everyone's part." Better to exercise the control you have over the food that comes into the house in a way that helps him lose weight. Then if you and other family members eat the same food, you'll all be doing well. This is one of the tenets of Weight Watchers. "One of the things we discourage is this idea of preparing food for yourself and providing different food for the family," says Miller-Kovach. "If you're feeding yourself well, you should be feeding your family well."

Whether you go into this as a joint undertaking with the aim of each losing weight, or you enlist as a support person in your husband's effort, it's critical to be clear on your goals and your roles, and that you make sure to keep talking with each other. Kelly Brownell, Ph.D., a weight-loss expert who directs the Yale Center for Eating and Weight Disorders at Yale University, says good communication is vital.

"Very often couples get into this mind-set where they think they should be able to read each other's minds," Dr. Brownell says. But of course we can't, so discussing expectations in detail will help avoid conflict. That means your partner needs to tell you how you can be helpful, and you need to tell him what you are—and are not—willing to do. Be specific. For example, find out from him when he wants your opinion, and when he'd rather you stay quiet. Ask him directly: "What should I say? What should I not say?"

One mistake many women make is to take on too much—too much responsibility, too much guilt, too much stress. "One thing the woman has to remember at all times is that his weight is not her responsibility," Dr. Brownell says. "She needs to know that if he's not losing weight, it doesn't reflect poorly on her as a wife. It doesn't mean he doesn't love her. Or that he's doing something nasty to her."

It's also important that your husband reward you for the help you give him. If all he does is scowl when you praise him for how well he is doing, you probably won't feel like giving him positive feedback for very long. So tell him it's a two-way street and that if he wants support, so do you. You need to know that your efforts at loving support are being recognized.

Weighty Problems for Your Relationship

Another problem that crops up for some couples is that one partner starts losing weight and it signals a change in the dynamic of the relationship, a change that can be frightening to the other partner. Sometimes just the thought of a partner getting healthy or changing in some way can provoke behavior that is intended to "sabotage" the other person's effort to improve.

Cornell's Dr. Jeffrey Sobal says noncooperation from family members can be one factor that keeps a whole family from moving toward healthier eating. Working with some of his colleagues to examine Dr. Dean Ornish's healthy heart program, they found that cooperation of a spouse was a key factor in the success or failure of the effort.

"People who had a very cooperative spouse started off on a positive trajectory," Sobal says. "Both spouses just switched their family food system, eating more whole grains, low fat, et cetera, and both got healthier. But one of the predictors of people dropping out of the program or being unsuccessful was having a spouse who wasn't interested or wasn't cooperative. People reported it was hard to eat a low-fat brown rice dish when the person sitting across from you was having a cheeseburger and then cheesecake for dessert."

Since every couple's relationship is unique, you'll need to tailor your approach to your individual personalities and your style as a couple. "No one approach is going to go for everybody," says Brownell. "There are some men who benefit from having a woman who's a policewoman, who makes note when he's not doing so well, praises him when he does do well, and acts kind of like a traffic cop with respect to the food he eats. Other men would find this far too intrusive and would prefer a woman who is supportive when he's doing well but doesn't bring attention to it when he's not."

Brownell, a psychologist, puts a person's relationships at the center of the weight-loss effort. The most recent edition of his book *The LEARN Program for Weight Management 2000* includes a section for the family and friends of the person who's trying to lose weight. As he points out in the book, "The burden falls to the person losing weight to express how he or she feels and how the family can help. This is sometimes difficult when the person resents the family's response to his or her weight." It is also important that the family members tell the overweight person how they feel: communication needs to go two ways.

HOW TO HELP SOMEONE LOSE WEIGHT

- *Do not hide food from the person losing weight.* He will only find it and feel resentful.
- *Do not avoid social situations because of the person's weight.* This will batter the self-esteem of the family member losing weight and will breed resentment in the family.
- *Do not expect perfection or 100 percent recovery.* Weight problems are something a person learns to control, not cure. There will be periods of misery, weight gain, and overeating. The individual's achievements should be appreciated and the setbacks met with compassion.
- *Do not lecture, criticize, or reprimand.* These rarely help. The person needs to feel better, not worse.
- *Do not play the role of victim or martyr.* Overweight has many causes, both psychological and physiological. It is unfair for the family to blame the overweight family member and to feel victimized. Support and encouragement will do more than guilt and shame.

Source: K. D. Brownell, Things the Family Should Avoid: The LEARN® Program for Weight Management 2000, pp. 156–57, Dallas, Texas: American Health Publishing Company, 2000. Adapted with permission. For ordering information, call 1-888-LEARN-41.

LOSING IT—TOGETHER

Trying to lose weight together can be a good approach for many couples. But it can also be complicated. If each partner is in a different place in terms of making this change, they may have different agendas and different levels of motivation.

Joining a weight-loss program together helps some couples, but it's not for everyone. Rena Wing, Ph.D., director of the Weight Control and Diabetes Research Center at Brown Medical School, says it can backfire on some couples. One of her studies found that joining a weight-loss program together was helpful for the woman, but not for the man. Wing isn't sure exactly why that was so, but she did notice that some of the men turned over to their wives many of their responsibilities, such as recording the food they ate. In other words, they abdicated control. "This made the husbands less careful about their own eating, less aware of their own eating," Wing says.

Still, for some couples, joining a program together could be a good move. If you're thinking about doing this, talk carefully about your expectations of each other and what roles each of you expect to play in the process. Leading your husband by the nose and doing all his work for him is not a good idea.

On the other hand, making a commitment together to a healthy lifestyle and deciding together how best to get there will help both of you stay on track. Remember to reward each other not only for changes on the scale but for changes in behavior (diet and exercise) and for changes in attitude (being positive and supportive). Always celebrate success together!

Going Forward

Once you've talked things through and agreed on your approach, you'll be ready to start making changes. The place to begin is at the dining table. As we pointed out earlier, when women who were taking part in a major health study started changing what they ate at home, nearly a third of their husbands lost weight and became healthier, too. With a minimum of cajoling and nagging, the whole family changed its ways.

Of course, it won't always be that easy. Many men are creatures of habit—like eating meat at nearly every meal—and aren't about to change. As one woman told me about her husband: "His mother made a steak and a baked potato for dinner every night, and that's what he wants me to do, though I know he needs to change."

One problem, of course, is that your husband doesn't get all his food from home. In order to plot the best course for losing weight, he'll need to have a good understanding of where his calories come from. Encourage your mate to write down what he eats for at least one week. He may be surprised when he realizes that the things he thinks are inconsequential actually turn out to be adding lots of calories. He may realize that eating healthy meals at home will go only so far if every morning on the way to work, he stops for a café latte and croissant. In chapter 11, we suggest how you can buy and serve healthy, nutritious food. (Also see chapter 10 on helping someone change.)

One of the best things you can do for a loved one who is trying to lose weight is to help him set a realistic goal for weight loss. Experts say a modest loss of just 5 percent to 10 percent is enough to bring significant health benefits. Yet most dieters want all or nothing when it comes to losing weight. When a goal is not met, many people throw up their hands and use it as an excuse to say "See, it doesn't work. I might as well eat what I want." Then, sure enough, the pounds come back on and the effort is dashed. It's important to know that lifestyle changes that lead to permanent weight loss don't happen overnight. Appreciation for slow but steady progress should be included in your encouragement.

Another reason people give up is because they deprive themselves of everything they like to eat. Then they can't take the lack of pleasure and find themselves right back where they started. Deprivation is not a good long-term strategy. If you remind your partner of that, it may help him feel better about his incremental progress, and also will help him stick to it.

BIG LEAPS MIGHT BE EASIER THAN BABY STEPS

If the conventional wisdom on weight-loss is that incremental change is the only sustainable way to go, Dean Ornish, M.D., has another view. Ornish is president of the nonprofit Preventive Medicine Research Institute and clinical professor of medicine at the University of California in San Francisco, as well as the best-selling author of *Eat More, Weigh Less*. He advocates radical change for those who already have heart disease but believes everybody is capable of making big changes—as long as they see results. He argues that the only thing that will motivate people to make difficult changes is if there's a clear payoff that can be seen fairly quickly. Abstract concepts like reducing risk factors or adding a theoretical 5.3 months to their life span simply don't have that effect. That's why he thinks people are better off making big changes and doing it quickly—revamping their diet, launching an exercise program.

"Sometimes it's actually easier to make big changes than small ones because people feel so much better so quickly," says Dr. Ornish. "When people make these changes, their brain literally gets more blood. So they think more clearly. They have more energy. They need less sleep. Even sexual organs may receive more blood flow, in the same way that Viagra works." And once people taste the benefits, it can help them avoid slipping back into their old ways. The reward is so worth the effort that people are willing to change.

Ornish also believes that one reason many people don't want to lose weight is because they think they'll have to eat tofu and birdseed for the rest of their lives. "There's this myth that you have to choose between a fun, interesting, sexy life—and you get sick and die early as a consequence. Or you eat boring food and you lead a boring life," Ornish says. He describes this attitude as "Am I gonna live longer, or is it just gonna *seem* longer? There's no point in giving up something you enjoy unless you get something back that's even better—and quickly. While fear of dying may not be a sustainable motivator, joy of living often is. When you make big changes in your diet and lifestyle, you may feel so much better, so quickly, the choices become clearer and, for many people, worth making. Not just to live *longer*, but also to live *better*."

DON'T BE A SOLE SUPPORTER

If you try to be your partner's only supporter in his effort to lose weight, that can put a lot of pressure on you. Maybe he'd be more motivated by the support of other men. One thing you can do is to encourage him or make it possible for him to exercise regularly with some of his pals. *Men's Health* magazine has taken the idea of mutual support among men and made a campaign out of it through its Belly-Off Club. What started as a magazine story about seven editors in search of "abdominal perfection" turned into one of the magazine's most popular features. It includes an

Internet component where men can share the successes and failures of their effort to lose weight. So far, the magazine says the club has helped motivate more than eighty thousand subscribers to trim down.

If all else fails, you might try getting your husband's doctor to say something to him about his weight and need for weight loss. For years, many doctors took a hands-off attitude toward their patients' weight. More recently, many in the medical community are waking up to the fact that they need to be more aggressive in counseling patients about their lifestyle. Studies are beginning to show that if doctors make recommendations to their patients about exercise and weight loss and then follow up with continued conversation, it can improve a patient's motivation.

THE BEST DIET TO LOSE WEIGHT

If you're seeking a silver bullet for weight loss, you can stop now. There isn't one. I've been a medical reporter for nearly ten years and I can tell you that any story that even hints at an easy solution to weight loss may generate a lot of coverage and attention, but it should be taken with a huge grain of salt. I don't want to denigrate the multibillion-dollar-a-year weight-loss industry, but I can honestly say that diets don't work and thinking you can get something (a healthy weight) for nothing is a fantasy. That doesn't mean that the solution to being overweight is complicated—it's not. You just have to stick to it. The best diet is the one that includes lots of fresh whole foods of the highest nutritional value that a person will actually eat.

For most people who are a bit overweight (but not clinically obese), the thing to do is shockingly simple. Eat less and move more! Virtually every legitimate weight-loss expert will tell you that the best strategies for losing weight are built around three pillars: reducing the calories you eat, increasing your physical activity, and getting support or therapy to help you change your habits. It's a package deal.

Government health experts suggest that people try this approach for six months, aiming to reduce their weight by about 10 percent, losing a pound or two every week. If you succeed, you can shift your efforts to maintaining your gains—or your losses, in this case—by trying to keep your weight steady.

But some people simply won't be able to follow this recipe or won't be able to lose as much weight as they need to. For those folks, weight-loss drugs may be an option. Government guidelines suggest that people try diet and exercise for six months first, then talk with their doctors about medications. And again, only people who really need to lose weight should consider taking weight-loss drugs. That means people who are seriously obese—they have a BMI of 30 or greater—or overweight people with a BMI of 27 who also have two or more risk factors such as high blood pressure or diabetes. Some seriously obese people who are suffering health problems may benefit from gastric bypass surgery. In the surgery, part of the stomach is closed off to make it smaller, and it therefore cannot hold much food. This is serious surgery with side effects and is not to be embarked upon lightly or without much thought beforehand.

THE CHOLESTEROL BATTLE

A few years ago, at a national conference on heart disease in San Francisco, Dr. John LaRosa, now of the State University of New York Health Science Center, got everyone's attention by projecting onto a large screen a picture of a bear and a man. "These are two mammals," Dr. La Rosa said. "Both eat diets high in fatty meat." The big difference, he said, is that bears have sharp teeth for tearing, short intestines, and cholesterol levels up to 600 while humans have flat, grinding teeth, long intestines, and cholesterol levels under 300. The other difference: Bears don't get clogged arteries.

Unlike bears, Dr. LaRosa declared, humans are natural vegetarians with the wrong anatomy for processing lots of animal fat. Animal fat and dairy products are the main sources of saturated fat and the cholesterol that comes with it. Saturated fat and cholesterol are the biggest problems with the American diet, and the biggest reasons why we have so much more heart disease than other countries where people eat less meat and fat.

There is great variation among people in how their bodies respond to fat and cholesterol. A person's genes, as well as his or her eating and exercise habits, have a lot to do with how much cholesterol hangs around in the blood and how much he or she is able to get rid of. It's simply a lot harder for some people to lower their cholesterol levels than others, just as it's harder for some people to lose weight. For these folks, it seems that no matter how hard they try, their genetic makeup limits how much change they can achieve.

That certainly is the case with my husband, Avery. He has, mostly from the luck of his own genetics, a very poor lipid profile—too much of the wrong kinds of fats and cholesterol. He works pretty hard to control what he eats, but can get only so far in pushing down his LDL number. He has had some success, though, in increasing his HDL, mostly through exercise, but it's a struggle. For Avery, and for other men and women like him, cholesterol will be a lifelong problem, something he—and I—will have to pay attention to and manage for the rest of his life. It's like having diabetes or asthma. The good news is that as he works to do things that lower his cholesterol levels, it also helps his overall health.

Still, no matter what's in their genes, most people can make some progress in lowering high cholesterol levels by making dietary changes and exercising. These changes can often be made quite quickly, though the real fight is often to maintain the changes over time. Powerful cholesterol-lowering medications are also available to help those who aren't able to control their levels by diet and exercise alone.

The trouble is that while most people today know to watch out for and manage their cholesterol, many are not doing it. Over 100 million Americans have cholesterol levels considered high or borderline high—enough to push up their risk of heart disease. A majority of these people are men, who tend to have higher cholesterol levels than women until menopause, when hormonal changes in women start to equalize their numbers.

Everyone who is twenty years or older should have their cholesterol measured at least every five years. This test should be done after a nine- to twelve-hour fast and include total cholesterol, HDL cholesterol, and LDL cholesterol as well as triglycerides. The general goal is a cholesterol level of less than 200 mg/dl. In addition, men who have an LDL of 130 mg/dl or above after dietary therapy should be on statin medications (more on that later). (See the section on cholesterol testing on page 335 for a full explanation of cholesterol and cholesterol levels.)

How High Is a Man's Risk?

Many men in their thirties, forties, and even fifties don't think they need to worry about heart disease—they figure they're too young. But they may be wrong. A study in the journal *Circulation* looked at the arteries of 760 teens and young adults who died of accidents, suicides, or murder and found that many had coronary arteries that were clogged badly enough to cause a heart attack. Two percent of males between fifteen and nineteen, and 20 percent of men between thirty and thirty-four had advanced fat-laden plaques, putting them well on their way to an early heart attack or stroke.

The risks keep growing with age, of course. By the time men reach their forties, half of them are destined to develop coronary artery disease in their lifetimes, according to the Framingham Heart Study, the famous fifty-year examination of more than five thousand volunteers from Framingham, Massachusetts. It was that study, of course, that gave researchers tremendous new insights into the process of heart disease, and led them to coin a new term—"risk factor."

You can get an idea of someone's chances of having cardiovascular problems by analyzing these risk factors. In general, the higher a man's LDL level and the more additional risk factors he has, the greater his chances of developing heart disease or having a heart attack.

Some people are at high risk for a heart attack because they already have heart disease—their arteries are already congested—or because they have diabetes or some combination of other health problems. If you want to get a sense of your husband's risk (or your own), you can check out the American Heart Association's website (*http://americanheart.org/presenter.jhtml?identifier=3003499*) and follow the instructions. The National Heart Lung and Blood Institute website (*http://www.nhlbi.nih.gov/chd/index.htm*) also has an excellent discussion on cholesterol as well as a risk calculator. Understanding your risk of having a heart attack over the next ten years will help you choose the course of treatment you should follow.

How to Help Lower Your Husband's Cholesterol

If your husband battles with his cholesterol level like mine does, every meal can be part of the problem or part of the solution. Eating even a single high-fat meal can increase a person's risk of having a heart attack for the next three or four hours. The bottom line is that if you and your husband want to work together to lower his chances of developing heart disease or suffering a heart attack, it's critical to lower his cholesterol levels. Reducing them even a little can go a long way toward improving his heart health. In fact, for every 1 percent drop in his cholesterol count, his risk of heart attack goes down by 2 percent, according to the National Heart Lung and Blood Institute. That's like doubling your investment!

When you embark on an effort to cut his cholesterol, the main thing you're trying to affect is that bad LDL level. You want to bring that baby down as much as possible. How low does it need to go? That depends on your husband's other risk factors. Remember that the optimal LDL level is under 100. If he doesn't have other risk factors that could predispose him to heart disease, he could afford for that LDL number to be somewhat higher—up to around 130. But if he already has heart disease—meaning his doctors have detected a significant buildup of plaque in his arteries—he should aim to get to 100 or lower.

Maintaining a healthy weight will help get cholesterol levels under control (see chapter 11).

A Little TLC

If your partner has high cholesterol numbers but doesn't have other risk factors for heart disease, most doctors would urge him to push hard to bring those numbers down by changing what he eats and how he lives. While there are many dietary approaches that will likely help, the U.S. Government has one called Therapeutic Lifestyle Changes. The TLC approach has three main parts:

- The TLC diet.
- Maintaining a healthy weight.
- Exercise.

The TLC Diet

The basic idea here is to reduce saturated fat from your diet so that you end up getting fewer than 7 percent of your calories from saturated fat and consuming less than 200 milligrams of dietary cholesterol per day. In addition to saturated fat, the other big evil to avoid is trans fat, a kind of fat created by food chemists and found in hydrogenated and partially hydrogenated vegetable oil, hard margarine, and many processed and packaged foods. The TLC diet has no particular calorie goal, other than managing calories to avoid weight gain. (Also see page 421 for the DASH diet.)

TLC SAMPLE MENU

Traditional American Cuisine
Male, 25 to 49 Years, Who Engages in Moderate-Intensity Physical Activity

Breakfast
Oatmeal (1 cup)
    Fat-free milk (1 cup)
    Raisins (¼ cup)
English muffin (1 medium)
    Jelly (1 Tbsp.)
Honeydew melon (1 cup)
Orange juice, calcium fortified (1 cup)
Coffee (1 cup) with fat-free milk (2 Tbsp.)

Lunch
Roast beef sandwich
    Whole-wheat bun (1 medium)
    Roast beef, lean (2 oz.)
    Swiss cheese, low fat (1 oz. slice)
    Romaine lettuce (2 leaves)
    Tomato (2 medium slices)
    Mustard (2 tsp.)
Pasta Salad (1 cup)
    Pasta noodles (¾ cup)
    Mixed vegetables (¼ cup)
    Olive oil (2 tsp.)
Apple (1 medium)
Iced tea, unsweetened (1 cup)

Dinner
Orange roughy (3 oz.) cooked with olive oil (2 tsp.)
    Parmesan cheese (1 Tbsp.)
Rice (1½ cups)

Foods low in saturated fat include dairy products that are fat-free or contain 1 percent fat, lean meats, fish, skinless poultry, whole-grain foods, and fruits and vegetables. Lay off butter and hard stick margarine and go instead for soft margarine that comes in a liquid or tub—they're low in saturated fat and contain little or no trans fat. Better still, look for ones that are trans fat–free. Limit meat, poultry, and cheese, as well as foods that are high in cholesterol such as liver and other organ meats and full-fat dairy products. Egg yolks are pretty much *verboten*, too: The new recommendations allow for only 200 milligrams of cholesterol a day, less than the amount found in one yolk.

Corn kernels (½ cup)
    Soft margarine* (1 tsp.)
Strawberries (1 cup) topped with low-fat frozen yogurt (½ cup)
Fat-free milk (1 cup)

Snack
Popcorn (2 cups) cooked with canola oil (1 Tbsp.)
Peaches, canned in water (1 cup)·
Water (1 cup)

Nutrient Analysis

Calories	2,523
Cholesterol (mg)	139
Fiber (g)	32
Soluble (g)	10
Sodium (mg)	1,800
Carbohydrates, percentage of calories	57
Total fat, percentage of calories	28
Saturated fat, percentage of calories	6
Monounsaturated fat, percentage of calories	14
Polyunsaturated fat, percentage of calories	6
Trans fat (g)	1
Omega-3 fat (g)	0.4
Protein, percentage of calories	17

No salt is added in recipe preparation or as seasoning. The sample menu meets or exceeds the Daily Reference Intake (DRI) for nutrients.

*Margarine may contain some trans fat but has less cholesterol-raising potential than butter and is preferable to butter. The trans fat in margarine is formed when vegetable oil is hardened to make margarine; the softer the margarine, the less trans fat it is likely to contain. There are now margarines available that contain no trans fats. Soft margarine is a suitable spread in a cholesterol-lowering diet, especially if it is the type that has no trans fat.

Source: Adapted from NHLBI Third Report of the National Cholesterol Education Program (NCEP) Expert Panel on Detection, Evaluation, and Treatment of High Blood Cholesterol in Adults (Adult Treatment Panel III), September 2002, NIH Publication No. 02–5215.

Eating food with a lot of soluble fiber such as oat bran, oatmeal, beans, peas, rice bran, barley, citrus fruits, strawberries, and apple pulp can help lower LDL levels. So can some of the new "functional food" margarines and salad dressings made with Benecol and Take Control. They contain substances derived from plants that can actually lower cholesterol.

So to see what one day on the TLC diet would look like, the National Heart, Lung, and Blood Institute, which developed the diet, has a web page that can help you figure out an eating plan. I went to that page to figure out a one-day diet for a hypothetical man who, let's say, is five feet ten inches tall and weighs 175 pounds. His goals on the TLC diet are to keep saturated fat to 17 grams a day while consuming up to 2,600 calories. The TLC Sample Menu on pages 410–11 is an example of a one-day diet that adds up to the right numbers from the National Heart, Lung, and Blood Institute.

Watch Your Weight

If you are overweight, shedding some pounds can help lower LDL levels. This is especially important for people who have a cluster of risk factors such as high triglyceride levels, low HDL levels, or having a large waist measurement (more than 40 inches for men and more than 35 inches for women).

Get Physical

Thirty minutes of physical activity on most, if not all, days of the week, is good for everyone. It can help raise your HDL and lower your LDL. Again, this is especially important for people with high triglycerides and/or low HDL levels who have large waistlines.

MAGIC POTIONS?

If your husband tries to cut his cholesterol by changing his diet and getting more exercise, but can't move the numbers enough, his doctor may suggest medications. Studies show that cholesterol-lowering medications for those who need them can prevent death from heart attacks and strokes. Many experts say that when the stakes are high, people should be on these medications. The most likely choice for a cholesterol-lowering medication is one of the statins—the cholesterol-lowering drugs that have become some of the best-selling prescription drugs in the country.

Statins work by blocking an enzyme (HMG-CoA reductase) that your liver uses to make cholesterol. This keeps extra cholesterol from going into your bloodstream, reducing your risk of a heart attack and angina. Studies have found that statins can lower LDL levels by up to 55 percent, cut triglycerides by up to 30 percent, and boost HDL levels by up to 15 percent. In short, they are enormously powerful. But because they're so powerful, they also present a danger—that many patients will prefer taking them to making changes in their lives, and that many doctors will prefer prescribing them to helping and encouraging patients to make those changes.

There are five different statin drugs now on the market (and more on the way): Lipitor (atorvastatin), the top-selling drug in America in 2001, Zocor (simvastatin), Mevacor (lovastatin), Pravachol (pravastatin), and Lescol (fluvastatin).

The first statin studies found that people with high cholesterol who took them cut their risk of heart attacks. Then came studies showing that even people whose cholesterol wasn't all that high could benefit as well. Then more studies suggested that statins helped people with diabetes avoid heart disease and that they might help prevent stroke and diabetes, and even dementia and bone fractures in women over sixty. At this point, though, these other benefits are not proven, and statins are only approved for lowering cholesterol in order to reduce the risk of heart disease.

Who Should Take Cholesterol-Lowering Drugs?

In 2001, a panel of experts convened by the government made sweeping changes in the official recommendations for how patients and doctors should deal with cholesterol. The new guidelines nearly tripled the number of Americans who should be taking cholesterol-lowering drugs from 13 million to 36 million people—that's 18 percent of the adult population. Almost one third of those eligible are under fifty-six, and 12 million are under forty-five years of age. Under the new guidelines 55 percent of statin takers would be men. Should your husband (or you) be among them?

Yes, the guidelines say, if he has heart disease, has had a heart attack, or has diabetes *and* has LDL levels over 100.

But even if he hasn't been diagnosed with these problems, the guidelines urge him to take medications if he has high LDL levels coupled with other risk factors that increase his chances of developing heart disease. What are these risk factors? You probably have them memorized by now. They include cigarette smoking, high blood pressure (140/90 or greater), a low HDL level, and a family history of heart disease and inactivity.

In many cases, the guidelines suggest that doctors begin treatment by urging their patients to make "lifestyle changes"—the TLC diet and regular exercise—and to try that for three months before prescribing medications. But drug treatment could be started at the same time as the diet, the guidelines say, if the doctor thinks that's best. And there, in the view of critics like Dr. Dean Ornish, lies part of the problem.

Statins: Are They All They Are Cracked Up to Be?

Dr. Ornish is probably the country's best known and most respected advocate of preventing or reversing heart disease by altering the way people live, eat, and exercise.

He worries that the government's call for increased use of statins, coupled with the huge marketing and media presence of these drugs, is making them into the first line of treatment, instead of a backup. For top-selling Lipitor, for instance, the Pfizer company spent more than $50 million per year on advertising in 1999–2000. In Ornish's view, the authors of the new government guidelines are sending a clear message to heart patients: "We know you're not going to change, and why would you want to when you can just go on statins?"

To Ornish, the recommendations play into the biases of many doctors who have only a few minutes to spend with a patient, don't know much about diet and lifestyle, and don't get reimbursed for it when their patients do go on a diet.

All statin drugs have some side effects, most notably muscle damage and pain as well as liver inflammation. One statin, Baycol (cerivastatin), was pulled from the market because muscle damage was possibly tied to the deaths of thirty-one patients. These side effects seem to be much more rare in the statins that remain on the market. Still, patients who take them need to have their livers checked periodically and to be tested for signs of muscle breakdown.

Statins are an important weapon in the fight against high cholesterol and heart disease, and when the stakes are high should be taken without reservation. However, people should not give up on improving their diets and getting more exercise. On this point I'm clear, and you should be too: If your husband starts taking a statin or other cholesterol-lowering agent, it doesn't mean he can eat whatever he wants and sit on the couch all day. I have seen this false security with statins in some close relatives. The "It's okay. I can have that burger and fries—I'm on a statin" thinking has me a bit worried. In fact, some people take their statin medication *only* after a high-fat meal in the false belief that it protects them. Nothing could be further from the truth! By exercising and watching what he eats, your husband can keep his dose of medicine as low as possible and lower his risk in other ways as well. And best of all, says Dean Ornish, he'll be able to feel the positive changes in his body that make all this sacrifice worthwhile.

Other Drugs

The statins are not the only drugs that can reduce troublesome cholesterol levels. Others include bile acid sequestrants, nicotinic acid (niacin), and fibric acids. The bile acid sequestrants (like cholestyramine, colestipol, colesevelam) lower LDL by 15 percent to 30 percent and raise HDL by 3 percent to 5 percent but have no effect on triglycerides. Fibric acids, like fenofibrate, lower LDL by 5 percent to 20 percent, raise HDL by 10 percent to 20 percent, and lower triglycerides by 20 percent to 50 percent. Nicotinic acid lowers LDL by 5 percent to 25 percent, raises HDL by 15 percent to 35 percent, and lowers triglycerides by 20 percent to 50 percent.

RISK FACTORS IN THE PIPELINE

In addition to the familiar risk factors we've just been discussing, scientists are investigating emerging risk factors that you may hear much more about in the future. Indeed, many doctors are already using some of these tests routinely. In general, less is known about them than is known about cholesterol. But that may change in the future.

Homocysteine

There is mounting evidence that people with abnormally high levels of the amino acid homocysteine have a greater risk of coronary artery disease, stroke, and blood clotting. A number of small studies have found links between homocysteine and heart disease, including one that found that the higher the level of homocysteine in a subject's blood, the more blockage there was in his coronary arteries. Excess homocysteine seems to harm the lining of blood vessels, contribute to blood clotting, and make LDL cholesterol even more dangerous. Excessive levels of homocysteine occur when the body is deficient in vitamins B_{12}, B_6, and folic acid. There is debate in the medical community about whether or not homocysteine actually causes the disease or is just a marker.

The best way to keep homocysteine from building up in your bloodstream, or to get rid of it if it does, is to get plenty of B_{12}, B_6, and folic acid, either in what you eat or in nutritional supplements (see page 315).

Infections

Believe it or not, some researchers believe that some cases of heart disease might actually be triggered by an infection. The idea is that a virus or bacterium somehow inflames or damages the wall of a blood vessel, beginning the process of atherosclerosis. Researchers are looking most closely at three germs: *H. pylori,* the bacterium that causes stomach ulcers; Chlamydia pneumonia, a bacterium that causes respiratory infections in young adults; and cytomegalovirus (CMV), a common virus. This topic is still being researched so it may be a while before we see results from studies that will help guide testing or treatment.

C-reactive Protein

This protein, which can be measured in the bloodstream, is a marker of inflammation and an important predictor of heart disease. Testing for c-reactive protein will likely become commonplace as studies show that high levels of this protein predict heart attacks at least as well as cholesterol. Experts don't understand yet why this protein is elevated in some heart patients, but there is evidence that people with elevated levels may benefit from statins.

Lipoprotein (a)

This fat molecule is like a smaller version of LDL and contains a lot of cholesterol. Researchers think it can be a big contributor to atherosclerosis in some people. Experts say this lipoprotein is largely controlled by genes and that neither diet nor medicine has much influence over it.

Cholesterol Particle Size

Cholesterol comes not only in a good form and a bad form but also in different sizes. Large cholesterol particles, which are "fluffy," may glide more easily through the blood stream and be less likely to stick to artery walls and build up compared to the smaller, denser cholesterol particles. Having smaller particles can increase the risk of heart attack and stroke as the buildup leads to plaque on the artery wall and then heart attack or stroke. While cholesterol level is an indicator of cardiovascular disease risk, it is not perfect. People with normal cholesterol levels have heart attacks and strokes. Some experts think that particle size is a better indicator of risk than cholesterol level. Currently, only a few labs test for particle size, but as more research is done it is likely to become a more common test for heart disease risk.

UNDER PRESSURE! HYPERTENSION

For ten years Bob*, a maintenance worker, slowly gained weight. By the time he was forty years old he weighed 210 pounds—on a five-feet-eight-inch frame. He never thought much about his weight gain until his physician told him that his blood pressure was 150/90 and that he needed to lose weight if he wanted to get it down. Bob, who loves pizza and beer, had no idea the two were connected. "What," he asked his wife, "does my weight have to do with my blood pressure?" Well, lots. Men (and women) like Bob are becoming the norm in this country. One consequence of the overweight and obesity epidemic is an increase in the number of people with high blood pressure. High blood pressure, or hypertension, is one of the most common serious health conditions in America. Well over half of all Americans over the age of sixty have hypertension. One in four adults—about 50 million people—have this condition, according to the National Heart, Lung, and Blood Institute. But nearly one third of them don't even know they have it. What's more the government recently designated a new category—called "prehypertension"—that is people whose blood pressure is in the higher range of normal. These people, according to experts at the National Heart, Lung, and Blood Institute are at risk for going on to develop high blood pressure. This adds 45 million people to the list of those who need to be concerned. That's because this disease has no symptoms until it has progressed so far that it has caused a serious problem like heart or kidney disease. And because of its association with extra weight, it is also increasingly common for people to have both hypertension and diabetes!

Men of Bob's age—and men of all ages up to sixty—are more likely than women to have high blood pressure. And once a person, man or woman, develops it, it rarely goes away, and becomes worse over time if it's not taken care of. Yet many people, perhaps up to 70 percent, are not getting treatment and when they do the treatment is adequate less than half the time. Altogether this translates into millions of people at risk for the long-term effects of high blood pressure, a fact not well understood by the public.

Over time, high blood pressure can seriously damage your organs. It can increase your risk for a whole host of diseases including stroke, heart disease, heart failure, and kidney disease—not to mention impotence. Deaths related to high blood pressure are in the hundreds of thousands annually. Yet few people think of high blood pressure as a leading cause of strokes or heart disease. And when a person has cardiovascular disease and any other risk factor like high cholesterol or diabetes, the risk of the blood pressure is magnified. So why is high blood pressure such a big killer? And what does blood pressure really mean?

A Short Primer on Blood Pressure

Blood doesn't flow through arteries in a steady stream like a river. Rather, it moves in spurts as the result of the heart muscle contracting and pumping blood. With each beat, about two ounces of freshly oxygenated blood is forced out of the main chamber of the heart—the left ventricle—and into the aorta, where it then travels through the body's 100,000 miles of blood vessels. Blood pressure is the tension or force exerted on the inside walls of arteries. Blood pressure doesn't stay steady; it can change moment to moment depending on how hard the heart is working. During exercise the heart can pump up to three times as fast as during periods of rest. Between heartbeats the heart muscle rests momentarily and gets ready for the next beat and the pressure eases. That's why two numbers are included in a blood pressure reading. The first number, your *systolic blood pressure,* measures that surge of blood when the heart contracts. The second, lower number, *diastolic blood pressure,* is the force on the artery walls during the relaxed period between heartbeats. So a blood pressure of 120/80 mmHg (millimeters of mercury) is called 120 over 80. Having blood pressure at or below that figure, is considered optimal. A consistent reading of 140/90 or higher is considered high blood pressure.

High blood pressure is like a heavy weight that your heart must continually lift to get blood to the body. Over time the constant strain on the heart can cause it to enlarge, then wear out. Greater pressure also takes a toll on your arterial walls, scarring them and making them less elastic. Eventually, these damaged blood vessels may be unable to deliver enough oxygen and nutrients to vital organs like the brain and kidney, thus leading to disease.

The good news about high blood pressure is that it largely preventable. (See chapter 11 on prevention.) It can be treated by a combination of lifestyle changes, including diet. If modifying your diet doesn't help, there are many medications that can. The bad news is that millions of people either don't know they have a problem or have the problem and ignore it. I can tell you from firsthand experience that many, many men (and women) simply don't take this problem seriously because they don't feel any symptoms.

If your husband has been told that his blood pressure is elevated, it is very important to follow up—whether he's twenty-something or seventy-something. (Don't ignore the warnings.) If you can encourage your husband to be aware of his blood pressure and to take steps to control it, you'll be helping him avoid getting those blood pressure–related diseases down the road.

Follow the Numbers: Understanding Blood Pressure

Blood pressure doesn't have to be that high to cause problems. In fact, experts now say that problems can begin when blood pressure is around 130 to 139/85 to 89. In one recent study, researchers took blood pressure readings from 10,000 young men aged eighteen to thirty-nine, then followed them for the next twenty-five years. When they compared the men's death rates, they found that the men whose blood pressure was classified in this borderline range—not high, but higher than the midlevel of normal—had a 34 percent greater risk of dying from heart disease than those whose blood pressure was lower.

The point is that even small elevations can make a difference, and the bigger your numbers, the greater your risk. Those in the prehypertension category (see below) still face increased cardiovascular risks. Furthermore, blood pressure is known to increase with age. So even if you and your husband are young, it is still important that you know what your blood pressure is, try to prevent it from getting high as you get older, and take care to address it now if it is high.

If the systolic and diastolic pressures fall into different categories, the higher category is used to classify blood pressure status. If either one is high, it is a predictor of disease that should not be ignored. And even if a man falls in the "prehypertensive category" that doesn't mean there's no room for improvement. He should still strive to get as close as possible to the optimal range of 120/80.

WHERE IS YOUR BLOOD PRESSURE?

Category	Systolic	Diastolic
Optimal	less than 120	less than 80
Prehypertension	120 to 139	80 to 89
High blood pressure		
Stage 1	140 to 159	90 to 99
Stage 2	160 and up	100 and up

Afraid of the Person in the White Coat?

Though so-called white-coat hypertension is a problem for more women than men, it is something to be aware of. White-coat hypertension basically means that a person's blood pressure goes up because he is consciously or subconsciously anxious around the doctor. While such a jump is usually not huge, it can be enough to move someone into the high-blood-pressure category.

Some doctors will recommend additional measurements that are done at home, but most likely if the pressure is high on three different visits, then the diagnosis of high blood pressure can be made.

White-coat hypertension may be less of an anomaly than it seems. Many doctors believe that high blood pressure in the office is a harbinger of things to come—including stroke and heart disease—and should be closely monitored if not treated. Studies back up this idea.

In general, stressful situations can make blood pressure go up temporarily but this isn't the real danger. To harm the heart, kidneys, and other organs, blood pressure would need to be up most of the time.

HELPING YOUR HUSBAND REDUCE HIS BLOOD PRESSURE

The very things that help keep people healthy and reduce other risks can also bring down your blood pressure. This includes managing weight, avoiding bad habits like smoking and heavy drinking, getting regular exercise, and, above all, eating right. One of the most important things you can do to control blood pressure is to reduce salt in the diet and be generous with fruits and vegetables. Many times, these things alone are enough to lower high blood pressure.

Unfortunately, men with high blood pressure also tend to have other problems: they're overweight, they smoke, or they have high cholesterol, for instance. If that's the case, he will need to do more than just control his blood pressure numbers if he wants to dodge heart disease. He'll need to get *all* those risk factors under control. That, experts say, is the only way to improve the odds of a long, healthy life.

Finally, know this: You're probably helping just by being with him—*if* you have a good relationship. Studies have shown that people's blood pressure tends to go down when they're with a spouse or significant other. However, if things are rocky and tense and you tend to argue, being around you could push his blood pressure up temporarily.

Drop the Pounds

This is one of the most important "treatments" for high blood pressure. Everyone who is carrying extra weight ought to lose some if they want to improve their pressure or avoid it in the first place. If an overweight person loses even ten to twenty pounds, it usually helps bring down their blood pressure. But weight loss alone may not be enough for many people with hypertension. You should also do the following.

Spare the Salt

No doubt you've heard conflicting things about the role of salt in high blood pressure. For many years it was common wisdom that a diet high in salt could contribute to high blood pressure. Then came some research suggesting that salt might be a problem only for those who are salt-sensitive. Then, in early 2001, came another study that put the issue to rest by proving quite conclusively the link between salt and blood pressure, even in people who did not have hypertension. Too much salt encourages the body to retain fluid, which increases blood pressure. Most Americans do eat too much salt, and this is one reason we have higher rates of hypertension than most other countries in the world. How much salt we eat matters!

Why do Americans use so much salt? It's an easy way to add flavor to food. In other countries, people tend to use more spices for seasoning. But here, when a dish lacks flavor, we dump salt on it. Little by little, our tastes adapt to this higher salt content and we expect it of all that we eat. The food industry fuels this trend by adding salt to processed foods to attract buyers. The result is a Catch-22 that pushes the salt content of food ever higher.

Reducing Salt Intake

- Modify recipes by omitting salt or cutting the amount of salt in half.
- Flavor foods with a variety of herbs, spices, wine, lemon juice, lime juice, or vinegar. Be creative!
- Choose fresh fruits and vegetables instead of salty snack foods.
- Get the saltshaker off the table or replace it with an herb substitute.
- Eat more whole, unprocessed foods.
- Choose fewer processed, canned, and convenience foods.
- Avoid condiments such as horseradish, ketchup, Worcestershire sauce, soy sauce, teriyaki sauce, and monosodium glutamate (MSG), or use low-sodium versions.
- Read food labels to become aware of high-sodium foods and select low-sodium varieties.
- Limit your intake of cured foods (such as bacon and ham) and foods packed in brine (such as pickles, pickled vegetables, olives, and sauerkraut).

DASH to the Produce Store

That pivotal 2001 study on salt and blood pressure, published in the *New England Journal of Medicine,* did more than point a finger at salt. It also proved that by eating more fruits and vegetables, more nonfat and low-fat dairy products, and less animal fat, people can achieve major reductions in their blood pressure—reductions as large as those people got from taking blood pressure medications. For years, experts have noted that vegetarians generally have lower blood pressure than meat eaters.

The eating plan followed by the study's more than four hundred volunteers came to be called the DASH diet, after the National Heart, Lung, and Blood Institute of the National Institutes of Health–sponsored diet called Dietary Approaches to Stop Hypertension. The DASH diet calls for:

- Seven to eight servings of grains and grain products a day (breakfast cereal, whole-grain bread, rice, pasta, et cetera).
- Four to five servings of vegetables a day.
- Four to five servings of fruit a day.
- Two to three servings of low-fat or nonfat dairy foods a day.
- No more than two servings of meat, poultry, or fish a day.
- Four to five servings of nuts, seeds, or legumes per week.
- Limited intake of low-fat sweets.

After spending a month eating this diet, along with about 3,300 mg of salt per day—somewhat below the amount of salt the average American consumes—the volunteers ate three different diets of varying salt levels. As salt level declined, so did their blood pressure. One problem for the volunteers was that many found the low-salt diet bland. Over time, though, their taste buds adjusted and many found that spices and herbs could make the low-salt versions of some foods quite tasty.

Learning to cook without salt is not as hard as you might think. (See the Resources section for a book and a website that can teach you about how to avoid salt and replace it with spices that add flavor.) The other important thing to know is that you don't need to have high blood pressure to benefit from this diet! The DASH diet is good for anyone who wants to maintain good health. For example, the DASH diet also lowers bad LDL cholesterol.

Other Ways to Lower the Pressure

What else can be done if you want to bring those numbers down? Watching how much you drink can help. Researchers estimate that for up to 11 percent of people with high blood pressure, the main cause is that they consume too much alcohol. Nobody is sure how alcohol increases blood pressure, but many studies show that it does. Keeping consumption to no more than two drinks per day can help keep the numbers down.

Exercise also helps. Several review studies have shown that regular physical activity such as brisk walking can lower blood pressure. Furthermore, regular exercise can help you stay healthy in many other ways by your lowering risk of heart disease and, of course, controlling your weight.

Finally, a diet that includes plenty of potassium—3,500 mg a day is recommended—leads to lower blood pressure. Bananas, prune juice, orange juice, and cantaloupe are good sources of potassium.

Beware the Restaurant Entrée!

Not long ago, Stephen Havas, M.D., one of the country's top experts in the prevention of heart attacks and strokes and a professor at the University of Maryland School of Medicine, finished working on a proposal he wanted the American Public Health Association—the largest group of public health professionals in the country—to endorse as official policy. The policy recommended that food manufacturers and the restaurant industry lighten up significantly on the added salt. He and other health experts say a 50 percent reduction in added salt in processed and restaurant foods over the next decade is essential in order to reduce the total number of deaths from high blood pressure.

Before leaving for the meeting in Philadelphia, Dr. Havas and his wife Susan Wozenski dined at their local country club. Salt being on his mind, Dr. Havas asked the chef just how much salt he added to the typical entrée. Havas was shocked when the chef, whose food he had been eating for ten years, told him, "Oh, about a teaspoon." Dr. Havas knew that was more added salt than he or any other American needed in a whole day. "It never occurred to me that he was adding that much salt." But that turns out to be typical. Dr. Havas says 75 percent of salt in the American diet comes from processed and restaurant food, 15 percent from the saltshaker, and only 10 percent occurs naturally in foods. When asked, the chef happily agreed to leave out the salt and Dr. Havas enjoyed his baked salmon very much.

Dr. Havas attended the meeting and the proposal was unanimously endorsed by the APHA—meaning that all major public health professionals agreed the food industry needs to make big changes—at least in the amount of salt they are adding to our food. Back in Maryland Dr. Havas dropped into his local Chinese eatery. He now realized that the only way to eliminate hidden salt was to specifically request that it not be added. So he asked the waiter to hold the salt in his chicken and broccoli. "Sure," the waiter replied eager to please. "We'll just cook it with soy sauce." Soy sauce, of course, is no better a choice—it, too, is loaded with sodium!

The lesson, according to Dr. Havas: It is not enough to simply avoid the saltshaker at home. Ask about salt in restaurants, then opt for the salt-free version. That's the best way to eliminate hidden sources of salt.

When Stronger Medicine Is Needed

No matter how they try, some people will be unable to cut their blood pressure enough by changing their diet, losing weight, and getting more exercise. In those cases, to lower the risk of stroke or heart disease medication will usually be necessary. This, of course, does not mean that people should give up on getting their weight under control or reducing salt. All people with high blood pressure should follow the nutrition and exercise guidelines outlined above. If you must take medication, sticking with a lifestyle changes might allow you to take fewer medications or at lower dosages than if they don't adopt the healthy lifestyle changes that are recommended.

Fortunately, there are many medications on the market to help: diuretics, beta-blockers, angiotensin converting enzyme (ACE) inhibitors, angiotensin receptor blockers, calcium channel blockers, alpha-beta blockers, nervous system inhibitors, and vasodilators, to name the most important types. Some people will need more than one at a time to get their numbers to safe levels. These medications can be life savers; though like all drugs, they can also have side effects. The most common are impotence, depression, and insomnia.

If your husband experiences a side effect that makes him want to stop taking the medication, encourage him to speak to his doctor. Because there are so many medications to choose from, it is usually easy to switch to another medication that may be more tolerable. Newer medications such as the angiotensin receptor blockers have fewer side effects than other medications. Over the years, I've heard many people complain that they didn't like the side effect of their blood pressure medicine, so they simply stopped taking it. This is not a good idea.

FOCUS ON A GOAL: GET COMPETITIVE

Experts are urging people to focus on a goal—the blood pressure number that you need to achieve to avoid complications. It may be up to you to push your doctor to get your pressure down to as close to normal as possible. Frankly, many doctors often neglect to treat blood pressure adequately (in fact, most patients are not well controlled). Some doctors hold to the mistaken belief that the pressure will go too low and harm the patient, or they believe that systolic hypertension (when the upper number is high) does not carry serious risk. It does. This is one time you may need to be aggressive in working with your doctor. In the meantime, make sure you are doing everything you can to help yourself through diet and weight control. Don't leave the doctor's office without a goal, and then do what needs to be done to get there!

If you want to encourage a man to get with the program, one way to do it is to get his competitive juices going. If your husband has a male friend who is in a similar predicament, maybe you can get the two into a friendly competition to see who can drop the pounds first and get the pressure under control.

Monitoring Blood Pressure at Home

If your husband or another loved one needs to check his blood pressure frequently, being able to do it at home is a good idea. With a little practice, you can use a stethoscope and inflatable cuff, just like the doctor does. Or you can choose one of the many digital home monitors that are simpler to operate.

One advantage of doing this at home is that it engages a man in his own health care (assuming you don't do it for him, which you shouldn't). This sort of involvement is vital because it helps him feel more in control of his treatment and his destiny. No doctor can be solely responsible for treating a man's high blood pressure, and you can't either. When people take on direct responsibility like this, it strengthens the connection between habits and health. If you decide to do home monitoring, take the machine to the doctor's office to compare it to his. Make sure the readings match. The doctor can also help make sure the cuff is the right size.

When you take the readings at home, do so after five minutes of relaxing. That way you can more easily compare readings from one day to the next. And be sure to set up a good system for recording the numbers so you can go over them with your doctor. A word of caution: Don't obsess over home blood pressure readings and don't overdo it. Keep track and discuss the results with your doctor.

A note about home monitors. Many experts think that the non-mercury home BP monitors are not as accurate as the old-fashioned ones that were used in the doctor's office. The Environment Protection Agency has urged hospitals and doctor's offices to eliminate mercury devices because of concerns about possible health effects of mercury exposure. In June 2003, *Consumer Reports* rated home blood pressure monitors. Check this report out before you make a purchase.

HOW SWEET IT ISN'T: DIABETES

These are the numbers of an epidemic: In 1958, less than 1 percent of Americans—about 1.5 million people—had diabetes. Today, some 17 million people—that's 6 percent of Americans and more than 8 percent of adults—have this disease. Diabetes, experts agree, is quickly becoming the most common chronic disease in the country.

Unfortunately, it gets even scarier. Nearly 6 million of the people with diabetes don't even know they have it and are getting no treatment as a result. And another 16 million people have a condition called prediabetes and are likely to develop full-blown diabetes within ten years.

The vast majority of people with this disease (up to 95 percent) have type 2 diabetes, what used to be called adult onset diabetes. It's not called that any longer because increasing numbers of children and teenagers are getting this disease, which, in years past, rarely struck anyone under the age of forty-five. Among young adults from thirty to thirty-nine the incidence of diabetes shot up 70 percent between 1990 and 1998. In this section, we will focus on type 2 diabetes (see page 141 for an explanation of the different kinds of diabetes).

My own dear husband was recently told that he has diabetes. This was not a surprise to me because there were hints along the way that he was headed for a problem with blood sugar. The good news is that getting a definitive diagnosis has spurred him to make some big changes in his life. I only wish he had taken those earlier hints a little more seriously. He's pretty typical though: Few people heed the early warning signs, and health experts say this has to change if we are going to get a handle on this growing epidemic.

Why are so many Americans, including children, developing this once-uncommon disease? It has a lot to do with some other discouraging trends we've been talking about—the fact that 61 percent of Americans are now considered overweight or obese, and the fact that fewer than half of Americans get regular exercise.

Men are no more likely that women to get diabetes; women reading this will have as much chance of developing diabetes as your husbands do. That means that preventing diabetes is not just something he needs to do and you need to support, but something you should tackle together. The good news is you can do a lot to avoid diabetes just the way you avoid high blood pressure and heart disease—eat right, exercise, and manage your weight.

One of the best ways to help someone with diabetes (or any disease, for that matter) is to get information. Learn as much as you can about how the disease develops, how it affects a person physically and emotionally, and how it is treated. There is much to learn, so what follows is an overview. Check out the Resources section because there are many wonderful books and websites that provide a wealth of helpful information.

UNDERSTANDING DIABETES

Diabetes is a complicated disease that occurs when the body fails to process carbohydrates (carbs) correctly. Most of the carbs you eat—from potatoes, rice, cereal, or vegetables—are turned into glucose, a sugar, that provides energy needed by all the cells in your body. Your body tries to keep a constant, even supply of glucose in the blood so it will be available whenever it's needed. After a meal, there's usually excess glucose, which your body stores for later use. How does the body do that? A hormone called insulin, produced in the pancreas, stimulates cells in the liver and muscles to absorb the extra glucose.

People with diabetes have problems with regulating or producing insulin. In some cases—5 percent to 10 percent—they don't produce it. This is called type 1 diabetes. In other cases, their bodies don't respond to it or can't use it. This is called type 2, and it's what the vast majority of people with diabetes have and what we are focusing on here. Type 1 and type 2 are different diseases. Nearly every person with type 2 diabetes is obese or seriously overweight. When insulin doesn't do its work of getting cells to store glucose, the glucose level in the bloodstream starts to rise. With no glucose going into your cells, your body thinks it's starving and another hormone triggers the release of stored glucose into the bloodstream. The end result: a whole lot of sugar— glucose—floating around in your blood.

All this sugar changes the way your body and organs function. It puts extra glucose into your urine, causing you to urinate more often. The extra glucose and more frequent urination make you thirsty. Over time, diabetes can damage small blood vessels, harming the retina of the eye and injuring the kidney. It can also cause water to be pulled out of your blood, making the blood thicker and less able to flow as it should. Other symptoms include unexplained weight loss, extreme hunger, frequent fatigue, blurred vision, very dry skin, sores that are slow to heal, and frequent colds and infections. People with diabetes are also prone to gum disease.

If diabetes is not treated and controlled, people who have it can experience a host of serious problems.

- They are two to four times more likely to have a heart attack or stroke. In fact, according to the American Heart Association, heart attack is the leading killer of people with diabetes. Some 80 percent of people with diabetes develop and die from cardiovascular disease, yet only one third of them consider themselves at risk for this problem!

- Many people with diabetes suffer nerve and blood vessel damage, and in some the damage is so severe it causes loss of adequate circulation in the feet or legs. In the worst cases, this can lead to amputation of a foot or leg.

- Diabetes is the leading cause of blindness and kidney failure in adults.

- Uncontrolled diabetes can cause metabolic imbalances that, in extreme cases, can trigger coma or even death.

- People with diabetes often have compromised immune systems and are therefore more susceptible to infections such as flu or pneumonia and are less able to fight them off when they get them.

Who Gets Diabetes?

Type 2 diabetes is a classic example of genes and environment combining to do terrible damage to people's health. It has a strong genetic component and it clearly does strike some groups of people more frequently than others. People with family histories of diabetes are much likely to develop it themselves and some ethnic groups—especially African-Americans, Hispanics, Asian Americans, and Native Americans—have especially high rates.

Among one group of American Indians, the Pima of Arizona, fully 50 percent of adults over thirty have diabetes, and 95 percent of those with diabetes are overweight. Many researchers believe that the Pima and other Indians may possess a so-called "thrifty gene"—a gene or genes that originally served to slow their metabolism to help them store fat in times of plenty so they could make it through the scarce times without starving. Such a gene enabled people to survive the harsh uncertainties of desert life. But in recent decades, the Pima and other tribes have adopted a Western lifestyle and so they eat more fat and calories and exercise less. The combination of their genetic history and their new lifestyle has been disastrous.

How can you tell if the man you love—or you, for that matter—might be on the road to diabetes? Here are a few things you can look for. Measure your waistlines. If his waistline is 40 inches or bigger or yours is 35 or bigger, you're increasing your risk of developing diabetes. Exercise is another big factor. If you don't get any, your risk goes up, but if you get some regular exercise, you can cut your risk substantially. Finally, people who eat a diet that is high in carbohydrates but low in fiber (processed foods such as cakes and cookies are a good example)—the kind of diet that boosts blood sugar—are also at risk. (See chapter 11 for a discussion of fiber and carbohydrates.)

"It's Not Diabetes—I Just Have a Touch of Sugar"

For many years, the father of a good friend of mine was under the care of a kindly small-town doctor in the Midwest. At one point, her father developed a sore on his foot. Though he did not remember injuring the area, the wound was stubborn and wouldn't heal. Several times he returned to the doctor, who each time cleaned and dressed the wound. Then one day my friend found her father at home, confused and disheveled. She took him to the emergency room, where doctors found that his blood sugar was very high and his wound had become infected. Fortunately, he recovered.

When she asked him if he knew he had diabetes, he said, "I don't have diabetes, I just have a little sugar in my blood."

"Why didn't you tell me?" my friend asked.

"There was nothing to tell," he replied. "The doctor told me I'm fine, I just need to watch sweets."

It turned out that for years his doctor had been telling him he had too much sugar in his blood. Trouble was, he neglected to explain exactly what that meant.

Unfortunately, this is all too common. Often physicians will tell people that they have a slight elevation in their blood sugar but offer little information about the effect that a "touch of sugar" can have. Telling patients that they have "borderline diabetes" does little good unless they are also given clear instructions and support to help them make critical changes in the way they live and eat. The stakes are high: Long before the classic symptoms of diabetes set in, excess blood sugar can be causing long-term, permanent damage.

This is why public health experts are now focusing on this "touch of sugar" and have given the condition a new name—prediabetes—and a public awareness campaign to warn people about it. Experts now urge all people aged forty-five and older who are overweight to have their blood sugar tested. Overweight people younger than forty-five should be tested if they have a family history of diabetes, have low HDL cholesterol and high triglycerides, have high blood pressure, or belong to a minority group such as African-Americans or American Indians known to be at an increased risk for diabetes.

Experts have also lowered the level of blood sugar that is considered acceptable or safe. To understand this, you need to know a little about how blood sugar levels are measured.

Blood Glucose Tests

There are a number of different blood tests used either to diagnose diabetes or prediabetes or to monitor the fluctuations in blood sugar of people who have the disease. (Urine tests do exist, but they are not recommended because they are so inaccurate.) The diagnostic tests are generally performed at the doctor's office. People diagnosed with diabetes must learn to do their own home testing so they can control their blood sugar levels and avoid complications. Two tests, both normally performed at your doctor's office, are used to diagnose your condition and, on occasion, to monitor a treatment regime. The other tests are used to monitor progress of the disease.

FASTING BLOOD GLUCOSE TEST

This measures your blood sugar after a fast of eight to twelve hours. If your level is 110 mg/dl (milligrams per deciliter of blood) or below, you're fine. That's considered normal. If your level is between 110 and 125 mg/dl, you have what doctors call "impaired fasting glucose." Under the new definitions, that means you have prediabetes. If your level is 126 mg/dl or above, you have full-blown diabetes.

ORAL GLUCOSE TOLERANCE TEST

Here, you fast for eight to twelve hours. Then your blood sugar is tested twice—once before and once after you drink a solution containing sugar. This is sometimes called a "glucose challenge." If your blood glucose rises no higher than 140 mg/dl two hours after the drink, that's considered normal. If it goes up to between 140 and 199 mg/dl, you are said to have "impaired glucose tolerance." Again, that's the threshold for prediabetes. If your glucose rises to 200 mg/dl or above, you have full-blown diabetes.

HOME TESTING

People who are diagnosed with diabetes need to test their blood sugar so they can make sure they are controlling it adequately. There are a number of home-testing products available for this purpose. All involve sticking your finger to collect blood and then using a machine to analyze the glucose level. Each test provides a snapshot of your glucose level at any given moment. Working with a health-care provider, patients will develop a daily schedule for testing and keep a log of their results. The most common time to test is just before meals.

HEMOGLOBIN A1C OR HBA1C TEST
(Also Known as Glycosylated Hemoglobin or Glycohemoglobin A1c Test)

To complement the snapshot image obtained through home testing, this is one other "big picture" test you may also need to take from time to time. This lab test reveals average blood glucose over a period of two to three months. Specifically, it measures the number of glucose molecules that have attached themselves to hemoglobin, a substance in red blood cells. The test takes advantage of the life cycle of red blood cells. Although they are constantly replaced, individual cells live for about four months. By measuring these attached glucose molecules, average blood sugar levels over the previous two to three months can be determined. HbA1c test results are expressed as a percentage, with 4 percent to 6 percent considered normal. Research shows that people with diabetes can best reduce complications if they maintain a level of less than 7 percent.

CHANGING THE ODDS, AVOIDING DISASTER

All these tests and numbers can be both overwhelming and frightening. If you and your husband get tested and find that either of you have "impaired" glucose levels, or prediabetes, you might feel upset. But really, you may be lucky. You got an early warning and caught on to a developing problem before it could become serious. You have an excellent chance of slowing down or reversing these numbers *if* you make some changes in how much you eat and how often you exercise. A recent study by the National Institutes of Health proved it can be done.

The Diabetes Prevention Program looked at ways of helping people with prediabetes prevent or delay the development of full-blown diabetes. The study participants used two different approaches. In one, people changed what they ate and exercised about thirty minutes a day. By doing this, they were able to lose an average of 5 percent to 7 percent of their body weight and reduce the risk of developing type 2 diabetes by 58 percent. In the second part of the study, volunteers took a commonly used oral medication called Glucophage (metformin) that helps keep blood sugars regulated. They found it cut their risk of developing the disease by 31 percent.

This is great news because it means that many people with prediabetes can shift the odds and avoid full-blown diabetes without taking medication. So how can you and/or your husband make these changes? Let's start by looking at what—and especially how much—you eat. If you have type 2 diabetes, or are on the verge, chances are you're overweight, so that's the place to begin (see chapter 11 and Resources).

COUNTING CARBS

Nutrition experts used to say that people with diabetes couldn't eat anything with sugar, but they've now changed their view. "With proper education and within the context of healthy eating, a person with diabetes can eat anything a nondiabetic eats," says Karen Chalmers, R.D., director of nutrition services at Joslin Diabetes Center in Boston.

Whether you're trying to prevent diabetes or you already have it, there are several important principles that you need to know. First of all, there is no such thing as a one-size-fits-all "diabetes diet." That notion went out of favor several years ago. But that doesn't mean that what you eat isn't critical in both preventing and managing diabetes. Your real enemy is excess—excess carbohydrates and excess sugar, both of which turn into glucose in your bloodstream.

Most foods other than meat and fat contain carbohydrates. Starchy foods such as rice, potatoes, and pasta are mostly carbs; vegetables and fruits contain them too, but in lower concentrations. If your husband or you have diabetes, or are at risk of developing the disease, you'll want to work with a nutritionist to develop an eating plan.

Based on how much you weigh, if you need to lose weight, how often you exercise, and other factors, you'll set a limit on the amount of carbohydrates you can consume in a day. If your husband is, say, six feet tall and weighs 185 pounds, he might be told he could eat 350 grams of carbohydrates, spread out over the course of the day so that his blood sugar never gets too high at any point. He can then eat pretty much whatever he wants—even some sweets—as long he doesn't exceed his daily carb quota.

There's been a lot of discussion in recent years about a concept called the glycemic index (see page 301). To review, the basic idea is that some carbohydrates break down into glucose more quickly than others. White flour has a very high glycemic index— it readily converts to glucose. Carbs that are more chemically complex like beans, or that contain more dietary fiber like vegetables, take longer to break down and have a lower glycemic index.

Does that mean that people with diabetes should worry about the glycemic index of the food they eat? Depends on who you ask. The American Diabetes Association recently released new dietary guidelines for people with diabetes and recommended against making the glycemic index of foods a major consideration. The basic thrust of the report is that people with diabetes should count their carbs and stay within their allowable total, but not worry about whether the carbs are coming from brown rice or from mashed potatoes. One reason for the ADA's recommendation is the belief by its experts that trying to figure out the glycemic index of every food item people might want to eat is enormously complicated and confusing.

Other experts disagree. In a paper recently published in the *Journal of the American Medical Association,* David Ludwig, M.D., director of the obesity program at Children's Hospital in Boston, reviewed a number of studies that examined the effects on people of following either high- or low-glycemic diets. He notes in the paper that "the glycemic index and glycemic load of the average diet in the United States appear to have risen in recent years because of increases in carbohydrate consumption and changes in food-processing technology." During those same years, obesity and diabetes have become virtually epidemic, and Dr. Ludwig believes these two trends are probably related.

He argues that it makes sense to urge people to aim for a diet that emphasizes low-glycemic food and limits high-glycemic food. Such a diet, he says, can probably help people avoid or control diabetes. He thinks experts shouldn't worry so much about confusing people.

"The concept of glycemic index may be complex from a food science perspective," he says, but "its public health application can be simple. Increase consumption of fruits, vegetables, and legumes, choose grain products processed according to traditional rather than modern methods—for example, whole-wheat pasta, stone-ground grains, old-fashioned oatmeal—and limit intake of potatoes and concentrated sugar." This is sound dietary advice, whatever the precise effect of higher or lower glycemic food.

Counting Calories

One of the biggest reasons people develop type 2 diabetes is because they are overweight, which makes it harder for their bodies to use insulin to convert food into energy. That's why many people with diabetes need to count their calories and fat, as well as their carbohydrates. And since people who are diabetic are also at high risk for heart disease, they usually need to mind their fat and cholesterol consumption, whether or not they're overweight.

If you or your husband is at risk for developing diabetes, it makes sense to start controlling the foods you eat and how much of them you consume. A number of health organizations, including the ADA on its website (www.diabetes.org), sell food lists that tell you the carbohydrate and fat content of most foods.

One of the best moves you could make would be to work with a nutritionist to design a menu and eating plan that works for you and your family. If your health insurance won't pay for it, consider paying yourself. Spending $70 or $80 for an hour's consultation could be a real bargain if it helps you develop a healthy and tasty eating plan. Studies show that people who educate themselves about their diets do better. For most people that means sitting down with a nutritionist and going over basic information about how to control diabetes.

Much of the diet advice we've presented in other chapters is relevant to people with diabetes, too. Meanwhile, keep in mind a few basic ideas that are especially relevant to diabetes.

- Stay away from fried foods.
- Make meat an ingredient instead of the main event. Eat little red meat and make sure it's lean. Opt for skinless chicken and fish instead. In general, people with diabetes should keep protein consumption at no more than 15 percent of calories because excess protein can contribute to kidney disease.
- Go easy on cheese and stay away from margarines made with trans fats.
- Make your plates colorful—load them with vegetables and fruit.

In addition to controlling blood sugar it is vital that people with diabetes control cholesterol and triglycerides if they want to reduce their risk of heart problems (see page 336).

Testing Blood Sugar

In some cases it will be necessary to regularly test the blood sugar level (see page 337) by getting a small drop of blood and having it analyzed by a small handheld meter. This gives an excellent picture of how things are going if carefully recorded and evaluated. The diabetes educator or doctor will let you know how often and what times of day to do it—though often it is before meals. The good news is that there are new products that make the process easier. One warning: Don't be the keeper of your partner's diabetes equipment—make sure he takes responsibility for himself!

Diabetes Medications

Some people with prediabetes will be unable to keep their blood sugar levels from rising further by changing their diet and exercising. For these people, medication may help and there are a variety available. Some, like metformin, lower blood sugar by blocking the liver from making too much glucose. Others stimulate your pancreas to make more insulin, make your body more sensitive to insulin, or slow the rate at which you absorb carbohydrates.

Around 40 percent of people with type 2 diabetes will eventually need to take insulin injections like people with type 1 diabetes. That's because over time, their pancreas will be unable to make enough insulin.

Finally, because people with diabetes are at very high risk of heart disease, experts now recommend they consider aspirin therapy. Speak to your doctor about whether or not it is right for your partner and at what dose. You should also speak to the doctor about drugs called ACE inhibitors that have been shown to prevent or delay kidney disease in people with diabetes. Also, ask about lipid-lowering medicines that control cholesterol levels and can reduce the risk of developing heart disease.

Whatever medications you may be taking, you'll still need to watch how much you eat and to get plenty of exercise. These are the most powerful weapons you have for keeping your blood sugar controlled.

Exercise

This is one area that often gets neglected when "treatments" for diabetes are discussed. Exercise helps because it can increase tissue sensitivity to insulin and that can reduce blood sugar levels. It can also increase levels of good cholesterol—HDL—and lower bad cholesterol—LDL—and help with

---

HYPOGLYCEMIA

Symptoms of hypoglycemia include:

- hunger
- nervousness and shakiness
- perspiration
- dizziness or lightheadedness
- sleepiness
- confusion
- difficulty speaking
- feeling anxious or weak

Hypoglycemia can also occur while you are sleeping. You might cry out or have nightmares, find that your pajamas or sheets are damp from perspiration, or feel tired, irritable, or confused when you wake up.

weight loss goals. Thirty minutes every day is a bare minimum. But be sure that your partner undergoes a thorough cardiac evaluation before embarking on a vigorous routine. The reason is that people with diabetes are at risk for heart disease. In addition, some people with diabetes can experience a drop in blood sugar (*hypoglycemia*) if they exercise (see box, page 433). Having a snack before exercise is a good idea to avoid this problem. And finally, make sure shoes fit well. An injury to the foot can be hard to heal in a person with diabetes.

GOING FORWARD

If someone you love has been diagnosed with diabetes, many things are likely to change in your lives and they probably should. My husband's diabetes has made me even more aware of the importance of eating the best diet possible. But I have also had to deal with a wide range of emotions: fear (something bad is going to happen to him); guilt (I should have done more to prevent it); even anger (why didn't he do more?). I have to catch myself often and make sure that I continue to encourage him rather than nag. I sure don't want my husband's diabetes to get worse. I therefore really want him to take control, lose that weight, and really watch what he eats. I also know that for better or worse, we are in this together and that I have to keep my emotions in check as we strive to do better. One thing I can do is help my husband with the logistics such as follow-up tests. Because diabetes can

THE ANNUAL DIABETES TO-DO LIST

Get a flu shot (October to mid-November).
Get a dilated eye exam to catch retinopathy early.
Get a foot exam (including check of circulation and nerves).
Get a kidney test:
 Have your urine tested for microalbumin.
 Have your blood creatinine measured.
 Get a twenty-four-hour test.
Get your blood fats checked:
 Total cholesterol.
 HDL.
 LDL.
 Triglycerides.
Get a dental exam at least twice a year (people with diabetes are prone to gum disease).
Talk with your health-care providers about how you can tell when you have low blood glucose and how you're treating high blood glucose.
Examine your feet daily. Call your doctor at the first sign of redness, swelling, or infection anywhere on your feet.

Source: Copyright © 2003, Redspring Communications, Inc. Reprinted with permission.

lead to a variety of complications he will need to have regular monitoring. This is one area that many folks with diabetes don't do so well. Although your diabetes control plan is geared to your personal concerns, there are a number of things that everyone with diabetes needs to do regularly (see box).

MEN AND DIABETES

As we mentioned earlier, diabetes is not a man's disease. In fact, in the African-American and Latino communities, women are more likely to be diabetic than men. But diabetes can affect men and women differently, both in their bodies and in the way they manage the medical and psychological aspects of their illness. It can also have a major effect on a relationship.

On the medical front, men with diabetes are more likely than women to experience vascular problems. One vascular problem is *claudication,* leg pain that occurs when you're walking, usually in the calf or thigh muscle. It goes away after a brief rest, but then comes back when you start walking again. Claudication occurs because not enough blood is flowing to meet the increased need of a muscle at work, and it's a symptom of peripheral vascular disease. Left unchecked, peripheral vascular disease can lead to cold, pale legs and feet; ultimately it can lead to amputation of a foot or leg. This happens much more commonly to men than women. Men are also more likely than women to die from a heart attack or suffer a stroke.

A diabetes-related problem unique to men is impotence, or erectile dysfunction. In fact, diabetes is one of the most common causes of erectile dysfunction. Between 50 percent and 60 percent of diabetic men over fifty suffer from it. Obviously, this is a major issue for diabetic men and their wives. It happens because diabetes makes it difficult for blood to flow into the penis to create an erection. The disease can also damage nerves in the penis. And then there's the psychological dimension. The rising and falling of glucose levels and the other symptoms of diabetes are stressful, and that in itself can make sexual performance difficult. If your husband is experiencing erectile dysfunction, make sure he gets a test for diabetes. And yes, Viagra works for many people with diabetes (see chapter 22 for more on impotence).

Men, Women, and Diabetes

A number of studies suggest that men handle the psychological impact and life changes of diabetes better than women do. One recent study by two researchers at Johns Hopkins University School of Medicine, Richard Rubin, Ph.D., and Mark Peyrot, Ph.D., reviewed more than one thousand patient surveys and made some interesting findings. They found that men tended to feel more confident about their ability to manage and control their diabetes, were more satisfied with their treatment and their diet, were less likely to be depressed, and generally felt they had a better quality of life than women. "Simply put," the authors write, "we found that men seemed to have an easier time living with diabetes that did women."

Another finding of the study may help explain why men feel so at ease, relatively speaking, with this disease. They get more support, logistically and emotionally, from their partners and from other family members than women with diabetes get, according to the surveys. The men got into fewer arguments and hassles related to diet, medication, and blood testing. Wives of male patients were more likely to attend education meetings about diabetes and even to respond to the survey than husbands of female patients . I guess this should come as no surprise. We're better at nurturing than men are, so they get better taken care of when they're sick.

But many men don't do well in the patient role. They suffer, and make us suffer along with them, because they have so much trouble accepting help and being cared for. "Diabetic men seem to shut out the women in their lives more often than diabetic women shut out their men," says Dr. Richard Rubin, who is also the coauthor of *Psyching Out Diabetes: A Positive Approach to Your Negative Emotions.* "Maybe that's because men have been trained in stoicism more than women have. Men are more likely to see diabetes as a weakness or a burden to be borne in silence. Some men stay closeted about their diabetes out of fear that loved ones may overprotect or police them."

In treating diabetes, doctors say, this gender gap becomes particularly evident. Authors Peter A. Lodewick, M.D., June Biermann, and Barbara Toohey have written books for both men and women with diabetes. But *The Diabetic Woman* outsells *The Diabetic Man* by more than 10-to-1 in online sales. And while they got lots of letters from women who have read *The Diabetic Woman,* they have never received a single letter from a male reader of *The Diabetic Man.* The only readers of that book that have written were women, who read the book to help the men in their lives.

The Disease of Denial

Men's tendency to avoid dealing with their health problems and to minimize the seriousness of having diabetes has many roots, notes Dr. Lodewick. "Some men fear diabetes will destroy their image of being strong and invulnerable," he says. "Still others would be willing to admit that they have diabetes, except that they don't want others to treat them differently, such as a hostess who goes out of her way to prepare them a special meal."

Here's how one woman described her husband's tendency to minimize and deny problems related to his condition. She made her comments in a 1997 survey conducted by *Diabetes Forecast* magazine.

My spouse (50+) thinks he can still do all the physical work he did in his thirties. He works too hard and is often pale, shaky, and disoriented with low blood sugar. When I express concern, he tells me he can "handle" it and knows when it's coming on. Ten years ago, he had a violent episode, thrashing around on the floor. I took him to the emergency room and the doctor on duty accused him of being drunk!! Now he accuses me of "watching him."

—WORRIED IN WISCONSIN

Source: Copyright © 1997 American Diabetes Association. From Diabetes Forecast, *July 1997. Reprinted with permission of the American Diabetes Association.*

Men's unwillingness to face up to the disease can create serious martial discord, says Rubin. "It's most often the wives who experience this kind of frustration when their husbands refuse to take care of their diabetes, ignoring it as if it didn't exist," he says. "These women go back and forth between screaming at their husbands and giving up completely."

Some people become paralyzed at the prospect of trying to manage their disease and leave all decisions about day-to-day care to their partners. This is much more likely to happen when a man, not a woman, is the diabetic, says Dr. Rubin.

"In our society, caretaking is a skill more highly developed in women than in men," Dr. Rubin points out. "Sometimes the diabetic is very open about wanting to have someone else manage his disease. One man told me he had turned his diabetes over to his wife because 'she does enough worrying for both of us.' Another said he took it for granted that his wife would carry his supplies when they went out, because 'she has a big bag that she takes everywhere anyway.'

"But this habit that couples get into is not healthy for either partner," Dr. Rubin goes on. "Women resent it. They begin to feel like the police and feel that if anything were to happen it would be their fault. And men never learn to take responsibility for their own disease."

Diabetes researcher Dr. Mark Peyrot says there is a tendency for women to "nag" their husbands about their diabetes—an approach that has good and bad sides. "The upside is perhaps it will work and somebody will do something that they wouldn't otherwise have done," Dr. Peyrot says. "The downside is it can create 'reactants'—people digging in their heels [and acting like] 'I don't want anybody bossing me around. I'll decide for myself what I'm gonna do.'"

Rather than nagging, Dr. Peyrot suggests saying things like "It's good to know you're checking your blood." The trick, he says, is to find ways to help the person feel they can be successful taking care of themselves. But let me tell you—it's not always easy.

Because denial is such a common problem among people who are at risk for diabetes, or who already have it, Rubin and his coauthors have developed a quiz they call the Denial Self-Test. Here it is:

- Do you have symptoms you can't explain, like frequent urination, chronic exhaustion or infections, pains in the arms or legs, or blurry vision?

- Do you avoid medical care for your diabetes?

- Do you feel uncomfortable acknowledging that you have diabetes or reading about the disease?

- Do you tell yourself that you can effectively treat your disease simply by taking pills or insulin shots?

- Do you ever say that you have "borderline diabetes" or "just a touch of sugar?"

If you're dealing with a man who is in denial about his need to deal with prediabetes or diabetes, this quiz could come in handy. Show it to your partner and maybe it will jar him into realizing that his disease is serious and needs attention. Good luck!

Other Things You Can Do to Help Someone You Love Who Has Diabetes

- Go with your partner to nutrition classes or to diabetes education classes so that you both hear and learn important information that could help with the disease. You know what they say: Two heads are better than one. If you both hear it, there will be less confusion later on.

- A diet for a person with diabetes is a healthy diet. Instead of trying to feed various members of the family many different diets, try sticking to one that your partner can eat. It will be good for the whole family.

- Incorporate physical exercise into the time you spend together as a couple: Go for walks or take bike rides together. If your routine is typically to have dinner and watch TV for a few hours, consider using one of those hours to take a walk.

- Do some research and check into the latest gadgets and gizmos to help people with diabetes manage their disease. Instead of "taking over" management, you could offer to be the informed consumer keeping an eye out for the newest ways to help with the disease.

- Be supportive, don't nag, and by all means take care of yourself. You will be setting a good example!

METABOLIC SYNDROME (SYNDROME X)

The term Syndrome X was first coined in the late 1980s by Gerald Reaven, M.D., of Stanford University who wanted to alert doctors to a group of patients who didn't have actual diabetes but were still at great risk of developing other problems that could cause them to develop heart disease. Syndrome X is now also called Metabolic syndrome. If there is a triple whammy in medicine this is it. Metabolic syndrome is not really a single illness but rather a cluster of problems—obesity (especially in the abdomen), high blood pressure, insulin resistance, high triglycerides, and low HDL levels. When a person has this syndrome—as some 60 million to 75 million Americans do—it puts them at great risk of heart disease. People with Metabolic syndrome are four times more likely to have a heart attack or stroke than those who do not have the condition.

The central problem for people with this disorder is that obesity and inactivity combined with genetic factors leads to insulin resistance—the cells of their body do not respond normally to insulin. Because of this, the pancreas pumps out lots of extra insulin in an effort to overcome this resistance by the cells. Eventually the cells in the pancreas that produce insulin become defective and die off, causing a drop in insulin production and a rise in blood sugar levels. For one in four people with insulin resistance, the result is full-blown diabetes.

Others never get diabetes, but they can still have big problems. Researchers are not exactly sure how this happens, but they do know that the excess insulin causes the liver to produce more triglycerides and keeps the kidneys from excreting salt, thus triggering high blood pressure. Other changes seem to make the blood more likely to clot, increasing the risk of heart attack.

Who Gets Metabolic Syndrome?

Like diabetes, Metabolic syndrome is a product of nature and nurture—genes and lifestyle. Sometimes you can recognize someone who's at risk just by looking at his belly. Big bellies, as we have said, cause big problems. Metabolic syndrome runs in families, but is exacerbated by a poor diet high in simple refined carbohydrates (breads, pasta, cakes, and so on) plus the fat and the sugar. These carbohydrates not only raise glucose and insulin to unhealthy levels, but they also lack many vitamins, minerals, and nutrients our bodies need. Dr. Reaven estimates that half of a person's insulin resistance stems from his or her genes and the other half from being obese and physically inactive. Smoking, he says, is also a minor factor.

So how do you know if your husband might have Metabolic syndrome? Men are considered to have it if they have three or more of the problems below:

- Triglyceride levels of 150 mg/dl or higher.
- HDL levels of less than 40 mg/dl (50 mg/dl for women).
- Blood pressure of 130/85 or higher.
- Blood glucose level of 110 mg/dl or higher.
- A waist measurement of 40 inches or more (35 inches for women).

If you or your spouse has this constellation of problems, do everything you can to get each risk factor under control. As always, the best place to start is by losing weight!

16

Alcoholism: The Hidden Epidemic

I grew up with every privilege a child could have. We had servants, cars, a lovely home, nice clothes, and private schools. We also had stature within the community. My father was a prominent judge. My brothers and sisters and I should have been the happiest kids in the world. But we were not. My parents were alcoholics, and there was much unhappiness in our home. At the time I did not understand the root of the problem. I only knew they drank, and often too much. I was over forty before I understood what much of my life had been about. And though I never drank—and do not now— my life has been about alcohol. Even when I left my parents' home, I did not leave alcohol behind. At age twenty-five I married an alcoholic. We've been married for nearly forty years.

—EVE*, SIXTY-FOUR YEARS OLD

Alcohol is the most abused drug in America and those most likely to abuse it are men. According to the American Medical Association 20 percent of men and 10 percent of women drink above recommended limits of alcohol use and are at risk for health problems as a result. What's more, according to the Substance Abuse and Mental Health Services Administration nearly 10 percent of men (but only 2 percent of women) are considered to be heavy drinkers.

For the drinker, heavy alcohol use can affect nearly every organ of the body and aspect of life. But the disease harms far more people than those who actually do the drinking. In 2000, nearly 17,000 innocent Americans were killed in alcohol-related auto accidents and some 300,000 more were injured. Children, friends, and coworkers of alcoholics all know the terrible pain of being involved with someone with a serious drinking problem. Perhaps no group is more affected over time than the women who share their lives with alcoholic men.

The wives and girlfriends of alcoholics suffer right along with the drinker. They're the abused caretakers who clean up their husband's social and financial messes and endure his angry rages. They're the targets of abuse, both physical and emotional. And because they live with nearly constant stress, they are prone to all kinds of physical and psychological ailments, from heart disease and obesity to anxiety and depression.

Far too many women in this kind of relationship feel helpless and demoralized, blaming themselves for their husband's problems and withdrawing from friends and family. Indeed, many women remain loyal to their partner, almost to a fault.

A Family Disease

Alcoholism runs in families, passed from one generation to the next by genes, environment, or both. Right now, researchers are hunting for the genes that may predispose a person to having problems with alcohol. But while there may well be genetic factors that make some people more susceptible to alcohol problems, having those genes doesn't necessarily mean that you'll become an alcoholic. By the same token, *not* having them doesn't mean you can drink as much as you want without consequence. Lifestyle and life stresses play a big role in who develops the disease. Once you have it, though, you have it for life. You cannot expect to drink "normally." Alcoholism is a chronic disease like any other. People who are successfully treated are considered nondrinking alcoholics.

Excessive alcohol consumption can have profound effects on a person's body. Long-term, chronic drinking can lead to serious medical problems such as cirrhosis of the liver and pancreatitis. It can precipitate or exacerbate high blood pressure and diabetes. It can also increase the risk of cancer of the liver, head, neck, and pancreas.

For some alcoholics the decline is almost imperceptible. Many never experience profound setbacks or hit rock bottom. Instead, they function for years without a moment of serious drama. In other cases, a drinker's life can completely unravel, says Joseph A. Pursch, M.D., a psychiatrist and addiction specialist in Laguna Beach, California, who has treated such high-profile patients as Betty Ford and Billy Carter. First, family problems arise: The drinker argues and fights more at home, and normal conflicts take on a harder edge. Then his social life changes so he's hanging out only with other men who drink. As time goes by, he finds himself in jail or in court on drunk driving charges; he has mounting financial problems from car wrecks, legal fees, or lost work time; and he's experiencing physical and mental problems such as liver damage, blackouts, amnesia, and depression. By the end, he's lost his job and may be estranged from his friends and family. His life is total chaos. This sort of dramatic decline doesn't always happen, for sure, but it certainly can.

So what can you do? Your primary goal is making sure that you don't follow him down the black hole. If you can also help him, that's fine. But it's critical to be clear about your goals and the limits of what you can do for him. As always, the first step in dealing with an alcohol problem is recognizing that it's there.

I Think My Husband Is an Alcoholic

Figuring out if you should be concerned about a loved one's drinking can be tricky. Although two thirds of American men and half of American women drink alcohol, three fourths of them experience no serious consequences from their alcohol use.

Of course, serious problems such as blackouts, drunk-driving arrests, increasing interpersonal conflict, or medical problems are hard to miss. Early on, the problem may be subtler and more difficult to define. Still, recognizing the early signs of trouble may save you years of problems; it may even save lives.

People usually decide that someone's drinking is a problem after there's been a serious event or consequence. In general, if a man is downing more than two drinks a day most days, that's not a good sign. But it is important to know that these guideposts are devised from large studies and are general statements about risk. Having more than two drinks a day does not definitely mean that a man is an alcoholic or will suffer physical consequences from his drinking. Nor do these guidelines help in distinguishing who will get into trouble with alcohol. While it's helpful to under-

---

WHAT IS A SENSIBLE DRINKING LIMIT?

If your husband doesn't have any health problems and hasn't had a history of addiction, it should be okay for him to drink a limited amount of alcohol.

According to the U.S. Government, a sensible drinking limit for men who don't have a problem with alcohol is two drinks per day. That's the upper limit of what experts define as "moderate drinking" for men. For men over sixty-five, one drink per day is the recommended limit.

What Is Problem Drinking?

At-risk alcohol use, or problem drinking, is defined as more than seven drinks per week or more than three drinks per occasion for women, and more than fourteen drinks per week or more than four drinks per occasion for men. Heavy drinking is often defined as more than three to four drinks per day for women and more than five to six drinks per day for men.

Source: Reprinted from American Family Physician, "Problem Drinking and Alcoholism," vol. 65 (3), Feb. 1, 2002. Copyright © 2002 American Family Physician. All rights reserved.

What Is a Drink?

Standard drink (U.S.) = 12 g of alcohol: one 12-oz. bottle of beer (4.5 percent alcohol); or one 5-oz. glass of wine (12.9 percent); or 1.5 oz. of 80-proof distilled spirits.

stand general drinking limits, you must look at each case individually to discern if there is a problem. For example, some men don't drink every day, reserving their drinking for binges in which they'll put away five or more drinks in a sitting. This, too, is a problem, and a serious one. Here are some other red flags to watch for in your husband or partner:

- He's screwing up a lot, failing to fulfill his responsibilities at work, school, or home.
- He becomes isolated from the family, paying less attention to you and the children.
- He is argumentative and irritable much of the time.
- He keeps drinking in hazardous situations such as driving.
- He gets into trouble with the police or other authorities and has conflicts with people around him.
- His tolerance for alcohol increases; he needs more alcohol to achieve the same "high."
- He experiences withdrawal symptoms when he doesn't drink or he uses alcohol to relieve or avoid these symptoms.
- He's constantly trying to cut down on his use of alcohol but never succeeds.
- He spends a lot of time using or recovering from the use of alcohol.

THE CAGE QUESTIONNAIRE

The CAGE questionnaire is a short set of questions that many experts use to determine if someone has an alcohol problem. While this questionnaire is really for the drinker, it may help you to be familiar with these questions.

1. Have you ever felt you ought to **C**ut down on your drinking?
2. Have people **A**nnoyed you by criticizing your drinking?
3. Have you ever felt bad or **G**uilty about your drinking?
4. Have you ever had a drink first thing in the morning to steady your nerves or get rid of your hangover (**E**ye-open)?

Experts say that one yes answer means you *may* have an alcohol problem and more than one yes means it's highly likely.

It may be difficult to decide whether or not someone you love has a problem. Making a decision will be especially difficult if your partner is a drinker whose drinking does not seem to affect other areas of his life. He may be frequently intoxicated but never drives while drunk, excels at his job, and takes good care of the children. He may drink heavily at parties but at no other time or drink every day after work without it affecting any other sphere of his life. You are worried because of the frequency of his drinking, but you don't know what to make of it because he doesn't "screw up" in other areas. You certainly don't want to accuse him when there is in fact no problem. Being nonjudgmental and as objective as possible is imperative when it comes to evaluating a loved one's drinking habit.

Look at the Pattern

It can be helpful to look at how your partner has changed over time. Usually there is a gradual transition from moderate drinking to problem drinking to alcoholism. There is often a tug-of-war between the alcohol and the alcoholic. Here's how writer Sean Elder described his experience in *Men's Health* magazine:

> I had certainly had my problems with alcohol—I'd ruined a few relationships, wrecked a few cars, had run-ins with a few magistrates—but that was mostly behind me. I didn't drink to excess now (except when I did, and then I tried to hide it). I certainly wasn't out on the street, endangering the general populace. I was married (again), helping to raise a young child (again), and was working fairly steadily. Except when I wasn't. Then I would get depressed and drink myself into a stupor. Until I got a good job, which I would celebrate by drinking myself into a stupor. Then there were those awful in-between times when absolutely nothing seemed to be happening—times I would get through by drinking myself into a stupor . . . Every drunk has his own story, as unique as that person, though each ends up the same: Either he quits or he dies. There's an old Japanese proverb that expresses it as well as anything I've ever heard. "First the man takes a drink," the saying goes. "Then the drink takes a drink. Then the drink takes the man."
>
> Source: Reprinted with permission from Sean Elder.

Most addicts try to conceal their use. They abandon family and friends and hang out with other drinkers. And they make excuses—all kinds of excuses—to rationalize their behavior and placate those around them. Here are some of the most common:

- "I'm not *that* bad!"
- "It wasn't my fault" or "It's not the way it looks!"
- "I'm not hurting anybody but myself!"
- "Trust me—I know what I'm doing!"
- "I can stop anytime I want to!"
- "It will never, ever happen again!"
- "Nobody is going to tell me what to do!"
- "I'd be okay if it weren't for you!"
- "I don't have time [or money] to get help."
- "I'll handle it myself!"

If your partner has a drinking problem, you probably recognize these excuses. They can be an obvious sign someone needs help. But pay attention to the things you're saying, too. Many spouses will adopt the same excuse-making strategy as a way to cover for their partner. That's one reason that the first place to start looking for answers may be with yourself.

LOOK AT YOURSELF

Looking inward can reveal much about what is going on in a family. Many women spend a lot of time trying to fix problems created by an alcoholic husband, covering up, making things right, denying there is a problem. Alcoholism is the pink elephant in the room that nobody acknowledges. It is the big secret that most families don't want anyone else to know, and that wives often deny to themselves. "I think women who are married to alcoholics pick it up very early," says Dr. Pursch. "But often they won't admit it."

Laurie* began to suspect that her husband, Brad*, had a drinking problem early in their relationship. But she always rationalized that some current stress kept Brad drinking and that as soon as it was resolved the problem would go away. "No matter what people said to me about Brad's habits, I always defended him," Laurie recalls. "I made sure he got to work even when he could barely get out of bed. I handled everything with the kids and made excuses for him when they asked where their daddy was."

But the more Laurie covered for Brad, the worse things got. "I walked on eggshells around him," she recalls. "When he drank, his personality changed. Things started to slide at his job. His boss was sick of the excuses. I took an extra job to make more money. Then I became ill with pneumonia and everything fell apart. I wish I had realized sooner what was going on because I could have spared our children years of heartache."

Spouses of drinkers need to know that they are people in their own right and are entitled to a life without the conflict caused by a spouse who drinks.

IS YOUR PARTNER'S DRINKING AFFECTING YOU?

The twenty questions below devised by Al-Anon can be a starting point. If the answer to some of these questions is yes, then it's likely alcohol is causing problems for someone you love—and for you.

1. Do you worry about how much someone else is drinking?
2. Do you have money problems because of someone else's drinking?
3. Do you tell lies to cover up for someone else's drinking?
4. Do you feel if the drinker loved you, he or she would stop drinking to please you?
5. Do you blame the drinker's behavior on his or her companions?
6. Are plans frequently upset or canceled, or meals delayed because of the drinker?
7. Do you make threats, such as "If you don't stop drinking, I'll leave you"?
8. Do you secretly try to smell the drinker's breath?
9. Are you afraid to upset someone for fear it will set off a drinking bout?
10. Have you been hurt or embarrassed by a drinker's behavior?
11. Are holidays and gatherings spoiled because of drinking?
12. Have you considered calling the police for help in fear of abuse?
13. Do you search for hidden alcohol?
14. Do you often ride in a car with a driver who has been drinking?
15. Have you refused social invitations out of fear or anxiety?
16. Do you sometimes feel like a failure when you think of the lengths you have gone to in order to control the drinker?
17. Do you think that if the drinker stopped drinking, your other problems would be solved?
18. Do you ever threaten to hurt yourself to scare the drinker?
19. Do you feel angry, confused, or depressed most of the time?
20. Do you feel there is no one who understands your problems?

Source: Al-Anon Family Group Headquarters, Inc., copyright © 1980.

WHAT SHOULD YOU DO IF YOU THINK YOUR HUSBAND IS AN ALCOHOLIC?

If you think that your husband's drinking is a serious problem, you must remember the goal: Helping him realize he has a problem, not forcing him to stop drinking forever. The only person who can stop a drinker from drinking is the drinker. In fact, one mistake many women make is to seek help to "get him to stop drinking."

But if you keep this more limited goal in mind, you may be surprised at how much influence you have. As with so many other health problems, it is often a wife or girlfriend who spurs a man to get help with his drinking. "When the male alcoholic comes in, nine times out of ten, it's the result of some external pressure of some sort," says Dr. Floyd Garrett, a psychiatrist and addiction medicine specialist in Atlanta. "Usually that pressure is from the partner. You know, 'My wife said if I don't get help, she's divorcing me.'" The point: Know your power and its limits. Use it well. And don't wait for your husband—or you—to hit rock bottom before acting.

Arm Yourself with Information

Whether you start at a program like Al-Anon or by doing your own research, you need to learn about this disease before you can help anyone. There are hundreds of books and websites that can offer information, and many of them are excellent (see Resources).

For many spouses, the first step is Al-Anon, a nationwide program that holds support groups for family members and friends of alcoholics. It was started more than fifty years ago by women whose husbands were recovering alcoholics. Realizing that they too needed help, they formed themselves into family groups and followed the principles of Alcoholics Anonymous. Today there are meetings all over the world.

The goal of Al-Anon is to help family members find positive ways to deal with the challenges of living with an alcoholic. Meetings are free and anonymity and confidentiality are guaranteed. Alateen, a related group, is geared toward children of alcoholics.

It is important to understand what Al-Anon is and what it is not. You will not learn how to "fix" your problem drinker at Al-Anon meetings, and you won't get advice or counsel. What you should get is support and the wisdom of others' experience. Joanne, a fifteen-year Al-Anon member, says Al-Anon taught her how to take care of herself.

"I didn't realize that I needed help as much as my husband did, [since] I did not have a drinking problem," she says. "Hearing the stories of others was a real eye-opener. When I first started to attend, I could not figure out how other members could laugh about what was happening in their lives. But I learned to detach from my problems. I learned about the disease of alcoholism, and I learned how to go on with my own life."

Al-Anon cautions against treating the alcoholic like a child. Do not preach, do not nag, do not cover up the messes made by the drinker. And do not try to check on how much the person is drinking. Avoiding these things can lift some of the burden of being married to an alcoholic. Al-Anon helps you remember that the only person you can change is yourself. Once you've started helping yourself, you'll be more able to help your husband. This doesn't mean that you are responsible for his recovery, only that you love him and hope for a better life for the whole family.

The Direct Approach

Talking to an alcoholic about his drinking is not an easy thing to do. And in many cases, it won't make him stop drinking. He might not be ready to listen or to admit that he has a problem. But there are cases in which a person has gone right into rehab after one simple conversation. So be sure to find out what kind of help is available in your area before you have your talk.

Choosing the right time and mood is essential. This is a conversation that must take place when the person is not drinking. The best time is often shortly after an alcohol-related problem has occurred, such as a serious family argument or a car accident. Choose a time when both of you are fairly calm and you have a chance to talk in private.

When you're ready, approach him with a loving discussion about what you are seeing and how it affects you. Be as gentle as you can; accusatory language won't help. Couch your message in caring language that explains how his drinking makes you feel and how you worry about his health. Let him know that you care about him and are concerned about his drinking.

"If you catch him at the right time after a bout of drinking the alcoholic is often remorseful and willing to do something, at least apologize," says Robert Morse, M.D., professor emeritus in psychiatry and former director of addictive disorders at the Mayo Clinic in Minnesota. "Maybe you can get your foot in the door and get him to go for an evaluation before the remorse has worn off and he reverses his stand."

If your spouse is willing, you can call immediately for an appointment to see a counselor or doctor, or to attend an AA meeting. Offer to go with him. If the gentle approach doesn't work—and chances are it won't—you can then call on a friend. A recovering alcoholic may be particularly persuasive, but any person who is caring and nonjudgmental may help.

Of course, many women have tried some variation on these approaches with little positive result. In a relationship where there is abuse, these types of confrontations can trigger an outburst of anger or physical violence. Becoming violent yourself in an effort to make your husband change won't work either. One thing to keep in mind: Making threats you don't intend to keep will backfire, so choose your words carefully.

If you say you are going to leave him and take the kids if he continues to drink, then you must be prepared to do just that.

Bring in the Doctor

One little-used approach that sometimes can help is enlisting your husband's doctor. If he or she is willing, a trusted doctor may be able to initiate a discussion about the implications of your husband's drinking, especially if there are signs of alcohol-related health problems. Sometimes a doctor is the perfect person to stimulate reflection on the part of a drinker. The doctor may do it by giving advice or just by having a conversation that explores a patient's awareness of the problem. Sometimes a simple examination at the doctor's office that includes questions about alcohol use can be enough to get a man thinking about his drinking habit and its effect on his life. Studies show that advice from a physician can be surprisingly effective in getting a drinker into treatment.

Another Option: The Intervention

If these conversations have no effect and your husband still can't see the light of day and seems headed toward physical, emotional, and financial ruin, you may want to try an intervention.

Many people wait too long to perform an intervention, says Dr. Morse. The time to consider one is *before* a person has a serious car accident, a drunk driving arrest, or a serious medical problem. It must also be held at a time when the person is not drunk or drinking.

An intervention consists of a group of friends, family, coworkers, or other important people in the alcoholic-addict's life who confront the individual with their feelings about his alcohol or drug use. This is done in a controlled, objective, and systematic fashion in order to overcome the addict's denial and minimization of the problem as well as to present a unified front of support and care as everyone encourages the addict to get some help.

Dr. Pursch says a pre-intervention meeting of all those who would participate is essential so that each person can rehearse what he or she will say. The other important point is that the family itself cannot be in denial. Everyone must agree that the problem exists. People who care about the person and agree that he has a problem can attend. That can include family, friends, and coworkers, even the boss. You should have someone there who is professionally experienced with interventions (see Resources).

When the time comes, the drinker is brought in and each person speaks about how his drinking has affected him or her. He or she must speak with love and without judgment, but must tell him there will be consequences if he doesn't change—anything from canceling social plans to moving out or divorce. Explain that you are not making these threats to punish him but to protect yourself from his problems. Do not make any threats you are not prepared to carry out. Telling a father that his alcoholism is hurting his children or putting the family in financial jeopardy may be the best way to make him see the effect his drinking is having on the family. Ideally, after the intervention, you'll be able to take the person directly to a treatment facility.

It may seem dramatic, but it can be quite effective if it's carefully planned and executed. If you're going to try one, you may be able to get advice from the National Intervention Network (NIN), which has local affiliates around the country. NIN is organized by the National Council on Alcoholism and Drug Dependence. They can be reached at 1-800-654-HOPE. Keep in mind that interventions can be expensive when you take into account the cost of a professional, the price of travel, or time off from work for participants. You should also know that there is little research proving that an intervention is better than other approaches at getting people to stop drinking. Interventions may also raise ethical and legal issues of patient confidentiality if the drinker has not given explicit permission to professionals to share his medical information. Nevertheless, interventions have been used with success in many anecdotal cases.

Of course, not all interventions work. No one can force another person to change. But even if the man you love is not ready to make a change, *you* can and must. Don't wait to seek help for yourself. If you can't save him, at least save yourself.

Many women want to know if it is possible to have their husbands "committed" because of their drinking. Having someone involuntarily committed for treatment is difficult to do. Even if a person is hospitalized for his drinking or arrested for a crime related to his drinking, he can leave as soon as he sobers up or makes bail. You need to consult the law in your state for more information.

17

Cancer

Steve Bishop* never got sick. The fifty-one-year-old accountant never caught the kids' flu, never complained of feeling bad, and never went to the doctor. That's why his wife, Melanie*, thought it was particularly strange one New Year's Eve when her husband came home from work, announced that he had a fever, popped two Advils, and went off to take a nap. Melanie immediately suggested they cancel their party plans for the evening, but Steve said he'd be fine, and indeed, he got up two hours later and danced his way into the new year.

But just one month later—during a routine physical Melanie had convinced him to get—doctors found evidence of non-Hodgkin's lymphoma, a cancer in the lymphatic system. Steve reacted to the diagnosis with shock, denial, and anger. Melanie reacted by devoting nearly all of her energy (apart from her full-time job) to taking care of Steve, by making sure he kept a positive attitude, by ensuring he got the best treatment, and by forgetting about her own needs. "My whole world revolved around Steve once he became ill," Melanie now says. "I didn't go out with my friends or take a day to go shopping or anything."

Although her intentions were golden, the way that Melanie cared for Steve ended up hurting both herself and her husband. Steve became overly dependent on his wife, Melanie fell into a state of depression, and their marriage suffered.

The Bishops' story is all too common. As cancer rates soar (one in two men will develop cancer in his lifetime)—along with other diseases affecting aging Baby Boomers—more and more spouses find themselves in the role of caregiver. According to a 2000 survey conducted by the National Family Caregivers Association (NFCA), more than a quarter of the adult population—about 54 million people—provided care for a chronically ill, disabled, or aged family member or friend during the year prior to the survey. And 61 percent of "intense" family caregivers (those providing at least twenty-one hours of care per week) have suffered from depression, according to the same association. The vast majority of these caregivers are women.

Medical professionals, while skilled at treating the patient, often neglect to help the spouses and other family members much at all. Add in the tendency of women to think they can "do it all," and you see why so many women encounter the same pitfalls as Melanie Bishop.

I sincerely hope that you will never have to help a spouse who has been diagnosed with cancer or any serious chronic disease, for that matter. But if you do, the approaches discussed here may give you a head start in knowing how to approach the problem. If you never have to play this role, you should at least gain an appreciation for those who do and be able to help support a friend who is a caregiver.

The goal of this section is not to spell out complicated treatment options or the latest diagnostic methods for all forms of cancer. There are many excellent resources for that type of information. Instead, I will point out some resources that can help you navigate the medical world as you care for your loved one. The information presented here can also help you when confronting any serious or life threatening illness.

GATHER INFORMATION

The most important way to support someone who is newly diagnosed with cancer is to gather information. It may also be the most empowering. There is a tremendous amount of valuable information available and helping to sort through it will be very important to the care your partner receives. Today's physicians have many effective options to choose from, and that's good. But it also makes the evaluation and treatment decisions more time-consuming and complex. The "best" treatment is not always cut-and-dried.

Harmon Eyre, M.D., chief medical officer of the American Cancer Society, encourages patients and their families to seek out their own medical information: "It's very clear in today's world that the person with the disease needs to participate and find the treatment that's best for them. And to do that, they have to know the stage of disease, know the kind of cancer that's present, and understand the ramifications of the different options and treatments. If they have good, reliable information, it helps them talk to their doctor, helps them find the right way to do it."

Before Starting Your Research

Before you start diving into websites and books, you'll need to know as much as possible about the nature of your partner's cancer and whether and how far it has spread. Here are some of the basic details you need to be clear on: What kind of cancer does your partner have? What is the stage and grade? How large is the tumor? Where is it located? Has it metastasized? If so, to where?

The Internet

The Net can be a powerful tool. Though I am not aware of any study showing that people who do medical research on the Internet get better care, I have heard from many people that they have used it to locate a doctor, a hospital, or a therapy that helped or even cured them. If you do not know how to use the Internet, there are many libraries that can help you get started. Better yet, ask a relative (most likely a young one) for some help.

The problem with the Internet, of course, is that there is plenty of bogus information, too. I recommend starting out at the website run by the National Cancer Institute. The basic information resource from the NCI is called the PDQ, which stands for Physician Data Query. This is an excellent source of accurate, detailed information about the ninety-plus forms of cancer. A panel of experts provides summaries that cover diagnosis, treatment, the psychological aspects of being diagnosed with cancer, alternative and complementary approaches, and much more. PDQ also includes an invaluable up-to-date list of ongoing clinical trials for a wide range of cancers. You can access PDQ and other information and links at the CancerNet website: *www.cancer.gov*.

I can't emphasize enough that information will be your best tool in helping your partner through the cancer experience. Try not to overload him with too much, however, especially if he seems overwhelmed or unsettled by it all.

Here are some other resources you might want to check out:

- The National Coalition for Cancer Survivorship: *http://www.canceradvocacy.org*
- Cancer Care (800-813-HOPE; *http://www.cancercare.org*)
- American Cancer Society (800-ACS-2345; *http://www.cancer.org*)
- Steve Dunn's Cancer Guide: *http://www.cancerguide.org*
- The R. A. Bloch Cancer Foundation: *www.blochcancer.org*
- *www.cancersupportivecare.com*

Books

I generally prefer books by individual authors with a lot of clinical experience to large, hefty reference books published by large (even the most revered) universities, which tend to be dull, dull, dull. It's not that the information in these books is bad; to the contrary, it's usually excellent. The trouble is these tomes are often hard to understand and relate to because the human element is missing. Here are a few books on cancer, the cancer experience, and medical research that I think you'll find helpful.

- *Diagnosis Cancer: Your Guide to the First Months of Healthy Survivorship,* by Wendy Schlessel Harpham, M.D., a physician and long-term cancer survivor who writes and lectures on surviving and thriving after a cancer diagnosis, is the place to start. It is a nuts-and-bolts guide that teaches the basics about the medical, practical, and emotional challenges in a comforting and hopeful way. The latest edition includes "Harpham's decision tool," a chart that helps patients understand their options and work with their physicians to decide on the best treatment. There are other books you may want to check out (see below), but this is an excellent first purchase and an essential book for a person recently diagnosed.

- *Guide for Cancer Supporters* can be obtained from the website *www.blochcancer.org*. It contains helpful information for caregivers and can help you understand your new role. This book is by Annette and Richard Bloch, who founded the R. A. Bloch Cancer Foundation years ago after Richard, cofounder of the H&R Block tax preparation service, survived lung cancer.

- *Supportive Cancer Care: The Complete Guide for Patients and Their Families,* by Ernest H. Rosenbaum, M.D., Isadora Rosenbaum, M.A., and Alan Glassberg. This addresses everything from the cellular mechanisms of cancer development to issues of religion and spirituality that confront all cancer patients. Practical information and advice are plentiful here.

- *When Life Becomes Precious: A Guide for Loved Ones and Friends of Cancer Patients,* by Elise NeeDell Babcock. An excellent emotional guide for family and friends of cancer patients.

- *Everyone's Guide to Cancer Therapy: How Cancer Is Diagnosed, Treated, and Managed Day to Day,* by Malin Dollinger, M.D., Ernest H. Rosenbaum, M.D., Margaret Tempero, M.D., and Sean Mulvihill, M.D.

- *After Any Diagnosis: How to Take Action Against Your Illness Using the Best and Most Current Medical Information,* by Carol Svec, which takes you through the intricacies of gathering information and is recommended for anyone unskilled at research.

FINDING THE RIGHT DOCTOR

Once cancer has been diagnosed, you will be referred to an oncologist to start planning treatment strategies. It's important to find a doctor you trust and feel comfortable with and who is experienced in treating your type of cancer. If your family doctor has a particular oncologist in mind, find out as much as you can about that person: his experience, areas of expertise, training, and whether he accepts your insurance carrier. Ask your doctor if he or she has referred other patients to this doctor and if those patients or their spouses might be willing to talk to you. Call any cancer support organizations in your area and see if you can find other people who have used this doctor.

When your partner goes to meet with the doctor, accompany him and be prepared to write down or tape record everything the doctor says. Bring an initial list of questions and see how the doctor responds to your questions. Ideally, you'll both feel comfortable and confident with this doctor so you can start moving forward on treatment. But if you don't feel that confidence, or don't relate well to this doctor, you may want to keep looking. Obviously, the nature of your partner's condition will be a big factor in how much time you can spend looking around.

GET A SECOND OPINION

There are many ways to treat cancer. In some cases, though certainly not all, there may be several ways to treat one particular type of cancer. For this reason there may be no single "right" way to treat yours. I can tell you firsthand from my years of working in hospitals and clinics that there is huge variability out there when it comes to the way medicine is practiced. That's why I strongly recommend you get a second opinion. Believe it or not, studies have shown that geography, rather than medical science, often determines what kind of treatment you're likely to get.

The *Dartmouth Atlas of Health Care,* produced by Dartmouth University, analyzed the Medicare records of nearly 40 million elderly people and found that the practice styles of physicians in particular areas of the country may have as much influence on treatment decisions as hard science. For example, if you live in certain parts of Texas and complain of back pain, you have a less than 2 percent chance of getting surgery to treat it. But if you have the same problem in Santa Barbara, California, the chance that you will be prescribed surgery increases by 300 percent. The same can be said for many diagnostic tests and procedures. Too many patients get treatment based on the opinion—or even the guesswork—of their doctor. This is not a good thing!

This wide variability in the practice of medicine is one reason why the profession is currently undergoing something of a quiet revolution. The revolutionaries are pushing an approach that you'd think would already be the norm—they call it *evidence-based medicine.* They advocate treatment based on scientific evidence, and press doctors to look at the best research available to make treatment decisions. In other words, it seeks to remove as much as possible anecdotal decision making and "intuition" from the practice of medicine. Though many physicians initially balked at using practice guidelines, it is now becoming clear that they are helping to streamline and improve patient outcomes.

Second opinions are extremely important, especially if the diagnosis is unclear or the illness is life-threatening. You should also get one if you're considering an experimental or highly toxic therapy, even if it means wading through the red tape of an HMO to get it.

One of the biggest obstacles to getting a second opinion is that many people don't want to offend their current doctor. Don't let this hold you back. It's your or your partner's life we're talking about here. Besides, good oncologists consider second opinions a routine practice and are not the least offended if you seek one. Make sure your second opinion is from an independent oncologist or doctor, not one your original doctor recommends. If possible, opt for a multidisciplinary second opinion, which is offered by many large hospitals. This is a meeting, which the patient's family and friends are welcome to attend, in which specialists from different types of cancer medicine—radiation, chemotherapy, surgery—are present to tell you how they propose to treat the cancer. The Bloch Cancer Hotline (1-800-433-0464) or *www.blochcancer.org* can help you find an institution that offers multidisciplinary second opinions.

Still worried about offending your doctor? Carol Svec, the author of *After Any Diagnosis,* recommends delivering one of the following tactful messages to let your doctor know you want a second opinion:

"I understand and respect what you are telling me, but for my own peace of mind, I would like to get a second opinion."

"I feel comfortable with the opinions you have described, but as an informed consumer, I feel it is important to get a second opinion."

"I may very well end up coming back here, but first I would like to get a second opinion."

Attend All Appointments with Your Partner

One thing you can do that is profoundly helpful is to accompany your partner to the doctor, and listen and ask questions alongside him if he is comfortable with that. Two sets of ears and two minds are better than one. "There are too many situations in which the family member is left as a passive person in the waiting room," says Laurel Northouse, Ph.D., a professor of nursing at the University of Michigan School of Nursing. When caregivers participate with the doctor, they can ask questions the patient may forget or pick up details that the patient overlooks. Still, some men may prefer to go alone; respect boundaries but be available if he changes his mind.

If you want to get the most out of a medical encounter, pick up a copy of *Surviving Modern Medicine: How to Get the Best from Doctors, Family & Friends,* by Peter Clarke and Susan Evans of the University of Southern California School of Medicine. This book can help you and your loved one better navigate the medical waters. It's a bit technical but incredibly well researched.

ORGANIZE YOUR SUPPORT NETWORK

Organizing your support network will be very important to you and your spouse. Start by enlisting family and friends to help out with tasks around the house, errands, or general emotional support. Jamie Von Roenn, M.D., a medical oncologist and professor of medicine at Northwestern University School of Medicine, says you need to go further than just family and friends. "Patients and their families newly diagnosed with cancer should be seen by a social worker who will help them address a variety of problems. They also need to consider how they are going to handle the finances." That there will be many things to consider when a spouse is diagnosed with cancer, and the adjustment is often easier and smoother if couples enlist the expertise and assistance early on of a social worker, psychologist, psychiatrist, psychiatric nurse, and clergy. The best time to reach out is when the diagnosis is made, says Dr. Von Roenn. But it is never too late.

CAREGIVING AND STRESS

A diagnosis of cancer throws you, your partner, and your entire family into one of the most difficult periods of your life. Men, women, and children will all face this challenge differently, and all will experience anger, stress, and resentment. But the stress level may be highest for women who care for their spouses. A University of Michigan study of male colon cancer patients and the women who cared for them found that the women suffered more emotional stress than their sick partners, more even than other women who were actually diagnosed with cancer themselves.

Dr. Laurel Northouse, one of the study's authors, says part of the stress comes from the fact that women caregivers often get little help from other family members, friends, or doctors because people assume that they know how to care for sick people. "People assume when the woman is the caregiver, she can handle it," says Dr. Northouse. "When a man becomes the caregiver, however, people assume, 'Oh my gosh this poor guy has to take care of his wife and manage the house.' So they bring a casserole."

Another finding of the study: Women caregivers tend to get caught up in taking care of their loved ones and forget to tend to their own needs.

HOW MEN APPROACH CANCER

Men often react quite differently to a cancer diagnosis than women. They may refuse to talk about the disease, act as if they don't have it, or start getting angry over seemingly small things. All of these reactions can be confusing and upsetting to their partners and family.

Jimmie Holland, M.D., a psychiatrist at Memorial Sloan-Kettering Cancer Center in New York and author of *The Human Side of Cancer: Living with Hope, Coping with Uncertainty,* says most men are reluctant to talk about how they're feeling. "When we looked at spouses of men with prostate cancer, the women were often highly distressed. And they would admit to it," says Dr. Holland. "The men would say, 'I'm fine. I don't have anything to talk about.'" This also explains most men's strong aversion to joining support groups, even though they are proven to help cancer patients cope. (For more on support groups see page 467.)

Anger is another common reaction to cancer among men especially, and one that often mystifies the patient's wife, especially if he never displayed such outbursts before the diagnosis. Melanie Bishop was taken aback by the anger her husband sometimes directed at her, something which was foreign to their relationship up to that point. She describes how Steve would get angry at her if he caught her talking to a friend or relative on the phone about how he was doing or which tests he'd had.

"It's a very difficult thing to deal with when you've been with someone for twenty years and then all of a sudden they're angry at you all the time," she says. Melanie solved that situation by passing the phone to her husband whenever someone called to ask how he was doing. Helping get at the root of the anger and discussing it is another way to dissipate angry feelings.

In households where the man is still able to work, the outbursts of anger may occur on the weekends, says Dr. Holland. "Men can often keep up their macho front at work. But when the weekend comes and they have to think about the illness is when they panic," Dr. Holland says. "The woman often is left to pick up the pieces."

The situation can be even more difficult for men who have to give up work and are forced to deal with an ego-shattering role reversal. Suddenly, instead of feeling like the chief provider of the family, they are now a dependent, being cared for by their family members. "I think it can be a demeaning role for men who've been used to being at work and doing things, " says Dr. Holland. The same can be true for men who continue to work but feel they have less strength than before; they may feel humiliated that they can't mow the lawn or shovel the walk anymore.

That Old River in Egypt

Another common reaction among men is to deny that they are sick and continue living their lives almost as though the doctor had never even uttered the "C" word. In some cases, this might not be a problem; in other cases it is, says Dr. Jimmie Holland. "If they are denying the seriousness of it and it is not negatively impacting their getting treatment, then I think you can go along with that. But if they're denying it to a point they're not going in and getting appropriate treatment, then you have to interfere and say, 'Whoa, this is serious business and you're missing the boat.'"

One of the most important things Dr. Holland does in her book is to dispel many of the myths that have sprung up around the causes of cancer. One important myth she takes on is the idea that a person is somehow to blame for their cancer; that unresolved psychological or psychic issues somehow brought it on and a negative attitude

will make it grow faster. These ruminations on the part of a cancer patient are negative and unhelpful and they can sap the energy a person needs for this fight.

Another book that might be helpful for your partner is John R. Cope's *A Warrior's
Way*, about his battle with breast cancer, beginning at age thirty-nine. Though breast
cancer in men is indeed rare (see chapter 18), Cope's approach to the disease can serve
as an inspirational model for men dealing with any form of cancer.

HOW TO HELP HIM COPE

Helping your partner cope with cancer means respecting his independence and
realizing that there are many ways to cope, and that he may cope in different ways at
different times. Some people seek psychological help; others don't want to talk about
it. Some distance themselves from friends and family, while others would like them
nearby. Some rediscover what is important to them while others escape through
behaviors such as overeating. When UCLA associate professor of psychology Christine Dunkel-Schetter, Ph.D., surveyed cancer patients, most said they would like their
loved ones to ask them what they want instead of trying to guess. Sometimes they'll
want to be left alone; other times they'll want something done for them.

"You need to recognize that one [coping style] is not good and the other is bad, but
that people have different styles of coping," says Dr. Northouse. For example, a wife
might deal with the disease by wanting to talk about it a lot, but her husband may
want to talk about it as little as possible. In this case, the couple will need to negotiate
a bit. "People need to be reminded that sometimes that desire to talk or not to talk can
be a source of tension," Dr. Northouse says. "Stand back, verbalize the tension, and say,
'I guess we have two ways of coping with it.'"

That said, most cancer patients will benefit from having a chance to talk from time
to time. If your partner is anxious or depressed, he may need some strong encouragement to join a support group or see a counselor. "You really have to push him to get
over these cultural barriers that keep men from getting help for psychological problems," says Dr. Holland. "You may have to say, 'Look, you need some medication for
your anxiety. You're not sleeping all night. You're so depressed you don't get out of
bed. You need to see somebody, and I have the names of three people. We're calling
tomorrow.'"

Be aware also that some cancer treatments such as steroids and interferon can
cause emotional problems, says Dr. Holland. If you think that may be happening,
you'll want to talk to his doctor about it promptly.

One of the most common mistakes female caregivers make is trying to do everything for their partners. They talk with the doctors, plan his treatments, and take care
of his other needs while continuing to do all the other things they did before he was

diagnosed. Trouble is all that doting can send the message to your loved one that he isn't capable of doing anything himself, exacerbating his feelings of powerlessness *and* his dependence on you. The trick is to help without crushing his own efforts to cope with and understand his disease.

In their *Guide for Cancer Supporters,* Annette and Richard Bloch suggest that you encourage your partner to take care of himself as much as possible as you also praise him on his progress. Also, don't treat him like he is first and foremost a cancer patient. Make sure to spend time doing fun things together so that all of your interactions are not about cancer. Above all, treat your partner as though he can recover and is going to live, the guide says.

DON'T PULL BACK

People react in many different ways to the news that their partner has cancer. We'd all like to think that our reaction would be heroic, that we'd rally around our lover and roll up our sleeves for the fight. But life is not so simple, and people's reactions are not always what they'd like them to be. For some people, the prospect of dealing with a life-threatening disease conjures up such fear and dread that they simply can't deal with it. They deny that it's happening and cope by pulling away, distancing themselves from their partners. Or they become so negative, and feel so guilty about it, that they are almost immobilized.

It's important to acknowledge these negative feelings and try to deal with them. The impulse to pull away is a common and natural one. You need to be understanding, to forgive yourself for your responses and come to the support of your partner. This is critical. Social support matters a great deal to a person's ability to cope with and recover from a serious illness. People who feel supported and loved do better and may live longer than those who don't. The bottom line is you need to get support yourself so you can provide it to your partner.

A LIST OF THINGS NOT TO DO

After cancer treatment life will go on—admittedly, in a new way—but planning for that is important. Here are some other suggestions the Blochs have for people facing the same problems they faced twenty-five years ago when Richard was diagnosed with lung cancer.

Sympathy for the sake of sympathy doesn't help anyone. Show your compassion followed by a positive constructive statement. An example would be, "I'm sorry you have to go through this ordeal, but be grateful that it was caught at this time and medical treatments have advanced so greatly."

- Tears and sorrow are for the dead, not the living. When you are with the patient, cry with the patient, not for the patient. It can lead to meaningful conversations.
- Never lie or state anything that is not a fact. It will ruin your credibility and come back to haunt you. For example, never say, "I know you are going to get well." You can't possibly know that and the patient realizes it. Therefore, anything else you said with that would be ignored. However, it is possible to state any negative comments in a positive and constructive vein. "It's very serious, but we're going to do everything in our power to beat it," is an example.
- There are no secrets from a cancer patient. Be totally open and honest, but with tact and optimism.
- Do not classify the patient as a statistic in your own mind. This can cause you to harbor false feelings and your feelings have a way of coming through.
- Do not encourage a feeling of futility. The patient's actions might make a difference in the outcome and will make a difference in the quality of his or her life.
- Do not discourage work, prayer, exercise, or diet.
- Do not make a prognosis.
- Do not make decisions for the patient that the patient is capable of making.
- Do not fail to express love, caring, and concern. Let the patient know how much you are hurting and the anger you are also feeling.
- To summarize, your friend or loved one is going through a traumatic time in his or her life. He or she doesn't need your sympathy. He or she needs your help, support, and direction. Do not say, "John, it is so terrible," or "John, it's such a shame." Do say, "John, we're going to do everything we can to try to get you healthy again."

Source: From Guide for Cancer Supporters *by Annette and Richard Bloch. Reprinted with permission.*

What to Expect As a Caregiver

A cancer diagnosis brings major change to the life of a family. In some cases, the change can be positive, bringing families closer together. In other cases, it may overwhelm a family's emotional and financial resources. In most cases, there will be elements of both. Whatever your family's situation, you can count on your new role as caregiver to cause major disruptions in your life.

A survey of 300 spouses of prostate cancer patients, completed in 2001, showed what a big role wives play in their husband's fight with cancer. The survey, conducted by Roper Starch Worldwide, found that 83 percent of spouses feel they help keep up their husband's morale, 67 percent accompany him to doctor's appointments, and 53 percent help make treatment decisions.

But their husband's cancer, and their own role as supporters, also took a big toll on them. The women experienced any number of problems themselves: Eighty-five percent said they were under stress, 44 percent said they had trouble sleeping, and 30 percent went through weight changes. Nearly half reported a sense of helplessness or anxiety, and one third reported depression.

No matter how experienced you are taking care of sick kids, your new role as a caregiver to your partner will be different. Melanie Bishop worked in the medical field for twenty-five years, but even that didn't prepare her for taking care of her husband after he was diagnosed with cancer. "It's way different when it's the person you love the most in life," Bishop says. What's more, you'll have to help all those around you adjust to the new roles as well. This task is not always so easy, though research into the caregiver role is pointing to new ways to improve the situation.

First, it's important to point out that the expectations placed on family members have changed dramatically in the past twenty years. "People are leaving hospitals much sooner and much sicker than they used to," says Laurel Northouse. "People used to leave the hospital when they were well. Now they're often discharged to the care of family members when they're still sick."

Caring for a loved one is no longer just changing a bedpan. You may have to learn how to give injections or change an IV, or watch for an untoward side effect from a medication, while also looking out for the changing needs of your family. The disease will also bring new financial and time burdens. You'll be scheduling appointments, ferrying the patient to them, and listening as doctors give advice or discuss a treatment plan. Your plans and dreams are put on hold along with the patient's. Is it any wonder that resentment, frustration, and extreme stress can creep into the picture? It would be abnormal if a caregiver did *not* feel the strain of her new role.

The important thing is to recognize your feelings, accept them, and find ways to work through them. Denying your own feelings can lead to anxiety and depression, as it did for Melanie Bishop. She survived on her tenacious energy through months of her husband's precarious battle with cancer, projecting a positive attitude and getting him through the hardest part of the treatment. Then Melanie's inner strength collapsed.

"I lost it. I just felt myself becoming depressed, which was a whole new feeling for me, and I started to lose my concentration," she recalls. She would wake in the middle of the night in a cold sweat, and she lost twenty-five pounds in three weeks. Fortunately, her boss finally forced her to take some time off to get back on her feet.

Studies have shown that three aspects of being a cancer caregiver are especially stressful.

1. Dealing with your fear of your partner's cancer and the possibility of his death.
2. Dealing with the emotional needs of the patient.
3. Managing the disruptions in family routines and daily living caused by the cancer.

The uncertainty of cancer's course leaves both the patient and the spouse feeling helpless. Learning to take the experience one day at a time and to set short-term goals can help, Dr. Northouse says.

Your partner's emotional needs will probably seem overwhelming to you at times. Many caregivers feel that they must be cheerful all the time, and this becomes very stressful, particularly if they have little help and no one to lean on for emotional support. Melanie Bishop recalls how draining it was to project a positive attitude 24/7 for her husband. Because she isolated herself and didn't initially ask for help from other family members and friends, Melanie had no outlet for her negative emotions. "I would just advise [caregivers] to talk to someone," she says. "Even if it's just three or four people you can count on, where you can call them day or night and say, 'I just need someone to talk to.'"

After Cancer

Surprisingly, another stressful time often occurs when the treatments are over, even if the cancer is cured or in remission. As things finally return to normal, many patients have a hard time getting back to their pre-cancer life and find it difficult to give up their dependent role. Some caregivers exacerbate this problem by being overprotective instead of encouraging the patient to reestablish control over his own life. Dr. Wendy Schlessel Harpham writes in *After Cancer* that some of the toughest times for her and her husband were during recovery. People expect stress and problems during treatment but not during recovery so they are unprepared for new bumps in the road. It is important to understand that the recovery is a separate phase of the cancer experience, one that you also need to prepare for.

In addition, studies have shown that the fear of recurrence is one of the most common and disruptive worries of both caregivers and patients. It is so common, in fact, that it is considered a normal part of the cancer experience. Caregivers and patients alike should expect to go through this.

Coping with Your Burnout

If many of the statements in the box on page 466 seem to describe how you're feeling and functioning, you could probably use some help to deal with the stress that you're under as a caretaker. In that case, I suggest you take the following four steps immediately. Remember, you can't be of any help to your loved one if you aren't well yourself.

First and foremost, acknowledge your feelings. All of your feelings—no matter how scary or unpleasant they might be—are legitimate. Recognizing and accepting them is the first step toward resolving your problems. A caregiver support group, a counselor, or a friend you can talk to can help you with this step. The important thing is to express your feelings to someone.

Second, ask others to help you. Most family members and friends will be glad to have a concrete way to help your partner and you. If you need to, insist that out-of-town or more reluctant family members come and pitch in—as long as their presence doesn't add more stress! Don't be afraid to delegate tasks and divide responsibilities: Ask someone else to take your partner to the doctor one day, or to make dinner, mow the lawn, or baby-sit the kids. Try preparing a list of tasks and asking for volunteers to help you complete them. The point is to give yourself a chance to relax and take a breather from your husband's illness. Make a conscious effort to get over that feeling that you should be doing everything yourself. Friends, neighbors, and members of your church or synagogue are also good candidates for helping you out.

Third, don't forget to do fun things with your partner so that all of your activities don't revolve around his illness. Think of the things you used to do together and foster that connection.

Finally, take care of yourself. Find time to do those things you enjoy doing on your own, and don't feel guilty about it! Again, you can't be a good caregiver if you are stressed and burnt out. If you need to, explain to your spouse the importance of these steps for both you and him. Also, be sure to exercise, eat right, and get plenty of sleep.

It took Melanie Bishop many months and a lot of stress and anxiety to learn that she needed to find time for herself. "You have to separate yourself from the cancer patient" to a certain extent, she advises. Steve resisted her attempts in the beginning, Melanie says, "but I forced myself to do it because I feel that I really am a better caregiver because of it."

Northouse agrees. "Women need to give themselves permission to take a break from the caregiver role. They need to say 'I'll do my best to help, but not at the expense of my own health,'" she says. "Because if she wears herself out, the caregiver of today may become the patient of tomorrow."

Clearly, caregivers can expect to be under a good deal of stress and anxiety. But how much is too much? *Informed Decisions: The Complete Book of Cancer Diagnosis, Treatment and Recovery* (American Cancer Society, 2001) contains this list of signs that a caregiver may be burnt out.

BURNOUT ALERT

Caring for someone who is sick, taking over his or her responsibilities, having to change habits and routines, and worrying about what will happen results in fatigue at the very least. At the most, the combined pressures lead to resentment, guilt, exhaustion, depression, even physical illness and an inability to care for your loved one or friend. This condition is sometimes called burnout.

- You're exhausted all the time.
- You can't fall asleep, sleep through the night, or get up in the morning.
- You've pulled away from your friends and lost interest in the activities that used to bring you pleasure.
- You feel guilty that you're not doing enough or that you don't want to do even more.
- You worry that you don't really care anymore for the person you're caring for.
- You are easily irritated by people who tell you that you should take care of yourself.
- You think the only relief you can get right now is from alcohol, drugs, food, or cigarettes.
- You don't feel well.
- You're sure that nothing good is ever going to happen again; you feel numb; and you don't care.

What to Do

Above all, you must recognize the importance of your own respite and resist feeling guilty for thinking of yourself. You may need to learn to delegate some of the responsibilities that you think you "should" be doing yourself. Insist if need be that out-of-town family members provide their share of the assistance.

Divide responsibilities. Ask friends and neighbors or members of the church or synagogue to help out. Allow yourself the chance to relax and be distracted from your spouse's illness.

Source: Reprinted with permission of The American Cancer Society.

Caregiver Support Groups

One of the best ways to find support is through a caregiver support group. Here, you can share your feelings and experiences, as well as get ideas about how to cope from other people going through exactly what you're experiencing. A group can help decrease the feelings of isolation that caregivers often feel and give you a forum to express what you're feeling. In addition, you may want to find out about Well Spouse, a national, not-for-profit membership organization that gives support to partners of chronically ill and/or disabled people. Well Spouse can provide practical information on everyday issues facing caregivers. Local Well Spouse groups are being formed in many areas of the country. The website is *www.wellspouse.org*.

Who knows? If you join a support group, it may help convince your reluctant spouse to join one as well, although many men may initially resist them because they think they're too touchy-feely. John Page, president and CEO of Us Too! INTERNA-TIONAL—Prostate Cancer Education and Support, says he sees it all the time. "Guys may be reluctant to join at first, but their wives agree to go and then they are the ones driving the men. Men will typically attend when the support group is organized to sound like an educational meeting rather than simply an emotional support group. 'Come and learn about radiation therapy for prostate cancer.' Then after the lecture the socializing that occurs becomes an informal support session." When men attend they almost always learn that they are not alone and want to come back. Us Too! maintains a website that can help you locate meetings in your area: *www.ustoo.org*.

To find a support group for you or your spouse, or that you can go to together, check with your local hospitals, members of your health-care team, the local chapter of the American Cancer Society, local religious organizations, and the YMCA or YMHA. Also contact the National Self-Help Clearinghouse at 212-817-1822 or their website *www.selfhelpweb.org*.

GUIDING FRIENDS AND FAMILY

It is very likely that you will do much of the interfacing with friends and family members on behalf of your ill spouse. They will probably ask you for details that they would not be comfortable asking the patient, and this can put you in a tough spot at times. As annoying and insensitive as it may seem, people will probably neglect to ask you how you are holding up. Try not to get frustrated, but if you do offer up some information about your own condition, chances are people will tune in and lend an ear.

CONNECTING WITH CANCER PATIENTS

Here are a few tips adapted from the Bloch Cancer Foundation's *Guide for Cancer Supporters* that you can offer to friends and more distant family members on good ways to approach and deal with your loved one.

- Visit the patient even if you feel uncomfortable. Let him know you're thinking about him.
- Be natural and open with the patient. Talk about the disease and call it what it is: cancer. Avoiding the subject only causes more strain and stress.
- Ask the patient how he's doing and *listen* to what he has to say. Ask what you can do to help.
- Make it clear that you are there to give support, not sympathy.
- Be totally honest yet remain optimistic. For example, never say, "I know you are going to get well." But you might say something like, "You have so many things going for you."
- Reminisce about good times and don't be afraid to laugh: Laughter is therapeutic. Let the patient know how he has been special and meaningful in your life. Don't be afraid to cry either. It can lead to meaningful conversations.

Source: Reprinted with permission from Bloch Cancer Foundation.

TALKING TO KIDS

Talking to children about any serious illness or death can be very difficult. Dr. Jimmie Holland says it's particularly hard for male cancer patients to talk to their children. She recalls how one father in his thirties, who was going to die of colon cancer, used to confide in her that he did not know how to tell his son about his disease. "'How will I tell my little boy? How will I tell him to remember me?' he used to ask. He finally used *The Lion King,* that wonderful story of how you can look up in the sky and I'll be looking down at you. It was a wonderful way of telling his boy that he'd always be there for him."

Breaking the news about cancer is only the first of many challenges. Dr. Wendy Schlessel Harpham, a physician, cancer survivor, and mother of three children, tackles this difficult topic in her book *When a Parent Has Cancer: A Guide to Caring for Your Children.* She advocates open and honest communication about what a parent is going through. "This is one area of dealing with children where I believe that there is a right and a wrong way: You must, without exception, tell the truth in order to establish and maintain a bond of trust," she says. Through her own experience, parenting children while going through years of cancer treatments, she says what helped most was simple honesty with her children. "When we told the children bad news couched in love and support, they knew we would get through whatever happened together; when we told them good news, they believed us and didn't worry unnecessarily because we'd been honest when things were bad. By always telling them the truth you open the opportunity to guide your children toward healthy and hopeful ways of coping," says Dr. Harpham. "This open communication has spilled over into the rest of our lives. My children [now teens] feel comfortable talking to us about anything including sex and drugs." Telling the truth eases the parents' burden, too, she says. They don't waste energy trying to protect a lie. And by looking for honest yet hopeful answers for their children, they often find answers for themselves. Her book comes with a companion children's book entitled *Becky and the Worry Cup,* which helps children express and deal with the full range of emotions they may experience when a parent has cancer.

SEX, INTIMACY, AND CANCER

Sex will probably be far from your mind when a diagnosis of cancer is first delivered. Even after the dust settles, many patients and their spouses find that their sex life has been seriously disrupted leaving them confused and frustrated. Treatments for a wide variety of cancers can impact libido; prostate treatments, in particular, often lead to some degree of erectile dysfunction. Fatigue, nausea, pain, grief, and emotional distress all inhibit sexual desire. Many cancer patients (and their spouses) see themselves as somehow more fragile than before, and this affects their ability to feel sensuous or attractive. Any problems with intimacy or sexuality that existed before the diagnosis of cancer will be exacerbated after. Even when a couple is able to resume sexual relations, they may hesitate out of fear, embarrassment, or ignorance. One compounding problem for many couples is that sexual issues are often not addressed by physicians and couples often are reluctant to bring up the issue with their doctors. For all these reasons many couples simply give up on a sexual life after cancer. Fortunately, there is new thinking about sexuality after cancer and the good news is that most people, with some guidance and encouragement from professionals, can resume a sex life—maybe one that is even better than before. Virginia and Keith Laken describe their journey to recapture their intimacy in their remarkably candid book *Making Love Again.* This book is a must for any couple struggling with sexuality after the diagnosis of cancer. It details the available treatment options and how those treatments impact upon intimacy. The American Cancer Society website has a discussion of sexuality after cancer and a list of resources. Be sure to check out *Couples Confronting Cancer,* by Joy Fincannon and Katherine Bruss, as well as *Sexuality and Fertility After Cancer,* by Leslie R. Schover. See also chapter 18.

SPECIFIC CANCERS
Lung Cancer

If someone you love is diagnosed with lung cancer and they smoke, you probably won't be shocked. You may feel angry or even vindicated—after all, you've been telling him to quit for years and now look at what's happened! Is it any surprise? Some people even believe that smokers who get lung cancer "deserve" it. And when people learn of the diagnosis of lung cancer, the first question they often ask is, "Did you smoke?"

The implication is that it's the smoker's own fault, which makes lung cancer extremely stigmatizing to both men and women. When you seek out help from the medical profession, you're likely to meet with some subtle and not-so-subtle discrimination as well. That attitude may be extended to the person supporting someone with lung cancer, too.

The stigma attached to lung cancer is one reason it receives little attention and even less funding for research, despite the fact that it's the number-one cancer killer of both men and women. If you think about it, it seems a little odd. Lung cancer claims more lives each year than colon, breast, and prostate cancer combined.

Relatively effective methods exist to find lung tumors when they are small, yet routine screening is not yet recommended by any of the major medical organizations in this country. Newer screening tools, such as helical CT scanners, can detect tumors in the earliest stages. Yet lung cancer is rarely detected before it is quite advanced—one reason the five-year survival rates are at only about 14 percent, though there are signs that they're slowly improving.

Why don't we look for lung cancer the way we do for other cancers? The basic reason given by most experts is that no U.S. studies have shown that screening for lung cancer decreases mortality. In other words, catching it early doesn't seem to help people live longer. But other experts say that screening and early detection *can* reduce death rates. In Japan, for example, where more people smoke than here, screening for lung cancer is routine and the five-year survival rate was 58 percent in 1992.

Screening for lung cancer is a growing topic of debate among health experts as new screening techniques become available. People who should pay special attention to this debate and may want to consider screening are smokers aged sixty and older. They can consider participating in a clinical trial evaluating the role of high-resolution, low-radiation CT or sputum cytology.

Claudia I. Henschke, M.D., chief of chest imaging at the New York Hospital–Cornell Medical Center, Peggy McCarthy, and Sarah Wernick have written the definitive book on lung cancer, *Lung Cancer: Myths, Facts, Choices and Hope for Patients.*

Another resource for lung cancer patients is the Alliance for Lung Cancer Advocacy, Support and Education (ALCASE). They have a website, *http://www.alcase.org,* and a Lung Cancer Hotline, 800-298-2436.

Colorectal Cancer

Cancer of the colon and rectum is the third most common cancer among both men and women in the United States. Slightly more women than men are diagnosed each year. In 2003, the American Cancer Society expects nearly 150,000 new cases and around 57,000 deaths.

The most important thing to know about colon cancer is that if it's detected and treated in its early stages, when it is confined to the colon, the five-year survival rate is about 90 percent. Unfortunately, only 37 percent of colorectal cancers are found at that early stage. If it's not detected until it has spread to nearby organs or lymph nodes, the survival rate drops to 65 percent. And if the cancer has spread to distant parts of the body, such as the liver or lungs, the five-year relative survival rate is only 9 percent. There are, however, exciting ongoing trials of new therapies for people with metastatic colon cancer that give more hope than these scary statistics suggest.

The bottom line: Screening saves lives. We discussed the various screening tests in chapter 11. Make sure that you and your husband get screened regularly. Also check out *www.ccalliance.org*, the Colon Cancer Alliance website.

18
Male Trouble:
A Gland That Doesn't Always Behave

Not so many years ago, if you mentioned the word *prostate*, many people, including men, would give you a blank look. Or they might think you wanted them to lie down. The good news is that the male prostate gland has become a lot better known in recent years. The bad news is that the gland's newfound fame is due mostly to the problems it can cause. Prostate cancer is the second most common kind of cancer to strike men. Prostate infections afflict millions of young men, and noncancerous enlargement of the prostate affects most men who live past the age of sixty.

So what exactly is the prostate, this thing that can cause so much trouble? It's a small gland, roughly the size and shape of a walnut, that surrounds the male urethra (see illustration on page 49). It has one primary function: to produce part of the semen that mixes with a man's sperm. When a man climaxes during sex, muscular contractions propel prostate fluid into the urethra, where it mixes with sperm made in the testicles. Because of its alkaline nature, prostate fluid helps protect the sperm as they journey through the acidic environment of the vagina and cervix, on their way to fertilize the egg.

The prostate gland goes through two growth spurts. The first occurs during puberty when testosterone levels rise, causing the prostate to double in size by age twenty. Then, for reasons that are not well understood, the gland starts growing slowly again somewhere around the age of forty. By age sixty half of all men have an enlarged prostate; by eighty-five, that number rises to about 90 percent. Thanks to the structure of the prostate and the urinary tract, this enlargement can spell big trouble for a man's ability to urinate normally and can interfere with his quality of life.

While the prostate is not technically part of the urinary system, it surrounds the upper portion of the *urethra*—the tube that carries urine from the bladder to the tip of the penis. A swollen prostate can press on the urethra and obstruct the flow of urine. This can happen as a result of a cancerous growth in the prostate, but it occurs much more frequently as a result of inflammation or the gland's natural swelling with age. A swollen prostate can also impinge on the nerve that triggers erections, making it hard for men to get or maintain them.

Because you can't see or easily feel a prostate, and because men are men, most men pay little attention to their prostates. Even if they start to have problems—like mild discomfort or repeatedly getting up to pee at night—a lot of men ignore them and hope these problems will go away on their own. And that, says Robert Salant, M.D., a New York urologist, is where women often need to step in. "Probably a quarter to a third of patients come in because they're dragged in by their wives," Dr. Salant says.

IF MEN HAD PMS, IT MIGHT BE CALLED PROSTATITIS

Most people know about prostate cancer, and a lot have heard of enlarged prostate, even if they don't quite know what it is. But very few people have heard of *prostatitis,* even though it is one of the most common urological problems affecting men. Prostatitis is inflammation of the prostate gland that can cause some pretty uncomfortable symptoms. Nearly one quarter of all visits to urologists are for prostatitis, and perhaps half of all men will have symptoms of prostatitis at some point in their lives, experts say. Though it is rarely discussed and often ignored, "Prostatitis is much more common than prostate cancer or an enlarged prostate that causes symptoms," Dr. Salant says. "You see many men in their twenties, thirties, or forties with prostatitis. Though the symptoms are not debilitating, they are bothersome and it really affects the quality of life."

It can cause sexual problems and even infertility. The symptoms of prostatitis range from mild but frequent groin ache to excruciating pain. Because it can also make it difficult for a man to urinate, it is often confused with an enlarged prostate (called *benign prostatic hyperplasia,* or BPH) or prostate cancer. But while those two ailments affect mainly older men, the prime time for getting prostatitis is between the ages of twenty-five and forty-five.

Prostatitis is poorly understood. One reason is that so many of the young men who get it won't tell anyone or seek help from a doctor. "Men don't talk about prostatitis," says Clark Hickman, an educator from the University of Missouri–St. Louis. "It's a sexual organ, and men are loath to discuss sexual issues."

Another reason is that prostatitis is difficult to treat or to explain, and it has attracted little attention from researchers or from health officials in Washington. This lack of attention has led men with prostatitis to form their own organization, the Prostatitis Foundation, as a way for men to share information about the disease and to lobby for more research and better treatment. The foundation has been instrumental in getting the National Institutes of Health to put more money into researching the condition.

Many women worry that prostatitis is a sign that their husband is fooling around. It's almost certainly not; chronic prostatitis is not considered a sexually transmitted disease. So if your husband gets it, don't jump to that conclusion.

Here's what is known about prostatitis.

Acute Prostatitis

Caused by a bacterial infection, it is the least common kind of prostatitis but the easiest to cure. It causes fever and pain and can usually be treated quite easily with a short course of antibiotics. Because it is so painful and can make a man very sick, it won't take much convincing to get him to see a doctor. Symptoms include:

- Burning or dribbling with urination.
- Difficulty starting the urine stream or total inability to pass urine at all.
- Cloudiness or blood in the urine.
- Pain felt above or below the penis, in or below the scrotum, or in the back or rectum.
- Fever and chills.
- Nausea and vomiting.
- Muscle aches, fatigue, or flulike symptoms.

Chronic Prostatitis

This is much more common than acute prostatitis but not as well understood. The symptoms can vary a great deal, but they generally come on slowly and linger for weeks or even months. Some men hardly notice their symptoms or find them only slightly annoying. Other men find that the symptoms interfere with work, leisure activities, and sexual enjoyment. What's it like to have chronic prostatitis? Clark Hickman, who suffered with it for many years, makes this analogy to help women understand: "Visualize having a heavy, crampy period that lasts for months. Then you'll have some idea of what your partner with prostatitis is feeling."

Symptoms of chronic prostatitis include:

- Burning during or after urination.
- Difficulty starting the urine stream.
- Dribbling after urination has been completed.
- A need to urinate frequently or urgently.
- A sensation that the bladder cannot be emptied completely.
- Pain felt above the penis, in or below the scrotum, or in the back or rectum.
- Pain experienced during or after orgasm.

If you're trying to figure out whether you have chronic prostatitis, take a look at the National Institutes of Health Chronic Prostatitis Symptoms Index (*www.prostatitis.org/symptomindex.html*) on the Prostatitis Foundation's website. It will give you a symptom score to help you analyze your own situation.

Researchers now think there are two main types of chronic prostatitis. *Chronic bacterial prostatitis* results from an unresolved bacterial infection that causes swelling and inflammation of the prostate. With *chronic nonbacterial prostatitis,* patients have much the same symptoms as chronic prostatitis but no bacteria in their urine. Chronic nonbacterial prostatitis is the most common type and the most mysterious. What could cause it? Doctors aren't sure. In all likelihood, there is not one single cause but several. One theory is that it's caused by tension in the nerves and muscles in the area around the prostate. Other theories include fungal or viral infection, a *urethral stricture* (a narrowing of the urethra as a result of infection or trauma), and food allergies. And still others include irritation from urine backing up into the prostate, from prostate stones, or from an autoimmune or chemical process. Or it could be any combination of the above.

Asymptomatic Inflammatory Prostatitis (AIP)

This category is for cases in which the man doesn't notice any symptoms but white blood cells are found in prostate secretions or in prostate tissue.

Diagnosis of Prostatitis

Many men put themselves in danger of getting chronic disease because they don't get help in the early stages. "Men tend to ignore the first symptoms, which is when it can be treated most easily," Hickman says. "By the time they force themselves to go to the doctor—or somebody that cares about them forces them to go—it's already in the chronic stage. Then they have a hard time."

Diagnosing prostatitis is usually done by testing urine specimens. In some cases urine is obtained after the prostate gland has been massaged by the doctor inserting his finger into the rectum (a digital rectal exam; see page 334).

Treating Prostatitis

Treating chronic prostatitis can be tricky, since the exact cause is often unknown. Chronic bacterial prostatitis can sometimes be successfully treated with antibiotics, taken for four to twelve weeks.

But this doesn't always solve the problem. Other medications such as alpha-blockers, muscle relaxants, and anti-inflammatories are also used, as are alternative therapies such as biofeedback and an herb called saw palmetto. Eliminating caffeine and alcohol helps some men, as does taking warm baths to relax the muscles. Some doctors recommend frequent ejaculation to reduce "congestion." But none of these treatments work for everyone, and some men suffer for many years and try many different approaches before they find something that works for them.

Are there risk factors that can predispose a man to get prostatitis? Probably, but again, there is little agreement among experts on what those risk factors are. Possibilities offered by doctors and patients include a recent bladder or urethral infection or a history of a sexually transmitted disease such as chlamydia or gonorrhea. Some think men who ride bicycles, drive trucks, or operate heavy equipment might also be at greater risk.

One possible risk factor is especially intriguing—the lack of regular sex. "When a man approaches sex from a feast-or-famine point of view, that really plays havoc with the gland," says Clark Hickman. "This happens to men on ships in the navy. They go out to sea for an extended period of time then they go into port and have sex and drink a lot of alcohol at the same time. They tend to get a lot of prostatitis."

Men who have chronic prostatitis may lose their sexual appetite or have trouble getting an erection or having sex without pain. Obviously, your sex life will also be affected, though your partner may not want to discuss it. "This is such an intimate problem that men are reluctant to talk about it," says Hickman. "Wives can help a man come out of that shell. He's frustrated, he's embarrassed, he doesn't know what's happening to his own body."

What he'll need from you is your patience and your support, and that's not always so easy. The website of the Prostatitis Foundation (*www.prostatitis.org*) gets about 130,000 visits a month as well as many phone calls. Half the phone calls come from women worried about men.

Women whose partners have chronic prostatitis should remember that the road to recovery can be long and that men with chronic prostatitis can become depressed, frustrated, or angry. The important thing is to find a way to support him and take care of yourself at the same time. Clark Hickman says, "Support without getting impatient is essential. This guy has gone from being a fun-loving athlete to a real dud. He lies on the couch, he's depressed. He's stopped going to doctors. Women want to know when the problem will go away."

Enlarged Prostate

When they hear the term *enlarged prostate*, or *benign prostatic hyperplasia (BPH)*, many men and women jump to a frightening conclusion: prostate cancer. There are two important things to know about an enlarged prostate. First, it has nothing to do with prostate cancer. Second, it does not lead to prostate cancer, though it is possible for a man to develop both problems at the same time.

Prostates grow with age. In some men, probably most, this growth will not cause any problems. But in 40 percent to 50 percent of men, the swelling of the prostate can make urinating a major and sometimes painful ordeal. It all depends on how the prostate grows. If it grows out, away from the urethra, the enlargement won't have much effect. But if it grows inward, the swollen prostate can push into and constrict the urethra, slowing the flow of urine.

To compensate, the muscular walls of the bladder may squeeze harder to push the urine out. Over time, this can thicken the bladder walls, decreasing the organ's storage capacity and elasticity. Not only does a man with BPH pee slowly, in dribs and drabs, his need to go is more intense, since his bladder can't hold as much as it used to and can never rid itself of all the urine it holds. If the bladder never fully empties, germs may grow in the stagnant urine, and these germs can lead to infection. As a result, some men with BPH get urinary tract infections, which can damage the bladder or kidneys. In rare cases, the prostate can grow so large, and the urethra can get blocked so completely, that no urine can flow out at all, and a man can find himself in great pain. This problem, known as *urinary retention,* can sometimes also be caused by allergy medications or other drugs, which can weaken the bladder muscles. If this ever happens to your husband or someone else you know, get immediate attention—this is a medical emergency.

If your partner has an enlarged prostate, it's likely to affect you as well. Just ask Ethel Stein*. After thirty years of marriage, her husband, Bob*, started getting symptoms from an enlarged prostate. Soon he was getting up many times every night to go to the bathroom. His nighttime awakenings soon began to exhaust Ethel.

"Every time he got up he woke me up and I have a hard time going back to sleep," she says. "I got so exhausted I had to take naps in the afternoon."

But it wasn't only at night that Bob's symptoms interfered with their life. Wherever they went, Bob needed to use the bathroom all the time. Driving was a hassle because he had to pull over so often. Their plans to travel the world were sidelined until Bob got help.

Many men with an enlarged prostate become less interested in sex, and some even have trouble getting an erection. "Not tonight, I've got a groin ache" can become the story of your sex life, just as lack of sleep can become the story of your nights. The bottom line here is that if your husband is suffering with BPH, you have lots of reasons to want to help him take care of it—for your sake as well as his.

The symptoms of an enlarged prostate are:

- A weak urine stream.
- A slowed stream (can't keep up with young men at the urinal).
- Getting up at night several times to urinate.
- Dribbling of urine.
- Increased frequency of urination.

The severity of symptoms is not always related to the size of the gland. Some men have very large prostate glands and few symptoms; others have moderately enlarged glands and intolerable symptoms.

The American Urological Association has developed a brief quiz to help men score their own symptoms. If your husband is complaining of some of these symptoms, or if you notice that he is getting up often at night to pee, encourage him to take this quiz. A high score on this quiz means that you should talk with the doctor to seek treatment.

The questions below are based on a questionnaire developed by the American Urological Association to help men score their own symptoms. For each question give a score of 0 for never; 1 for less than one in five times; 2 for less than half the time; 3 for about half the time; 4 for more than half the time; and 5 for almost always. For question 7, add the appropriate number of times.

RATE YOUR SYMPTOMS

Over the Past Month, How Often Have You . . .

1. Had a sensation of not emptying your bladder completely after you finished urinating?
2. Had to urinate again less than two hours after you finished urinating?
3. Found you stopped and started again several times when you urinated?
4. Found it difficult to postpone urination?
5. Had a weak urinary stream?
6. Had to push or strain to begin urination?
7. Over the past month, how many times did you most typically get up to urinate from the time you went to bed at night until you got up in the morning?

A score of 7 or less indicates only mild symptoms and probably no need for treatment. A score of 8 to 19 (moderate symptoms) and 20 to 35 (severe symptoms) means your husband should talk with a doctor, especially if his symptoms are affecting his lifestyle.

Treating Enlarged Prostate with Medication

There are a number of different treatments that a man with BPH can discuss with his doctor. If the symptoms are mild and are not very bothersome, he might choose to do nothing and see how things go. Doctors call this "watchful waiting."

His doctor may suggest medication. There are two major kinds used for BPH: finasteride (Proscar) and alpha-blockers such as Hytrin, Cardura, and Flomax.

Alpha Blockers

First released to treat high blood pressure, alpha blockers had an unexpected side effect: They also helped ease urinary symptoms. Doctors began to prescribe them to men with BPH, with pretty good success. Up to 70 percent of men with enlarged prostates see improvement on alpha blockers. They work by relaxing muscles in both the bladder and the prostate and increasing the flow of urine. Alpha blockers can cause a number of side effects including lightheadedness, dizziness, fainting, headaches, low blood pressure, and erection problems.

Finasteride

Finasteride relieves symptoms by helping to shrink a swollen prostate by up to 30 percent. It acts by blocking an enzyme that converts testosterone into dihydrotestosterone (DHT), a male hormone that spurs prostate gland growth. It can take a while to work, as long as six to twelve months before men feel the full benefits.

Finasteride has been on the market since 1992 for BPH treatment (it is also used to treat baldness) and seems to help about 60 percent of the men who take it. Some men who take it find they have less sexual desire or more trouble getting an erection. Since it can lower PSA levels, doctors must take this into account when screening a man on finasteride for prostate cancer.

Treating Enlarged Prostate with Surgery

If a man's symptoms are severe, surgery can be helpful, though it also carries risks of side effects.

Transurethral Resection of the Prostate (TURP)

This is one of the most common procedures used to treat the problem. Doctors send tiny instruments through the urethra and cut out portions of the prostate that are obstructing the flow of urine. Patients usually stay in the hospital at least overnight and then may need up to a month to recover at home. Between 10 percent and 30 percent of men who have this surgery will have problems with sexual function.

Open Prostatectomy

This is major surgery to remove the obstructing portion of the prostate gland through an incision in the abdomen. It is used for BPH patients only if the gland is extremely large and causing major problems. It carries a risk of impotence between 16 percent to 32 percent, depending on surgical approach.

Transurethral Incision of the Prostate (TUIP)

This alternative to TURP involves making several slits in the prostate near the opening of the bladder without removing any tissue. Advocates of this surgery believe it will provide the same benefit but with less risk of side effects. At this point it is too early to know for sure.

Minimally Invasive Surgery

Minimally invasive surgery is becoming much more common in the treatment of BPH. One major benefit is that no incision is made. Men with BPH can also choose from a number of new treatments including laser surgery; the use of microwave or radio frequency waves to "cook" the prostate and eliminate tissue; and prostatic stents, which hold the urethra open to relieve obstruction.

Things That Can Help

Many men can avoid or postpone these treatments by making a few changes in their habits. Suggest he try some of these simple changes.

- Drink lots of water during the day. It will keep you urinating steadily and help prevent the collection of stagnant urine in the bladder.
- Stop drinking water in the evening before going to bed.
- Stay away from spicy food, alcohol, and coffee, since they can irritate the bladder and make men urinate more often.
- Avoid medications such as antihistamines and decongestants, which can block the flow of urine. Men with BPH should check with their doctors about all over-the-counter and prescription drugs they are taking.
- Take warm baths. They relax the muscles, draw blood to the area, and help relieve discomfort.
- Some health specialists advocate the use of an herb called saw palmetto to help shrink the gland. If your partner decides to try it, be sure he checks with his doctor, especially if he's taking other medications.
- Avoid constipation. It can aggravate symptoms of enlarged prostate.
- Stay active!

MEN AND FERTILITY

For many years, doctors assumed that if a woman couldn't get pregnant, it was her problem. So women would get checked out by doctors, obsess about their ovulation cycle, and suffer the guilt and pain of thinking—or being told—that they alone were at fault. In truth, nearly half the time, men are solely or partly responsible for a couple's inability to conceive a child.

There are many reasons why a man might be infertile. His sperm ducts could be blocked. He could have a *varicocele,* a dilated vein in his scrotum that causes blood to pool and impedes sperm production. Some studies suggest that up to 20 percent of men have varicoceles—and up to 40 percent of infertile men. He could have abnormally thick seminal fluid, which keeps sperm from swimming freely. He could smoke, take drugs, or drink alcohol—he might even do all three!—which can reduce his sperm count and quality. He might be taking medications or steroids that damage his ability to make sperm.

If a couple is having trouble making a baby, the easiest place to start looking for problems is with *him.* Checking a man's sperm quality turns out to be easier and cheaper than doing a fertility workup on a woman. If he checks out okay, then it makes sense to move on and start examining the woman.

Men Have Biological Clocks, Too

Life isn't fair. Women in their late thirties and forties struggle to get pregnant, while geriatric men like seventy-seven-year-old Tony Randall, or slightly younger guys like Michael Douglas and Julio Iglesias, become fathers.

Many people chuckle at the idea of old Tony Randall becoming a dad in his seventies. They seem to believe the notion that mothers ought not be too old, but fathers can become fathers whenever they're willing and able. But it turns out that becoming an older dad is riskier for babies than most people probably realize. The newest evidence of this risk comes from researchers at Columbia University who found that men over fifty are three times more likely than men under twenty-five to father children who later develop schizophrenia. Men in their forties are twice as likely.

Just as older eggs increase the risk of Down's syndrome, older sperm push up the chances of a baby being born with dwarfism, prostate cancer, Marfan syndrome (see chapter 6), Apert syndrome (which causes malformations of the skull, hands, and feet), and retinoblastoma, an eye cancer.

Now urologist Harry Fisch, M.D., and fellow researchers at Columbia University in New York have even linked older dads with Down's syndrome. Looking at more than three thousand babies born with Down's syndrome they found that a combination of advanced maternal age and advanced paternal age contribute to the development of this genetic disorder. "This should relieve women from the stress of believing they are solely responsible for this genetic abnormality," says Dr. Fisch. "When couples come in they often blame the other or themselves, but in truth it's most often a combination effect. I think we should coin a new term—advanced *parental* age—and stop saying advanced maternal age. They shouldn't approach it as individuals but rather as a team."

Another study finds that as men age, their sperm accumulates DNA damage much as the eggs of women do. In fact, according to the study presented at a recent meeting of the American Society of Reproductive Medicine by Dr. Narendra Singh from the University of Washington, the longer a man lives, the more likely his sperm-producing mechanism is to be exposed to things like pesticides, cigarette smoke, and radiation—each of which can damage DNA. Though the effect may be small, it could explain why some illnesses are linked to older fathers.

All this new information challenges another bit of conventional wisdom—the idea that men stay equally sturdy and fertile late into life. Research shows that men's ability to procreate starts to fall off as early as their twenties. It's not as quick or as steep a slide as women go through, but it's a clear decline nonetheless. Researchers in England found that about 8 percent of men under twenty-five will fail to get a woman pregnant after a year of trying. By age thirty-five 15 percent of them will fail.

What is for sure is that how a man takes care of himself can affect his sperm quality. Stress, smoking, drugs (including marijuana), obesity, exposure to certain chemicals, and sexually transmitted disease can affect sperm number and quality.

Boxers or Briefs?

Here's a burning question that's not just a question of style: Does your fellow wear boxers or briefs? And could it affect his ability to get you pregnant? The debate on this one has been raging for several years. Some say that brief-wearing men might be less able to conceive because sperm don't like it hot. When a man's testicles are too warm, they produce fewer sperm. Since briefs hold a man's testicles closer in to his warm body, his testicular temperature will rise.

Most studies have found no difference in sperm quantity or quality as it relates to choice of underwear. The bottom line: Under normal circumstances, briefs are not likely to cause any problems. So if you and your partner are having trouble conceiving, switching to boxers probably won't help. He should stay out of the hot tub and saunas, though. That much heat really could make a difference.

The Perils of Bike Riding

Men who spend lots of time riding bicycles seem to have more urological problems than other men, problems such as tingling or numbness in the penis. Some men who ride very long distances may even have trouble getting erections. The key to preventing these problems is to wear padded shorts that reduce the pressure and to use the proper seat, perhaps one of the newer seats that are specially designed to minimize pressure on the groin.

"FEMALE PROBLEMS" THAT MALES GET, TOO
When Men Have Breasts

Men have breast tissue just like women do—well, not *just* like women, obviously. Actually, men's breasts are a lot like the breasts of preadolescent girls. There is a small amount of tissue that can respond to hormones or drugs, which can spur the tissue to grow. When this occurs, and males "grow breasts," it's known as *gynecomastia* and can occur briefly during puberty. Usually it quickly regresses (see page 175).

In adult men, breast enlargement most often happens in response to certain medications, as a result of various diseases, or when men are overweight. Excess weight on a man can cause the body to produce more of the female hormone estrogen, which can stimulate breast tissue growth. This is not the same as when an overweight man has extra fat on his chest, giving him the appearance of having breasts.

Drugs that can cause enlarged breasts in men include steroids, anti-ulcer medications such as cimetidine, anti-epilepsy drugs such as phenytoin, cardiac drugs such as digitalis, the prostate drug finasteride, and others that act on the hormonal balance between estrogen and testosterone. The most common cause of gynecomastia in men, however, are the drugs used to treat prostate cancer that reduce testosterone.

Liver disease, cancer of the testes or adrenal glands, kidney dialysis, and a chromosomal disorder known as Kleinfelter's syndrome (see page 36) are among the conditions that can trigger the growth of breast tissue.

For a lot of adult men, this condition can be a source of embarrassment and humiliation. Increasingly men are opting for plastic surgery to correct the problem. The number of breast-reducing surgeries increased nearly 50 percent from 1997 to 2001 when 16,500 cosmetic surgeries for gynecomastia were performed on men.

Why Do Men Have Nipples?

Though men and women are very different, we have a great deal in common. In the earliest part of our embryonic development, we start out basically the same. Males have nipples as a "default," because if they are not exposed to testosterone in the womb (see page 22), they develop with the capacity to be female. Females call upon this capacity when they hit puberty and their breasts develop. Later, if they become pregnant, they call upon it again as milk is produced in their breasts.

For men, of course, nipples serve no important function.

Breast Cancer

Since men have breast tissue and nipples, can they also get breast cancer? The answer, unfortunately, is yes, although it is fairly rare. Every year around 1,500 men will discover a cancerous lump in their breast—slightly less than 1 percent of all breast cancer cases. And each year, some 400 men will die from this "woman's disease."

Typically a man will discover a firm, painless lump beneath his nipple. Sometimes the nipple will be inverted or will have a small discharge of fluid, which can sometimes be bloody. In some cases the breast can be painful. Nearly half of men with breast tumors will have enlarged lymph nodes under the arm of the affected side.

Breast cancer tends to strike men about ten years later than women; on average, men are around sixty-five when they get diagnosed. But men often ignore their initial symptoms. Studies show that men with breast cancer wait more than ten months before calling a doctor about their symptoms. As a result, by the time they get diagnosed, the cancer has already spread to surrounding tissues or organs in 41 percent of men, compared to 29 percent of women. That may be why the male's five-year survival rate is a bit lower than women's, though it is still quite high—81 percent for men, compared to 85 percent for women.

As with women, a family history of breast cancer or ovarian cancer appears to increase the risk. Men with a history of gynecomastia and Klinefelter's syndrome may also have a higher risk, as do men (and women) with a genetic mutation of the BRCA2 gene (a rare mutation that greatly increases the risk of breast cancer). Some experts think men with a strong family history of breast cancer might want to learn whether they have this mutation.

Because men tend to ignore breast cancer symptoms—and because they may be embarrassed to call their doctor about a lump in their breast—you can be a big help. If you know a man who has any of the complaints listed above, make sure he checks in with the doctor. It could save his life!

Osteoporosis

As women age, osteoporosis becomes a major concern. They worry about fractures, keep track of how much calcium they're getting, and, if they're smart, spend time doing weight-bearing exercise that can strengthen their bones. And they're encouraged in all these efforts by doctors, health advocates, and pharmaceutical companies.

So what about men? They don't get this disease, do they? Considering how little you hear about men and osteoporosis, you'd think for sure they did not. But while women are four times as likely to get osteoporosis as men, some 5 million men have this disease and millions more are at risk.

According to the National Osteoporosis Foundation, men suffer one third of the hip fractures in this country, and one third of those men will die within a year after suffering a broken hip. After age fifty, 6 percent of all men can expect to have an osteoporosis-related fracture.

A few years ago, when I was an intern in the hospital, I was called to the emergency room late one night to admit an elderly man who had fallen and broken his hip. The X rays showed that he had greatly decreased bone density.

The conversation went something like this: "Doctor, how could I have broken my hip? I fell only a few inches from the bed to the floor. How could such a little fall cause a bone to break?"

"Mr. Rosen*," I explained, "your bones have become so thin from osteoporosis that even a minor fall could fracture them."

"What?" he exclaimed. "That's ridiculous. Can't you see I'm a man?"

As the conversation continued, Mr. Rosen expressed his disbelief. After all, he said, his doctor—a very fine doctor—had never told him he had osteoporosis, and surely he would know. Later I heard from that doctor how angry Mr. Rosen was at him for not telling his patient that he was at risk.

I have no doubt that this scenario is played out every day. The sad thing is that as the population continues to age, more men like Mr. Rosen will learn they have osteoporosis only after they've broken a hip or fractured a vertebra.

So why do men get osteoporosis? For many of the same reasons as women. They may smoke, drink too much alcohol, and consume too little calcium. They may get too little exercise or have spent years taking certain medications, including steroids for asthma or arthritis, anticonvulsants, some cancer drugs, and even aluminum-coated antacids. They may have unusually low levels of testosterone, which can lead to bone loss. As with women, Caucasians and Asians are at greater risk, as are men who have a family history of the disease. Chronic diseases of the kidneys, lungs, or stomach can also cause bone density loss in men.

The trouble for men is that when they have osteoporosis it often goes undiagnosed. Male osteoporosis receives little media attention or research funding. One result is that symptoms and warning signs are ignored by many men.

> **WARNING SIGNS OF OSTEOPOROSIS IN MEN**
>
> - He breaks a bone.
> - He's shorter and maybe thinner than he used to be.
> - His posture gets noticeably worse.
> - He suddenly starts having back pain (fracture of the vertebrae is the most common result of this disease in men).

Treatment for men includes the class of drugs called bisphosphonates (alendronate and risedronate). None of the other drugs used by postmenopausal women are approved for use in men, however. Doctors may also prescribe testosterone therapy or calcitonin to help slow bone loss in men.

To protect themselves and prevent osteoporosis, men should:

- Get plenty of calcium (1,000 mg/day until age fifty and then 1,200mg/day after age fifty). You can get it from milk and other dairy products, as well as from tofu, soybeans, sardines, salmon, and vegetables such as kale, turnip greens, and okra. Orange juice is often fortified with calcium, and mineral supplements are another easy source.

- Get enough vitamin D. Most people get their D by spending a little time in the sun, which triggers your body to make the vitamin. The trouble is that cloud cover, northern climates, smog, and sunscreens can limit the body's ability to produce it. That's why vitamin D, which helps maintain calcium in bones, is also found in fortified milk and dairy products. It's also found naturally in some fish such as herring. Vitamin supplements can also provide vitamin D. The recommended dose is 400 IU a day for men over 50, and 600 IU a day for men over seventy.

- Get regular weight-bearing exercise. This helps men as well as women keep their bones strong.

Hormonal Dips and Shifts

The vast majority of men won't ever have the pleasure of experiencing a hot flash, sore breasts, or a period that just won't end, not to mention a serious, unexplained crying jag. Still, many researchers believe that men can be buffeted by hormonal winds all their own. The culprit—and the hero—in this story is testosterone. The hormone experienced quite a surge of attention a few years back when a spate of articles and books about its power were featured in the popular press, including the cover of *Time* magazine. The FDA had just approved a new testosterone gel that promised to revolutionize treatment for low testosterone. It was a heady time for a hormone that has often been maligned.

But as these things often go, things did not pan out in quite the way the breathless articles predicted. Most men don't seem to be clamoring to get their hands on testosterone gel to boost their sex drive or make them into men of steel. In fact, the vending of testosterone has gone back, almost, to the boring days before its fifteen minutes of fame. And so much the better. The only good reason for men to take testosterone is if they actually have a clinically documented deficiency and are experiencing symptoms as a result.

At one time or another, most of us have blamed testosterone for bad male stereotypes: on the aggressive overachiever, the womanizer, the power-hungry businessman, the man who drives too fast, yells, and muscles in on everything. Every now and again I find myself accusing some man of having "testosterone poisoning."

I remember in anatomy class during medical school, I barely got my hands on the cadaver. That's because the two guys also assigned to my cadaver were so aggressive in their cutting and dissecting I couldn't get a scalpel in edgewise. Of course, on the day we were to dissect the genitalia (we had a male cadaver), those two guys didn't show up. Figures. I hear they are both surgeons now—more guys with too much testosterone.

I'm kidding, of course. Sort of. There's no doubt, though, that testosterone takes the rap for lots of men behaving badly . Does it really deserve that reputation? When, if ever, should a man worry about his testosterone level? Can you really tell if somebody has too much or too little? And is there really such a thing as "male menopause"?

It's time for a brief review of testosterone and its impact on male development. Testosterone is produced in the testes and released during development in two big surges. The first occurs in the early weeks of gestation, when the tiny testes start churning out testosterone, triggering the development of male genitals and "sexing" the male fetus's body and brain (see chapter 1). The second surge (see chapter 7) occurs at the onset of puberty, triggering the growth of facial and pubic hair, the deepening of the voice, and the sexual maturation of the adolescent (not to mention the onset of acne).

Testosterone does more than turn a boy into a man. It maintains him. It helps regulate muscle mass, bone density, and even mood. It helps produce red blood cells, which is why men with extremely low levels of the hormone can become anemic. It is interesting to note that testosterone is converted to the female hormone estradiol in fat cells, giving most obese men higher levels of this female hormone than lean men.

A small amount of the testosterone supply—about 5 percent—is made in the adrenal glands, which convert cholesterol into a testosterone precursor called DHEA. While testosterone is the most famous and most important male hormone (male hormones are called androgens), it's not the only one. The testes also produce small amounts of *androstenedione*—the stuff Mark McGwire was so famously taking as a supplement during his record home run year. Andro, as it's called, is quickly converted into testosterone, which is why male athletes want it.

Testosterone can also be converted into another androgen called dihydrotestosterone (DHT). You may have heard of this hormone because it's the villain in male-pattern hair loss, and there are several products that claim to counter its effect (see chapter 23). A more serious problem from a health standpoint is that DHT also stimulates cells within the prostate gland to grow, leading to enlargement of the prostate and perhaps contributing to the development of tumors.

In any case, for most men testosterone will level off after puberty and stay constant until around age forty, when it starts to decline slowly at a rate of about 1 percent a year. Despite this drop-off, the vast majority of men have testosterone levels that are well within a normal range into their sixties, seventies, and even eighties, which explains older men fathering children in their golden years.

Testosterone can rise and dip to its own rhythm. A study a few years ago by social psychologist James Dabbs, Ph.D., of Georgia State University found that testosterone went up among sports fans before a big game and stayed high if the fan's team won, but took a dive if the team lost. "It is possible that such changes also occur in other situations that are competitive but do not involve sports, as in the political, legal, business, and social arenas," Dr. Dabbs writes.

Periods of stress can also cause temporary dips in testosterone: A bad review from the boss or a fight with the wife can send it falling. Levels also wax and wane over the course of a normal day, though they are generally highest in the morning and lowest in the late evening.

The big question, of course, and the one that is so endlessly debated by scientists, researchers, and testosterone boosters, is how much does testosterone influence male behavior? We cannot deny that it separates the men from the boys and the men from the women. And it seems absurd to think that it has no influence over human behavior. But the degree to which testosterone influences male behavior is notoriously hard to tease out.

People who have taken testosterone for medical purposes often report that it does give them a newfound confidence and sense of strength. But is it at the root of all things male? Is testosterone, for instance, the reason that the vast majority of contestants and winners on *Who Wants to Be a Millionaire?* are men? Anthropologist Helen Fisher, Ph.D., of Rutgers University thinks so. In an interview with ABC's Diane Sawyer, Dr. Fisher explained that testosterone helps men focus on the task at hand and tune out extraneous details.

Imagine one of our ancestors trying to hunt a beast in the savanna. It's not going to help him if he's distracted by the noise of the grasshoppers or birds flying overhead. He needs singular focus to kill the beast and keep himself out of danger in the process. To assist in this, men have evolved to see the world spatially, in other words, to instinctively feel what's coming at them from all sides. It is also this quality that helps a male *Millionaire* contestant list four countries going from east to west faster than most females. "That's totally spatial, visual, and it's associated with levels of testosterone," Fisher told Sawyer. "Men with more testosterone are more spatially talented."

Georgia State's James Dabbs is an unabashed believer in the power of testosterone. In his book *Heroes, Rogues, and Lovers: Testosterone and Behavior,* Dr. Dabbs pulls together research on testosterone to argue for its primacy in regulating male behavior. He links high levels of testosterone with everything from criminality and wife abuse to spatial skills and boldness. Trial lawyers, he says, have 30 percent higher testosterone levels than other attorneys. On the other hand, men with high testosterone levels tend to be lower achievers in the professional world, more likely to have blue-collar jobs or be unemployed.

Frankly, reading this book made me want to reach out and punch someone (it must have sent *my* testosterone surging). If you believe Dr. Dabbs, it's a miracle any man under the unrelenting influence of the big T could accomplish anything other than the most rudimentary and base human functions. And while his book makes for a compelling read, focusing on testosterone quantity is an overly simplistic approach.

Fascinating as the subject is, Dr. Dabbs's research on the impact of testosterone on behavior is largely of theoretical interest. Most men who think about taking the hormone care less about modifying their behavior; they want to increase the size of their muscles or the performance of their penises. And most doctors who prescribe testosterone are doing so because their patients are suffering from a serious testosterone deficit that needs to be treated.

Is There Really Such a Thing As "Male Menopause?"

Your normally sweet, unassuming husband arrives home one day from work on a brand-new Harley-Davidson motorcycle. Should you:

a. Hop on the hog, wrap your arms around him, and yell, "Get this thing movin'," baby!"
b. Insist he take it back and grow up.
c. Grab the kids and go home to your mother for a while.
d. Call the nearest psychiatric ward and have him committed.

Men's midlife crisis has long been the subject of discussions and jokes, but no one ever seriously talked about it as the equivalent of menopause in women. But now that's exactly the way some experts are viewing "male menopause." It's clear that the vast majority of men never undergo the dramatic and relatively sudden hormonal changes that women go through when they reach a "certain age." On that nearly everybody agrees. What the experts don't agree about is whether there is such a thing as male menopause, or andropause, as some like to call it. It has even been called IMS—Irritable Male Syndrome! Jed Diamond, author of *Male Menopause,* says not enough serious attention is given to this part of a man's life, and so millions of men suffer needlessly. He says middle age in men brings a drop in hormone levels that lead to other changes—weight gain, decreased physical endurance, slower recovery from injuries, reduced interest in sex, and feelings of irritability and depression. Because men don't understand the aging process, they try to overcompensate for the decline with extramarital affairs, and, yes, the purchase of sports cars and motorcycles. Diamond seems to have hit a nerve not only with men but also with women. In response to the many questions from women he received after his book was published, he wrote a second, *Surviving Male Menopause: A Guide for Men and Women.*

There's no doubt that as men age they experience physical changes, including a slow loss of muscle mass (up to 20 pounds), bone density (averaging 15 percent), and height (around 2 inches). Most men's sex drive takes a slow downward spiral as they lose some of the interest and stamina they had in their youth. But are all these changes caused by declining testosterone levels? And is this experience so universal and so significant that we should be calling it "male menopause"? And most critically, should most men consider taking testosterone as they begin to round the last bend of life? In my opinion, the answer to all these questions is no. I know of no expert who advocates across-the-board testosterone replacement for aging men—no matter how much attention testosterone gets from the media.

Clearly, however, some men's testosterone levels decline more than they should and cause problems that ought to be treated. But those levels must truly be low to be the cause of these problems. There is a tendency among many men to blame low testosterone for problems that have other causes. Diabetes, vascular disease, and heart problems are much more likely than low testosterone to be responsible for a reduced sex drive or general fatigue. If men want to avoid the symptoms they probably associate with declining testosterone, the best thing they can do in most cases is exercise, eat right, drink in moderation, and avoid smoking. If they do, most men won't need to spend a single day worrying about "male menopause."

That said, true testosterone deficiency, *hypogonadism,* is a real medical problem that can cause troubling symptoms in some men. It can be treated with prescription testosterone in shot, patch, or gel form. (A pill form is available in Canada but not in the United States.) Some 4 million to 5 million men are thought to have this problem, but only about 5 percent receive treatment.

Signs and Symptoms of Low Testosterone

- Loss of sex drive.
- Difficulty getting or maintaining an erection.
- Lethargy or fatigue.
- Irritability or depression.
- Sleep disturbance.
- Loss of motivation or self-esteem.
- Weakness.
- Loss of muscle mass.
- Trouble with memory or concentration.
- Mood swings.
- Reduced testicle or penis size.

If your partner is experiencing any of these symptoms, see if he'll take the Androgen Deficiency in Aging Men (ADAM) questionnaire.

ADAM Questionnaire

1. Do you have a decrease in libido (sex drive)?
2. Do you have a lack of energy?
3. Do you have a decrease in strength and/or endurance?
4. Have you lost height?
5. Have you noticed a decreased "enjoyment of life"?
6. Are you sad and/or grumpy?
7. Are your erections less strong?
8. Have you noticed a recent deterioration in your ability to play sports?
9. Are you falling asleep after dinner?
10. Has there been a deterioration in your work performance?

If your husband answers "yes" to questions 1 and 7, or "yes" to three or more questions overall, he should talk to a doctor.

If You Have Concerns

What should you or your partner do if you believe he may have low testosterone? What your partner should *not* do without talking to his doctor is use any over-the-counter product that claims to diagnose low testosterone or to replace or enhance testosterone levels.

You can't walk into a health food store these days without seeing shelves full of products that claim to boost male performance or stamina. The Internet is flooded with sites selling products such as DHEA, "andro," even "deer antler velvet" that are supposed to boost a man's testosterone the natural way. Take these supplements, their come-ons boast, and you'll be sexier and stronger, with more muscles, more energy, and better sexual stamina. Are they too good to be true? Yes.

For men who are on the downhill side of middle age and are starting to question their own vitality, such messages have an undeniable appeal. But it's tricky enough for doctors to diagnose and treat low testosterone; the risks of self-treatment are just too great. There's a reason testosterone is available only by prescription. It is a potent medication with serious side effects, including birth defects if a woman is exposed to it during pregnancy. Other side effects of too much testosterone include liver toxicity, stroke, breast development, infertility, acne, and baldness. It can also boost levels of bad cholesterol and, most ominously, fuel the growth of prostate cancer.

The only good thing about many of these products is that they don't actually contain anything that can have much of an effect, good or bad. "Half of the DHEA products on the market don't have bio-available DHEA in them," says John Morley, M.D., an expert in testosterone therapy and the director of geriatric medicine at St. Louis University Health Sciences Center. "So you're taking nothing and even if you get the right stuff, it hardly works."

In fact, the biggest danger probably comes when these products actually provide what they advertise. The same side effects that can occur with testosterone can occur with these products if they're used at high doses over a long period of time. Among the side effects are ones men will surely want to avoid: shrunken testicles, abnormal hair growth, acne, and infertility, not to mention behavioral problems such as aggression, mood swings, and even psychosis.

Testing for low testosterone must be done carefully and involves a blood test. Men's testosterone levels rise and fall throughout the day, which presents another problem in trying to link testosterone to behavior. Within any given age range, testosterone levels can vary widely and still be considered normal. In fact, researchers simply do not know whether variations within the normal range have any clinical significance. And testosterone replacement therapy is not without risks, including the possibility that it will increase the risk of prostate cancer. Long-term risks associated with testosterone replacement therapy have not been studied. Many experts, however, believe that in the right patient testosterone can help improve stamina and outlook as well as reverse lethargy.

So when should a man consider testosterone replacement therapy? First, a cautionary tale. For years women were told that the benefits of hormone replacement therapy (HRT) after menopause far outweighed any risks. Millions of women were placed on HRT and kept on it for years. In fact, many doctors essentially prescribed it for the duration of a woman's life. The idea that HRT was good for everything from osteoporosis to maintaining mental acuity was accepted as medical gospel and repeated so often in both medical literature and the popular press that few questioned whether it was really supported by good science. I must have received fifty books over the years written by well-meaning physicians touting hormones as the cure for just about everything.

Eventually, however, cracks started to appear in this rosy picture, and it now turns out that many of the beliefs about HRT for women were wrong. The full story is yet to be known, leaving millions of women and their doctors in doubt about whether they should be taking hormones and for how long.

If after decades of research, we're still not sure about the advisability of HRT for women, how could we possibly recommend widespread use of testosterone replacement for men? Clearly, we cannot. But just as clearly, there are men with clinically low levels of testosterone who are experiencing problems as a result, and these men can benefit from taking testosterone.

"The whole secret," says Dr. Morley, "is that you don't treat people just on symptoms. You don't treat people just on a biochemical measure. You try and treat people when they have both."

If a man does begin testosterone therapy, it is important that his doctor follow him closely, monitoring his progress and looking out for side effects, especially changes in the prostate gland.

For most men, it can take from two to three months on testosterone to see results. But if you're holding your breath waiting for your tired couch potato partner to turn into a virile animal—well, don't. The effects are much subtler than that.

19

The Emotional Male

THE STRESSED MALE

To say that we live in a stressful time would be an understatement. Think for a moment about the things that have happened in the two years since we began researching and writing this book. Domestic terrorism, war abroad, financial insecurity, a looming recession, and current events—from the work of unknown snipers to the tragedy of the Space Shuttle *Columbia*—can fuel our anxiety and stress.

Of course, this list of high-stress events doesn't even include the things that may be most stressful—the press of obligations and problems most of us face on a daily basis. The pressure to work more hours, to get a second or third job, or to find any job; the growing crush of traffic congestion, the mounting piles of bills on the kitchen table, the worries about crime, health problems, health insurance, our kids, and their education. And let's not mention the fact that the *!#$*!! computer just crashed for the fifth time today, and that you can't eat dinner without three unsolicited phone calls from credit card companies or mortgage brokers!

Stress is such a part of our lives that no adult (or child or adolescent, for that matter) is immune from it. And that means that everyone ought to think about how they will deal with it and have a strategy for coping.

Acute stress can have a very immediate and direct effect on our health. We've all heard the stories about people dropping dead of a heart attack after getting a distressing piece of news. When the Northridge earthquake struck the Los Angeles area in 1994, sixteen people suffered fatal heart attacks within an hour of the initial tremor. On the day that Iraq lobbed its first Scud missiles at Israel during the first Gulf War, deaths among Israeli adults were 58 percent higher than usual, excluding those killed by the missiles. Most of the excess deaths were due to cardiovascular causes, according to the *Harvard Heart Letter*.

Even sporting events can cause acute stress reactions. In December 2002, the British Medical Journal reported a 25 percent spike in hospital admissions in England for heart attacks and strokes immediately after the last-minute defeat of the British soccer team by Argentina in the 1998 World Cup. Millions of Britons had watched the heartbreaking loss; it was the most widely watched TV program in England that year. "These findings support the view that heart attacks can be triggered by emotional upset, such as watching your football team lose an important match," the journal reported.

Why does this happen? Experts say it's a question of simple physiology. Stress triggers an increase in adrenaline levels, boosting blood pressure and increasing the tension in the coronary arteries. In those who are vulnerable, this can cause plaque within the artery to rupture, breaking off particles of fat that can surge into the bloodstream. If these floating particles of fat get lodged in the wrong place, they could cause a blockage that leads to a heart attack or stroke.

Even superstition can increase stress and cause trouble. In Japanese, Cantonese, and Mandarin, the word for the number four and the word for *death* are pronounced almost the same, so the number four evokes superstitious stress among this group. A study in the *British Medical Journal* found that Chinese Americans and Japanese Americans are more likely to die from heart disease on the fourth day of the month than on any other. The authors term this phenomenon the "Hound of the Baskervilles" effect, because in that Sherlock Holmes novel, Charles Baskerville dies of a heart attack induced by extreme psychological stress.

MEN AND STRESS

There's no particular evidence that men are under more stress than women; in fact, many researchers think the opposite is true. But I suspect that women tend to be more aware of the effects of stress and have more conscious strategies for dealing with it than men do. Men and women have very different ways of both experiencing and coping with stress, differences that may well contribute to men's shorter life span. The female response to stress may actually protect us biologically and help us live longer than our men.

One key difference in coping styles has been uncovered by Shelley Taylor, Ph.D., a social psychologist at UCLA. She has found that when women are stressed, they "tend and befriend"—that is, they protect and nurture their young (tend) and reach out to others, talk about what's bothering them and seek support, mostly from other females (befriend). Men tend to either battle back against the source of the stress or run from it—the famous "fight-or-flight" response.

More commonly perhaps, men try a strategy that might be called "deny and hide." "Men tend not to talk about emotions or about worry. You'll see silence, withdrawal, avoidance, and irritability in men," says Allen Elkin, Ph.D., a stress expert who directs the Stress Management and Counseling Center in New York and is the author of *Stress Management for Dummies*. Men will also withdraw sexually, he says, and their stress will often be felt in the form of muscle tension and fatigue.

Like most personality characteristics, these gender differences are a product of biology and culture. Women have higher circulating levels of the hormone oxytocin, and we know that animals and humans with high levels of oxytocin are more relaxed, more social, and more maternal. Oxytocin levels rise, for instance, when women breast-feed. Men secrete oxytocin, too, but the effects are blunted by testosterone. Culturally, men are expected to be tough, to be able to handle anything that comes their way without complaint. Anything less is unmanly.

When men come home from work, Taylor points out, they often want to be left alone to enjoy a little peace and quiet. If job stress was really bad, a man might come home and create conflict with his wife and kids or drink to cope with the stress. When a woman comes home from a bad day, she's more likely to fuss over the children.

Oxytocin is not the only hormone implicated in stress reactions. We know stress also triggers the release of cortisol and adrenaline. When cortisol remains at high levels over long periods of time, it seems to impair the effectiveness of our immune systems, as it also boosts blood pressure, including within the coronary arteries. There is also mounting evidence that sustained high levels of cortisol increase appetite (presumably as a way to help the body replace the carbohydrates that were burned off fighting or fleeing). When stress and cortisol levels stay high, insulin levels do, too, and that can cause fat gained from this stress-induced hunger to accumulate in the worst possible place—your middle. Bottom line: Stress can make you fat. And here's one more problem men should consider: Acute stress can cause testosterone levels to fall, says Gerald Lincoln of the Medical Research Council's Human Reproductive Sciences Unit in Edinburgh.

Stress and how we respond to it is increasingly understood to have biological roots. According to Jeff Friedman, M.D., of the Department of Psychiatry at Harvard Medical School, "We now know that stress has certain associations to brain anatomy and function. For example, in the past five years, researchers have discovered that the hippocampus, part of the brain responsible for memory and emotion, is abnormally small in people suffering from depression and who were victims of abuse." Moreover, Dr. Friedman says, stress hormones called glucocorticoids released in association with depression or abuse may lead to nerve cell death and shrink the hippocampus. This new understanding tells us that many people may be biologically primed to deal with stress by developing mood disorders and impaired memory. It may also lead to new treatments for stress, anxiety, and depression.

Men are more likely to respond to stressful situations by developing certain stress-related disorders such as high blood pressure, aggressive behavior, and substance abuse. One common style of reacting to stress was summed up succinctly by Susan Nolen-Hoeksema, Ph.D., a psychologist and researcher at the University of Michigan: "Women think and men drink." She and a colleague surveyed some 1,300 adults in the San Francisco Bay Area to find out whether they were stressed or depressed and how they coped when they were. They discovered that women were more likely to ruminate or stew about how bad they felt or how upset they were, while men were more likely to drink alcohol. "The gender differences in both rumination and drinking to cope were quite pronounced," she said.

Interestingly, she also noted that while alcohol tends to fuel rumination in women, possibly because they feel more guilt or shame about their drinking, men may use it try to cut off their ruminations. "Men may get more negative social feedback for ruminating than they do for drinking, because ruminating violates male gender roles, but drinking does not," Dr. Nolen-Hoeksema says.

Other Sources of Stress for Men

Work and stress go hand in hand, for men and women alike. Nearly one in four workers say they've been driven to tears by workplace stress, 29 percent admit to yelling at coworkers while under stress, and 42 percent say their workplace is a place where yelling and verbal abuse take place, according to a national survey of American workers conducted by the Opinion Research Corporation in 2000.

Because job stress is such a big part of our lives, it can easily become a chronic health problem, making it hard to sleep and making us more prone to illness, back problems, and accidents. Chronic stress can also put a tremendous strain on the heart and circulation. The Japanese even have a word for sudden death caused by overwork, *karoshi*.

In some respects, the work environment can be more stressful for women because researchers have found that workers who have the least power and control—for instance, waitresses and secretaries—tend to be the most stressed. Sexual harassment on the job can add enormously to the stress levels faced by women, but is rarely encountered by men. And despite all the changes in the work world, men still are more likely than women to be in positions of power.

On the other hand, far more men work in jobs where they face real physical danger. Men account for 93 percent of people killed on the job, they're three times more likely to be a victim of homicide in the workplace, and they're also much more likely to be injured. Yet danger on the job is not the main reason that men get stressed out about work. As we said, the biggest source of stress on the job is not how many hours people must work, or even the type of work they do, but how much control they have over their work and their time. Despite their generally higher position in the pecking order, most men still have bosses telling them what to do. Assembly-line workers or waiters have a lot of job stress because they have little control over what they must do compared to, say, repair men or computer programmers.

Control and autonomy are important to everyone, but our culture makes it especially so for men. Men who feel under the thumb of their boss, with little influence over their own work, are more likely to be stressed than men who have more autonomy. (Just think of all those stressed-out postal workers.) Men who lack social support or feel alienated by coworkers also have more stress.

Technology adds its own stresses. Cell phones, faxes, and e-mail make it harder than ever to leave work at the office. Evening and weekend work can interfere with family relationships. We all know the man who can't really take a vacation—he spends the day at the beach talking to his office while his wife and kids play in the sand. And finally, though more women then ever are in the workforce, there is still a sense that a man's identity is more wrapped up in how successful he is on the job.

Like women, many men face the challenge of filling dual roles within the family— breadwinner and parent. And while men increasingly say they want to be more involved with their families, and find it satisfying when they are, there's not a whole lot of support for them to do so. Most occupations and workplaces offer little flexibility, which means that if a child is sick, it's usually Mom who can arrange to stay home. The result: Men can be involved with their families as long as it doesn't interfere with their jobs. This creates stress and tension for men and women.

Many men are so invested in their roles as breadwinners that they actually work more hours after they have a new baby. In the *Review of Economics and Statistics* in May 2002, two University of Washington economists reported on a survey that showed that men logged about 118 more hours per year at work after the birth of their firstborn son and 54 more hours after a firstborn daughter. It seems that having a child, and especially a son, makes men more committed to their kids and their families—so they spend more time earning money at work, *away* from their kids and families. A less generous interpretation may be that some men are made anxious by the birth of the baby, become jealous of the attention paid to the baby by their wives, and retreat into their work, other activities, and even affairs.

God help the man whose work life is so stressful that it interferes with his home life, leading to separation or divorce. Researchers reporting in the *Archives of Internal Medicine* in February 2002 found that the combination of chronic high stress at work and the dissolution of a marriage caused an increase in mortality among men.

Secondhand Emotions

When a family member is stressed out or moody, it can infect the whole family, like a nasty virus or secondhand smoke. A study in the *Journal of Marriage and the Family* looked at the ways these "secondhand emotions" are transmitted within the family. It found that negative emotions such as anger, depression, and anxiety are more infectious than positive emotions and have longer-lasting effects. These "bad vibes" are also more likely to be passed from husband to wife and from parents to children.

One of the most frequent patterns was for stressed-out men to bring their worries and frustrations home from work and transmit them to the rest of the family, kind of

SIGNS OF STRESS

- General irritability, hyperactivity, or depression.
- Pounding of the heart. Dryness in the mouth and throat.
- Trembling, nervous tics.
- Impulsive behavior.
- Emotional instability, such as an overpowering urge to cry or run.
- Inability to concentrate. Confusion.
- Feelings of weakness or dizziness.
- Fatigue.
- Floating anxiety or panic feelings for no known reason.
- Emotional tension, alertness, or feelings of being keyed up.
- High-pitched, nervous laughter.
- Grinding teeth.
- Sleeping problems.
- Stomach and bowel problems, indigestion, pain, nausea, constipation, or diarrhea.
- Frequent need to urinate.
- Migraine or tension headaches.
- Neck or lower back pain.
- Loss of or excessive appetite.
- Increased smoking.
- Accident proneness.
- Alcohol or drug problems, including tobacco (nicotine), tranquilizers, and caffeine.
- Nightmares.

Source: Reprinted from The Stress of Life *by H. Selye. Copyright © 1978 McGraw-Hill Companies. Reproduced with permission of the McGraw-Hill Companies.*

like the old cliché about the man who comes home and kicks the dog. "We all have bad days and negative interactions," says David Almeida, Ph.D., a University of Arizona researcher who coauthored the study. "This work brings a new awareness that being in a negative mood, being inaccessible or generally grouchy can have a noxious effect on the well-being of our families."

What You Can Do

For all of these reasons, it's important to have ways to relieve stress. Women tend to be better at this. Our ability to tend and befriend helps us get support when we need it. Since men don't seem to come by these skills naturally, it's in our interest to help them, to share our knowledge and experience. It can make life easier and more pleasant for all of us, including our children.

Men rarely say they're under stress, but we can usually tell. Perhaps he's more irritable, sullen, or withdrawn. He may have an extra drink or look for a way to be alone. One thing he's not likely to do is start a conversation that uses a lot of emotional language, even though talking about his stress may actually help him and make him more receptive to talking things over the next time he's feeling this way.

Don't hound him or nag him to talk if he's resistant; that isn't likely to work. Instead, use your intuition to throw out a specific question that might get at the source of his angst. "Is Johnson on your case again?" "Is Walker up to his old tricks?" "Traffic bad?"

Go for a walk together. Encourage him to open up about whatever is going on. Maybe ask one of his friends to try talking to him. "People do feel better when they talk about it. Men just need a little more encouragement and direction," Dr. Elkin says.

The Stress Scale

Everyone experiences stress differently and reacts differently to different stressors. Still, there are some things we all find stressful. The following is a list of fifty major life events, ranked according to the amount of stress they tend to cause. Officially called the Social Readjustment Rating Scale, it was developed by T. H. Holmes and R. H. Rahe and was first published in 1967 in the *Journal of Psychosomatic Research*. These kinds of experiences add to each other, of course. The more problems we experience, the greater the chances we'll have trouble coping.

THE TOP 50 STRESSFUL EVENTS

- Death of spouse or mate.
- Death of a close family member.
- Major injury or illness.
- Detention in jail or other institution.
- Major injury or illness in a close family member.
- Foreclosure on a loan or mortgage.
- Divorce.
- Being a victim of crime.
- Being a victim of police brutality.
- Infidelity.
- Domestic violence or sexual abuse.
- Separation or reconciliation with a spouse or mate.
- Being fired, laid off, or unemployed.
- Experiencing financial problems or difficulties.
- Death of a close friend.
- Surviving a disaster.
- Becoming a single parent.
- Assuming responsibility for a sick or elderly loved one.
- Loss or major reduction in health insurance or benefits.
- Self or a close family member being arrested for violating the law.
- Major disagreement over child support, custody, or visitation.
- Experiencing or being involved in an auto accident.
- Being disciplined or demoted at work.

- Dealing with unwanted pregnancy.
- Having an adult child move in or moving in with an adult child.
- Having a child with a behavior or learning problem.
- Experiencing discrimination or sexual harassment at work.
- Attempting to modify addictive behavior.
- Discovering or attempting to modify addictive behavior in a close family member.
- Employer reorganization or downsizing.
- Dealing with infertility or miscarriage.
- Getting married or remarried.
- Changing employers or careers.
- Failing to obtain or qualify for a mortgage.
- Pregnancy of self or of spouse or mate.
- Experiencing discrimination or harassment outside the workplace.
- Release from jail.
- Spouse or mate begins or ceases work outside the home.
- Major disagreement with boss or coworker.
- Change in residence.
- Finding appropriate child care or day care.
- Experiencing a large unexpected monetary gain.
- Changing positions (transfer or promotion).
- Gaining a new family member.
- Changing work responsibilities.
- Having a child leave home.
- Obtaining a home mortgage.
- Obtaining a major loan other than a home mortgage.
- Retirement.
- Beginning or ceasing formal education.
- Receiving a ticket for violating the law.

Source: Reprinted from Journal of Psychosomatic Research, vol. 11, T. H. Holmes and R. H. Rahe, Social Readjustment Rating Scale, copyright © 1967, with permission from Elsevier.

The Toxic Emotions: Anger and Hostility

One of the most damaging messages that our culture delivers to males, starting from a very early age, is that they must be strong and self-sufficient, and that to admit weakness is unmanly. Boys and men learn that certain emotions—such as anger—are acceptable, while others—sadness and hurt—are not. The legacy of this message is powerful. It means that when men are faced with pressure and stress, they have a hard time seeking help but an easy time getting in touch with their rage.

In this area more than almost any other, differences between men and women come into sharpest focus. If emotions were colors, men would be trying to paint with nothing but black and white, while women were choosing from a whole palette, expressing their emotional state in a rich variety of hues. For all too many men, the result is predictable: They feel hurt or put down, and they lash out in anger. They feel sadness, and they just get mad. Men pay a high price for their limited emotional repertoire and so, unfortunately, do the women and children in their lives.

One of the costs of being frequently angry is that it endangers the health of the heart. In one study published in the journal *Circulation*, researchers assessed thousands of people free of heart disease to see how prone they were to anger. Over the next six years, the people who ranked highest on the anger test were nearly three times more likely to have a heart attack than the people who ranked as the mellowest. The high scorers were about twice as likely to have developed coronary heart disease.

In two other studies, John Barefoot, Ph.D., a research professor of behavioral psychiatry at Duke University, found that medical and law students who scored high in hostility on a personality test were four to five times more likely to die of heart disease over the next twenty-five years than their less hostile schoolmates. Among the law students, for instance, nearly 20 percent of those who scored at the top of the hostility scale were dead by the age of fifty. Hostility seems to be an even bigger predictor of heart disease than physical factors such as high cholesterol, smoking, and excess weight, according to a study in the journal *Health Psychology.* And for older men, the greater their level of hostility, the greater the chances of developing heart disease.

Why does this happen? Researchers speculate that anger boosts those stress hormones, cortisol and adrenaline. "We think . . . these hormones can damage the arteries and heart muscle itself and can also cause the heart to beat irregularly," says Janice Williams, the lead author of the *Circulation* study. Another explanation comes from a study at Ohio State University. It found that hostile, angry people have higher levels of homocysteine, a chemical that circulates in the bloodstream and has been linked to heart disease.

Experiencing or expressing anger and hostility is not the same as being a type A personality, as those hard-driving, fast-talking, alpha-male types were called by researchers in the 1970s. It turns out that being a type A doesn't seem to put people at higher risk for heart disease after all *unless* they're also hostile. (Many type As are fidgety, nervous, competitive, and high-energy but *not* angry or hostile.)

It seems to me there's another commonsense reason why hostile people would have heart problems. They alienate people and push them away, and that can leave them without something that's really important in keeping people healthy—good friends that provide social support. Hostility doesn't just make people more prone to having heart attacks, it frequently goes along with a host of other unhealthy habits such as smoking, drinking alcohol, and overeating.

The Venting Myth

Credit Sigmund Freud with helping start a popular misconception that continues to this day. His ideas about the importance of emotional catharsis became part of what psychologists now call the "hydraulic model of anger." In essence, this model holds that frustration leads to anger, and that anger then builds up until it is released in some way. The implication is that if someone is angry, he needs to vent his anger verbally or physically, or he may "explode."

Fritz Perls, the prominent psychiatrist, argued that if a person "bottles up his rage, we have to find an outlet. We have to give him an opportunity for letting off steam." This idea has permeated popular culture for many years. "Youngsters should be taught to vent their anger," wrote famed advice columnist Ann Landers in a column some years ago. And pop self-help books advise people to punch pillows or punching bags or to smack couches with plastic bats to get rid of their pent-up anger.

But this kind of venting, says Brad Bushman, Ph.D., an associate professor of psychology at Iowa State University, "is like using gasoline to put out a fire—it only makes matters worse." The reason, he says, is that venting anger keeps people aroused, increasing the chance that that they will say or do something that may be harmful or violent. In a series of fascinating experiments, Bushman angered students by showing them negative comments—for example, "this is one of the worst essays I have ever read"—about something they had written. He then gave them the chance to whale on a punching bag and then to zap an opponent with a loud, obnoxious noise. He found that the more the students had liked punching the bag, the more aggressive they were in sound-blasting their opponents. The point, says Bushman, is that when people express their anger physically by yelling, slamming doors, or hitting things (or people), it keeps their anger alive and allows them to rehearse being angry.

Coping Without Venting

So what's a more productive way to deal with frustration and anger? Bushman and other experts say the goal should not be to withhold or repress the anger, but rather to manage it by finding ways to cool off that don't keep you aroused and upset. Rather than thinking about anger as a pressure cooker from which people have to let off stream, he suggests a different metaphor. "An electronic capacitor builds up charge and then shocks you if you touch it," he writes in an online discussion. "But wait for the charge to dissipate and you won't get shocked. Anger works in a similar way. When you become angry over something, you build up a charge, but if you wait, the anger will decrease over time until it is gone."

In this section, I'll talk about some ways people can manage their anger. It might be helpful for you, of course, if you have problems with anger, but the real challenge will be to find ways to share these ideas with your partner—without prompting him to blow his stack! So even though I present some ideas that "you" can try, I'm really trying to talk to your partner through you.

One technique that allows for anger to dissipate is that old notion of counting to ten before responding to something that's made you angry. You can also take a walk or take deep breaths to help you calm down. In *Stress Management for Dummies*, Allen Elkin, Ph.D., a stress-management expert, suggests the following method for deep breathing to calm your anger.

1. Take a deep breath, inhaling through your nostrils.
2. Hold that breath for three or four seconds.
3. Slowly exhale through your slightly parted lips.
4. Let a wave of relaxation spread from the top of your head, down your body, to your toes.
5. Wait a little bit, and then take another deep breath.
6. Repeat the process.

Source: Reprinted from Stress Management for Dummies *by Allen Elken. Copyright © 1999 by Wiley Publishing, Inc. All rights reserved. Reproduced here by permission of the publisher.*

Another technique is to rehearse—when you're calm, of course—how you might respond in a situation that's likely to make you angry. You might want to choose an incident that has made you angry in the past and think about how you might have responded differently.

You can also use humor to defuse your anger—or somebody else's. John Gottman, Ph.D., a psychologist at the University of Washington and one of the most influential marriage researchers in the country, tells a story about a time when his future wife, whom he was then dating, made a grouchy, critical comment to him. He fell to the floor, clutching his chest, then moaned, "Nice shooting, partner, you got me." The tension was broken, and both partners had a good laugh.

There are plenty of anger-management programs available, many of them affiliated with local hospitals. At least some of these programs have the potential to reduce people's anger and their risk for heart disease. In one recent small study, Karina Davidson, Ph.D., a researcher at the Mount Sinai School of Medicine, tested a hostility reduction program on twenty-two heart attack survivors from Nova Scotia. Ten of the patients took part in the cognitive-behavioral program that, in eight ninety-minute sessions, taught people to understand their hostile behavior and to reframe their thinking to reduce their edginess and tendency to respond with anger. After the sessions ended, the participants had much lower blood pressure and were rated by evaluators and by themselves to be significantly less hostile than before *and* less hostile than the patients who didn't take part. One reason the strategy helps, Dr. Davidson believes, is because "as hostile men become less hostile, they spend less of their time being vigilant to threats from others, and as a result are more 'relaxed' physiologically." When the study was over, four of the people in the control group asked to receive the training.

There are plenty of other anger-management techniques that you can find in books. Of course, it's a lot easier to talk about any of these techniques than to actually practice them. It's especially hard to suggest these ideas to a spouse who has problems with his anger and have him be receptive as opposed to getting agitated or upset. (Watch your timing!) But if your partner does have problems with anger and managing stress, it can have serious health implications for both of you. Let him know that his anger is not only unpleasant but could actually be life-threatening. Let him know that anger boosts his blood pressure and can damage his heart, that it may also push people away, leaving him without social support. If you can, enlist some help from someone else that he listens to—his mother or father, a best friend or coworker. See if one of them would be willing to talk to him about getting some help. You might also bring your concerns to his doctor.

"Hostility flares like a beacon, a risk factor that needs to be tempered," writes Redford Williams, M.D., the director of the Behavioral Medicine Research Center at Duke University and author of *Anger Kills.* "If people who have excessive anger learn to control it, it may have beneficial effects." He suggests that if you feel your fury rising over something that's happened, ask yourself some questions, which you can remember from the mantra "I am worth it."

> **I**: Is this *important* to me? If you answer no, you are wasting your time thinking further about the situation.
>
> **A**: Are my thoughts and feelings *appropriate*, given the facts?
>
> **M**: Can the situation be *modified*? Can you change things, or should you just save your energy?
>
> **Worth It**: All things considered, is taking any kind of action worthwhile, or would it be better to just let things go?

DEPRESSION IN MEN: A COVERT OPERATION

In many men, anger is also a mask for another serious problem, one that most people consider more of a woman's problem—depression. Most research has found that about twice as many women as men suffer from depression—about 20 percent of women and 10 percent of men. But a number of psychologists who work with men are starting to question that estimate. They argue that mental health professionals often fail to recognize depression because it can look so different in men from the traditional "female" model they've been trained to recognize. A 1991 study by the RAND institution showed that doctors failed to diagnose depression in men 67 percent of the time.

"In the traditional model, depressed people are tearful and sad and withdrawn and they have rather low energy," says Sam Cochran, Ph.D., an associate professor of counseling psychology at the University of Iowa, and the editor of *Psychology of Men & Masculinity,* a journal of the American Psychological Association. "I don't think it's quite that picture for men. The male manifestation is irritability and anger, withdrawal from relationships and connections, alcoholism, and substance abuse. And there's a real clear connection between depression and violence in men, especially interpersonal violence."

Where women in our culture have learned to internalize their pain, by thinking obsessively and self-critically, blaming themselves, and feeling bad, men have learned to externalize their pain by blaming others and disconnecting from their feelings. Ask a man how he's feeling, how he's *really* feeling, and he often won't know because he's so cut off from that part of himself. "The capacity to externalize pain protects some men from *feeling* depressed," says Terrence Real, a Massachusetts therapist and author of *I Don't Want to Talk About It.* "It does not stop them *being* depressed."

Real says many depressed men act out what he calls "the holy triad of covert depression." They self-medicate with drugs and alcohol. They isolate themselves from their partners, other family members, and friends. And too often, they strike out in rage, often against the people they love.

"Look at all the men that are depressed that are also alcoholic," says Dr. Cochran. "Look at all the men that are into domestic violence, that are murderers, that perpetrate all this violence and wreak havoc all over the place—these men are depressed. It's clear as a bell." That is not to say that depression is at the root of all murders or violent behavior, or that depression can be used as an excuse for this behavior. In the end, some men also strike out against themselves. A whopping 80 percent of all the suicides in this country are committed by men.

Rachel Rabinowitz* knows all about the anger of a man with untreated and unacknowledged depression. Her father, an immigrant to the United States, was an irritable, angry man who took out his frustrations by verbally abusing his wife and yelling at his children. "My father doesn't like to talk about what's bothering him and when it does come out, it's rage," she told reporter Laurie Udesky in 2002. "He's also at least fifty pounds overweight. When everyone goes to bed, he pigs out on junk food. That's his way of suppressing those unwanted feelings."

Suspecting that her father was depressed, and worried about the health of both of her parents, Rabinowitz took her concerns to her father's physician. "I told my dad's doctor, 'My father has high blood pressure, a horrible temper, and verbally abuses his wife. Do you think he could use antidepressants?' " The doctor broached the issue with Rabinowitz's father by bringing up his problems with anger rather than depression, and he agreed to take them.

The doctor's prescription was not just a ruse to get Rabinowitz's father to take antidepressant medication for his depression. It is, in fact, often difficult to distinguish anger from depression. And some recent studies have suggested that lower than normal levels of serotonin in the brain can cause hostility as well as sadness, and that drugs used to treat depression by boosting serotonin levels may help some heart patients with their depression.

Depression in men can also take the more traditional form, the kind that fits the classic definitions. But many men try to keep it hidden. In 1984, a libel trial against CBS News and Mike Wallace, the famed correspondent for *60 Minutes,* opened in a Manhattan courtroom. Wallace and CBS were being sued by General William Westmoreland for a critical documentary on Vietnam. Every day, for nearly five months, Wallace had to sit in the courtroom and listen as his integrity, fairness, and journalistic accuracy were attacked. The experience triggered a despondency in Wallace that he'd never known before, and he began to doubt himself and the journalism he was known for.

"You just feel utterly hopeless—you don't want to get out of bed, you're spacey, you don't want to eat, you're not interested in very much," Wallace remembers. "The fact of the matter is you're losing control of your mind, and for a fellow like me, who thinks himself in charge of his mind, it was a very discouraging process."

Each night after the day's proceedings in court, Wallace would sit down at the dinner table with his wife, Mary, and she'd reassure him that he'd done nothing wrong. But Wallace could not be reassured so easily. "I'd say 'Then why in the hell am I feeling the way I'm feeling,'" Wallace remembers. "And I really didn't know what I was feeling. I did not want to acknowledge the fact of depression."

At Mary's insistence, Wallace went to see his longtime internist to try to figure out what was going on. He asked about the possibility of depression, but the doctor dismissed it. "My own doctor said, 'Come on, Mike, you're not depressed. I've seen you through tougher times than this. You're too strong, you're too tough.' He did not diagnose it as depression." The doctor also warned Wallace not to let his emotional problems become known publicly because it could damage his reputation.

Mary Wallace didn't believe the doctor and felt he was minimizing the problem, but Mike soldiered on, convinced he could lick whatever the problem was. But a few weeks later, Wallace caught a flu bug and collapsed in exhaustion. He was admitted to a New York hospital where, for the first time, a psychiatrist diagnosed his depression. As the trial continued, Wallace began to take antidepressants and to see a psychotherapist three times a week during lunch breaks from the trial.

With the help of the medication and therapy, and the support of his wife and a couple of friends, Wallace got through the trial (Westmoreland finally dropped the case) and eventually the depression lifted. He kept taking the antidepressants for a couple more months, but then stopped. A week later, he broke his wrist playing tennis and plunged back into the darkness.

Wallace kept his depression secret from everyone but his family and his doctor. When he was supposed to appear on *The Phil Donahue Show,* he made an excuse that he had the flu. "It was a great secret," says Wallace. "I didn't want it known among our friends or in the office. It's crazy to think about it twenty years later—for Christsakes, you're not Typhoid Mary. But the stigma of being depressed—you didn't want to talk about it."

In the nearly twenty years since his first brush with depression, Wallace has had a few relapses, usually when he went off his medication. But he's always had the help of his wife, his psychiatrist, and his good friends, humorist Art Buchwald and writer William Styron, both of whom have also suffered from depression. During the tough times, Wallace says, "Art would get in touch with me every single night on the telephone, no matter where he was in the country, or where I was."

Several years ago, Wallace went public with his condition, and he has since discussed it in a number of articles and documentaries. The response, he says, has been enormously gratifying. He's gotten hundreds of letters from readers and viewers who say that hearing about his depression has helped them get through theirs. Wallace has learned that most other people don't think less of him because he has battled depression. He has a message for men and the women who love them: "Depression is a disease, not a weakness," he says. And with the help of medication and therapy, it usually can be overcome.

Recognizing Depression in Men

The classic symptoms of depression include the following, though not every depressed person experiences all of these symptoms. Remember also that the severity of symptoms can vary greatly from one person to another, and from one episode to the next.

CLASSIC SYMPTOMS OF DEPRESSION

- Sleep problems—insomnia, waking up early, or oversleeping.
- Feeling frequently sad, anxious, or "empty."
- Feeling hopeless or pessimistic.
- Feeling guilty, worthless, or helpless.
- Losing interest in activities that were once enjoyed, including sex.
- Decreased energy, fatigue, being "slowed down."
- Trouble concentrating, remembering, and making decisions.
- Loss of appetite and maybe weight, or overeating and weight gain.
- Thinking about death or suicide; attempting suicide.
- Feeling restless or irritable.
- Frequent physical problems that don't go away with treatment, such as headaches, digestive disorders, and chronic pain.

Other Symptoms Often Suffered by Men

Many mental health professionals say that while men may suffer from some of the traditional symptoms listed above, they often have some of these problems as well:

- Is frequently angry, edgy, or irritable.
- Is easily and frequently frustrated.
- Is verbally or physically abusive.
- Often gets in fights or lashes out violently.
- Uses alcohol or drugs in an effort to mask pain.
- Works long hours frequently and seems consumed by work.
- Takes risks and engages in reckless, sometimes dangerous behavior.

Treating Depression

There are several treatment options for people with depression. Finding the right approach for your partner may take some time, some trial and error. It will definitely take some tolerance and understanding.

The most commonly used treatment for depression by far is medication. It's the only treatment most people use, the only one many doctors prescribe. And while it helps millions of people, it is not a panacea or a cure-all. In fact, while many articles and media reports suggest that antidepressant medications work for 75 percent to 90 percent of people who try them, this may be an overstatement. In recent years, outcome reviews that look at large numbers of studies have suggested that antidepressants alone provide significant relief from the symptoms of depression in about 50 percent of patients, compared to about 30 percent of those taking placebos. The good news is that by switching medications or by combining different medications and/or psychotherapy, 80 percent of patients will be successfully treated.

Though there are many classes of antidepressants, the most commonly used by far are the SSRIs (selective serotonin reuptake inhibitors). These drugs block the reabsorption or reuptake of the neurotransmitter serotonin by neurons, leaving more of it circulating in the brain. Contrary to popular opinion, the SSRIs are no more effective than older classes of antidepressants, but they do have significantly fewer and milder side effects and are nearly impossible to overdose on. Still, during most clinical trials, 10 percent to 20 percent of patients stop taking the drugs because of unwanted side effects. The most common side effects include nausea, diarrhea, sleep problems, headache, nervousness, restless agitation, and decreased sexual desire.

One of the biggest issues for men is that SSRIs cause sexual problems such as loss of desire and difficulty with erections or orgasms in as many as 30 percent to 70 percent of people who take them, according to a study in the *Journal of the American Medical Association.* For this reason, many men take Viagra in addition to their antidepressant, and the *JAMA* study found that more than half of the men that took the two drugs had an improved sex life. The combination was not found to have any serious negative interactions. Another antidepressant, bupropion, causes far fewer sexual side effects than the SSRIs, and most people who have sexual side effects on SSRIs can take bupropion (or the combination) without problems.

These antidepressants generally take three to six weeks to have an effect, and if they're going to work, a patient will usually know by the end of that time period. Often, a patient who does not respond to one medication will respond to another. Because of their relative safety and ease of use, most doctors will start patients on one of the SSRIs and will usually try a second SSRI if the first is unsuccessful. There are now several new non-SSRI antidepressants and some of them appear to be more effective for cases of serious depression than the SSRIs, though they may also cause more serious side effects.

One of the biggest mistakes that many people who take antidepressant make is that they stop taking the drug too quickly and relapse. Most experts suggest that patients should remain on an antidepressant for at least six months after the acute symptoms of depression fade. People who have had a history of previous episodes of depression may be advised to continue on an antidepressant indefinitely.

Many men prefer taking medications to working with a therapist for the same reasons that men tend to hide from depression: They don't like to talk about their problems or feelings. Medication allows them to treat their problems as a medical condition, and that feels less invasive and stigmatizing to many people. If that's the case with your husband, be glad that there is a treatment that works for many people who *don't* want to talk about it.

For men that do, there are a number of different kinds of "talk" therapy available. Some forms have been shown in outcome research to be just about as effective as medication, helping just over 50 percent of patients to feel significantly better. One advantage of therapy over medication is that people are more likely to relapse back into depression when they stop taking medication, compared with ending therapy. For example, in a study by researchers at Vanderbilt University and the University of Pennsylvania, 25 percent of patients who took part in a form of treatment known as cognitive behavior therapy for four months suffered a relapse when they stopped, compared to 40 percent of patients who continued on medication and a whopping 81 percent who stopped taking medication.

Therapy also allows patients to gain more confidence in their ability to handle their problems themselves, without becoming dependent on medication. For instance, some people improve while they're taking medication, but then feel like the good things they accomplish are due to the medication and not their own efforts. The gains made through therapy, on the other hand, are often more enduring. That's because people learn through therapy to understand the cause of their depression or to mentally reframe their issues so that they can deal with them in a better way.

For many people, the best option may be a combination of medication and therapy. Antidepressants often start working more quickly than therapy does, allowing a person to feel better and relax. Then, in a less agitated or depressed state, people can take a more active part in therapy, developing skills that will allow them to function without medication down the road.

Finally, though infrequently used as a first-line treatment, with modern techniques *electroconvulsive therapy* (ECT) can be an effective and safe treatment for people whose depression is life-threatening or fails to respond to medication and therapy and who are disabled by their symptoms. Entertainer and broadcast host Dick Cavett is among those who have publicly attested to the benefit they received from ECT.

Real, Cochrane, and other psychologists who work with men, including Harvard's William Pollack, Ph.D., argue that male depression goes unrecognized and undiagnosed so often by medical and mental heath professionals that it needs to be looked at in a new light. They'd like to see some changes in the official diagnostic criteria to account for some of the differences between the male and female versions of depression. But mostly, they'd just like to see more public and media attention paid to depression in men.

That may, finally, be starting to happen. In April 2003 the National Institutes of Health launched a national campaign called "Real Men, Real Depression" to raise awareness of the problem. According to the NIMH, there are 6 million American men with depression, and they're far less likely to seek treatment and four times more likely to commit suicide.

THE REAL STORY: A CONVERSATION WITH TERRY REAL

Terrence Real spent years trying to bury the pain he felt from growing up with a violent and abusive father. He used drugs and alcohol to hold the pain at bay and fell into depression when he was no longer able to do so. Then he became a therapist, in large part, he says in retrospect, so he could help heal his father—and himself. Today, he works to heal other men as a senior therapist with the Family Institute of Cambridge in Massachusetts. We talked with Real about men and depression and how women can help the men they love.

You have argued that there is a big difference in the way depression looks in women and men and that, as a result, men's depression is underdiagnosed. Tell us about that.

I call male depression a hidden epidemic, and I believe it affects millions of American men. The conventional wisdom is that depression is really a woman's disease. I disagree with that. I think men tend to express depression differently than women. There are men who experience it in the same manner as women, and they're the ones who are counted as depressed in the statistics. But I believe that for every one of them, there are two more who have what I call covert depression. I think it's underreported because depressed men often experience the depression as unmanly. It goes against the stoic code to be brought down and in some ways disabled by your own feelings. It's shameful.

When men go to the doctor and try to talk about their depression, it's usually about their physical complaints. Then they'll move from there and say 'well, I feel kind of blah.' But they don't generally come out and say they're depressed. The first line of defense for this is the family physician, the internist. But depression in men is missed upwards of 70 percent of the time.

So what's the difference between these two forms, the male and female forms of depression?

Overt depression is the kind of depression that you think of as depression. It looks exactly the same in both sexes, but it tends to be predominantly female. In covert depression you don't get the depression explicitly, what you get is what I call depression's footprint—the defensive moves that the man is making to escape the depression. When women are in pain, they have a tolerance for it, they acknowledge it, they reach out for help. When men have pain, emotional pain, we have about a millisecond's worth of tolerance and then we try to fend it off and move into action. That's not all bad, but we also move into forms of escape that fuel many of the problems we think of as typically male.

You talk about the unholy triad of covert depression. What are the elements?

The first is self-medication. Are you or your partner using some form of enhancement to deal with a baseline state that's not very comfortable? The most common form is substance abuse. You can also self-medicate with things like gambling, sex addiction, or risk taking.

The second is what I call radical isolation. Are you or the person you love withdrawing from life, withdrawing from pleasure, becoming more and more internally isolated and apathetic?

Third and most troublesome is rage or lashing-out behavior. And that can run the spectrum from increased irritability all the way to physical violence. I'm not saying that every alcoholic or batterer is depressed necessarily, but that the great many of these men have a masked, covered-over core of internal dysphoria [sadness] or discomfort. This whole issue is routinely missed by both the man and his doctor and even mental health professionals. They're not really looking for it.

What do you think accounts for these differences in the ways men and women act when they're depressed?

Our culture raises girls in ways that produce one kind of depression, and it raises boys in a way that produces a uniquely different kind. We have never raised boys to be intimate and psychologically connected, and we understand now how injurious that is. Girls tend to be wounded on issues of disempowerment and the healing move is to help them reempower themselves. With boys and men, the wound is about disconnection. We equate masculinity with numbness, with not feeling, not caring, with ultra-toughness. We basically toughen up our boys and beat the sensitivity out of them.

Women have worked to heal themselves over the last generation by reclaiming their wholeness and by understanding that they can be assertive and they can be sexy and they can be loving—the total woman thing. Men need to do the same, we need to heal from the wound of disconnection that happens as early as three, four, five years old. Prekindergarten boys are already putting aside those qualities of expressiveness, dependency, and vulnerability because they know the rules. Before our boys have learned to read, they've read the stoic code of masculinity.

Boys are shamed for their own humanity, their own dependency and vulnerability. I used to think that violence was a by-product of boy's socialization, and I now have come to believe that violence *is* boyhood socialization. The way we teach boys to become men is by teaching them to cut off. The price of disconnection in boyhood is a cut-off adult and now we're in trouble. The result is a man who may create pain but doesn't admit it. It feels very out of his control. And that is coupled with permission to rage or to drink.

Women often hold back from naming what's going on with their man and insisting that he get help. Because it's almost cruel to tell a man how vulnerable he is. Our culture is very protective of distressed men, and women are raised to be caretakers. So they move to protect the guy, to protect his fragility and not deal with the issue.

Are you saying that women consciously deny the problem? Or are they just blind to it?

There's a kind of cultural collusion to keep this issue in the closet. Partners are always involved in that collusion. Partners aren't stupid; they live with the guy. Everybody always knows what's going on in relationships. She may not want to admit it to herself, or she's intimidated or afraid. When women tell men the truth, they're afraid that the man will retaliate, or withdraw, or fall apart. Real men don't get depressed.

How can men who are hiding from their depression and are acting out in these ways be helped?

A lot of therapies ignore the issues of self-medication and go right to the under-lying wound and that doesn't work. Or they ignore the rage or the acting out. I'm saying that covert depression has to be a two-pronged treatment. The lashing out, the substance abuse, the withdrawal—these have to be confronted and treated in their own right. Once the man stops acting out, once he sobers up, or is brought out of that intense isolation and his defenses calm down, then the overt depression comes right to the surface. And then treatment isn't that dif-ferent: You look for medication and you talk about the pain. But people miss this two-step process. The flip side is you take a guy like this to an addiction coun-selor and he'll get thrown into a rehab, but his underlying core issues won't be dealt with. The closest thing to what I'm calling covert depression is now called a dual diagnosis.

So if you didn't self-medicate or do these other things, the depression would be so intolerable as to become overt?

That's right. I suffered from covert depression and I self-medicated—anybody in their right mind would do what they needed to do to get out of that state 24/7. It's painful. Trying to treat a covertly depressed man for the underlying depres-sion while he's still drinking or drugging or womanizing is spitting in the wind. It just ain't gonna happen.

How can a woman recognize that her man is depressed?

You ask yourself: How healthy is this guy, how happy is this guy? How comfortable is he in his skin? How intimate is he, how shut down is he, how emotionally aloof and isolated or withdrawn or passive? Freud said the two signs of healthy functioning are love and work, and I think that's true. A lot of women either don't trust their instincts about the disconnection that she's feeling with the guy, or she feels like it's her fault and she has to fix it.

What can women do if they're married to or involved with men who are struggling with covert depression?

I'm beginning to do some thinking about this very issue, of women as an untapped resource in the health of men. Quite often the men get treatment—guess when? When the woman insists they do. My message to women who are partners to depressed males is deal with it. You have the right to insist on health in your marriage and your family, and this is not a negotiable item. If your partner won't go into individual therapy, then I counsel women to get into couple's therapy, to say to their partner, 'Look, you may not have a problem, but *we* have a problem and I'm going to book this appointment and I expect you to be there.' That's what women can do with depressed husbands.

I call the work I do relational recovery therapy. Because one of the things we know about healthy human functioning is that there's a very solid correlation between health and rich social connections. People recover faster from surgery, people have fewer incidents of cancer remission, et cetera. So all of these behaviors are detrimental to a man's health partly because in doing them, he withdraws from the nurturant support of human relationships.

How does covert depression and the ways men act it out affect their health?

The foundation of traditional masculinity is the denial of vulnerability. Part of the code is that you're tough and stoic. The reason men live less long than women is because they don't take care of themselves physically. There's nothing genetic about it. They don't take care of themselves, they don't go to the doctor when they need to, and they're less compliant when the doctor tells them what to do. Also they're prone to more accidents because of their addiction to intensity and their delusions of grandeur. So they're dangerous to themselves, and I haven't spoken about male violence. Men die—they die in wars, they die in dangerous jobs, they die inflicting violence on one another. There's a lot that's toxic about the traditional male role, as well as a lot that's good about it. But it needs to be reconfigured.

Source: Reprinted with permission from Rob Waters.

20

Tossin', Turnin', Cuttin' Zs

TOO MUCH NOISE, TOO LITTLE SLEEP

Consider the case of Bruce Menia age fifty-one. His snoring was so loud he was threatened with eviction from the Albany, New York, apartment he shares with his wife and stepdaughter. Complaints from his neighbors pushed the managing agent to send him a letter saying he either get the snoring fixed or he's out. Poor guy. It's bad enough when your wife is irritated, but it's downright embarrassing when your neighbors complain. Snoring is the basis for lots of jokes and laughter, and there are lots of funny terms that we use to imitate or describe the sound—sawing logs, needs a new muffler, or sounds like a foghorn. But for lots of women out there, it's also a nightly nightmare.

What makes it worse is that most men who snore seem to ignore or flat out deny it. After all, they don't hear themselves snore, and somehow, they don't quite believe their bedmates. A lot of times it seems to take someone else making the same observation— a child or a tent partner on a camping trip—for a man to believe it. And even if he finally admits to snoring, he's likely to make a joke or two, but do little else about it.

I should probably stop here and say that, of course, it's not only men who snore. Plenty of women saw logs as well, and many no doubt do it at great volume. But sleep experts and wives agree on this point: Men are far more likely than women to snore.

But here's where snoring really stops being funny: No matter who's doing it, snoring can be a sign of a serious sleep disorder called *sleep apnea.* The term comes from the Greek word *apnoia,* meaning "absence of breath," because people who have it literally stop breathing for short periods of time.

Let's be clear, though: Lots of people snore regularly, and just about everyone snores once in a while. It happens when the *uvula,* the fleshy flap of tissue that hangs down at the back of the throat, and sometimes the tonsils relax during sleep and vibrate against the soft palate, creating noise.

Not all snorers have sleep apnea, though sleep apnea is one of the most common sleep disorders, affecting around 4 percent of adult men and about half as many women. The most common form, *obstructive sleep apnea,* happens when the muscles of the soft palate at the back of the tongue and the uvula relax so much that they block the airway. The airway can also be blocked in obese people when excess tissue in the area causes it to be narrowed. People who are overweight, have a structural abnormality in their throat or nose, or have high blood pressure are also prone to sleep apnea.

A much rarer kind of sleep apnea, known as *central sleep apnea,* occurs when the brain fails to signal muscles in the chest and diaphragm to inhale and exhale as they should.

Typically, a person with obstructive sleep apnea snores, then falls silent briefly until the lack of oxygen and buildup of carbon dioxide is so great the brain signals the sleeper to awaken, usually with a loud gasp. Usually the sleeper has no idea that he is being aroused repeatedly throughout the night. These interruptions of breath can happen as many as sixty times an hour, ruining a person's ability to get the deep, restorative sleep we all need and leaving the troubled sleeper exhausted during the day. Drinking alcohol or taking sleeping pills can make the airway more likely to collapse and the breathing pauses last longer.

Because people with sleep apnea are so chronically and deeply sleep deprived, they run the risk of falling asleep at the wheel or on the job, putting their lives and the lives of others at risk. Sleep apnea also helps trigger high blood pressure and increases the risk of heart attack and stroke. It can cause irritability as well as learning and memory difficulties. And a recent study in the journal *Neurology* found that 80 percent of men with cluster headaches also suffered from sleep apnea. Cluster headaches are more likely to occur in men.

If you suspect that your partner suffers from sleep apnea, point out to him some of these health problems that can result. If none of them is enough to convince your partner that he should see a doctor, try this one. A 1999 study at the National Naval Hospital found that chronic sleep deprivation caused by sleep apnea can sap a man's sexual energy and hinder his ability to get an erection.

If your husband refuses to believe that he has sleep apnea, there are a couple of things you can do. One is to make a tape recording of his nighttime concerto, then play it back for him. It may be quite convincing, even if it's a bit embarrassing. The tape can also help a doctor make at least a preliminary diagnosis.

A doctor can also order other tests, including an overnight sleep test called a *polysomnograph,* in which the sleeper is wired up with electrodes to the scalp, face, chin, chest, and legs to

SIGNS OF SLEEP APNEA

People often tend to deny that they have sleep apnea. Here are some of the most common symptoms:

- Loud snoring, often accompanied by gasping and sputtering that briefly rouse the sleeper and allow him to take a breath.
- Morning headache.
- Daytime sleepiness.
- Poor memory, inability to concentrate.
- Irritability, anxiety, and depression.

measure brain activity, eye movement, heart rate, muscle activity, blood oxygen levels, and other functions.

TREATING SLEEP APNEA

Some mild cases of obstructive sleep apnea can be managed without any major medical intervention by avoiding alcohol and sleeping pills or sleeping on one's side. Losing weight may also help. If these approaches don't work, there are several treatment options, depending on the nature of the patient's anatomy and the severity of the apnea. Here are the major ones:

Continuous Positive Airway Pressure (CPAP)

This is the most common treatment for sleep apnea. The patient wears a mask over the nose (and sometimes the mouth) and a blower forces air into the nasal passages. This constant air pressure keeps the airway from collapsing and so prevents any interruption in breathing. There are two major problems to this approach. It works as long as it's in use, but it doesn't alter the patient's airway anatomy, so it must be used every night or the symptoms of apnea will return. Also, many people find it uncomfortable and awkward.

Dental Appliances

People who snore or have mild to moderate apnea are sometimes helped by a dental device that repositions the tongue and jaw.

Surgery

Surgery to increase the size of the airway can help some patients. This can be accomplished in different ways: by removing adenoids and tonsils, especially in snoring children; by trimming excess tissues of the mouth and throat; by using laser treatment to excise unwanted tissue; by using a radio frequency device called Somnoplasty to shrink some of this excess tissue. This device has been approved by the FDA for snoring, obstructive sleep apnea, and nasal obstruction. Unfortunately, these procedures are rarely covered by health insurance and can be quite expensive.

ASLEEP AT THE WHEEL . . . OR THE DESK

Millions of people find themselves nodding off during the day, even after getting— or seeming to get—enough sleep. They find the urge to doze almost overwhelming and may fall asleep in situations where they really need to be fully awake and alert, like when they're driving. This can happen as a result of several different sleep disorders, including sleep apnea or *narcolepsy,* a neurological problem that keeps the central nervous system from properly regulating sleep and wakefulness.

The most frightening thing about these problems is that they so often cause drowsy driving. Some 100,000 crashes and 1,500 deaths every year result from drivers falling asleep at the wheel, according to the National Highway Traffic Safety Administration. The drivers in these crashes are most often young men who stay up late, sleep too little, and drive at night. One study in North Carolina found that 78 percent of drivers causing fall-asleep crashes were males, and more than half were twenty-five or under.

Don't Let Him Shrug It Off

If your partner, son, or father (or anyone else you care about) has a significant sleep problem, don't let him yawn and shrug it off. Sleep disorders can be not only dangerous, they can also affect a person's mood and morale and be a prelude to depression, not to mention serious health problems like heart disease. Push him to see a doctor. If he resists and you're really concerned, don't get in the car when he's driving, at least on any long trip. Maybe, just maybe, that will help convince him that you think it's serious and that he ought to, too.

21

Boomeritis

"Go Out for One—Ouch!"

We all know the middle-aged man who simply doesn't realize that he's not in high school anymore and thinks that twenty years of relative inactivity won't affect his ability to perform great athletic feats. He works at his office job all week and doesn't get to the gym all that often. He doesn't stretch or stay conditioned. Then some Saturday, he tells his wife that some guys are getting together to shoot some hoops or play a little touch football. Next thing you know, he's limping in the front door on crutches. Or calling from the emergency room.

This scenario has become so common that the American Academy of Orthopaedic Surgeons has even adopted a name for it—"boomeritis." "Boomeritis is the disease that happens to the overzealous baby boomer who wants to stay active yet doesn't know the safest way to do it," says Nicholas A. DiNubile, M.D., the Philadelphia orthopedist who actually coined the term and has become the world's expert on this phenomenon. And—big surprise—Dr. DiNubile believes it's mostly men who are suffering boomeritis injuries.

Just how big a problem is this? The U.S. Consumer Product Safety Commission crunched the numbers a couple of years ago and found a whopping 33 percent increase in sports injuries among boomers—people born between 1946 and 1964—from 1991 to 1998. More than 1 million boomers needed medical attention for sports-related injuries in 1998, compared to three quarters of a million in 1991. And nearly 370,000 of the boomers injured in '98 had to go to the ER for treatment.

In 1998 some 65,000 boomers were injured while bicycling and some 48,000 while playing basketball, the two sports that racked up the greatest number of injuries. Boomers were nearly twice as likely to die in a bicycle accident as children, probably because they were much less likely to be wearing a bike helmet while riding.

But a lot of men don't make it into the statistics because they suffer in silence. According to DiNubile, the most common boomer injury is an overuse injury, the nagging low-grade hurt that happens when a person does subtle damage—what doctors call micro-trauma—to a muscle, ligament, tendon, or joint. These injuries start slowly, usually from sports with lots of repetitive motion such as running or cycling. The pain builds gradually until you can no longer work through it. Examples are *plantar fasciitis* (heel spur pain), shoulder rotator cuff, tendinitis, and osteoarthritis of the knee. These can improve over the short term, says DiNubile, but are prone to recur unless the athlete changes the way he exercises.

Then there are the acute injuries—the broken ankles, the torn hamstrings, the blown-out ligaments in the knee—that so often strike weekend warriors. The recipe for these injuries is quite simple, according to DiNubile. Go to a tennis match or a softball game having done no recent conditioning. Arrive late and don't warm up or stretch. Then go out and start hitting the ball. At some point, you dig hard to return that passing shot hit along the sideline or to beat a throw into third base and—voilà—instant pulled hamstring.

Why do boomers get into so much trouble when they're really just trying to stay young? In fact, that's part of the problem. Boomers are notoriously unwilling to admit that they're aging and that they might need to change how they do things. But the reality is that we all start to lose muscle in our forties (unless we spend hours lifting weights and conditioning). Tendons and ligaments lose elasticity over time, limiting range of motion and causing joints to stiffen. Add to this natural decline the fact that many men just don't stay in shape. (Of course, lots of women don't either—the difference is we know it.)

The result for a lot of men is that when they try to get out there and recapture the magic they once had on the basketball court they don't have the strength, the flexibility, or the endurance and are primed for injury. And when they do get injured, it takes forty-somethings a lot longer to heal than it did when they were still in their twenties.

Slow healing can be maddeningly frustrating for many boomer men. Some succumb to what DiNubile calls "fix-me-itis." These are the men who have had an injury, yet find it impossible to believe that no doctor can return them to their preinjury state. "They've been to five specialists, they've had three MRIs," DiNubile says. "They've already had their knee scoped two or three times. They want it fixed and they want it fixed now. They want it back to the way it was. And they want to go on forever. This 'fix-me-itis' drives a lot of unnecessary health care. Because more is not always better when it comes to health care. More surgeries aren't always better. More MRIs aren't always better."

So how can men avoid the "boomeritis syndrome," and how can we help? It's mostly a matter of common sense. Here are some suggestions to help your boomer avoid the big pitfalls and enjoy being a middle-aged man who's in shape and injury-free.

Problem: He starts out with a sprint instead of a jog, though he hasn't run for twenty years. A lot of men tend to push too hard and go too fast when they decide to start working out. You've probably seen the forty-five-year-old man who goes into the gym acting like he's still in his twenties. DiNubile describes it like this: "They're bouncing the weight. They don't pay attention to form. They're there to demonstrate strength more than to build it, so they're probably using too much weight. They do old-fashioned sit-ups, though we realize now they're not good for the body. A woman will look for instruction, whereas a guy will say, 'Oh no, I know how to do that. I don't need instruction.'"

Solution: Encourage you partner to plan his workout routine in advance. Warn him about the risk of injury from starting too fast or too hard. Better yet, get one of his male friends to make the warning—he'll probably be more likely to listen. Best of all, give him a present of two or three sessions with a personal trainer.

Problem: Overworking some muscle groups while ignoring others. A lot of boomers can get into trouble this way. "Guys like to lift weight," say DiNubile. "But their weight training is not balanced. They favor the upper body. They favor what I call the mirror muscles—the ones you see when you're looking in the mirror. They're doing bench presses, they're doing curls. They're building up their chest and biceps. And that kind of workout can actually create imbalances." One example is the shoulder. An unbalanced workout can overdevelop the front of the shoulder at the expense of the rear—the upper back and deltoids—and lead to a rotator cuff malfunction.

Solution: Encourage your husband to exercise regularly, and to include a mix of cardiovascular activity, strength training, and flexibility exercises. We're all better off if our workout routines are balanced, and we're more likely to avoid injury if we exercise during the week as well as on the weekend. Varying an exercise routine can also help avoid overuse injuries. So instead of always running, try alternating between running and an elliptical machine or swimming. And again consider a gift of a personal trainer.

Other Tips

Make gifts to your husband of gear that might improve his safety or help prevent injuries such as a helmet or knee pads. If he's injured himself but isn't getting good medical attention, consider getting him an appointment with a sports medicine specialist who can help him develop a treatment plan, as well as an exercise program that will do him more good than harm. If an injury does occur remember the PRICE rule:

> **P**rotection: Don't reinjure the area by continuing to play.
> **R**est: Stay off it.
> **I**ce: Every twenty minutes or so for the first twenty-four to forty-eight hours.
> **C**ompression: Wrap the area with an ACE bandage using light pressure.
> **E**levation: Keep the injured area higher than the heart to reduce swelling. And when in doubt seek medical attention.

22

Men and Sex

SEX AND THE HEALTH OF YOUR RELATIONSHIP

Few things are more important to the health of your relationship than sex. To a greater extent than many people imagine, sexual contentment in a marriage (or long-term partnership) is a harbinger of the long-term strength and happiness of the marriage, and even the physical and mental health of a husband and wife. So in the pages that follow, we're going to talk frankly about sex. And though this is a book about men's health, we're going to talk about women's sexuality, too. We'll discuss issues and problems both sexes face, along with some ways to address them. The reason, I think, is obvious: Sex is an interactive experience, and the nature of a couple's sex life has a profound effect on the marriage and the partners. If either person in a relationship feels sexually disconnected or is having sexual problems or concerns, both people will be intimately affected. After all, it does take two to tango.

WATCHING AMY, JUDGING OURSELVES

As anyone who watches television, goes to the movies, reads magazines, or looks at advertising knows, Americans are bombarded with sexual images, sexual innuendo, and talk about sex. The media's preoccupation with sex forces us all to compare our own sex lives to the sexpots and studs we see in the media. Imagining that others are doing it better or doing it more can leave us feeling inadequate, as if we're somehow abnormal if we're not having sex 24/7.

Part of the reason we tend to make these comparisons is that we don't really know what's normal. Maybe it will help people feel better to know that the average married couple has sex just six times per month, and that the average for single people is even lower. A full third of Americans have sex just a few times a year or less. Even some married couples simply don't have sex at all (a situation we'll talk about a bit later).

Yet despite the cultural obsession with sex, it is a topic that often goes undiscussed among American couples, especially those who most need to talk about it—couples who are having sexual problems. And since most people don't talk much about sex outside their relationship either—other than to gossip, chortle, or boast—sexual myths, misinformation, and stereotypes abound.

The result is that many of us figure that everybody else is having a lot more sex than we are, and that it's way more exciting. Most men probably think that other men last longer than they do and give their partners orgasms more often. And most women probably make the same assumptions—that other women have sex and orgasms more often. After all, sex is always wilder on the other side of the street. Isn't it? Such notions are among the many myths that can undermine our sexual self-esteem and the health of our relationships. In fact, there are probably more myths perpetuated about sex than just about any other subject. Here's a small sampling:

Myth 1: Swinging Singles Have More Fun

Getting married is the beginning of the end of your sex life. Slowly but steadily your sex life will decline and you'll have less and less sex that's more and more boring. Right?

Well, no. The surprise is that married people have more sex, not less, than their single counterparts, and by a good margin. Singles may talk a lot about sex, but it's mostly to plot how they're going to get some. Married people don't have to hunt, since they've got a generally available sex partner. Indeed, this is one of the reasons people get married—to have sex with the man or woman they love.

Married people are also more content with their sex lives, according to sex researchers from the University of Chicago. In a 1992 study of more than 3,000 adult Americans, the most satisfied respondents were the people who were married. A whopping 88 percent of married folks said they experienced great physical pleasure from their sex lives, and 85 percent said they were satisfied emotionally. That study, technically called the National Health and Social Life Survey, but better known as the Sex Survey, is widely regarded as the most accurate American sex survey to date.

It is true that married people spend less time in each sexual encounter than singles do, at least according to the Chicago survey. Maybe that's because married sex is more predictable and less adventurous, as lots of people probably assume. But maybe it's also because married people know each other's bodies, so they spend less time with awkward fumbling. Or because those singles don't have kids and so are less harried and pressed for time.

Myth 2: Everybody Else Is Having More Sex Than We Are

Unless you're a voyeur, you don't really know how often the people across the street have sex. But that doesn't stop us from speculating, and from thinking that others do it more often and have more fun. The truth is that while everyone talks about hot, hot sex, Americans are rather tame when it comes to bedroom activity. Most Americans do have sex, especially if they're in a couple, but they don't have a whole lot of it. Depending, of course, on what you think of as a lot.

So if you really want to know how you stack up, compared to Jim and Jane Average American, here's a sort of "box score" taken from the University of Chicago Sex Survey.

Myth 3: The French Are Sexy, Americans Are Dull

Few stereotypes are more pervasive. The French, we're all convinced, are always and forever having sex. The truth is Americans and Frenchmen (and women) are far more similar in their sexual habits than most of us would ever have believed—especially those smug Parisians. At least that's the word from researchers who compared survey results on sexual behavior in both countries in *The Journal of Sex Research*.

"In contrast to common stereotypes of sexuality in the United States and France— one a mythic bastion of sexual Puritanism, the other the most sexually celebrated of Western cultures—we found quite similar patterns of sexual conduct . . . from young adulthood to late middle age," write the researchers. "Overall, adults in France and in the U.S. are remarkably alike in their sexual behavior."

Despite the stereotype that all French men have mistresses, the French are just as likely to be monogamous as we are—which means very likely. In both countries, more than 90 percent of married or cohabiting men and women said they had only one sexual partner in the past year. And among those who are not living with a partner, the French were actually *more* likely to be monogamous.

AVERAGE NUMBER OF TIMES PER MONTH THAT AMERICANS HAVE SEX		
Age	Married	Single
18–29	9	6
30–39	7	5
40–49	6	4
50–59	4	3
60–69	3	1

Two thirds of French men, but fewer than half of American men, had only one bed partner in the past year. The trend was similar with women.

Americans also report having more sex partners through the course of their lifetime. American men said they'd bedded, on average, sixteen women in their lives, compared to thirteen for French men. American women claimed about six sexual partners to French women's four.

There is one place where the French come closer to living up to stereotype: They generally have sex more often than Americans. Around half of French men and women had sex two to three times per week, compared to about one third of American men and women. And one great thing about being a French woman is that they continue to have sex as they age. Ninety percent of French women and men in their fifties reported having had a sexual partner in the past year, about the same number as among American men. In contrast, just over one quarter of American women in this same age group reported having a sexual partner in the past year.

"It appears as if older women in the U.S. are less desirable sexually or are themselves less interested in sexual activity than French women of a comparable age," write the researchers. In other words, the cult of youth worship in America means that here, older women are not seen as sexy. In France, they are. Something's got to change.

THE THINGS THAT GO WRONG

Given how important your sex life is to the health of your marriage, it's surprising how often couples who experience sexual problems or disconnection simply ignore it. Trouble is that when you ignore this one, it really can go away, leaving a great void in your relationship. Sooner or later, nearly every man and woman will have some kind of sexual difficulty or concern. If that sounds like an exaggeration, consider these recent studies:

- A survey from the University of North Carolina at Chapel Hill found that a whopping 99 percent of 14,000 women of all ages said they had at least one sexual concern. Topping a long list of worries, 87 percent felt they should be more interested in sex, 83 percent had trouble reaching orgasm, 69 percent didn't think they were attractive enough, and 67 percent felt some of their sexual needs were not being met.

- A similar survey of men of all ages conducted through family physicians' offices in Germany found that 93 percent of the men suffered at least occasionally from one or more sexual problems. As with the North Carolina women's survey, low sexual desire was the most common concern, experienced sometimes by 73 percent of men. In addition, 66 percent of the men had problems with premature ejaculation, 50 percent worried about sexual failure, and 38 percent had problems getting or maintaining erections.

- A 1999 study from the University of Chicago became front-page news with its finding that 43 percent of American women and 31 percent of American men suffered from some sexual dysfunction. While some experts believe this study overstated the extent of major sexual problems, it did bring these issues to public attention and got people talking about them.

IT'S NOT HAPPENING . . .

So what should you do if you're feeling unhappy with your sex life or think your husband is? If you're like a lot of people, this is an area of your life that the two of you have rarely discussed, yet you know that things could be better than they are. The first step is to talk about it and try to figure out how you both feel about your sexual relationship. Because a continuing mismatch between the expectations either of you have and the reality of your intimate life can spell trouble.

"The first thing you want to find out is if anyone is distressed," says Megan Fleming, Ph.D., a psychologist specializing in sexuality at Beth Israel Medical Center in New York. "Many partners have sexual desire discrepancies that they need to negotiate and resolve. That's where you start."

Some problems you'll be able to solve that way—by talking things through and coming to some agreements that can help you both to better satisfy your needs and desires. Other issues may be harder or impossible to resolve just by talking, though that is still the way to begin. Below we've tried to identify some of the major problems that men and then women experience in their sex lives. Later we discuss how you can begin to change some of the things that might be troubling you.

You're Hot, He's Not

As the television columnist for the *San Francisco Chronicle* is fond of saying, "Everything we know we learned from television." And what I say is thank God for those *Sex and the City* girls. They've taught lots of us some important lessons—about putting ourselves out there as seekers and initiators of sex, instead of being passive. And how even crushing, humiliating rejection can be survived. We even get some free sex therapy tips. In one episode, Charlotte's future husband can't seem to perform in bed. Not one to be easily put off, Charlotte gives him the "stamp test," which he passes, proving that his problems are psychological. It's a great relief to Charlotte and great comedy for us. (And, yes, we'll explain this later and why the *City* girls may be intimidating many men.)

There is actually a real lesson here—a reminder of how wrong and unfortunate it is for women to assume that when a man has trouble getting an erection it's either her fault or a signal that she's not attractive to him. This, says sex researcher Pepper Schwartz, Ph.D., is one of the most erroneous and harmful assumptions that women make. "I think women overestimate men's physiological capacity," says Dr. Schwartz, a sociologist at the University of Washington. "They take it personally when men don't function well, and men can't explain that their body isn't this [ever-ready] hammer. [There's] this expectation that men are just basically sexual machines, and they are not. They're not even close. I think it sets up a lot of disappointment on both sides."

The point is this: We have to give the men a break, and ourselves as well. Things don't always work perfectly, and we shouldn't blame our partners or ourselves when that happens.

How Men Work

If we want to understand more about the problems men can have, it helps to have some understanding of how they work under normal circumstances. So here's a brief lesson about how the penis and the rest of the male sexual apparatus work.

Depending on how you count, there are four or five stages to the male sexual cycle. The first thing that must occur is desire or libido—the feeling of being interested in sex. Sexual desire is made possible by the action of testosterone in the brain. It's the feeling that causes men to fantasize about sex, to look at attractive women, and to try to seduce you. Nearly all men have this desire to a greater or lesser degree, though it does fade somewhat with age. Men who have little or no sexual desire may have low testosterone levels and might want to check in with a doctor (see page 486).

The next phase, excitement, is the physical reaction to this desire, the flame that comes from striking the match. To use a different metaphor, people often talk about sexual electricity or chemistry, and it turns out that both are actually involved in sex. When a man becomes sexually excited, the portion of his brain that controls sexual response sends electrical impulses to nerves in the pelvis. These nerves release chemicals—neurotransmitters—that cause the smooth muscle tissue in the penis to relax, letting more blood flow in. Normally, when a man does not have an erection, blood flows out as fast as it flows in. But as he becomes sexually aroused, his heart starts beating more rapidly, bringing blood more quickly into the penis. As the blood rushes in, it fills two chambers (called the *corpora cavernosa*) that run the length of the penis and contain tissue that's much like a sponge. As the little holes and spaces in the tissue fill with blood, the chambers expand and push out against a sort of membrane or sheath (the *tunica albuginea*) that surrounds them. This pressure seals off the veins that normally let blood flow out of the penis. The result: Blood flows in but can't flow out. The man has an erection. As the penis hardens, the head swells, deepens in color, and becomes warmer. The scrotum thickens, and the muscles holding the testicles tighten, lifting them up toward the body. The penis is ready for action.

In the next stage of the sexual act, the plateau phase, a man is poised at a high level of sexual arousal. His heart races, his muscles tense, and his blood pressure rises still more. As the head of his penis increases in size, a small amount of fluid emerges. It's not semen, though it can contain some sperm. How long this phase lasts can vary a great deal. In general, if a man can stay at this phase for a while and delay the next one, it can make the sexual experience more pleasurable for him as well as his partner.

The fourth phase, orgasm or climax, is the promised land, the part of the sexual act that brings that intense rush of pleasure. Physiologically, several things happen almost at once. As the man senses that ejaculation is imminent, semen produced in both the seminal vesicles (behind the prostate) and the prostate itself gets mixed together with sperm as muscles of the prostate and seminal vesicles squeeze. This is called emission. At the moment of climax, muscles at the bottom of the penis contract repeatedly, propelling the semen out through the urethra. All this happens very quickly, in mere seconds.

The final phase is a little time-out—the refractory, or resolution, period. After a man has climaxed, things go quickly back to normal. Blood pressure drops, blood drains from the penis, and the heart rate slows as nerves signal the body to relax. The body needs a rest and won't produce another erection for a while. Exactly how long depends on the age of the man. A twenty-something may need only to catch his breath; a man of seventy may need a couple of days.

Problems Under the Hood

So now that we know how things work, let's talk about what happens when they don't. There are, of course, lots of things that can go wrong with a man's complex sexual process. And there's lots of pressure on men to perform—more, in some ways, than there's ever been. An article in *New York* magazine in the summer of 2002 provided a glimpse of that pressure and the effect it can have on many men. The writer, a twenty-something fellow named Ben Kaplan, was, for the first time in his young life, having problems getting an erection. As he called around to urologists and sex therapists in New York City, he found that they were seeing more young male patients than ever before.

One urologist, Laurence A. Levine, M.D., told Kaplan he had seen an 800 percent increase in patients under forty over the past four years. Another urologist attributed the rise to Viagra, which both raised awareness of erection problems and gave young men who might be having problems a reason to call a doctor.

Kaplan had a more interesting theory: He blames it on *Sex and the City* and especially Samantha. "The *Sex and the City* vixen's craving for size, for novelty, for frequency, for orgasm on demand raised—or actually lowered—the bar for New York men like me," he writes. "Faced with a city of women who now consider satisfaction to be their birthright, many of us have developed chronic performance anxiety."

With that in mind, here is a quick overview of some of the problems men face.

Don't Call It Impotence

A curious thing happened just a few years ago in the way people talk about the most famous of all male sexual problems. The word *impotence,* a rather harsh word that seemed to sum up and put down not just a man's sexuality but his very being, suddenly went out of favor. Was it because the research, pharmaceutical, and medical communities suddenly became more sensitive? Well, that may have happened with some, but the big reason had a lot more to do with selling a drug.

Instead of impotence, the marketers of Viagra made use of the recently coined term *erectile dysfunction.* Where impotence sounds difficult if not impossible to treat, the new term of choice, erectile dysfunction, sounds more clinical, like a problem that can be solved with the right wonder drug. Like Viagra. And in fact, this blockbuster erection drug has helped lots of men while bringing a once-hidden problem out of the closet. Perhaps the best thing about Viagra is that millions of men who had been suffering silently suddenly began flocking to their doctors. For many of them, their inability to get an erection turned out to be a symptom of another medical problem that needed to be addressed.

Erectile dysfunction is defined as the persistent inability to have an erection sufficient for sexual intercourse. It affects anywhere from 10 to 30 million men in the United States, becoming increasingly common as men age. So while about 5 percent of forty-year-old men have this problem, so do 15 percent to 25 percent of men over sixty-five. An important thing to remember is that most men will have trouble with erections at some point.

It used to be thought that if a man had trouble getting an erection, the problem was all in his head, the result of anxiety or some other psychological issue. That is, of course, one reason that men get ED, and it's probably the biggest cause of ED among young men. Stress, anxiety, depression, guilt, and fear of sexual failure can all take their toll on a man's confidence and ability to perform sexually. If there's a lot of tension or problems in your relationship, that can also be a factor. And if a man has had any history of being sexually abused or traumatized, that can double or triple the chances that he will have ED or other sexual problems. Sadly, the abuse of boys is far more common than many people realize, in part because men are so reluctant to talk about it.

With the majority of men, especially older men, ED is much more likely to be the result of a health problem. It can be an early warning sign of heart disease, because the same process that clogs heart arteries can clog small blood vessels in the penis, preventing blood from flowing in as it should. It can be a side effect of a number of medications including tranquilizers, antidepressants, antihistamines, or drugs used to treat ulcers or high blood pressure. Here are some of the other medical problems that can cause erectile dysfunction.

- diabetes
- high cholesterol
- high blood pressure
- smoking
- pelvic surgery
- radiation therapy
- pelvic or spinal injuries
- hormonal problems (low testosterone levels, thyroid disease)
- bicycle riding
- alcohol and drug abuse

Not So Fast

Trouble with erections may be the most famous problem men face in bed, but it's far from the only one. In fact, it's not even the most common, according to the 1999 survey from the University of Chicago. No, the problem that more men report than any other is their tendency to reach orgasm and ejaculate before they (or their partner) want them to. In other words, premature ejaculation. Nearly one third of men in every age group said they'd had this problem in the past year.

Of course, it's important to recognize that there is no rule or precise definition about what constitutes a "premature" ejaculation. In one sense, any ejaculation that happens before you want it to is premature. The goal here is sexual pleasure for both partners and if that happens, it doesn't really matter how long a man lasts. In other words, sexual intercourse isn't an Olympic endurance event where a man needs to outlast the pack. Seeing it that way only adds to the pressure and, perversely, makes it more likely that a man will come quickly. On the other hand, sex isn't a sprinting event either.

Premature ejaculation is often confused or lumped together with erectile dysfunction. In fact, they are quite different, though they can share a common cause—anxiety, stress, or worries about performance. As we mentioned earlier, erection problems sometimes stem from psychological issues. Premature ejaculation almost always does.

Almost every man will have an orgasm sooner than he (or you) would like once in a while. If that's all it is, don't worry about it. After all, nobody's perfect; men, as Pepper Schwartz says, are not sex machines. But if it's happening fairly often or all the time, and it's frustrating one or both of you, then it's important to find a way to talk about it without your partner feeling threatened or blamed. Remember, this is sensitive ground for him. While he may not admit it, he probably is more upset about it than you are.

One thing for you or him to notice is whether he tends to ejaculate quickly under certain conditions: for example, using certain sexual positions, after an argument, or when you haven't had sex for a while. Most women know that the conditions need to be right for them to feel sexy. But men tend to think that they should always be ready for sex, that if a woman is ready and willing, he should be, too. That, after all, is what it means to be a real man.

Fortunately, premature ejaculation is one of the easier sexual problems to address, and sex therapists have developed a number of techniques that can usually help men overcome it. Your husband and you can see a sex therapist to work on these techniques, but they can also be practiced by men on their own, or, preferably, with your help and involvement. A number of books can help guide you in dealing with ejaculatory and other problems. Probably the best of them is *The New Male Sexuality,* by the late Bernie Zilbergeld, Ph.D. Here, in brief, are the two most commonly used techniques for improving ejaculatory control.

The Stop-Start Technique

In this technique, developed by the appropriately named Dr. James Semans in the 1950s, the man practices having sex and being stimulated until he feels that he is close to orgasm, then stops for anywhere from ten seconds to one minute before starting again. The idea is to stop long enough to prevent ejaculation but not so long that he loses interest—and his erection. As men practice this technique, they learn to detect the middle range of arousal before the point of no return and stop at that point, then continue. Many therapists recommend that men first learn to use this technique while masturbating, then move on to being stimulated by a partner manually. Once he has mastered things at that level, he can stop and start during intercourse.

The Squeeze Technique

In this variation on the stop-start approach, the man again stops when he senses that he is about to reach orgasm. Then he or his partner squeezes the head of his penis, just under the tip, between a thumb and two fingers, applying light pressure for a few seconds—again, you'll learn how long as you practice—before resuming stimulation. This can be repeated as often as necessary to delay ejaculation.

If these techniques don't work for you, you should definitely consider seeing a sex therapist. Another option to think about is using low doses of antidepressants. When doctors realized a few years ago that one side effect of antidepressants is that they tend to delay ejaculation, they began using them as a treatment for this problem. But you should also realize that another common side effect of these medications is a reduced sexual drive.

Other Sex Problems
No Heat, No Fire

Another common sexual complaint men make, according to the sex surveys, is that they don't have much of a sex drive. In the 1999 University of Chicago survey, 15 percent of men said they lacked interest in sex. This was slightly more common among older men, but amazingly, 14 percent of men in the eighteen-to-twenty-nine set had this complaint. There are a number of reasons why men might yawn at the idea of sex. It can be caused by low testosterone levels, especially in older men (see page 486). It might come from a man feeling bored or unhappy in a relationship, or from suppressing sexual interest as a result of being traumatized or abused. Some men who have had traumatic sexual experiences may even show dramatic physical reactions to the prospect of sex such as sweating, trembling, dizziness, or nausea. Depression can often dampen men's and women's sexual interest, as can some antidepressants and other medications. If your partner seems to have lost interest in sex, try to talk to him about it, and get him to get some professional help, including a check on his testosterone levels.

I Can't Get No ...

Some men come too quickly, a few can't seem to come at all. They get an erection, they have intercourse with their partner, but they can't seem to ejaculate or have an orgasm. It's frustrating, uncomfortable, and can be a real turnoff. It's usually caused by depression, anxiety, or from using alcohol or drugs. Doctors call this orgasmic disorder. If it persists, he should definitely get some help.

Peyronie's Disease

Many men have a slight curve in their penis when it's erect. If it causes no pain and doesn't interfere with sex, there's no real problem. But when the penis is curved or bent in a way that causes pain or interferes with sex, it is known as Peyronie's disease. It happens when hard scar tissue forms under the skin on the upper or lower side of the penis, where the tissue should be elastic and flexible. It can be caused by trauma from rough sex or even by banging an erect penis against a wall or bedpost. In other cases the problem develops slowly and the cause is not clear. If your partner has symptoms of Peyronie's disease, he should see a urologist as soon as possible. And if a sudden or major injury occurs to the penis, he should get medical attention immediately. There is no clear treatment for Peyronie's disease, though a number of different approaches are being studied. Some doctors say they've gotten good results by giving patients vitamin E orally to promote healing of the scar tissue, according to the National Institutes of Health. Surgery can often correct the problem, but it is not recommended except in serious cases that prevent intercourse. That's because the surgery itself can sometimes cause side effects, including impotence. Fortunately, the problem sometimes goes away on its own.

Pain During Sex

Sex should be fun; it should never be painful. But it can be, for any number of reasons, including prostatitis, tight foreskin or infection in uncircumcised men, STDs, and allergic reactions to gels, foams, or creams used for pleasure or contraception. Doctors call pain during sex *dyspareunia*. If sex hurts your partner, he should call his doctor to figure out why.

DEALING WITH PROBLEMS IN THE BEDROOM

Several years ago, Virginia and Keith Laken of Winona, Minnesota, had to face a medical and sexual crisis. Forty-nine-year-old Keith had prostate cancer and would need surgery that would likely leave him impotent. He told his wife Virginia that he would rather die. Initially, Virginia discounted Keith's feelings as irrational and ridiculous. She insisted that sex was unimportant compared with life. Keith felt that impotence was the worst thing that could happen to him. His ability to get an erection was an inherent part of his identity as a man, and the prospect of losing it was devastating.

The issue became the subject of heated arguments between them. He told Virginia, "This is not just about sex. It's about *life*. What kind of life would I have if I couldn't make love to you anymore? If I thought people didn't respect me?" Being impotent, to him, meant being weak, useless, ineffective, powerless in the eyes of his wife and others. He believed that others would be able to detect his loss of virility.

Eventually Keith changed his mind and in 1995, he had a radical prostatectomy. For months afterward, he and his wife waited to see if Keith would recover to the point where a normal sex life was possible. As it became clear that Keith could not have a normal erection, their marriage deteriorated and almost ended.

Viagra didn't help him, but penile injections did. For a while, the couple had a sex life again. But he grew tired of using the injections and told his wife that he no longer wanted to have sex. The Lakens grew distant and stopped touching each other or connecting physically. Hurt and rejected, Virginia realized that she really did miss their sexual intimacy.

Eventually, with the help of a sex therapist, they also realized that Keith still had a sex drive and that their sexual life could continue if they were willing to redefine it. Keith began using the injections again, and the couple now has sex that is deep and satisfying, even if it lacks spontaneity.

In the midst of their crisis, the Lakens often wished for a book that could help them understand how to confront such a major sexual problem. So they wrote their own, *Making Love Again,* a first-person account of how they dealt with sexual dysfunction and rebuilt a sexually intimate life. This book can help couples create their own road map for recovery and sexual healing, whether the problem is erectile dysfunction as a result of prostate cancer or any other sexual problem that gets in the way of two people making love.

DEALING WITH ERECTILE DYSFUNCTION

When a man has trouble with erections or another sexual problem, it doesn't affect only him. So it makes sense that efforts to solve the problem will work best when both partners are willing to work together. Of course, some men will prefer to seek help on their own, but they are more likely to succeed if their spouse is involved in a supportive way. Here are ways you can help your partner—and yourself—when he's having erectile problems.

Step 1: Communication

For a couple to deal with any crisis—sexual or otherwise—they need to be able to communicate. "The only really great tool you have is communication and honesty," says Dr. Pepper Schwartz. Where things get tricky is that even though your partner is the one having the problem, he often will be too afraid or embarrassed to even want to talk about it. If you want to see things change, it may be up to you to start the conversation. So how do you do that?

Gently. Very gently. This is tender ground for most men, says sex therapist Megan Fleming. So you want to pick the right time and place. One time *not* to bring things up is when you're in the midst of having sex. Or just before or after. Instead, Fleming says, try to talk about it at a quiet time when you're both relaxed and feeling affectionate, and are in a place other than the bedroom. Tell him you're still attracted to him and want to improve your relationship. Tell him that he's not alone, that ED, premature ejaculation, and other sexual problems affect *millions* of other men. And tell him also that many sexual problems are due to things that are easily treated and that his doctor may be able to help figure out the problem. Think about what you're going to say in advance and don't say too much. Give him plenty of time to speak.

"I think you have to be very careful about how you communicate dissatisfaction or distress," says Dr. Fleming. Tell him you miss him and want to have more affection in your relationship. Begin with "I" statements ("I feel sad"; "I miss your sexy body") rather than accusatory ones. Reassure him that you love and desire him and will support him in any way he wants.

"You don't want to be critical," says Dr. Fleming. "You don't want to be applying pressure. You don't want to imply that he's not fulfilling your needs. You want him to recognize that this sexual concern in no way affects how you love him or feel about his role as a husband or father. You need to support his sense of self-esteem and confidence."

Never underestimate the importance of sexual performance to a man's self-esteem. It's hard for many of us to understand that a man's self-worth is often rolled up in his ability to perform in the bedroom and that erection problems can be among the most stressful a man faces. This fear can be downright paralyzing. Many men start to feel that they are fundamentally inadequate and to fear that their wives will leave them. A man may avoid physical contact with his partner because he's afraid she'll want intercourse and he'll be unable to perform.

But the fears and guilt don't belong solely to the men. When a man has trouble getting erections, many a woman starts to feel that she is somehow to blame, that she's not attractive or sexy, or that he's having an affair.

So how do you both overcome these fears? Again, the first step is to talk to each other and share your fears. "There's a lot that you can do for each other by just focusing on it and saying, honestly, 'You know, I miss when we used to . . .'" says Dr. Pepper Schwartz.

Step 2: Do Try This at Home

Many sex therapists who work with couples will suggest they try an approach called *sensate focus therapy,* developed by famed sex researchers Masters and Johnson. There's no reason why couples can't try this on their own, before spending money on sex therapy. Many books describe this process, including Bernie Zilbergeld's *The New Male Sexuality,* though he calls it nongenital body rubs.

The technique is designed to help couples in which the man is having problems getting an erection. The idea is to help the partners connect sensually and intimately without the stress of the man having to perform on demand. It can also be used by any couple who wants to increase their understanding of how they each like to be touched.

Each partner take turns stroking, massaging, and caressing the other in a pleasurable way for a set amount of time, say twenty to thirty minutes. In the most common form of this exercise, the person who's being touched calls the shots as a way for the toucher to learn how the touchee likes to be touched. So as you pleasure each other, you tell your partner what you like, using positive language such as "I like it like this" rather than "Don't do that." In one variation, you can also have the toucher be in charge, choosing how and where to touch the other. The only other rule is that nobody should touch or be touched in ways that feel bad or painful.

The first few times you do this, avoid touching your partner's genitals. Later, you can move on and touch your partner's sexual organs, but not to orgasm. The goal here is to learn about your partner's body, not to make him have an orgasm. There will be plenty of time for that later.

Step 3: Get Professional Help

One of the first things you and your partner need to know is whether his erection difficulties are due largely to physical or to psychological problems. How can you tell? It's usually not all that difficult.

If a man gets erections from masturbating, or if they pop up spontaneously during the day or night, that's a sign that the problem is psychological and not physical. If he's unsure or doesn't recall getting erections recently, you can check further by performing the "stamp test," as Charlotte did on *Sex and the City*. You simply loop five to eight postage stamps around the base of the penis and seal them end to end. If they're broken in the morning, it means the plumbing works and the problem probably stems from stress or psychological issues. If the stamps remain intact, try it one more night to be sure. Then, if the result is the same, it's time to get medical attention. But don't panic: If there is a physical problem, it doesn't mean that your partner is permanently challenged. It simply means he needs to check in with a doctor for a more thorough evaluation.

Of course, in many cases a medical or physical problem may be compounded by anxiety. So if a man has circulatory problems—and intermittent trouble with erections as a result—he may start worrying that he's not going to be able to get an erection. And that can almost guarantee that he won't. A man in this situation needs to do two things: get medical attention for the underlying problem and avoid pressuring himself (or being pressured by you, his partner) to solve the problem and perform.

... From a Doctor

If the problem seems to be largely physical, or if you just can't tell, encourage your husband to talk to his doctor. Offer to go with him if you think that would help. Depending on the cause of the problem, there are a number of different ways to treat the problem, from Viagra to penile injections to hormone therapy to penile implants. We'll discuss some of these treatments a little bit later.

... From a Sex Therapist or Psychologist

If a man's erectile problems don't stem from a medical condition, and if you can't seem to take care of them on your own, you may benefit from the help of a sex therapist. Ideally, you would meet with a sex therapist as a couple, tackling the problem together. A sex therapist will usually spend a little bit of time getting to know you as a couple and identifying the source of the anxiety causing problems. Usually, the major focus of sex therapy is to solve the problem rather than get to the psychological roots of it. So the sex therapist will generally lead you through various exercise like the ones we mentioned earlier aimed at helping you overcome the difficulties.

In some cases, especially if a man has been sexually abused in the past, deeper psychological work may be needed for him to get past the trauma that has caused him to fear sex or to shut down.

"If there is any anger or any depression about sexuality, then seeking help from a therapist is essential," says Dr. Pepper Schwartz. "Anger and depression are both big flashing lights that something is not where it ought to be, and that is dangerous to the relationship or to the person."

Viagra: The Hard Facts

If I had a dollar for every time I said the word *Viagra* on national television, I would be—well, I'd have a lot of extra money. When Viagra was launched in 1998, the excitement of men—including those who control the newsroom where I worked— could not be contained. For two weeks straight, I talked about Viagra every day on TV, no doubt helping sell more than a few of those little blue pills. Pfizer, the maker of Viagra, didn't even bother to advertise the drug until long after it was on the market— they didn't need to, because we in the media were doing it for them.

As you probably know by now, Viagra works by increasing blood flow to the penis and has helped tens of thousands of men—many of whom hadn't had erections in many years—to have sexual intercourse. But it doesn't work for everyone. A recent review of studies found that Viagra helps men with mild or moderate ED to get erections hard enough to have sex about 60 percent of the time. Men with more severe symptoms are less successful; they're able to get erections and have sex 47 percent of the time. And men with diabetes, probably the most common physical cause of ED, were successful with Viagra only 44 percent of the time. It doesn't work well after a man has eaten a meal or had a drink—two things people frequently do before getting in the romantic mood.

Viagra seems to lose some of its effectiveness over time. A small study released in 2001 found that nearly 40 percent of men who were initially helped by the drug either stopped taking it because it no longer worked or had to double their dose to continue to get help.

For some men, Viagra can even be dangerous. In its first year on the market, more than one hundred thirty men died after taking the drug. As a result, the FDA required Pfizer to alter its warning label to advise people taking nitrates such as nitroglycerin or isosorbide for heart disease to stay away from the drug. Thousands of other men quit using it because of side effects that may include headache, lightheadedness, dizziness, flushing, or distorted vision.

What about men with prostate cancer who have surgery to remove the gland? As we discuss on page 479, many men who have prostatectomies lose their ability to get erections. That's even true of men who have so-called nerve-sparing surgery designed to leave intact the pelvic nerves that control erections. But some recent studies have found that for men who have nerve-sparing surgery, Viagra can greatly improve their chances of getting an erection.

One other thing you should know about Viagra is that it's not an aphrodisiac. It can't create desire where none exists. Men who take Viagra still have to be stimulated in some way to get an erection.

One downside to all the upbeat news about Viagra is that many women find that it increases their partner's phallus fixation. "Sexuality is a lot more than intercourse, particularly to women," says Dr. Pepper Schwartz. "Often one of the things women like about men as they get older is they get less penis centered and [pay more attention to] hands, mouth, and emotions."

For women, this can make Viagra a double-edged sword: It can help reawaken a couple's dormant sex life, but it also leads to men pressuring their wives for sex more often than the women would like. "When Viagra first came out, all these men thought, 'Wow! I've got a new toy! Look what I can do,'" says Dr. Schwartz. But many women are not interested in suddenly entering the sexual Olympics. They want to have sex, sure, but they are at least as interested in being emotionally intimate with their partners. Viagra also fuels a tendency among many men and couples to avoid getting to the bottom of their sexual and interpersonal issues, the very issues that can fuel anxiety and keep a man from getting an erection.

Still, Dr. Schwartz says, "I think overall Viagra has had a positive effect. In general, men want very much to please their partners and they think it's important to have a penis to do it. I think it's helped many relationships because a man can feel proud of himself. He can feel confident, and then maybe they can both relax and try other things."

As the first drug to help men get erections, Viagra tapped into a huge market, a market that Pfizer has had to itself for the last few years. But that has changed. The Bayer Corporation has developed a similar drug, vardenafil (brand name Levitra), and is now on the market. Lilly Corporation and ICOS are coming out with taldenafil (brand name Cialis), which already has European approval and is now also waiting FDA approval. Another new drug, apomorphine (brand name Uprima), has been approved in some European countries and was, at one point, expected to gain FDA approval in 2000. But concerns about its side effects—especially fainting and severe nausea—have kept it off the U.S. market as of this writing. Unlike Viagra, Uprima acts on the brain to inhibit smooth muscle contractions, allowing more blood to flow to the genitals. Because it is dissolved under the tongue, Uprima acts more quickly than Viagra and might allow for a bit more spontaneity.

But what about women? Does Viagra work for us? And if not, is there another magic pill that can help women reclaim their faded desire or reliably have orgasms? Don't hold your breath. While Viagra does seem to increase blood flow to a woman's pelvic region, it doesn't seem to have a great deal of impact on the sexual experience for many women. Some researchers say it seems to cause more side effects in women, like headaches—not exactly the best way to get in the mood.

HE'S HOT, YOU'RE NOT

When we think of sexual tension in a marriage, we usually think of the man begging for sex and the woman holding him off, nail file in hand, exclaiming that she has a headache. They want it; we want to be left alone. That's also the cliché immortalized in the Woody Allen film *Annie Hall* in which Diane Keaton and Woody Allen talk to their respective therapists in split screen about their sexual relationship. Asked how often they are having sex, Woody replies, "Almost never, only three times per week." Keaton, responding to the same question, says, "Constantly. I'd say three times per week." Sexist? Maybe. But let's face it, many women can relate! Dr. Pepper Schwartz says men are indeed more likely to complain that their sex life is lacking. But she also says that while men complain, it's usually women who get the couple into therapy when there are problems.

If *Annie Hall* were seeing a therapist nowadays, she'd probably be asked about more than the number of times per week she's having sex. For years the holy grail for sex researchers (most of them men, of course) was to come up with a cure or treatment for erection problems. Nothing wrong with that goal, of course; I'm all for men having erections. But what about women's sexual problems and issues? Listen to this description of a conference for science writers sponsored by the American Foundation for Urologic Disease in 2000. The conference, the description said, "will feature an update in the field of male sexual dysfunction and introduce female sexual dysfunction to the medical media"—as if they had just discovered that women might have sexual issues or problems.

THE NEW SEXUAL REVOLUTION

The good news is that this conference reflected a dramatic shift in the attention of researchers. It's almost as if everyone is finally realizing that—shock of shocks—there are two people in the sex equation. So now, for the first time, real dollars are flowing into research on female sexuality. Drug companies are working frantically to develop pills and potions to enhance women's sexual experience. Women like Jennifer and Laura Berman are pioneering investigations into the biology and psychology of female sexuality and searching for new ways to treat women's sexual problems. It all amounts to a new sexual revolution that seeks to claim sexual satisfaction and fulfillment for women as a birthright too long ignored.

The bad news is that when the medical and pharmaceutical communities pay attention to an issue, it's usually to throw pills or treatments at it. Every problem or issue becomes a "disorder" or "dysfunction" that requires diagnosis and treatment from properly trained medical practitioners. This approach, say some critics, turns all things sexual into medical and biological issues, matters of blood flow and neurological response, in need of pharmacological intervention.

If women like Erica Jong symbolized the first sexual revolution, the Berman sisters have come to symbolize the new one. Young, photogenic, smart, and sexy, Jennifer and Laura Berman have turned women's sexual satisfaction (and dissatisfaction) into a cottage industry worth millions.

Jennifer Berman, M.D., a urologist by training, and sister Laura, Ph.D., a sex therapist, run the Female Sexual Medicine Center at UCLA and are coauthors of *For Women Only: A Revolutionary Guide to Overcoming Sexual Dysfunction and Reclaiming Your Sex Life.* With their frequent TV appearances they have brought the issue of female sexual satisfaction into the open. They have shown that there are physical reasons that many women have little sex drive, that the problem isn't always in their heads. Why is this important? Because many women still assume either that they're psychologically messed up—"frigid" was the old-fashioned epithet—or they accept the mistaken notion that losing desire is a normal and inevitable part of aging. The Berman sisters are working to prove the falsity of this notion, to put good science in the service of women, and to point the way to good diagnosis and management of women's sexual problems.

A rather different take on women's sexuality comes from Leonore Tiefer, a New York University Ph.D. and sexologist who is fiercely critical of the "medicalization" of women's sexual problems. She expressed this viewpoint well in an essay posted on the online sexuality site Nerve.com. The new attitude toward sex, she wrote, "can be seen today in a rapidly growing industry of hospital-based sex clinics, first for men, now for women, hell-bent on giving every last sexual complaint some medical explanation and expensive medical treatment, funded by a massive advertising budget."

Tiefer and her colleagues also question the assumption that men and women are sexually equivalent and that the answer to women's problems is a "female Viagra." They argue that sex researchers are trying to squeeze women's sexuality into a framework that looks at sex as a biological and mechanical activity that functions well if the sexual parts work and poorly if they don't. The real key to good sex for women, they say, is intimacy and connection with their partner.

Of course, women can and do have real medical problems that interfere with their sexual pleasure, and they should by all means get treatment or help for those problems. But generally, when women lose interest in sex, it may have more to do with their overburdened lives or the fact that their relationships are less fulfilling than they'd like. Women who have sex under these circumstances may feel they are fulfilling an obligation or appeasing their partner—guaranteed turn-offs.

I think an overemphasis on the medical model hurts men as well as women and that intimacy and connection are more important to men than many men or sex researchers will admit. "People are not just medical drawings," says Dr. Pepper Schwartz. "We are complex things of emotions and reactions." In my view, the most overlooked need that men and women have is the need to communicate and understand each other.

Another danger of the new efforts to address "women's sexual dysfunction" is the idea that there is a magical solution that will free women and allow them to be sexually fulfilled—meaning they can and should have lots of orgasms. This threatens to place a new layer of pressure and stress on women to live up to some new social expectation of the sexually liberated woman.

The surge of interest into women's sexuality comes largely from two events. First, the phenomenal success of Viagra for men made it abundantly clear how women have been ignored. And second, the 1999 Chicago Sex Study not only demonstrated that sexual problems among women were much more widespread than anybody realized, but also put it on the front page.

Below is a rundown on some of those problems. Many of them are quite similar to the problems we talked about with men. Others, of course, are unique.

Lack of Desire

Over 30 percent of the women surveyed in the 1994 National Health and Social Life Survey complain that they have little desire for sexual activity, what doctors call *sexual desire disorder.* Since sex is about the body *and* the mind, a lack of sexual desire can have roots in anxiety, depression, poor self-esteem, or other psychological issues. It can also reflect anger or conflict with a partner. But there are also physical causes such as menopause, pregnancy, breast-feeding, illness, pelvic or abdominal surgery, or side effects of antidepressants or other medication. In many cases, both physical and psychological factors combine. As with men, some women have had such negative experiences from trauma or abuse that they avoid sex or become agitated at the prospect of sexual contact. Doctors call this *sexual aversion disorder.*

No Sparks, No Flame

Some women have a desire for sex, but when it comes to actually doing it, they don't get turned on. They don't lubricate, they don't feel much in their clitoris or labia. This problem, *sexual arousal disorder,* can happen as a result of psychological issues or problems in the relationship, but it can also result from the use of medications, pelvic trauma, or surgery. It can also be related to menopause or painful intercourse.

Sex Without Climax

In surveys, around 10 percent of women say they've had lifelong difficulty having an orgasm. And at least half report having this problem on occasion. It is, in short, a very common sexual complaint among women. And as with the other problems, *orgasmic disorder* can be caused by a variety of factors including surgery or trauma, and the use of certain medications. Psychological issues or a history of unpleasant sexual experiences may also contribute to lack of orgasm. Male partners often feel responsible for women not getting an orgasm, and that can contribute to difficulties in a relationship.

Pain with Sex

Again, sex is not supposed to be painful. Yet some women experience painful sex, or *dyspareunia,* quite often. In some cases, contractions in the muscles around the vagina close, making penetration difficult or impossible—as well as painful. This is called *vaginismus.*

TREATMENT FOR WOMEN

The sudden interest in female sexuality and "female sexual dysfunction" has created a burgeoning industry of sexual aids and love potions as well as a feverish hunt for new drugs. Viagra has not proven to be of much help to women and so far, there's no female equivalent, though pharmaceutical companies are spending lots of money to try to find one. The Internet is full of websites hawking products aimed at enhancing women's sexual experience. New York urologist Jed Kaminetsky, M.D., promotes his Dream Cream as "the exciting new cream that enhances female sexual sensation." Another site promotes "ViaGirl, a natural sexual enhancer just for women." Then there's Vitara, Viacreme, Euphoria, and my personal favorite—the name, I mean—Clitoria.

All of these products are nonprescription supplements, which are not regulated and don't need FDA approval. Most contain L-arginine, an amino acid said to increase blood flow to the genitals generally and the clitoris specifically. Some also contain naturally occurring testosterone precursors like DHEA and androstenedione, which signal the body to increase testosterone production, or more exotic-sounding substances such as yohimbe, which is only suspected to raise testosterone levels. Why testosterone? Because men are not the only ones with natural testosterone in their bodies; women produce it too, though in much smaller quantities. It is now being tested as a way to boost sexual desire among women.

Testosterone may increase a woman's libido, but it may also enlarge her clitoris and spur the growth of body or facial hair, significant downsides, to say the least. Increasingly, doctors are giving testosterone to women in creams, pills, or patches as a way to help pick up a flagging sex life. This remains controversial, though many experts including the Berman sisters champion its use by women with low sexual desire and low testosterone levels. Keep in mind that the long-term effects of testosterone have not been studied.

Medications and creams are not the only products out there. In 2000, the FDA approved a small suction device known as Eros-CTD (clitoral therapy device). Produced by the U.S. company Urometrics and available by prescription at a cost of around $400, the Eros-CTD is designed to fit over the clitoris and provide gentle suction to increase blood flow and improve sensation. Studies suggest that it may help women who are often dry, or who don't seem to have much sensation, become better lubricated, with improved sensation and better orgasms.

23

Narcissus—What a Guy!

We are all familiar with the Greek myth of Narcissus, the beautiful young man who fell in love with his own reflection in a pool. He died of sorrow because he could not bear to leave his own image. In his place grew a flower that now bears his name. Your guy may not have as big a problem with his own appearance as Narcissus, but these days he is likely to be feeling increased pressure about his looks. It's a new world out there—a youth-obsessed culture that affects women, as we know, but also increasingly men. Guys today cannot get by on a good shave, a nice trim, and a few slaps of Old Spice. Oh no. To succeed in today's competitive environment men need much, much more.

Weight loss researcher Kelly Brownell of Yale sees it firsthand. "Back in the '60s and '70s a man who was thin and muscular was considered the ideal for attractiveness. But now you get these images of guys that are incredibly well designed. And so words like *cut* and *buff* are now part of the language. Think about the abdominal business, for example. You've got this incredible pressure on people that's so precise to an area of the body, that's about six square inches. Just being overall fit is no longer good enough. You have to have sculpted abs. If you add it all up, what it means is intense pressure that's basically relentless. And it shows that nobody's good enough." Brownell adds, "If you go in search of a woman who's happy with her body, you're gonna have a long search without much payoff. Because even if a woman is happy with her weight, she's not gonna like her nose, or her feet, or her butt, or something. And now, the same thing's happening with men."

I have only one thing to say: "Welcome to the club, guys!"

THE NEW MALE VANITY

Get ready to shop, boys. There are hundreds of new products, procedures, and pills aimed at helping you look your best. Guys, it seems, are buying into it, shelling out the dough in hopes of a more lovely appearance. Companies can't come up with new marketing plans fast enough to cash in. So "Are Men the New Women?" as *New York* magazine asked in a 2001 cover story. The upshot of the article was that men are now indulging in everything from plastic surgery to manicures and pedicures, hair high-lights and even—for God's sake—wearing makeup!

Sales of beauty products packaged to appeal to men have also jumped. One product line called Zirh Skin Nutrition experienced a 307 percent increase in sales according to the *New York* article after the product was featured in a *Sex and the City* episode and during the Tom Cruise movie *Eyes Wide Shut*. A large number of cosmetic and personal care companies that are now producing and marketing products for men—encouraging them to cleanse, exfoliate, tone, and moisturize.

Whether or not you think this sort of thing should be left exclusively to women, there is one definite health benefit—moisturizers with sunscreens. Men in general tend to avoid sunscreen, thinking (incorrectly) that they are immune to the damaging and potentially cancer-causing rays of the sun or preferring that weather-beaten look. If you encourage one beauty trend that's guaranteed to produce results, make it sunscreen, good sunglasses, and a hat! If you notice a suspicious mole or growth, encourage him to get it checked out. For men, though, there may be more at stake than just looking good. Job security could be on the line. Staying young-looking and improving one's professional image may be the only way to keep the kids coming up the ladder from taking your office. Not only does a guy need an Ivy League education to make it on Wall Street, he also needs a strong jaw line. Hence the chin implant. It is no longer the norm that dad works for the company for thirty years then retires. Nowadays men are likely to switch jobs several times in their lives. All the while they need to battle an ever-growing younger pool of competitors.

Some of this objectification of men is leading them to some of the same unhealthy extremes that women have indulged in for decades. In their book *Making Weight: Healing Men's Conflicts With Food, Weight, and Shape*, authors Arnold Andersen, M.D., Leigh Cohn, and Thomas Holbrook, M.D., examine this new phenomenon and point out that at least one in six people with eating disorders are men. Few people, including health providers, understand that men are at risk for these problems. Further, men are much less likely than women to talk about it and much more likely to use exercise rather than diet to control their shape. Increasingly, images of impossibly buff guys raise the bar ever higher for men (see chapter 6).

WHEN MEN GO UNDER THE KNIFE

According to the American Society for Aesthetic Plastic Surgery, men had over 1 million cosmetic surgical and nonsurgical procedures in 2001, amounting to nearly 12 percent of the 8.5 million cosmetic procedures preformed during that year. That's a nearly 300 percent increase from 1997! The top five surgical procedures for men were lipoplasty (liposuction), nose reshaping, eyelid surgery, breast reduction (treatment of gynecomastia), and face-lift, according the American Society of Aesthetic Plastic Surgery. Baby Boomers between thirty and fifty had the most procedures—44 percent of the total.

Gerald Imber, M.D., a plastic surgeon in New York City and author of *For Men Only: Looking Your Best Through Science, Surgery, and Common Sense* sees an ever-growing number of men in his office seeking procedures such as liposuction for love handles and double chin repair. "They are delighted to have gray hair and wrinkles that make them look powerful and distinguished, but bags under their eyes make them look dissipated," says Dr. Imber. "They want vitality. They are CEOs who play two hours of tennis a day and they want to look vital." Though men rely on women for almost every other medical decision, when it comes to plastic surgery the partner gets cut out of the picture, according to Dr. Imber. "Men always come in alone [and] have done a lot of introspection before they see me."

But the macho façade fades once the actual knife gets waved around according to Dr. Imber. "They push themselves, but they are terrible patients. They ask no questions, they have done no homework, no research. They faint when we put in the IV and then afterwards it's as if it never happened and I never see them again."

Women, on the other hand, are much less secretive, according to Dr. Imber. "They talk to everyone about it. They talk before; they talk afterwards. For men it didn't happen."

While a face-lift may provide a temporary boost in self-esteem and make a man feel more competitive, there is no research that shows that it will actually help him secure another job or beat out a man twenty years younger for a better position.

If your partner is considering going under the knife, you can help him by making sure he (or you) has done the research and sought the skills of a qualified surgeon.

HOLD THE COMB-OVER PLEASE!

Except for bulging biceps and a square jaw, nothing says "masculine" like a thick head of hair. It was all over for Samson when the hair went. Despite Michael Jordan's efforts, baldness is still the number-one vanity complaint for nearly 50 million American adult males. Male pattern baldness is completely normal, the result of genetics and the hormone testosterone. While many men like to blame their mother's side of the family, male pattern baldness can be inherited from either side of the family. The genetics of male pattern baldness are complex and there is a great deal of variability. Both parents can have great heads of hair well into old age, but their son can begin balding at twenty. At any rate it's time to let Mom's family off the hook where baldness is concerned. Testosterone is essential for the process, but the actual culprit is an enzyme called 5-alpha reductase, which converts testosterone to dihydrotestosterone, or DHT. DHT stimulates growth in hair follicles in the beard and body. Here's the heartbreak for millions of men. DHT has the opposite effect on scalp hair. Were it not for this offending enzyme, there would be no multibillion-dollar hair-loss industry.

Men try all sorts of things to disguise a balding pate, and let's be honest, very few of them actually work. We can spot 'em a mile away—the weaves, the comb-overs, the toupees, the transplant plugs, and on and on. If I were to give men one piece of beauty advice it would be to forget about trying to fool us (or yourself) about the status of your hair. Most of us could not care less! (Of course, I know this pep talk will have little effect on men's feelings about their hairline.)

Hair transplants have improved over the years, but many men still come away with a less than natural look. Before your partner plunks down a small fortune (as steep as $60,000) for a new head of hair, try telling him about the Tsavo lions of western Kenya. These lions are unique. They have a bad reputation for eating humans, and they live in harems (one male with seven females—usually male lions have to share the females with other males). Finally, the Tsavo males have no manes because they have more testosterone than any other kind of lion. Who says bald guys aren't virile?

Afterword

We began this book by pointing out some of the ways that men ignore and subvert their own health. What's encouraging is that this subject is finally getting more attention, that small changes are indeed taking place. A growing men's health movement is raising awareness about these issues and looking for ways to improve the health and longevity of men. Men's health issues are getting more coverage in the media. And many new parents are trying to raise their sons with a different set of attitudes toward their bodies and their health.

Then there's this encouraging sign: In the year 2000, according to the CDC, the life expectancy of American men reached 74.1 years, a record high. That means that men, on average, lived two tenths of a year longer than they did in 1999. The longevity gap—the difference in life expectancy between men and women—narrowed slightly as well.

Since we began this project in the summer of 2001, much has happened in the world as well. Fear of a kind unknown to most Americans came into our lives, and it lives on in color-coded terror alerts, endless airport security lines, and in a general unease and anxiety that is especially prominent here in New York. At times like these, the support and love of friends and family has never been more important.

How fitting, then, that as we researched this book—talking to doctors, interviewing experts, and reviewing key studies—one theme in particular kept coming up. What helps us all stay healthy is not so much having access to the latest drugs and the newest medical technology but rather the way we live. I'm not just talking about what we eat and drink, and how much exercise we get, though these things are vitally important. I'm thinking also about the way we communicate and connect with the people and world around us.

The health and well-being of all people, including boys and men, depends a great deal on the importance of what psychologists call "support systems" and the rest of us call friends and family. People who are in enduring relationships or have rich social connections get sick less often, are less prone to chronic diseases, and recover better from surgery and illness. As women, we lead the way in forging these kinds of connections and providing attention and care to all the people in our lives—to sons and daughters, partners and parents. The more men learn about the importance of these connections, the better off they—and we—will be.

Resources

PART ONE: SONS

1: It's a Boy! (But First It's a Girl)

American Academy of Pediatrics
This professional pediatrician organization's website has a section, "You and Your Family," that contains information on immunizations, pediatric subspecialties, children's health, and other topics.

141 Northwest Point Boulevard
Elk Grove Village, IL 60007-1098
847-434-4000
www.aap.org

Brott, Armin A., and Jennifer Ash. *The Expectant Father: Facts, Tips, and Advice for Dads-to-Be.* Abbeville Press, 2001.

Davis, Ian. *My Boys Can Swim: The Official Guy's Guide to Pregnancy.* Prima Publishing, 1999.

Hill, Thomas. *What to Expect When Your Wife Is Expanding.* Andrews McMeel Publishing, 1993.

Pruett, Kyle. *Fatherneed: Why Father Care Is As Essential As Mother Care for Your Child.* Broadway Books, 2001.

Reuben, Carolyn. *The Healthy Baby Book: A Parent's Guide to Preventing Birth Defects and Other Long-Term Medical Problems Before, and After Pregnancy.* Greensland Publishing Co., 1992.

Sussman, John R., and B. Blake Levitt. *Before You Conceive: The Complete Prepregnancy Guide.* Bantam Doubleday Dell, 1989.

Boy Anxiety

Bassoff, Evelyn S. *Between Mothers and Sons: The Making of Vital and Loving Men.* Dutton, 1994.

Caron, Ann F. *Strong Mothers, Strong Sons: Raising the Next Generation of Men.* Perennial, 1995.

Karlin, Elyse Zorn, and Muriel Warren. *Sons, A Mother's Manual.* Avon Books, 1994.

Stevens, Patricia. *Between Mothers and Sons: Women Writers Talk About Having Sons and Raising Men.* New York: Scribner, 1999.

The Weaker Sex

The National Institutes of Health website is loaded with information on the various diseases discussed in this chapter. Visit the government agency's main page at *www.nih.gov/icd* to link to its many institutes, such as the National Heart, Lung, and Blood Institute, the National Institute of Arthritis and Musculoskeletal and Skin Disease, and the National Institute of Child Health and Human Development. The publications list under this last institute, found at *www.nichd.nih.gov/publications/pubskey.cfm,* features downloadable reports regarding the latest research on many childhood and genetic diseases.

March of Dimes (Birth Defects Foundation)
This national nonprofit foundation works to combat birth defects; its website contains information on genetics and pregnancy and prevention techniques.

1275 Mamaroneck Avenue
White Plains, NY 10605
888-MODIMES or 888-663-4633
www.modimes.org

Duchenne's Muscular Dystrophy
Muscular Dystrophy Association—USA
This group's website contains a wealth of information on Duchenne's muscular dystrophy, ranging from basic informational articles to current medical research to ongoing clinical trials.

National Headquarters
3300 East Sunrise Drive
Tucson, AZ 85718
800-572-1717
www.mdausa.org

Parent Project Muscular Dystrophy
This nonprofit organization's website offers a message board and information on treatment and research for Duchenne's and Becker Muscular Dystrophy.)

1012 North University Boulevard
Middletown, OH 45042
800-714-5437
http://parentprojectmd.org

Emery, Alan E. H. *Muscular Dystrophy: The Facts.* Oxford University Press, 2000.
Siegel, Irwin M. *Muscular Dystrophy in Children: A Guide for Families.* SCB Distributors, 1999.

Hemophilia
National Hemophilia Foundation
This foundation's web page has information about all bleeding disorders, blood safety, treatment guidelines, new treatment, and insurance issues.

116 West 32nd Street, 11th Floor
New York, NY 10001
800-424-2634
www.hemophilia.org

World Federation of Hemophilia

This international nonprofit's website has an "About Hemophilia" section with general information, frequently asked questions, and an "ask-the-doc" section, as well as a history and timeline of hemophilia.

1425 René Lévesque Boulevard West, Suite 1010
Montreal, Quebec
H3G 1T7 Canada
514-875-7944
www.wfh.org

Fragile X Syndrome

Carolina Fragile X Project

This project's site features summaries of current research, information on how to care for children with FXS, and case studies of families of children with the disease.

FPG Child Development Institute
Campus Box 8180
University of North Carolina at Chapel Hill
Chapel Hill, NC 27599-8180
919-966-2622
www.fpg.unc.edu/~fx

FRAXA Research Foundation

This private organization's website contains general information about Fragile X, treatment, and research.

45 Pleasant Street
Newburyport, MA 01950
978-462-1866
www.fraxa.org

The National Fragile X Foundation

This foundation's web page offers support to families affected by the disease as well as links, research, and a quarterly newsletter.

P.O. Box 190488
San Francisco, CA 94119
925-938-9300
www.fragilex.org

Hagerman, Randi Jenssen, and Paul J. Hagerman, eds. *Fragile X Syndrome: Diagnosis, Treatment, and Research.* Johns Hopkins University Press, 2002.

Parker, James N., and Philip M. Parker, eds. *The 2002 Official Patient's Source Book on Fragile X Syndrome.* Icon Group International, 2002.

Weber, Jayne D., ed. *Children with Fragile X Syndrome: A Parents' Guide.* Woodbine House, 2000.

XXY Males (Klinefelter's Syndrome)

Klinefelter's Syndrome and Associates

This nonprofit's website features basic information, a newsletter, and information on Klinefelter's syndrome support groups around the country.

P.O. Box 119
Roseville, CA 95678-0119
888-XXY-WHAT (888-999-9428)
www.genetic.org/ks

Parker, James N., and Phillip M. Parker. *The Official Parent's Sourcebook on Klinefelter Syndrome: A Revised and Updated Directory for the Internet Age.* Icon Health Publications, 2002.

Cleft Lip and Cleft Palate

Children's Craniofacial Association

This nonprofit's website provides information on financial assistance and support groups for people with facial differences and their families.

13140 Coit Road, Suite 307
Dallas, TX 75240
800-535-3643
www.ccakids.com

Cleft Palate Foundation

This group's website provides lot of information on cleft lips and palates, surgery and treatment options, and support services.

104 South Estes Drive, Suite 204
Chapel Hill, NC 27514
919-933-9044 or 800-24-CLEFT
www.cleftline.org

The Smile Train Headquarters

This international children's charity has a "public library" on its website with extensive, easy-to-understand information on all aspects of cleft lip and cleft palate.

245 5th Avenue, Suite 2201
New York, NY 10016
877-KIDSMILE (877-543-7645)
www.smiletrain.org

Gruman-Trinker, Carrie T., and Blaise Winter. *Your Cleft-Affected Child: The Complete Book of Information, Resources, and Hope.* Publishers Group West, 2001.

Circumcision

Circumcision: A Lifetime of Medical Benefits

A website run by Dr. Edgar J. Schoen, a proponent of circumcision who presents information on the medical benefits, science, and history of circumcision.

http://www.medicirc.com/

Circumcision Information and Resource Pages

An objective website that covers both sides of issues.

www.cirp.org

Circumcision Resource Center

An anticircumcision nonprofit group.

P.O. Box 232
Boston, MA 02133
617-523-0088
www.circumcision.org

National Organization of Circumcision Information Resource Centers (NOCIRC)

An anticircumcision nonprofit group.

P.O. Box 2512
San Anselmo, CA 94979-2572
415-488-9883
www.nocirc.org

Fleiss, Paul M., and Frederick M. Hodges. *What Your Doctor May Not Tell You About Circumcision: Untold Facts on America's Most Widely Performed and Most Unnecessary Surgery.* New York: Warner Books, 2002.

Gollaher, David L. *Circumcision: A History of the World's Most Controversial Surgery.* New York: Basic Books, 2001.

Kimmel, Michael. "The Kindest Un-Cut: Feminism, Judaism and My Son's Foreskin," *Tikkun,* May/June 2001, pp. 41–44.

Family Jewels

American Foundation for Urologic Disease

A nonprofit group working to prevent and cure urologic disease through patient education, research, and advocacy.

1128 North Charles Street
Baltimore, MD 21201
410-468-1800
www.afud.org

American Urological Association
The professional group sponsors an excellent website for patients.

1120 North Charles Street
Baltimore, MD 21201
410-727-1100
http://www.urologyhealth.org

Intersex

Intersex Society of North America (ISNA)
An advocacy group against shame and unwanted surgery for intersex people.

4500 9th Avenue NE, Suite 300
Seattle, WA 98105
206-633-6077
www.isna.org

Preves, Sharon E. *Intersex and Identity: The Contested Self.* Rutgers University Press, 2003.

Boys Versus Girls

Morris Shaffer, Susan, and Linda Perlman Gordon. *Why Boys Don't Talk and Why We Care: A Mothers' Guide to Connection.* Mid-Atlantic Equity Consortium, 2000.

Pyloric Stenosis

Hypertrophic Pyloric Stenosis
The Yale University Department of Surgery offers a primer on this condition.

http://yalesurgery.med.yale.edu/surgery/sections/ped_surg/pyloric.htm

G6PD

An Introduction to G6PD Deficiency
A personal website with lots of information and links on G6PD.

www.rialto.com/g6pd

G6PD Deficiency
KidsHealth, a project of the Nemours Foundation, offers an informational page on G6PD deficiency.

http://kidshealth.org/parent/general/aches/g6pd.html

Autism

Autism Society of America
This society, formed by parents of autistic children in 1965, now has 200 chapters and 20,000 members nationwide. The website contains helpful articles on the diagnosis, treatment, research, and education methods for both autism and Asperger's disorder.

7910 Woodmont Avenue, Suite 300
Bethesda, MD 20814-3067
301-657-0881 or 800-3-AUTISM
www.autism-society.org

The CDC's Autism Page
The National Center on Birth Defects and Developmental Disabilities, part of the U.S. government's Centers for Disease Control and Prevention (CDC), offers basic information about autism, information on state and federal programs concerning autism, and countless links to other information sources about the condition.

National Center on Birth Defects and Developmental Disabilities
Centers for Disease Control and Prevention
1600 Clifton Road
Atlanta, GA 30333
404-498-3800
http://www.cdc.gov/ncbddd/dd/ddautism.htm

Siegel, Bryna. *The World of the Autistic Child: Understanding and Treating Autistic Spectrum Disorders.* Oxford University Press, 1998.

Tourette's Syndrome
Tourette's Syndrome Association
The website of this nonprofit volunteer group provides information on support services nationwide as well as information on Tourette's for the newly diagnosed and recent news on research and treatment. Call for a free information packet.

42-40 Bell Boulevard
Bayside, NY 11361
718-224-2999
www.tsa-usa.org

Tourette's Syndrome Plus
This award-winning website is put together by Leslie Packer, Ph.D., a New York psychologist who specializes in Tourette's and whose husband and two children have the disorder. It contains hundreds of articles on all aspects of the syndrome and of other conditions commonly associated with it, like ADHD.

www.tourettesyndrome.net

The National Institutes of Health's Tourette's Syndrome Page
Provides links to many government sites about Tourette's research, clinical trials, and treatment.

http://www.nlm.nih.gov/medlineplus/tourettesyndrome.html

Hearle, Tracy, ed. *Children with Tourette Syndrome: A Parent's Guide.* Special Needs Collection. Woodbine House, 2003.

Mental Retardation/Developmental Disabilities

The Arc of the United States

This national nonprofit organization has one thousand local chapters and 140,000 members and focuses on advocating for the rights and adequate support services for people with mental retardation and related developmental disabilities and their families. The website provides basic information on mental retardation as well as on support services and topics like education, employment, and self-determination.

1010 Wayne Avenue, Suite 650
Silver Spring, MD 20910
301-565-3842
www.thearc.org

The National Institutes of Health's Developmental Disabilities Page

Provides links to many government and nongovernment sites about developmental disabilities research, treatment, and advocacy.

http://www.nlm.nih.gov/medlineplus/developmentaldisabilities.html

Trainer, Marilyn. *Differences in Common: Straight Talk on Mental Retardation, Down Syndrome and Your Life.* Woodbine House, 2003.

Environmental Concerns

Natural Resources Defense Council (NRDC)

A nonprofit environmental group whose website has information on everything from global warming to pesticides.

40 West 20th Street
New York, NY 10011
212-727-2700
www.nrdc.org

U.S. Department of Agriculture (USDA)

The federal agency responsible for the safety of meat and agricultural products.

Room 416-A, Whitten Building
Washington, DC 20250-1330
202-720-2791
www.usda.gov

U.S. Environmental Protection Agency (EPA)

The federal agency responsible for protecting human health and the environment—air, water, and land.

Ariel Rios Building
1200 Pennsylvania Avenue NW
Mail Code 3213A
Washington, DC 20460

202-260-2090
www.epa.gov

U.S. Food and Drug Administration (FDA)
The federal government's consumer protection agency which oversees the safety of all food products sold in the country.

5600 Fishers Lane
Rockville, MD 20857-001
888-INFO-FDA
www.fda.gov

2: Snips and Snails

New York University Child Study Center maintains a website AboutOurKids. They also have a resource section for books on a variety of issues.

www.aboutourkids.org/books/index.html

The Parents Place
An iVillage website with articles and message boards on all aspects of parenting.

www.parentsplace.com

Brazelton, Berry T., and Joshua D. Sparrow. *Discipline: The Brazelton Way.* Perseus Publishing, 2003.
Elium, Don, and Jeanne Elium. *Raising a Son: Parents and the Making of a Healthy Man.* Celestial Arts, 1996.
Gurian, Michael. *The Wonder of Boys: What Parents, Mentors, and Educators Can Do to Shape Boys into Exceptional Men.* J. P. Tarcher, 1997.
———. *The Good Son: Shaping the Moral Development of Our Boys and Young Men.* J. P. Tarcher, 2000.
Kindlon, Daniel J., and Michael Thompson. *Raising Cain: Protecting the Emotional Life of Boys.* New York: Ballantine Books, 2000.
Pollock, William S. *Real Boys: Rescuing Our Sons from the Myths of Boyhood.* Owl Books, 1999.
Thompson, Michael, and Teresa Barker. *Speaking of Boys: Answers to the Most-Asked Questions About Raising Boys.* New York: Ballantine Books, 2000.

Violence
Talking with Kids About Violence
A website by Children Now and the Kaiser Family Foundation.

www.talkingwithkids.org/violence.html

Cappello, Dominic. *Ten Talks Parents Must Have with Their Kids About Violence.* New York: Hyperion, 2000.

Boys and School

No Child Left Behind
President George W. Bush's education policy website features tips for parents.

www.nclb.gov/parents/index.html

U.S. Department of Education
U.S. government site has information and tips on education and learning.

http://www.ed.gov/index.jsp

Greene, Ross W. *The Explosive Child: A New Approach for Understanding and Parenting Easily Frustrated, Chronically Inflexible Children.* HarperCollins, 2001.

Gurian, Michael. *Boys and Girls Learn Differently!: A Guide for Teachers and Parents.* Jossey-Bass, 2002.

Levine, Mel. *A Mind at a Time.* New York: Touchstone Books, 2003.

Turecki, Stanley, and Leslie Tonner. *The Difficult Child.* New York: Bantam Doubleday Dell, 2000.

Learning Disabilities

LDOnline
Nonprofit group's website with tons of general and detailed information on learning disabilities for parents, kids, and teachers.

www.ldonline.org

Shaywitz, Sally. *Overcoming Dyslexia: A New and Complete Science-Based Program for Reading Problems at any Level.* Alfred A. Knopf, 2003.

Levine, Mel. *Keeping a Head in School: A Student's Book About Learning Abilities and Learning Disorders.* Educators Publishing Service, 1991.

Rimm, Sylvia B. *Dr. Sylvia Rimm's Smart Parenting: How to Raise a Happy, Achieving Child.* Crown Publishers, 1996.

Child Mental Health

American Academy of Child and Adolescent Psychiatry
The web page of this top professional organization of child and adolescent psychiatrists offers fact sheets for parents on the various mental illnesses and mental health issues affecting children today.

3615 Wisconsin Avenue NW
Washington, DC 20016-3007
202-966-7300
www.aacap.org

The National Institutes of Health's Child Mental Health Page
Provides links to many government and nongovernment sites about research, treatment, and advocacy for children with mental disorders.

http://www.nlm.nih.gov/medlineplus/childmentalhealth.html

The U.S. Department of Health and Human Service's Child Mental Health Page
This web page provided by the DHHS's Center for Mental Health Services provides information about government services and a variety of links to programs for children's mental health. Free pamphlets may also be ordered.

www.mentalhealth.samhsa.gov/child/childhealth.asp

Koplewicz, Harold S. *It's Nobody's Fault: New Hope and Help for Difficult Children and Their Parents.* New York: Times Books, 1997.

American Academy of Child and Adolescent Psychiatry (AACP)
The Facts for Families section of this website contains descriptions of various mental illnesses.

3615 Wisconsin Avenue, NW
Washington, DC 20016-3007
202-966-7300
www.aacap.org

SOS Fires: Youth Intervention Programs
Website contains helpful articles, FAQs, and links about fire-setting by children and teens.

449 S.E. 15th Street
Gresham, OR 97080
503-805-8482
www.sosfires.com

Obsessive-Compulsive Disorder
American Academy of Child and Adolescent Psychiatry
The children's OCD web page of this top professional organization of child and adolescent psychiatrists offers basic facts for parents of children and adolescents with OCD.

3615 Wisconsin Avenue NW
Washington, DC 20016-3007
202-966-7300
http://www.aacap.org/publications/factsfam/ocd.htm

Anxiety Disorders Association of America
The web page of this national nonprofit organization provides basic information about OCD and other anxiety disorders, as well as an OCD self-test and a list of treatment providers by geographic area.

8730 Georgia Avenue, Suite 600
Silver Spring, MD 20910
240-485-1001
http://www.adaa.org

The National Institutes of Health's Obsessive-Compulsive Disorder Page
Provides links to many government and nongovernment sites about diagnosis, research and treatment for obsessive-compulsive disorder.

http://www.nlm.nih.gov/medlineplus/obsessivecompulsivedisorder.html

Obsessive-Compulsive Foundation
The web page of this nonprofit organization provides basic information on OCD in adults and children as well as a newsletter, links to support groups, and a list of mental health professionals who specialize in OCD.

337 Notch Hill Road
North Branford, CT 06471
203-315-2190
www.ocfoundation.org

Chanksy, Tamar E. *Freeing Your Child from Obsessive-Compulsive Disorder: A Powerful, Practical Program for Parents of Children and Adolescents.* Three Rivers Press, 2001.
Waltz, Mitzi. *Obsessive-Compulsive Disorder: Help for Children and Adolescents.* Patient-Centered Guides, 2000.

Boys and AD/HD

Barkley, Russell. *Taking Charge of ADHD, Revised Edition: The Complete, Authoritative Guide for Parents.* Guilford Press, 2000.
Zeigler Dendy, Chris A. *Teenagers with ADD: A Parent's Guide.* Woodbine House, 1995.

FOR CHILDREN

Moss, Deborah M. *Shelly, the Hyperactive Turtle.* Woodbine House, 1989.
Quinn, Patricia O., and Judith M. Stern. *Putting on the Brakes: Young People's Guide to Understanding Attention Deficit Hyperactivity Disorder.* Magination, 2001.

Bullying

Bully-Free Living
An individual's website with articles for parents of both the bullies and the bullied.

www.bullyfreekids.com

Colorado Anti-Bullying Project
The state's campaign site includes lots of useful information for parents, teachers, and kids.

http://no-bully.com

The Safe Child Home Page's Bully Page
A nonprofit group's site with lots of advice and links to research on bullying.

www.safechild.org/bullies.htm

Coloroso, Barbara. *The Bully, the Bullied, and the Bystander: From Preschool to High School, How Parents and Teachers Can Help Break the Cycle of Violence.* HarperResource, 2003.

3: Boys and Accidents and Injuries

National Center for Injury Prevention and Control (NCIPC)
The U.S. government's Centers for Disease Control and Prevention site on preventing accidental injuries.

Mailstop K65
4770 Buford Highway NE
Atlanta, GA 30341-3724
770-488-1506
http://www.cdc.gov/ncipc

National SAFE KIDS Campaign
A national nonprofit group dedicated to preventing accidental injuries among kids. Website features many tips and articles.

1301 Pennsylvania Avenue, NW, Suite 1000
Washington, DC 20004
202-662-0600
www.safekids.org

Widome, Mark D. *Ask Dr. Mark: Answers for Parents.* National Safety Council, 2003.

4: Boys and Body Control

Dr. Spock
A website of advice put together by doctors who follow in the footsteps of the legendary pediatrician Dr. Benjamin Spock. The "Infant" and "Toddler" sections are especially helpful.

www.drspock.com

Stuttering Foundation of America
This nonprofit's website provides information and resources for those who stutter and their families.

3100 Walnut Grove Road, Suite 603
Memphis, TN 38111-0749
800-967-7700
www.stutteringhelp.org

American Academy of Pediatrics and Steven P. Shelov, ed. *Caring for Your Baby and Young Child: Birth to Age 5.* New York: Bantam Doubleday Dell, 1998.

Brazelton, Berry T., and Joshua D. Sparrow. *Calming Your Fussy Baby: The Brazelton Way.* Perseus Publishing, 2003.
————. *Sleep: The Brazelton Way.* Perseus Publishing, 2003.
Ferber, Richard. *Solve Your Child's Sleep Problems.* New York: Fireside, 1986.
Kirby, Amanda. *Dyspraxia: The Hidden Handicap.* Souvenir Press, 2002.

5: The Care and Feeding of Boys

FOR YOUNG BOYS

Children's Hospital Medical Center of Akron
   Hospital website contains great information for kids and parents.

   www.akronchildrens.org

FOR TEENS

HealthFinder
   The U.S. Department of Health and Human Service's special health website has a section for teens under the "Just for You" categories.

   www.healthfinder.gov/justforyou

On the Teen Scene
   The U.S. Food and Drug Administration's website for teens.

   http://www.fda.gov/opacom/7teens.html

TeenGrowth
   A physician-reviewed website for teens about all their health questions.

   www.teengrowth.com

TeensHealth
   The Nemours Foundation website offers nutrition and health information for teens; interactive format features quizzes and graphics.

   www.teenshealth.org/teen

FOR PARENTS

KidsHealth Parents' Site
   The Nemours Foundation website offers nutrition and health information for parents.

   www.kidshealth.org/parent

Lopez, Ralph I. *The Teen Health Book: A Parents' Guide to Adolescent Health and Well-Being.* New York: W. W. Norton & Company, 2002.

Marks, Andrea, and Betty Rothbart. *Healthy Teens, Body and Soul: A Parent's Complete Guide.* New York: Fireside, 2003.

Slap, Gail B., and Martha M. Jablow. *Teenage Health Care: The First Comprehensive Family Guide for the Preteen to Young Adult Years.* New York: Pocket Books, 1994.

6: When Things Go Wrong

Obesity

Centers for Disease Control and Prevention's Obesity Information

The U.S. government disease prevention agency offers information on obesity trends among children and adults.

www.cdc.gov/nccdphp/dnpa/obesity

Brownell, Kelly, and Katherine Battle Horgen. *Food Fight: The Inside Story of the Food Industry, America's Obesity Crisis & What We Can Do About It.* McGraw-Hill Books, 2003.

Sothern, Melinda S., and T. Kristian von Almen. *Trim Kids: The Proven 12-Week Plan That Has Helped Thousands of Children Achieve a Healthier Weight.* HarperResource, 2001.

Stature and Status

Human Growth Foundation

This nonprofit organization's website contains information on human growth disorders, clinical trials, and treatments.

997 Glen Cove Avenue
Glen Head, NY 11545
800-451-6434
www.hgfound.org

The Magic Foundation

This nonprofit organization's website offers information on all syndromes, clinical trials, a page for kids, and a listserv.

6645 W. North Avenue
Oak Park, IL 60302
708-383-0808
www.magicfoundation.org

National Marfan Foundation

This organization's website offers general information on Marfan syndrome, a newsletter, and resources.

22 Manhasset Avenue
Port Washington, NY 11050
800-8-MARFAN
www.marfan.org

Eating Disorders

National Association of Anorexia Nervosa and Associated Disorders (ANAD)

This volunteer advocacy group's website provides information on the disorders, resources, and support.

P.O. Box 7
Highland Park, IL 60035
847-831-3438
www.anad.org

National Eating Disorders Association (NEDA)

Website contains lots of information on all eating disorders, treatment options, and support.

603 Stewart Street, Suite 803
Seattle, WA 98101
206-382-3587
www.nationaleatingdisorders.org

Steroids and Supplements

Adolescents and Anabolic Steroid Use

The American Academy of Pediatrics' position paper on adolescents and steroids.

www.aap.org/policy/970601.html

National Institute on Drug Abuse (NIDA): Steroids

This U.S. government web page offers the most recent research and tips for parents and teens.

www.drugabuse.gov/drugpages/steroids.html

Steroid Abuse

A website of the National Institute on Drug Abuse.
www.steroidabuse.org

Steroids: Play Safe, Play Fair

The American Academy of Pediatrics' information sheet on the dangers of steroid and supplement use.

www.aap.org/family/steroids.htm

Monroe, Judy. *Steroid Drug Dangers.* Enslow Publishers, 1999.
Yesalis, Charles E., and Virginia S. Cowart. *The Steroids Game.* Human Kinetics Publishers, 1998.

Things Only Boys Get

American Foundation for Urologic Disease (AFUD)

This nonprofit organization's website provides information on various conditions, clinical trials, research, and resources.

1128 North Charles Street
Baltimore, MD 21201
410-468-1800
www.afud.org

Gynecomastia.org
An individual's website with basic information, discussion boards, and treatment options.

www.gynecomastia.org

7: *Sturm und Drang?* The Teen Years

About.com's Parenting Adolescents Website
http://parentingteens.about.com/mbody.htm

Gianetti, Charlene C., and Margaret Sagarese. *The Roller-Coaster Years: Raising Your Child Through the Maddening Yet Magical Middle School Years.* New York: Broadway Books, 1997.
Panzarine, Susan. *A Parent's Guide to the Teen Years: Raising Your 11- to 14-Year-Old in the Age of Chat Rooms and Navel Rings.* Checkmark Books, 2000.

Boys and Cars
American Automobile Association. *AAA's Teaching Your Teens to Drive.* Order a copy from the AAA by calling 800-327-3444.

Mothers Against Drunk Driving (MADD)
This drunk-driving victims' organization's website has information for parents, teens, and teachers.

511 E. John Carpenter Freeway, Suite 700
Irving, TX 75062
800-GET-MADD
www.madd.org

Students Against Destructive Decisions (SADD) a.k.a. Students Against Drunk Driving
P.O. Box 800
Marlboro, MA 01752
877-SADD-INC
www.sadd.org

Teen Drivers
The National Center for Injury Prevention and Control's statistics sheet on teen drivers.

www.cdc.gov/ncipc/factsheets/teenmvh.htm

Boys, Smoking, Drinking, and Drugs

Alcohol and Drug Information

The U.S. Department of Health and Human Services offers a great site full of articles and interactive guides about drugs and alcohol and how to talk to your children; also has a section for youth.

www.health.org

National Institute on Drug Abuse

This U.S. government website has many different interactive sites about drugs for parents, youth, and teachers.

www.drugabuse.gov

Capello, Dominic, and Xenia G. Becher. *Ten Talks Parents Must Have with Their Children About Drugs and Choices.* New York: Hyperion, 2001.

Mannion, Michael T. *How to Help Your Teenager Stop Smoking.* Welcome Rain, 2000.

Schwebel, Robert, and George D. Comerci. *Keep Your Kids Tobacco-Free: Smart Strategies for Parents of Children Ages 3 to 19.* Newmarket Press, 2001.

———. *Saying No Is Not Enough: Helping Your Kids Make Wise Decisions About Alcohol, Tobacco, and Other Drugs—A Guide for Parents of Children Ages 3 to 19.* Newmarket Press, 1998.

Boys, Depression, and Suicide

American Foundation for Suicide Prevention (AFSP)

National organization's website provides general information and statistics on suicide and depression as well as links and resources.

120 Wall Street, 22nd Floor
New York, NY 10005
888-333-AFSP
www.afsp.org

National Youth Violence Prevention Resource Center

The Centers for Disease Control and Prevention's youth website for teens about suicide has tons of great information and links to other resources.

http://www.safeyouth.org/teens/topics/teen_suicide.htm

Cobain, Bev. *When Nothing Matters Anymore: A Survival Guide for Depressed Teens.* Free Spirit Publishing, 1998.

Oster, Gerald D., and Sarah S. Montgomery. *Helping Your Depressed Teenager: A Guide for Parents and Caregivers.* John Wiley & Sons, 1994.

William, Kate. *A Parent's Guide for Suicidal and Depressed Teens: Help for Recognizing If a Child Is in Crisis and What to Do About It.* Hazelden Information Education, 1995.

Boys and Boot Camp

Boys & Girls Clubs of America

The web page for this national center providing after-school support for boys and girls provides information on the services available.

1230 W. Peachtree Street NW
Atlanta, GA 30309
800-854-CLUB
www.bgca.org

Girls and Boys Town

This national organization helps boys and girls in crisis in nineteen centers throughout the United States. Residential living for victims of abuse or neglect and family counseling offered.

14100 Crawford Street
Boys Town, NE 68010
800-448-3000
www.girlsandboystown.org

Bernstein, Neil I. *How to Keep Your Teenager Out of Trouble and What to Do If You Can't.* New York: Workman, 2001.
Riera, Michael. *Uncommon Sense for Parents with Teenagers.* Celestial Arts, 1995.

Boys and Work

Child Labor Coalition

The National Consumers League's website about protecting minors in the workforce.
1701 K Street, NW, Suite 1200
Washington, DC 20006
202-835-3323
www.stopchildlabor.org

TeenWorkers

The Occupational Safety and Health Administration's (OSHA) website on teen workers' rights and responsibilities for parents, teens, and employers.

200 Constitution Avenue, NW
Washington, DC 20210
800-321-OSHA
www.osha.gov/SLTC/teenworkers/index.html

Young Worker Safety and Health

The National Institute for Occupational Safety and Health's (NIOSH) web page about adolescent workers.

Hubert H. Humphrey Building
200 Independence Avenue, SW, Room 715H

Washington, DC 20201
800-356-4674
www.cdc.gov/niosh/topics/youth/

8: Boys and Sex

TODDLERS

Krasny, Laurie, and Mark Brown. *What's the Big Secret? Talking About Sex with Girls and Boys.* New York: Little Brown & Company, 2000.

Nilsson, Lennart, and Lena Katarina Swanberg. *How Was I Born?* New York: Bantam Double-day Dell, 1996.

ADOLESCENCE

Gravelle, Karen. *What's Going On Down There: Answers to Questions Boys Find Hard to Ask.* Walker & Company, 1998.

Harris, Robie H. *It's Perfectly Normal: Changing Bodies, Growing Up, Sex, and Sexual Health.* Candlewick Press, 1996.

Madaras, Lynda. *The What's Happening to My Body? Book for Boys, A Growing Up Guide for Parents and Sons.* Newmarket Press, 1997.

Mayle, Peter. *What's Happening to Me?* Lyle Stuart, 1981.

TEENS

Akagi, Cynthia. *Dear Michael: Sexuality Education for Boys Ages 11–17.* Gylantic Publishing Company, 1996.

Ayer, Eleanor H. *It's OK to Say No: Choosing Sexual Abstinence.* Rosen Publishing Group, 2000.

Basso, Michael J. *The Underground Guide to Teenage Sexuality: An Essential Handbook for Today's Teens and Parents.* Fairview Press, 1997.

Bell, Ruth. *Changing Bodies, Changing Lives: A Book for Teens on Sex and Relationships.* New York: Times Books, 1998.

Columbia University's Health Education Program. *The Go Ask Alice Book of Answers: A Guide to Good Physical, Sexual, and Emotional Health.* Owl Books, 1998.

Daldry, Jeremy. *The Teenage Guy's Survival Guide: The Real Deal on Girls, Growing Up, and Other Guy Stuff.* Little Brown and Company, 1999.

Moe, Barbara A. *Everything You Need to Know About Sexual Abstinence.* Rosen Publishing Group, 1998.

Sex, Etc.

The nonprofit Network for Family Life Education hosts this website written for teens by teens. Very objective and open.

www.sxetc.org

Sexuality Information and Education Council of the United States (SEICUS)
This national nonprofit organization's site offers a Parents and Teens section, and all the latest news on sexuality policy from Capitol Hill.

www.siecus.org

Teenwire
Planned Parenthood Federation of America's sex and relationship information website for teens.

www.teenwire.com

Boys and Homosexuality

OutProud
The National Coalition for Gay, Lesbian, Bisexual & Transgender Youth's website provides online brochures and many resources for youth and their families.

369 Third Street, Suite B-362
San Rafael, CA 94901-3581
www.outproud.org

Parents, Families and Friends of Lesbians and Gays (PFLAG)
This national nonprofit's website offers much information for gays and lesbians as well as their families and friends; also find local chapters and support on this site.

1726 M Street NW, Suite 400
Washington, DC 20036
202-467-8180
www.pflag.org

Youth Resource
A website created by and for gay, lesbian, bisexual, transgender, and questioning youth. Lots of information on sexual health and advocacy as well as first-person essays.

Advocates for Youth
1025 Vermont Avenue NW, Suite 200
Washington, DC 20005
202-347-5700
www.youthresource.com

Heron, Ann, ed. *Two Teenagers in Twenty: Writings by Gay & Lesbian Youth.* Alyson Publications, 1995.
Jennings, Kevin. *Always My Child: A Parent's Guide to Understanding Your Gay, Lesbian, Bisexual, Transgendered or Questioning Son or Daughter.* New York: Fireside, 2002.
Parents, Families and Friends of Lesbians and Gays. *Our Daughters and Sons: Questions and Answers for Parents of Gay, Lesbian, and Bisexual People.* Available to order on PFLAG's website (*www.pflag.org*) under Publications.

9: Boys and Sports

American Youth Soccer Organization (AYSO)
Nonprofit promoting fun, fair leagues nationwide with the philosophies of "everyone plays" and "balanced teams."

12501 S. Isis Avenue
Hawthorne, CA 90250
800-872-2976
www.soccer.org

Little League Online
The complete history, rules, and news about Little League in America.

www.littleleague.org

National Alliance for Youth Sports
This nonprofit organization's website provides information and news on youth sports safety for parents and volunteer coaches.

2050 Vista Parkway
West Palm Beach, FL 33411
800-729-2057
www.nays.org

National Youth Sports Safety Foundation
A nonprofit dedicated to reducing the number and severity of injuries in youth sports. Newsletter and fact sheets available to purchase online.

http://www.nyssf.org

MomsTeam.com
A private site that lists advice for mothers on all kinds of youth sports, including safety information and nutrition.

www.momsteam.com

Physical Activity and Health
The Centers for Disease Control and Prevention's fact sheet on the benefits of physical activity for youth.

www.cdc.gov/nccdphp/sgr/adoles.htm

Andersonn, Christopher, and Barbara Andersonn. *Will You Still Love Me If I Don't Win?: A Guide for Parents of Young Athletes.* Taylor Publishing, 2000.
Burnett, Darrell. *It's Just a Game! Youth, Sports, & Self-Esteem: A Guide for Parents.* iUniverse.com, 2000.
Wolff, Rick. *Good Sports: The Concerned Parent's Guide to Competitive Youth Sports.* Sports Publishing, 1998.

PART TWO: HUSBANDS, PARTNERS, LOVERS

10: Husbands, Partners, Lovers

National Screening Days/Months

January

National Diet Month: Promotes the importance of getting back on a healthy eating plan after the winter holidays.

February

Cardiac Rehabilitation Week (second week): Sponsored by the American Association of Cardiovascular and Pulmonary Rehabilitation, 312-321-5146, *www.aacvpr.org.*

National Condom Day (Feb. 14): Sponsored by the American Social Health Association, 919-361-8400, *www.ashastd.org.*

National Heart Month: Sponsored by American Heart Association, 800-242-8721, *www.americanheart.org.*

March

National Alcohol and Other Drugs Awareness Week (March 1–7): Sponsored by the National Clearinghouse for Alcohol and Drug Information: 800-729-6686 or *www.health.org.*

American Diabetes Alert (fourth Tuesday in March): Sponsored by the American Diabetes Association. This is a one-day "wake-up-call" for the 8 million Americans who have diabetes and don't know it; *www.diabetes.org.*

National Colorectal Cancer Awareness Month: Sponsored by Cancer Research and Prevention Foundation, 800-227-2732, 703-836-4412, *www.preventcancer.org/colorectal/.*

National Nutrition Month: Sponsored by the American Dietetic Association, 800-877-1600, *webdietitians.org/Public/index.cfm* or *www.eatright.org.*

National Kidney Month: Sponsored by the National Kidney Foundation: 800-622-9010 or *www.kidney.org.*

April

National Sleep Awareness Week (first week): Sponsored by the National Sleep Foundation, 202 347 3471, *www.sleepfoundation.org*

National Alcohol Screening Day (April 10): Screening for Mental Health, 781-239-0071.

Alcohol Awareness Month: Sponsored by the National Council on Alcoholism and Drug Dependence. This month focuses attention on America's number-one (but often overlooked) drug problem. *www.ncadd.org.*

Cancer Control Month: Sponsored by the American Cancer Society, 800-227-2345, *www.cancer.org.*

Stress Awareness Month: Designed to promote public awareness of the dangers of stress and coping strategies, *www.mentalhealthscreening.org.*

May

National Suicide Awareness Week (May 4–10): Sponsored by the American Association of Suicidology, the National Hopeline Network is 800-SUICIDE or 202-237-2280, *www.suicidology.org.*

National Anxiety Disorders Screening Day (May 7): Sponsored by Freedom from Fear, 718-351-1717, *www.freedomfromfear.org.*

National High Blood Pressure Education Month: Sponsored by the National Heart, Lung, and Blood Institute, 800-575-WELL, *www.nhlbi.nih.gov/index.htm.*

National Melanoma/Skin Cancer Detection and Prevention Month: Sponsored by the American Academy of Dermatology, *www.aad.org.*

National Mental Health Month: Sponsored by the National Mental Health Association, 800-969-6642, *www.nmha.org.*

National Arthritis Month and Annual Arthritis Walk: Sponsored by the Arthritis Foundation, 800-283-7800, *www.arthritis.org.*

National Stroke Awareness Month: Sponsored by the National Stroke Association to alert the public about strokes' warning signs and prevention, 800-787-6537, *www.stroke.org.*

June

National Men's Health Week (the week preceding Father's Day): Sponsored by the National Men's Health Foundation. This week is designed to promote the benefits of preventive health care among men, *www.menshealthweek.org.*

National Safety Month: Sponsored by the American Society of Safety Engineers. This month is designed to increase the public's awareness of the critical role safety and health professionals play in preventing accidents, eliminating hazards, reducing insurance costs, and saving lives, *www.asse.org.*

September

Prostate Cancer Awareness Week (second or third week): Sponsored by the American Foundation for Urological Disease, *www.afud.org.*

Healthy Aging Month: Sponsored by the Educational Television Network, Inc. The goal is to focus national attention on the positive aspects of growing older in the areas of physical, social, mental, and financial fitness, 610-793-0979, *www.healthyaging.net.*

National Cholesterol Education Month: Sponsored by the National Heart, Lung, and Blood Institute, *www.nhlbi.nih.gov/index.htm.*

National Sickle Cell Month: Sponsored by the Sickle Cell Disease Association of America, *www.sicklecelldisease.org/default.htm.*

October

National Depression Screening Days: Sponsored by Screening for Mental Health, Inc., 781-239-0071, *www.mentalhealthscreening.org.*

Healthy Lung Month: Sponsored by the American Lung Association, 800-586-4872, *www.lungusa.org.*

National Liver Awareness Month: 800-GO-LIVER, *www.liverfoundation.org.*

November

National Alzheimer's Awareness Month: Sponsored by the Alzheimer's Association, 800-272-3900, *www.alz.org/mainpage.htm.*

National Diabetes Month: Sponsored by the American Diabetes Association, 800-342-2383, *www.diabetes.org.*

11: An Ounce—or Two—of Prevention

American Dietetic Association
The nation's largest organization of food and nutrition professionals. ADA promotes optimal nutrition, health, and well-being.

120 South Riverside Plaza, Suite 2000
Chicago, IL 60606-6995
312-899-0040 or 800-366-1655 (recorded messages)
www.eatright.org

FDA's Center for Food Safety
Includes updates on dietary supplements and regulatory actions related to food.

http://www.cfsan.fda.gov/

Food Information Line
To report an adverse reaction to a food supplement, call 800-FDA-1088.

www.cfsan.fda.gov/~dms/supplmnt.html

Government website on nutrition, food products, and food safety

www.nutrition.gov

Federal Trade Commission
"For Consumers" section provides advice on avoiding scams and rip-offs.

600 Pennsylvania Avenue NW
Washington, DC 20580
202-326-2222
www.ftc.gov

American Heart Association (AHA)
A national voluntary health agency whose mission is to reduce disability and death from cardiovascular diseases and strokes.

7272 Greenville Avenue
Dallas, TX 75231-4596
800-242-8721
http://www.americanheart.org

Center for Science in the Public Interest
A nutrition advocacy organization with a widely circulated health newsletter, *Nutrition Action Healthletter.*

1875 Connecticut Avenue NW, Suite 300
Washington, DC 20009
202-332-9110
http://www.cspinet.org/

President's Council on Physical Fitness and Sports
www.fitness.gov

American College of Sports Medicine
A professional organization whose website has information on exercise and sports medicine.

P.O. Box 1440
Indianapolis, IN 46206-1440
317-637-9200
www.acsm.org

Healthfinder
Gateway to reliable consumer health and human services information developed by the U.S. Department of Health and Human Services.

www.healthfinder.gov

MedLinePlus
Up-to-date, quality health care information from the National Library of Medicine at the National Institutes of Health.

www.medlineplus.gov

Immunization Action Coalition (IAC)
This website includes a quick quiz that can help determine which shots a person needs.

1573 Selby Avenue, Suite 234
St. Paul, MN 55104
651-647-9009
http://www.immunize.org

National Coalition for Adult Immunization (NCAI)
A network of some 130 organizations that support public health and provide information on immunization against the major vaccine-preventable diseases in adults and adolescents.

4733 Bethesda Avenue, Suite 750
Bethesda, MD 20814
301-656-0003
http://nfid.org/ncai

National Center for Complementary and Alternative Medicine Clearinghouse (NCCAM)
One of the twenty-seven institutes that comprises the National Institutes of Health (NIH), their mission is to support research on complementary and alternative medicine, to train researchers, and to disseminate information to the public on which alternative healing practices work, which do not, and why.

P.O. Box 7923
Gaithersburg, MD 20898
http://nccam.nih.gov/

National Cancer Institute

The National Cancer Institute (NCI) is part of the National Institutes of Health and is the federal government's principal agency for cancer research and training.

NCI Public Inquiries Office
Suite 3036A
6116 Executive Boulevard, MSC8322
Bethesda, MD 20892-8322
800-422-6237
http://cancer.gov
http://www.nci.nih.gov

The Centers for Disease Control Screen for Life Campaign

The CDC has developed materials and provides resources to promote increased knowledge of colorectal cancer and to emphasize the importance of screening.

www.cdc.gov/cancer/screenforlife

American Medical Association. *American Medical Association Complete Guide to Men's Health.* John Wiley & Sons, 2001.

Keene, Nancy. *Working with Your Doctor: Getting the Healthcare You Deserve (Patient-Centered Guides).* O'Reilly Publishers, 1998.

Korsch, Barbara M., and Harding, Caroline. *The Intelligent Patient's Guide to the Doctor-Patient Relationship: Learning How to Talk So Your Doctor Will Listen.* Oxford University Press, 1998.

12: Bad Habits

Centers for Disease Control and Prevention (CDC) Office on Smoking and Health
Tobacco Information and Prevention Source (TIPS)
4770 Buford Highway NE, Mailstop K-50
Atlanta, GA 30341-3724
800-CDC-1311
http://www.cdc.gov/tobacco/

National Spit Tobacco Education Program (NSTEP)

Oral Health America's National Spit Tobacco Education Program (NSTEP) educates the baseball family and the American public about the dangers of smokeless or spit tobacco.

Oral Health America
410 N. Michigan, Suite 352
Chicago, IL 60611
312-836-9900
http://www.nstep.org/nstep.shtml

The American Cancer Society (ACS)

The ACS publishes a series of pamphlets with helpful tips and techniques for smokeless tobacco users who want to quit. The White Pages of the telephone book may have the phone number for the local ACS office, which can also provide referrals to smokeless tobacco–cessation programs.

1599 Clifton Road NE
Atlanta, GA 30329.
800-227-2345
http://www.cancer.org/docroot/home/index.asp

The American Lung Association (ALA)

ALA is an organization dedicated to fighting smoking-related diseases, and provides referrals to local smokeless tobacco–cessation programs. They have an online smoking cessation program called Freedom from Smoking. Many local ALA offices also have self-help materials.

61 Broadway, 6th Floor
New York, NY 10006
800-586-4872 or 212-315-8700
http://www.lungusa.org/

Nicotine Anonymous

A twelve-step program to end smoking.

419 Main Street, PMB #370
Huntington Beach, CA 92648
415-750-0328
http://www.nicotine-anonymous.org

National Highway Safety Traffic Administration (NHTSA)

Part of the Department of Transportation, NHTSA provides information on vehicles and safety equipment, recalls, crash statistics, and traffic safety issues.

400 7th Street SW
Washington, DC 20590
888-327-4236
http://www.nhtsa.dot.gov/

Leon, James, and Diane Nahl. *Road Rage and Aggressive Driving: Steering Clear of Highway Warfare*. Prometheus Books, 2000.
Dr. Leon's website:

http://www.soc.hawaii.edu/leonj/leonj/leonpsy/leon.html

13: Dealing with Emergencies

American College of Emergency Physicians (ACEP)

ACEP is a professional organization with some 22,000 members.

1125 Executive Circle
Irving, TX 75038-2522
800-798-1822 or 972-550-0911
http://www.acep.org/

National Institute of Neurological Disorders and Stroke (NINDS)

Part of the National Institutes of Health, NINDS conducts research on the causes and treatment of neurological disorders and stroke, supports research, and disseminates research information related to neurological disorders.

BRAIN
NIH Neurological Institute
P.O. Box 5801
Bethesda, MD 20824
800-352-9424 or 301-496-5751
http://www.ninds.nih.gov
For a booklet on stroke by NINDS:

http://www.ninds.nih.gov/health_and_medical/pubs/stroke_hope_through_research.htm

American Heart Association/American Stroke Association

National directory of resources related to heart health and disease. Resources include medical information and contacts.

7272 Greenville Avenue
Dallas, TX 75231
AHA: 800-242-8721
ASA: 888-478-7653
http://www.americanheart.org/

National Stroke Association (NSA)

A national organization, the NSA considers itself "the voice for stroke," and works to create greater awareness for stroke prevention and urgent symptom recognition.

9707 East Easter Lane
Englewood, CO 80112-3747
800-STROKES or 303-649-9299
www.stroke.org

National Institute of Mental Health (NIMH)

The mission of the National Institute of Mental Health (NIMH) is to diminish the burden of mental illness through research.

6001 Executive Boulevard, Room 8184, MSC 9663
Bethesda, MD 20892-9663
866-615- 6464 or 301-443-4513
www.nimh.nih.gov

American Association of Suicidology (AAS)

The goal of the AAS is to understand and prevent suicide. A nonprofit organization, AAS promotes research, public awareness programs, public education, and training for professionals and volunteers.

4201 Connecticut Avenue NW, Suite 408
Washington, DC 20008
202-237-2280
www.suicidology.org
The National Hopeline Network, 1-800-SUICIDE, provides access to trained telephone counselors, twenty-four hours a day, seven days a week.

American Foundation for Suicide Prevention

The foundation's activities include supporting research projects that help further the understanding and treatment of depression and the prevention of suicide, providing information, promoting professional and supporting programs for suicide survivor treatment, research, and education.

120 Wall Street, 22nd Floor
New York, New York 10005
888-333-AFSP or 212-363-3500
www.afsp.org

14: "Houston, We've Had a Problem"

The American Association of Cardiovascular and Pulmonary Rehabilitation (AACVPR)

The AACVPR can help you locate a cardiac rehabilitation center in your area.

312-321-5146
http://www.aacvpr.org/

The Mended Hearts, Inc.

A national nonprofit organization affiliated with the American Heart Association offers hope to heart disease patients, their families, and caregivers through visiting programs and support group meetings.

7272 Greenville Avenue
Dallas, TX 75231
Information: 888-HEART99 (888-432-7899)
National Office: 214-706-1442
http://www.mendedhearts.org

Levin, Rhoda, Rachael Freed, and David V. Keith. *Heartmates: A Guide for the Spouse and Family of the Heart Patient.* Fairview Press, 2002.

800-544-8207 to order
http://www.heartmates.com

15: The Usual Suspects

Mayo Clinic Books

The Mayo Clinic publishes a series of books that are researched, written, and reviewed at Mayo Clinic. These include:

Mayo Clinic Family Health Book
Mayo Clinic Heart Book
Mayo Clinic Complete Book of Pregnancy & Baby's First Year
Mayo Clinic / Williams-Sonoma Cookbook
Mayo Clinic on Alzheimer's
Mayo Clinic on Arthritis
Mayo Clinic on Chronic Pain
Mayo Clinic on Depression
Mayo Clinic on Digestive Health
Mayo Clinic on Healthy Aging
Mayo Clinic on Healthy Weight
Mayo Clinic on High Blood Pressure
Mayo Clinic on Managing Diabetes
Mayo Clinic on Prostate Health
Mayo Clinic on Vision and Eye Health

Mayo Clinic book website: *http://www.mayoclinichmr.org/products/books.cfm*

National Heart, Lung, and Blood Institute (NHLBI)

Part of the federal government's National Institutes of Health, The NHLBI has many helpful websites.

General website *http://www.nhlbi.nih.gov/*

Girth of a Nation

The LEARN Program for Weight Management 2000

A company that specializes in weight loss, stress management, and healthy eating.

PO Box 610430, Department 80
Dallas, TX 75261
888-LEARN-41
www.Thelifestylecompany.com

Shape Up America!

A nonprofit organization dedicated to helping people to achieve healthy weight for life.

c/o Webfront Solutions Corporation
15757 Crabbs Branch Way
Rockville, MD 20855
301-258-0540
http://www.shapeup.org/

Aim for a Healthy Weight
Information about obesity is available on the NHLBI website.

NHLBI Information Center
P.O. Box 30105
Bethesda, MD 20824-0105.
http://www.nhlbi.nih.gov/health/public/heart/obesity/lose_wt/index.htm

Harvard Men's Health Watch
Harvard publications brings the most current authoritative health information, using the expertise of the eight thousand faculty physicians at the Harvard Medical School, to the public.

www.health.harvard.edu

Cholesterol
National Heart, Lung, and Blood Lifestyle Changes Website
Fun interactive website shows how changes in your lifestyle help you to lower cholesterol and reduce your chance of having a heart attack.

http://www.nhlbi.nih.gov/chd/lifestyles.htm
Figure out your cholesterol level from this National Heart, Lung, and Blood website: *www.nhlbi.nih.gov/guidelines/cholesterol/.*

Blood Pressure
Your Guide to Lowering High Blood Pressure:
www.nhlbi.nih.gov/hbp

American Heart Association. *American Heart Association Low-Salt Cookbook: A Complete Guide to Reducing Sodium and Fat in Your Diet,* 2nd edition. Clarkson & Potter, 2001.
Moore, Thomas, ed., et al. *The DASH Diet for Hypertension: Lower Your Blood Pressure in 14 Days Without Drugs.* Free Press, 2001. This website tells how to follow the DASH diet, along with many tips on foods and food products: *http://www.nhlbi.nih.gov/health/public/heart/hbp/dash/.*

How Sweet It Isn't: Diabetes
National Diabetes Education Program (NDEP)
The NDEP is a nationwide initiative of the CDC and the NIH and some two hundred public and private organizations whose goal is to reduce the morbidity and mortality of diabetes.

NDEP c/o NIDDK
Building 31, Room 9A04,
31 Center Drive, MSC 2560
Bethesda, MD 20892-2560
http://www.cdc.gov/diabetes/projects/ndeps.htm
National Diabetes Information Clearinghouse: 301-654-3327
For free pamphlets on diabetes call: 800-GET LEVEL or 800-438-5383

National Eye Institute (NEI)
2020 Vision Place
Bethesda, MD 20892-3655
301-496-5248 or 800-869-2020 (to order materials)
http://www.nei.nih.gov

Educating People with Diabetes
The Diabetic Eye
http://www.nei.nih.gov/nehep/ded.htm
Sponsored by the National Eye Institute

Office of Minority Health Resource Center
U.S. Department of Health and Human Services
P.O. Box 37337
Washington, DC 20013-7337
800-444-6472
http://www.omhrc.gov/

American Association of Diabetes Educators
Includes catalog of educational products, legislative updates, "Ask the Expert," continuing education seminars and medical articles.

100 West Monroe, Suite 400
Chicago, IL 60603-1901
800-338-3633 for names of diabetes educators
312-424-2426 to order publications
http://www.aadenet.org

American Diabetes Association
1701 North Beauregard Street
Alexandria, VA 22311
800-342-2383
http://www.diabetes.org

American Dietetic Association (ADA)
The ADA is the nation's largest organization of food and nutrition professionals. ADA promotes optimal nutrition, health, and well-being.

120 South Riverside Plaza, Suite 2000
Chicago, IL 60606-6995
800-366-1655 (recorded messages) or 312-899-0040
www.eatright.org

Joslin Diabetes Center
Affiliated with Harvard Medical School, Joslin is a nonprofit organization dedicated to finding a cure for diabetes and improving the lives of people with diabetes through its research, patient care programs, and publications.

One Joslin Place
Boston, MA 02215
617-732-2400
http://www.joslin.harvard.edu/index.shtml

16: Alcoholism: The Hidden Epidemic

National Institute on Alcohol Abuse and Alcoholism (NIAAA)
NIAAA provides leadership in the national effort to reduce alcohol-related problems. Its website provides printable pamphlets and answers many frequently asked questions.

6000 Executive Boulevard, Willco Building
Bethesda, MD 20892-7003
www.niaaa.nih.gov

Substance Abuse and Mental Health (SAMHSA)
An agency of the U.S. Department of Health and Human Services, SAMHSA's goal is to improve the quality of prevention, treatment, and rehabilitative services in order to reduce illness and cost to society resulting from substance abuse and mental illnesses.

Room 12–105 Parklawn Building
5600 Fishers Lane
Rockville, MD 20857
800-789-2647 or 301-443-8956
www.samhsa.gov
www.mentalhealth.org/suicideprevention

National Clearinghouse for Alcohol and Drug Information (NCADI)
NCADI is the nation's one-stop resource for information about substance-abuse prevention and addiction treatment.

800-729-6686
www.health.org

About.com Alcoholism Guide
Excellent comprehensive resource about alcoholism and substance abuse.

http://alcoholism.about.com/

Referral Service
Call the National Drug and Alcohol Treatment Referral Routing Service (Center for Substance Abuse Treatment) at 800-662-HELP for information about treatment programs in your local community and to speak to someone about an alcohol or substance abuse problem.

Al-Anon/Alateen
Helps families and friends of alcoholics recover from the effects of living with the problem drinking of a relative or friend. Alateen is a recovery program for young people.

1600 Corporate Landing Parkway
Virginia Beach, VA 23454-5617
888-4AL-ANON (weekdays, 8:00 A.M. to 6:00 P.M., EST) for meeting information
757-563-1600
http://www.al-anon.alateen.org/

Alcoholics Anonymous (AA)

AA is a fellowship of men and women who share their experience, strength, and hope so that they may help themselves and others to recover from alcoholism. The only requirement for membership is a desire to stop drinking.

Grand Central Station
P.O. Box 459
New York, NY 10163
212-870-3400
www.aa.org

National Council on Alcoholism and Drug Dependence (NCADD)

NCADD provides education, information, help, and hope. It advocates prevention, intervention, and treatment of alcoholism and substance dependency.

20 Exchange Place, Suite 2902
New York, NY 10005
212-269-7797
Hope Line: 800-NCA-CALL (24-hour affiliate referral)
http://www.ncadd.org

Domar, Alice D., et al. *Self-Nurture: Learning to Care for Yourself As Effectively As You Care for Everyone Else.* Penguin, 2001.

Drews, Toby Rice. *Getting Them Sober, volumes 1, 2 and 3.* Recovery Communications, 1998.

How Al-Anon Works for Families & Friends of Alcoholics. AFG (Al-Anon Family Group), 1995.

Johnson, Vernon E. *I'll Quit Tomorrow: A Practical Guide to Alcoholism Treatment,* rev. ed. Harper San Francisco, 1990.

Miller, Joy. *Addictive Relationships: Reclaiming Your Boundaries.* Health Communications, Inc., 1989.

West, James W. *The Betty Ford Center Book of Answers: Help for Those Struggling with Substance Abuse—and for the People Who Love Them.* Pocket Books, 1997.

17: Cancer

Us Too! International

A nonprofit prostate cancer education and support organization with hundreds of local support group chapters, publications (including a monthly newsletter and a biweekly e-mail–based newsletter), and educational programs for men with prostate cancer, their families, and men at risk.

5003 Fairview Avenue
Downers Grove, IL 60515
630-795-1002
support hotline: 800-808-7866
http://www.ustoo.org/

American Prostate Society
A nonprofit organization dedicated to the fight against prostate diseases.

P.O. Box 870
Hanover, MD 21076
800-308-1106
http://www.ameripros.org/index.html

CancerTrialsHelp.org
Cancer Research: A Guide to Clinical Trials is an online service designed to educate and empower cancer patients and caregivers. This easy-to-use program enables users to educate themselves about cancer clinical trials through a step-by-step interactive curriculum. Part of the Coalition of Natural Cancer Cooperative Groups.

1818 Market Street, Suite 1100
Philadelphia, PA 19103
877-520-4457 or 215-789-3610
www.CancerTrialsHelp.org

National Family Caregivers Association (NFCA)
NFCA is a grassroots organization created to educate, support, empower, and speak up for the millions of Americans who care for chronically ill, aged, or disabled loved ones.

10400 Connecticut Avenue, #500
Kensington, MD 20895-3944
800-896-3650
http://www.nfcacares.org/

American Association for Marriage and Family Therapy (AAMFT)
AAMFT is the professional association for the field of marriage and family therapy, which represents the professional interests of more than 23,000 marriage and family therapists.

112 South Alfred Street
Alexandria, VA 22314-3061
703-838-9808

Lyon Howe, Desiree. *His Prostate and Me: A Couple Deals with Prostate Cancer.* Winedale Publishing, 2002.
Walsh, Patrick C., and Janet Farrar Worthington. *Dr. Patrick Walsh's Guide to Surviving Prostate Cancer.* New York: Warner Books, 2001.
———. *The Prostate: A Guide for Men and the Women Who Love Them.* New York: Warner Books, 1997 (reissue).

18: Male Trouble: A Gland That Doesn't Always Behave

The Johns Hopkins Prostate Bulletin
The bulletin uses the knowledge of doctors at the Brady Urological Institute at Johns Hopkins, world-class prostate experts.

Subscription Department
P.O. Box 420148
Palm Coast, FL 32142
386-447-6313
http://www.hopkinsprostate.com/

American Foundation for Urologic Disease
This nonprofit organization promotes the prevention and cure of urologic disease through the expansion of patient education, public awareness, research, and advocacy.

1128 North Charles Street
Baltimore, MD 21201
800-242-2383 or 410-468-1800
http://www.afud.org/

Prostatitis Foundation
This foundation promotes prostatitis research, collects data on the disease, and provides information to men who are suffering from the disease.

1063 30th Street, Box 8
Smithshire, IL 61478
888-891-4200
http://www.prostatitis.org/

Osteoporosis

National Osteoporosis Foundation
A nonprofit, voluntary health organization dedicated to promoting lifelong bone health, reducing the widespread prevalence of osteoporosis and associated fractures, and working to find a cure for the disease through research, education, and advocacy.

1232 22nd Street NW
Washington, DC 20037-1292
800-223-9994 or 202-223-2226
http://www.nof.org/index.html

Lane, Nancy. *The Osteoporosis Book: A Guide for Patients and Their Families.* Oxford University Press, 2001.

19: The Emotional Male

National Institute of Mental Health (NIMH)
The mission of NIMH is to diminish the burden of mental illness through research.

6001 Executive Boulevard, Room 8184, MSC 9663
Bethesda, MD 20892-9663
866-615-6464 or 301-443-4513
www.nimh.nih.gov

Real Men, Real Depression
Interesting website where men tell personal stories about how they hid their depression. Also information on signs and signals of depression, and available treatments.

http://menanddepression.nimh.nih.gov/

Mental Help Net
A comprehensive source of online mental health information, news, and resources.

570 Metro Place
Dublin, OH 43017
http://mentalhelp.net

International Society for Mental Health Online (ISMHO)
Promotes the understanding, use, and development of online communication, information, and technology for the international mental health community.

P.O. Box 331339
Miami, FL 33233-1339
http://ismho.org/

National Mental Health Association
Provides information on a variety of mental health topics. Find a local mental health association or browse news and events.

2001 N. Beauregard Street, 12th Floor
Alexandria, VA 22311
Mental Health Resource Center: 800-969-NMHA or 703-684-7722
http://www.nmha.org/

20: Tossin', Turnin', Cuttin' Zs

American Academy of Sleep Medicine (AASM)
A professional organization dedicated to the advancement of sleep medicine and related research.

One Westbrook Corporate Center, Suite 920
Westchester, IL 60154

708-492-0930
http://www.aasmnet.org/

American Sleep Apnea Association (ASAA)
The ASAA is dedicated to reducing injury, disability, and death from sleep apnea and to enhancing the well-being of those affected by this common disorder.

1424 K Street NW, Suite 302
Washington, DC 20005
202-293-3650
http://www.sleepapnea.org/

National Center on Sleep Disorders Research (NCSDR)
Part of the National Heart, Lung, and Blood Institute (NHLBI) of the National Institutes of Health (NIH), the NCSDR combats the sleep problems that affect some 70 million Americans.

6705 Rockledge Drive
One Rockledge Centre, Suite 6022
Bethesda, MD 20892-7993
301-435-0199
http://www.nhlbi.nih.gov/about/ncsdr/

National Sleep Foundation
A nonprofit organization dedicated to prevention of catastrophic accidents caused by sleep deprivation and excessive sleepiness.

1522 K Street NW, Suite 500
Washington, DC 20005
202-347-3471
http://www.sleepfoundation.org/

21: Boomeritis

American College of Sports Medicine (ACSM)
ACSM's website provides state-of-the-art research and information on sports medicine and exercise science.

401 W. Michigan Street
Indianapolis, IN 46202-3233
317-637-9200
http://www.acsm.org

American Academy of Orthopaedic Surgeons (AAOS)
The AAOS provides education and practice management services for orthopedic surgeons and allied health professionals.

6300 N. River Road, Suite 200
Rosemont, IL 60018

847-823-7186 or 847-346-AAOS
http://www.aaos.org

American Physical Therapy Association (APTA)

APTA is a national professional organization representing more than 63,000 members whose goal is to foster advancement in physical therapy practice, research, and education.

1111 N. Fairfax Street
Alexandria, VA 22314
800-999-2782
http://www.apta.org

The association has published a free brochure titled *Taking Care of Your Knees.* It may be ordered via APTA's website or at the address above.

Arthritis Foundation

A national not-for-profit organization that supports the more than one hundred types of arthritis and related conditions with advocacy, programs, services, and research.

P.O. Box 7669
Atlanta, GA 30357-0669
800-283-7800 or call your local chapter (listed in the local telephone directory)
http://www.arthritis.org

The Foundation has several free brochures about coping with arthritis, taking nonsteroid and steroid medicines, and exercise. A free brochure on protecting your joints is titled *Using Your Joints Wisely.* Other free brochures include *Walking with Arthritis* and *Exercise and Arthritis.* The foundation also provides doctor referrals.

American College of Rheumatology/Association of Rheumatology Health Professionals

The American College of Rheumatology is the professional organization of rheumatologists and associated health professionals who share a dedication to healing, preventing disability, and curing the more than one hundred types of arthritis and related disorders of the joints, muscles, and bones.

1800 Century Place, Suite 250
Atlanta, GA 30345
404-633-3777
http://www.rheumatology.org

National Arthritis and Musculoskeletal and Skin Diseases Information Clearinghouse (NAMSIC)

NAMSIC supports research into the causes, treatment, and prevention of arthritis and musculoskeletal and skin diseases, the training of scientists to carry out research, and the dissemination of information on research progress in these diseases. NAMSIC offers a free brochure: *Questions and Answers About Knee Problems.* September 1997. NIH Publication No. 01-4912 (*http://www.niams.nih.gov/hi/topics/kneeprobs/kneeqa.htm*).

National Institutes of Health
1 AMS Circle
Bethesda, MD 20892-3675
301-495-4484
http://www.nih.gov/niams

Boomeritis

For more on Boomeritis, check out: *http://www.drnick.com.*

22: Men and Sex

American Foundation for Urologic Disease

1128 North Charles Street
Baltimore, MD 21201
800-242-2383
http://www.afud.org/

Impotence

Information on impotence from the American Foundation for Urologic Disease is at *www.impotence.org.*

www.newshe.com

Website of sisters Jennifer Berman, M.D., and Laura Berman, Ph.D. The website discusses women's sexual health, and the community billboard offers professional answers to e-mail questions, live chats with experts, frequently asked questions, and an archive of questions and answers.

American Society of Sex Educators, Counselors and Therapists (AASECT)

AASECT is a not-for-profit, interdisciplinary professional organization whose members share an interest in promoting the understanding of human sexuality and healthy sexual behavior.

P.O. Box 5488
Richmond, VA 23220-0488
http://www.aasect.org/about.cfm

Alterowitz, Ralph and Barbara. *The Lovin' Ain't Over: The Couple's Guide to Better Sex After Prostate Surgery.* Health Education Literary Publisher, 1999.

23: Narcissus—What a Guy!

Midlife Wives Club

A website that offers midlife crisis support for both men and women, including a twenty-four-hour chat line where people discuss common problems.

www.midlifewivesclub.com

American Academy of Dermatology
The American Academy of Dermatology is a professional organization with a membership of some 13,700 practicing dermatologists in the United States.

P.O. Box 4014
Schaumburg, IL 60168-4014
847-330-0230
To find a dermatologist: 888-462-3376
http://www.aad.org/

American Society of Plastic Surgeons (ASPS)
ASPS is composed of board-certified plastic surgeons who perform cosmetic and reconstructive surgery.

444 E. Algonquin Road
Arlington Heights, IL 60005
For plastic surgeon referral: 888-475-2784
http://www.plasticsurgery.org/

American Society for Aesthetic Plastic Surgery (ASAPS)
ASAPS, with some 1,900 members in the United States and Canada, is the professional organization of plastic surgeons certified by the American Board of Plastic Surgery, who specialize in cosmetic plastic surgery.

36 West 44th Street, Suite 630
New York, NY 10036
212-921-0500
Find-a-Surgeon referral service: 888-272-7711 or
    the Find-a-Surgeon locator on the website.
http://www.surgery.org/default.htm

Anderson, Arnold, et al. *Making Weight: Healing Men's Conflicts with Food, Weight and Shape.* Gurze Designs & Books, 2000.
Courter, Gay, and Pat Gaudette. *How to Survive Your Husband's Midlife Crisis: Strategies and Stories from the Midlife Wives Club.* Perigee, 2003.

Selected Bibliography

Abramson, Edward. *Marriage Made Me Fat!* New York: Kensington Books, 1999.

Adler, Robert, Sandra Ottaway, and Stacey Gould. "Circumcision: We Have Heard from the Experts, Now Let's Hear from the Parents." *Pediatrics* 107, no. 2 (2001): E20.

American Academy of Child and Adolescent Psychiatry. *Your Adolescent: Emotional, Behavioral, and Cognitive Development from Early Adolescence Through the Teen Years.* Edited by David B. Pruitt. New York: Harper Resource, 1999.

American Academy of Orthopaedic Surgeons. *Care of the Young Athlete.* Edited by J. Andy Sullivan and Stephen J. Anderson. Rosemont, IL: American Academy of Pediatrics, 2000.

The American Academy of Pediatrics. *Caring for Your Baby and Young Child: Birth to Age 5.* Edited by Stephen P. Shelov, et al. Rev. ed. New York: Bantam Books, 1998.

The American Academy of Pediatrics. *Caring for Your School-Age Child: Ages 5 to 12.* Edited by Edward L. Schor. Rev. ed. New York: Bantam Books, 1999.

American Medical Association. *American Medical Association Complete Guide to Men's Health.* Edited by Angela Perry. New York: John Wiley & Sons, 2001.

Bae, Yupin, Susan Choy, Claire Geddes, Jennifer Sable, and Thomas Snyder. *Trends in Educational Equity of Girls and Women* NCES 2000–030. Washington, DC: U.S. Department of Education, National Center for Education Statistics, 2000. *http://nces.ed.gov/pubs2000/2000030.pdf* (July 7, 2003).

Bassoff, Evelyn. *Between Mothers and Sons: The Making of Vital and Loving Men.* New York: Dutton, 1994.

Beal, Carole R. *Boys and Girls: The Development of Gender Roles.* New York: McGraw-Hill, 1993.

Berman, Jennifer, Laura Berman, and Elisabeth Bumiller. *For Women Only: A Revolutionary Guide to Overcoming Sexual Dysfunction and Reclaiming Your Sex Life.* New York: Henry Holt, 2001.

Blum, Nathan J., Bruce Taubman, and Nicole Nemeth. "Relationship Between Age at Initiation of Toilet Training and Duration of Training: A Prospective Study." *Pediatrics* 111, no. 4 (2003). 810–14.

Braus, Patricia. *Marketing Health Care to Women: Meeting New Demands for Products and Services.* Stamford, CT: Intertec Publishing Group, 1997.

Brazelton, T. Berry, and Stanley I. Greenspan. *The Irreducible Needs of Children: What Every Child Must Have to Grow, Learn, and Flourish.* Cambridge, MA: Perseus Publishing, 2000.

Brody, Leslie. *Gender, Emotion, and the Family.* Cambridge, MA: Harvard University Press, 1999.

Brownell, Kelly D. *The LEARN Program for Weight Management 2000: Lifestyle, Exercises, Attitudes, Relationships, Nutrition.* Dallas, TX: American Health Publishing Company, 2000.

Carey, William B., with Martha M. Jablow. *Understanding Your Child's Temperament: A Revolutionary Approach to Parenting.* New York: Macmillan, 1997.

594 | Selected Bibliography

Christensen, Andrew, and Neil S. Jacobson. *Reconcilable Differences.* New York: Guilford Press, 2002.

Colapinto, John. *As Nature Made Him: The Boy Who Was Raised As a Girl.* New York: Harper-Collins, 2000.

Coltrane, Scott. *Family Man: Fatherhood, Housework, and Gender Equity.* New York: Oxford University Press, 1997.

Courtenay, Will. "Behavioral Factors Associated with Disease, Injury and Death Among Men: Evidence and Implications for Prevention." *Journal of Men's Studies* 9, no.1 (2000): 81.

Dabbs, James McBride, and Mary Godwin Dabbs. *Heroes, Rogues, and Lovers: Testosterone and Behavior.* New York: McGraw-Hill, 2000.

Deutsch, Francine M. *Halving It All: How Equally Shared Parenting Works.* Cambridge, MA: Harvard University Press, 2000.

DeVault, Marjorie L. *Feeding the Family: The Social Organization of Caring As Gendered Work.* Women in Culture and Society, ed. Catharine R. Stimpson. Chicago: University of Chicago Press, 1994.

Diamond, Jed. *Surviving Male Menopause: A Guide for Women and Men.* Naperville, IL: Sourcebooks, 2000.

Diller, Lawrence. *Running on Ritalin: A Physician Reflects on Children, Society, and Performance in a Pill.* New York: Bantam Books, 1998.

Elkin, Allen. *Stress Management for Dummies.* Foster City, CA: IDG Books Worldwide, 1999.

Epstein, Leonard. *Stoplight Diet for Children: An Eight-Week Program for Parents and Children.* Boston: Little, Brown, 1988.

Freed, Rachael, and Rhoda F. Levin. *Heartmates: A Survival Guide for the Cardiac Spouse.* New York: Prentice Hall, 1987.

Friedman, Richard C., and Jennifer I. Downey. *Sexual Orientation and Psychoanalysis: Sexual Science and Clinical Practice.* New York: Columbia University Press, 2002.

Frontline. "Inside the Teenage Brain," first broadcast January 31, 2002 by PBS. Written, produced, and directed by Sarah Spinks. *http://www.pbs.org/wgbh/pages/frontline/shows/teenbrain/* (June 17, 2003).

Gagnon, John H., Alain Giami, Stuart Michaels, and Patrick de Colomby. "A Comparative Study of the Couple in the Social Organization of Sexuality in France and the United States." *Journal of Sex Research* 38, no. 1 (2001): 24–34.

Garrity, Carla, Kathryn Jens, William Porter, and Nancy Sager. *Bully-Proofing Your School: A Comprehensive Approach for Elementary Schools.* Longmont, CO: Sopris West, 2000.

Geary, David C. *Male, Female: The Evolution of Human Sex Differences.* Washington, DC: American Psychological Association, 1998.

Giannetti, Charlene, and Margeret Sagarese. *The Roller-Coaster Years: Raising Your Child Through the Maddening Yet Magical Middle School Years.* New York: Broadway Books, 1997.

Gilbert, Susan. *A Field Guide to Boys and Girls.* New York: HarperCollins, 2000.

Gollaher, David L. *Circumcision: A History of the World's Most Controversial Surgery.* New York: Basic Books, 2000.

Gonzales, Edmond T., and Stuart B. Bauer, eds. *Pediatric Urology Practice.* Hagerstown, MD: Lippincott Williams & Wilkins, 1999.

Gottman, John Mordechai, and Nan Silver. *The Seven Principles for Making Marriage Work.* New York: Crown, 1999.

Greenberg, Sindy, Elyse Kroll, and Hillary Grill. *Dreaming for Two: The Hidden Emotional Life of Expectant Mothers.* New York: Dutton, 2002.

Grunbaum, Jo Anne, Laura Kann, Steven A. Kinchen, Barbara Williams, James G. Ross, Richard Lowry, and Lloyd Lolbe. "Youth Risk Behavior Surveillance—United States, 2001." *Morbidity and Mortality Weekly Report* 51, no. SS04 (2002): 1–64. *http://www.cdc.gov/mmwr/preview/mmwrhtml/ss5104al.htm* (June 17, 2003).

Gurian, Michael. *The Wonder of Boys: What Parents, Mentors, and Educators Can Do to Shape Boys into Exceptional Men.* New York: Putnam, 1997.

Harrison, James B. "Warning: The Male Sex Role May Be Dangerous to Your Health." *Journal of Social Issues* 34, no. 1 (1978): 65–86.

Heber, David, and Susan Bowerman. *What Color Is Your Diet?* New York: Regan Books, 2002.

Hofman, Adele, and Donald E. Greydanus. *Adolescent Medicine.* 3d ed. Stamford, CT: Appleton & Lange, 1997.

Howland, J., R. Hinson, T. W. Mangione, N. Bell, and S. Bak. "Why Are Most Drowning Victims Men?: Sex Differences in Aquatic Skills and Behaviors." *American Journal of Public Health* 86, no. 1 (1996): 93–96.

Institute of Medicine (U.S.). Committee on Understanding the Biology of Sex and Gender Differences. *Exploring the Biological Contributions to Human Health, Does Sex Matter?* Edited by Theresa Wizeman and Mary-Lou Pardue. Washington, DC: National Academy Press, 2001.

James, Leon, and Diane Nahl. *Road Rage and Aggressive Driving: Steering Clear of Highway Warfare.* Amherst, NY: Prometheus Books, 2000.

Jovanovic-Peterson, Lois, Barbara Biermann, and Barbara Toohey. *The Diabetic Woman.* New York: Putnam, 1996.

Karlin, Elyse Zorn, and Muriel Warren. *Sons: A Mother's Manual.* New York: Avon Books, 1994.

Kaschak, Ellyn, and Leonore Tiefer. *A New View of Women's Sexual Problems.* New York: Haworth Press, 2001.

Kindlon, Daniel J., and Michael Thompson. *Raising Cain: Protecting the Emotional Life of Boys.* New York: Ballantine Books, 1999.

Kirkendall, Donald T., S. E. Jordan, and W. E. Garrett. "Heading and Head Injuries in Soccer." *Sports Medicine* 31, no. 5 (2001): 369–86.

Klein, Carole. *Mothers and Sons.* Boston: G. K. Hall, 1985.

Kotin, Joel. *How to Change Your Spouse and Save Your Marriage.* Franklin Lakes, NJ: New Page Books, 2000.

Kraemer, Sebastian. "The Fragile Male." *British Medical Journal* 321 (December 2000): 1609–12.

Krause, Carol. *How Healthy Is Your Family Tree?: A Complete Guide to Tracing Your Family's Medical and Behavioral Tree.* New York: Simon & Schuster, 1995.

Laken, Virginia, and Keith Laken. *Making Love Again: Hope for Couples Facing Loss of Sexual Intimacy.* Sandwich, MA: Ant Hill Press, 2002.

Lane, Nancy E. *The Osteoporosis Book: A Guide for Patients and Their Families.* New York: Oxford University Press, 2001.

Levant, Ronald F., and William S. Pollack, eds. *A New Psychology of Men.* Basic Books, 1995.

Levine, Mel. *A Mind at a Time.* New York: Simon & Schuster, 2002.

Levine, Suzanne Braun. *Father Courage: What Happens When Men Put Family First.* New York: Harcourt, 2000.

Levinson, Daniel J. *The Seasons of a Man's Life.* New York: Ballantine Books, 1986.

Lodewick, Peter A., June Biermann, and Barbara Toohey. *The Diabetic Man: A Guide to Health and Success in All Areas of Your Life.* 3d ed. Chicago: McGraw-Hill/Contemporary Books, 1999.

Maccoby, Eleanor E. *The Two Sexes: Growing Up Apart, Coming Together.* Cambridge, MA: Belknap Press of Harvard University Press, 2000.

Medical Department, United States Army. *Urology.* Surgery in World War II, ed. John F. Patton. Washington, D.C.: Office of the Surgeon General and Center of Military History, United States Army, 1987.

Michael, Robert T., John H. Gagnon, Edward O. Laumann, and Aina Kolata. *Sex in America: A Definitive Survey.* New York: Warner Books, 1995.

Moore, Sheila, and Roon Frost. *The Little Boy Book: A Guide to the First Eight Years.* New York: Ballantine Books, 1986.

Moore, Thomas J., Laura P. Svetkey, Pao-Hwa Lin, Njeri Karanja, and Mark Jenkins. *The DASH Diet for Hypertension: Lower Your Blood Pressure in 14 Days—Without Drugs.* New York: Free Press, 2001.

MTA Cooperative Group. "A 14-Month Randomized Clinical Trial of Treatment Strategies for Attention-Deficit/Hyperactivity Disorder." *Archives of General Psychiatry* 56, no. 12 (1999): 1073–86.

National Research Council and Institute of Medicine. "Risks and Opportunities: Synthesis of Studies on Adolescence." *Forum on Adolescence.* Michele D. Kipke, ed. Board on Children, Youth, and Families. Washington, DC: National Academy Press, 1999. *http://books.nap.edu/books/030906791X/html/index.html.*

Newberger, Eli H. *The Men They Will Become: The Nature and Nurture of Male Character.* Cambridge, MA: Perseus Publishing, 1999.

Notzon, Francis C., Sven Cnattingius, Per Bergsjo, Susan Cole, Selma Taffel, Lorentz Irgens, and Anne Kjersti Daltveit. "Cesarean Section Delivery in the 1980s: International Comparison by Indication." *American Journal of Obstetrics and Gynecology* 170, no. 2 (1994): 495–504.

Ornish, Dean. *Eat More, Weigh Less: Dr. Dean Ornish's Life Choice Program for Losing Weight Safely While Eating Abundantly.* New York: Quill, 2000.

Peth-Pierce, Robin. (2000). *A Good Beginning: Sending America's Children to School with the Social and Emotional Competence They Need to Succeed* (The Child Mental Health Foundations and Agencies Network (FAN) monograph). Bethesda, MD: The National Institute of Mental Health, Office of Communications and Public Liaison. *http://www.nimh.nih.gov/childhp/monograph.pdf* (July 3, 2003).

Pipher, Mary B. *Reviving Ophelia: Saving the Selves of Adolescent Girls.* New York: Putnam, 1994.

Pollack, William S. *Real Boys: Rescuing Our Sons from the Myths of Boyhood.* New York: Henry Holt & Company, 1999.

Ponton, Lynn E. *The Romance of Risk: Why Teenagers Do the Things They Do.* New York: Basic Books, 1998.

Pope, Harrison G. Jr., Katherine A. Phillips, and Roberto Olivardia. *The Adonis Complex: The Secret Crisis of Male Body Obsession.* New York: Free Press, 2000.

Prochaska, James O., John C. Norcross, and Carlo C. DiClemente. *Changing for Good.* New York: Avon Books, 1995.

Real, Terrence. *I Don't Want to Talk About It: Overcoming the Secret Legacy of Male Depression.* New York: Scribner, 1997.

Risman, Barbara J. *Gender Vertigo: American Families in Transition.* New Haven, CT: Yale University Press, 1998.

Rogers, Lesley J. *Sexing the Brain.* New York: Columbia University Press, 2001.

Ruben, David. "What Makes a Child Violent?" *Parenting,* August 1998, 97–102.

Rubin, Richard R., June Biermann, and Barbara Toohey. *Psyching Out Diabetes: A Positive Approach to Your Negative Emotions.* Chicago: McGraw-Hill/Contemporary Books, 1999.

Sacks, Frank M., Laura P. Svetkey, William M. Vollmer, Lawrence J. Appel, George A. Bray, David Harsha, Eva Obarzanek, Paul R. Conlon, Edgar R. Miller III, Denise G. Simons-Morton, Njeri Karanja, and Pao-Hwa Lin, for the DASH-Sodium Collaborative Research Group. "Effects on Blood Pressure of Reduced Dietary Sodium and the Dietary Approaches to Stop Hypertension (DASH) Diet." *New England Journal of Medicine.* 344, no. 1 (2001): 3–11.

Sandman, David, Elizabeth Simantov, and Christina An. *Out of Touch: American Men and the Health Care System: Commonwealth Fund Men's and Women's Health Survey.* New York: The Commonwealth Fund, 2000.

Savard, Marie. *The Savard Health Record: A Six-Step System for Managing Your Healthcare.* New York: Time Life, 2000.

Sax, Leonard. "Reclaiming Kindergarten: Making Kindergarten Less Harmful to Boys." *Psychology of Men and Masculinity* 2, no. 1 (2001): 3–12.

Schmaling, Karen B., and Tamara Goldman Sher, eds. *The Psychology of Couples and Illness: Theory, Research, & Practice.* Washington, DC: American Psychological Association, 2000.

Schmitt, R. Larry, Deborah J. White, and Marsha T. Wallace. "Injuries from Dog Bites." *Journal of the American Medical Association* 279, no. 15 (1998): 1174.

Sheehy, Gail. *Understanding Men's Passages: Discovering the New Map of Men's Lives.* New York: Ballantine Books, 1999.

Shettles, Landrum B., and David M. Rorvik. *How to Choose the Sex of Your Baby: The Method Best Supported by Scientific Evidence.* New York: Doubleday, 1997.

Silverstein, Olga, and Beth Rashbaum. *The Courage to Raise Good Men.* New York: Viking Press, 1994.

Small, Eric, and Linda Spear. *Kids & Sports.* New York: Newmarket Press, 2002.

Sommers, Christina Hoff. *The War Against Boys: How Misguided Feminism Is Harming Our Young Men.* New York: Simon & Schuster, 2000.

Sothern, Melinda S., T. Kristian von Almen, and Heidi Schumacher. *Trim Kids: The Proven 12-Week Plan That Has Helped Thousands of Children Achieve a Healthier Weight.* New York. Harper Resource, 2001.

Strasburger, Victor C., ed. *Adolescent Medicine: State of the Art Reviews* 1, no.1 (1990)—14, no. 1 (2003); Official Journal of the Section on Adolescent Health of the American Academy of Pediatrics. Philadelphia: Hanley & Belfus.

Thomas, Alexander, Stella Chess, Richard Lerner, and Jacqueline Lerner. *New York Longitudinal Study: 1956–1988.* New York: Murray Research Center, Radcliffe Institute for Advanced Studies.

Thompson, Michael. *Speaking of Boys: Answers to the Most-Asked Questions about Raising Sons.* New York: Ballantine Books, 2000.

Tremblay, Richard E. "The Origins of Youth Violence." *Isuma* 1 (Autumn 2000): 19–24.

Tudiver, Fred, and Yves Talbot. "Why Men Don't Seek Help." *Journal of Family Practitioners* 48, no. 1 (1999): 47–52.

2002 CASA National Survey of American Attitudes on Substance Abuse VII: Teens, Parents and Siblings. New York: The National Center on Addiction and Substance Abuse at Columbia University, 2002. *http://www.casacolumbia.org/usr_doc/TeenSurvey2002.pdf* (July 3, 2003).

U.S. Department of Health and Human Services. *Physical Activity and Health: A Report of the Surgeon General.* Washington, DC: U.S. Department of Health and Human Services, 1996.

Waite, Linda J., and Maggie Gallagher. *The Case for Marriage: Why Married People Are Happier, Healthier, and Better Off Financially.* New York: Doubleday, 2001.

Willcox, Bradley J., Craig D. Willcox, and Makoto Suzuki. *The Okinawa Program: How the World's Longest-lived People Achieve Everlasting Health—and How You Can Too.* New York: Three Rivers Press, 2002.

Willett, Walter C., and P. J. Skerrett. *Eat, Drink, and Be Healthy: The Harvard Medical School Guide to Healthy Eating.* New York: Simon & Schuster, 2001.

Zilbergeld, Bernie. *The New Male Sexuality.* Rev. ed. New York: Bantam Books, 1999.

Acknowledgments

This book could not have been written without the help and support of literally a few hundred people. Whether it was emotional support and encouragement, expert opinion, thoughtful reviewing, or detailed fact checking, we owe a huge debt of gratitude to a large number of busy, hardworking professionals—doctors, professors, psychologists, sociologists, and staff members at academies and other institutions. Their kindness and willingness to share their knowledge and expertise, as well as their enthusiasm for the project, helped make this book become a reality.

A few people deserve special thanks. Literary agent Richard Abate was enthusiastic about this project from the very start. His encouragement and counsel helped bring the book to fruition. Editor Beth Wareham kept the faith with us through the long process of birthing this book and lent us her patient reassurance and wise editorial eye. Paige Bierma, Jennifer Barefoot, Joan Kruckewitt, and Arielle Zibrak spent hours digging up details and fact checking. Joan Fitzsimons and Leslie Kuizema in the CBS library were always kind, competent, and willing to help.

The people at the Men's Health Network—especially Tracie Snitker—offered help and support throughout. Drs. Jean Bonhomme, Eli Newberger, Joshua Sparrow, Stephen Havas, William Pollack, Randolph Smoak, and Steven Parker read parts or all of the manuscript and offered excellent suggestions. Gina Steiner at the American Academy of Pediatrics and Mara Greengass at the American Psychological Association provided much cheerful and valuable assistance.

A few people deserve special thanks from each of us.

From Emily: Without my husband Avery's constant support, and his willingness to do his share and much, much more at home, this book would never have been written. He was an unflappable force who never let the pressure get to him. My sister Caroline Senay reviewed the manuscript over and over again and helped out with many of the technical details while at the same time providing constant encouragement for the worth of the project. My father, Edward C. Senay, M.D., reviewed chapters and offered constant support for the idea. My producer at CBS News, Matthew Geers, picked up the slack while I worked away on this book; his quiet competence allowed me to focus on the task at hand and still get on the air.

From Rob: The support of my partner, Lenore Goldman, and her willingness to take care of so many things on the home front helped free me up for the many long hours of work this project required. My friend Diana Hembree's wise counsel and editorial advice helped improve the quality of our writing. My office mate, Thea Bellos, put up with my constant interviews as well as my mounting stress level as this book moved toward deadline. And finally, my son Joshua gave me a constant, loving reminder of what this book is all about: nurturing the sweet, irrepressible energy of boys.

Finally, we'd like to thank the scores of other people who shared with us their stories, their perspectives, or their expertise. Many of them are mentioned or quoted in the book; others are not, but their thoughts and ideas helped guide us in important ways. Here are some of those who helped, with apologies to others we may have unintentionally omitted.

Larry Alexander, M.D., Teena Austin, David Bell, M.D., Richard Bloch, Jean Bonhomme, M.D., Leslie R. Brody, Ph.D., Armin Brott, Kelly D. Brownell, Ph.D., James Cameron, Ph.D., William B. Carey, M.D., Cheryl Chase, Andrew Christensen, Ph.D., Sam Cochran, Ph.D., Scott L. Coltrane, Ph.D., Bridget Conrad, Ross Coulter, Todd Dezen, Lawrence Diller, M.D., Nicholas A. DiNubile, M.D., Joy G. Dryfoos, Allen Elkin, Ph.D., Leonard H. Epstein, Ph.D., Marty Ewing, Ph.D., Harry Fisch, M.D., Kurt W. Fischer, Ph.D., Baruch Fischhoff, Ph.D., Marty Fisher, M.D., Megan Fleming, Ph.D., Warren Foster, Ph.D., Rachel Freed, Jeffrey Friedman, M.D., Betty Gallo, Om Ganda, M.D., Floyd Garrett, M.D., Julie Gilchrist, Ken Goldberg, M.D., Robin Goodman, Ph.D., Enoch Gordis, M.D., David Gremillion, M.D., Rev. Debra Haffner, Daniel Halperin, Ph.D., S. Sutton Hamilton, M.D., Wendy Schlessel Harpham, M.D., Mike Hennenfent, Terry Hensle, M.D., Clark Hickman, Jimmie Holland, M.D., Ian Holzman, M.D., Gerald Imber, M.D., Mary Lloyd Ireland, M.D., Wendy Isett, Leon James, Ph.D., Marion Johnson, Christine Kennedy, Ph.D., Michael Kimmel, Ph.D., Paul D., Kligfield, M.D., William Klish, M.D., Barry Kogan, M.D., Joel Kotin, M.D., Carol Krause, Judy and Ray LaCour, Virginia and Keith Laken, Alice Leeds, Gretchen LeFever, Ph.D., Jacqueline Lerner, Ph.D., Simon LeVay, Ph.D., Bennett E. Leventhal, M.D., Suzanne Braun Levine, Matthew Longnecker, M.D., Mary Lou, Patrick Lyden, M.D., Lynn Macken, R.N., Eileen J. Masciale, Mary McGorry, Angela Mickalide, Ph.D., Ann and Larry Miller, Eric Miller, Karen Miller-Kovach, M.S., R.D., George Molzen, M.D., John Morley, M.D., Barbara Morrongiello, Ph.D., Robert Morse, M.D., Lori Mosca, M.D., Karen Murray, Diane Nahl, Ph.D., Phillip F. Nasrallah, M.D., Robert Needleman, M.D., Eli Newberger, M.D., Laurel Northouse Ph.D., Eva Obarzanek Ph.D., Roberto Olivardia, Ph.D., Dean Ornish, M.D., Tagni Osentowski, John Page, Marisa Peacock, Ora Peskovitz, M.D., Craig Peters, M.D., Mark Peyrot, Ph.D., Stuart Plante, Jodie Plumert, Ph.D., Lynn E. Ponton, M.D., James O. Prochaska, Ph.D., Joseph A. Pursch, M.D., Terry Real, Ph.D., Edward Reiter, M.D., Cindy and Rick Reynolds, Joyce Rock, Jamie Von Roenn, M.D., Walter Rogan, M.D., Michael Rohrbaugh, Ph.D., Don Sabo, Ph.D., Frank Sacks, M.D., Robert Salant, M.D., David Sandman, Ph.D., Richard A. Schieber, M.D., Richard Schlussel, M.D., Edgar Schoen, M.D., Bob Schwadron, Pepper Schwartz, Ph.D., David Schwebel, Ph.D., Suzanne Seitz, Tamara Sher, Ph.D., Roger Sherman, James Shikany, Ph.D., Georganne Small, Eric Small, M.D., Bernie Smith, Jeffery Sobal, Ph.D., Freya Sonenstein, Ph.D., Melinda Sothern, Ph.D., Richard Stock, M.D., Shelley Taylor, Ph.D., Jonathan Trager, M.D., David Tseng, Mike Wallace, Abigail Wallis, MS.PH, Steven Warach, M.D., Marilyn Weeks, Merle James York, Andrea Zaldiver, Douglas Zipes, M.D.

Subject Index

Note: See separate symptoms index for specific symptoms.

abdominal fat, 371–372, 440
AboutOurKids.org, 76
Abraham, 39–40
abstinence-only sex education, 211–213, 223
accidents and injuries, 108–120
    bikes, 110, 111–112, 188, 520
    bodies of water, 110–111
    car accidents. *see* car accidents
    dog bites, 114–115
    falls, 114
    gender gap in, 108–110, 118–120
    guns, 110, 115–118
    on-the-job, 2, 110, 208–209, 497
    from sleep deprivation, 516, 518–519
    sports injuries, 242–253, 520–522
    traffic, 112–113
ACE inhibitors, 381
action stage of change, 281
active boys, 82–83
Adderall, 103
AD/HD. *see* attention deficit hyperactivity
    disorder (AD/HD)
adolescence
    alcohol use during, 179, 186, 193–197, 224
    car accidents in, 186, 187–190
    depression in, 199–202, 234
    drug use during, 186, 193–197, 224
    employment during, 192, 208–209
    gender gap in health care during, 11, 133, 134
    growth spurts, 139, 146, 154, 156, 181, 251
    mortality rates in, 1
    as normal transition, 183–185
    nutrition in, 138–139
    physical checkups, 134–138
    risk-taking behavior in, 179–180, 184–197,
        224–225
    sex education in, 218–220
    sexuality in, 210–234
    smoking during, 179, 186, 190–193
    sports in, 237–239
    suicide and, 179, 180, 203–205, 234
    warning signs of violence in, 88
    see also puberty
Adonis Complex, 160–161, 165–166

Adonis Complex, The (Pope et al.), 160–161,
    165–166, 240
adrenal glands, 483, 487
adrenaline, 502
advertising, 153
African Americans
    diabetes and, 142, 427, 428, 435
    glucose-6-phosphate-dehydrogenase (G6PD)
        and, 61
    life expectancy of, 8
    prostate cancer and, 340
    school readiness and, 90
    stroke in, 8
    testicular cancer and, 173
After Any Diagnosis (Svec), 455, 457
After Cancer (Harpham), 464
aggression
    in road rage, 354–356
    rough boys, 83–85
    stress and, 501–505
    see also anger
AIDS, 42–43, 194, 211, 223
air pollution, 73
Al-Anon, 448–449
albumin, 25
alcoholism, 441–451
    as family disease, 442–443
    impact on family, 446–447
    stress on spouse and, 441–442, 448–451
    warning signs of, 443–446
alcohol use
    during adolescence, 179, 186, 193–197, 224
    during adulthood, 314–315, 421–422,
        496–497
    driving and, 179, 180, 187, 189, 190, 315, 357,
        443, 444
    high blood pressure and, 421–422
    sexual activity and, 224
    in young adulthood, 266–267
aldosterone, 54–55
Alexander, Larry, 262
All Kinds of Minds, 95
Almeida, David, 499
alpha-beta blockers, 423

alpha blockers, 475, 479
Always My Child (Jennings and Shapiro), 232
Alzheimer's disease, 380
ambiguous genitals, 54–58, 230
American Academy of Pediatrics (AAP)
    ambiguous genitals and, 55
    annual checkups, 134–135
    circumcision and, 40–41, 42, 45–46, 47
    falls and, 114
    infant sleep patterns and, 39
    obesity and, 140–141, 143
    position on phthalates, 71
    sexuality and, 210
    sports and, 237, 249, 250
    television and, 153
    violence prevention tips, 85–87
American Indians. *see* Native Americans
amniocentesis, 27, 28
anabolic steroids, 137, 160, 162–163, 165, 176
Anaxagoras of Clazomenae, 24
Andersen, Arnold, 546
Androgen Deficiency in Aging Men (ADAM)
    questionnaire, 491
androgen insensitivity syndrome (AIS), 55
androgens, 23, 54, 176, 487
androstenedione, 162, 163, 165, 487, 543
anger, 68, 501–505
    in adolescence, 200
    cancer and, 459
    heart disease and, 502
    road rage and, 354–356
    rough boys and, 83–85
    stress and, 501–505
    strokes and, 386
    venting, 386, 503–504
angina pectoris, 362, 370
angiogram, 382
angioplasty, 382
angiotensin converting enzyme (ACE) inhibitors,
    423
angiotensin receptor blockers, 423
animal bites, 114–115
annual checkup, 11, 134–135
anorexia, 160, 161
antidepressants, 64, 507–508, 509–511
antihistamines, 480
antimalarial drugs, 61
antioxidants, 310, 317–318
Apgar scores, 33
armpit hair, 181
Armstrong, Lance, 172, 173
ascended testicles, 174
Asians and Pacific Islanders
    circumcision and, 41
    cleft lip and cleft palate and, 38

diabetes and, 142, 427
    osteoporosis and, 485
    testicular cancer and, 173
As Nature Made Him (Colapinto), 56–57
aspirin, 61, 361, 379, 380
asthma
    environmental toxins and, 72, 73
    of infants, 33
    of mother during pregnancy, 28
    obesity and, 140
    obesity/overweight and, 397
atherosclerosis, 318, 415
athletic supporters and cups, 171, 252–253
Atkins Diet, 302
atrial fibrillation, 386–387
attention deficit hyperactivity disorder (AD/HD),
    64, 98–104, 132
    treatment of, 98, 100–102, 103–104
    warning signs of, 99–100
Austin, Laurie, 105
autism, 33–34, 61–63
autosuggestion, 27–28

baby boomers, 276, 452, 520–522
BabyCenter.com, 24, 25, 27
Bailes, Julian, 250
balanitis, 167, 168
baldness, 547–548
Barefoot, John, 502
baseball, 193, 239, 242, 244–246, 254, 348–349
basketball, 239, 242, 243, 249, 254, 520
Bayer, 14
Beal, Carole R., 32, 84, 228
beauty products, for men, 545–546
Bechler, Steve, 164
bedwetting, 123–126
behavioral modification, 206–207
behavioral therapy, 82, 102–103
Beidel, Deborah, 81, 82
Bell, David, 269
Belly-Off Club, 405–406
benign prostatic hyperplasia (enlarged prostate),
    473, 476–480
Berman, Jennifer and Laura, 540–541
beta-blockers, 379, 381, 423
Biermann, June, 436
bigorexia, 160
bike riding, 238, 253
    accidents, 110, 111–112, 188, 520
    sexual problems and, 476, 482
bile acid sequestrants, 414
binge drinking, 315
binge eating, 161
biofeedback, 475
Birch, Leann, 147

birth control, 213, 222–224
birth defects, 28, 34–39, 73, 481–482
Bishop, Melanie, 459, 463–464, 465
bisphosphonates, 485
Blacks. *see* African Americans
bladder exstrophy, 53
Bloch, Annette and Richard, 455, 461–462
Blood Chemistry (Metabolic Panel), 333, 342
blood pressure
    measuring, 332, 335
    see also high blood pressure
blood tests, 333, 342, 407, 428–429, 432–433
Bloom, David, 5
blue balls, 178
Blum, Robert, 218
body control, 121–132
    clumsiness, 131–132
    encopresis, 126–127
    night terrors, 131
    night training, 123–126
    sleepwalking, 131
    snoring/sleep apnea, 129–131
    stuttering, 127–129
    toilet training, 121–123
body dysmorphic disorder (BDD), 160–161
body image
    Adonis Complex and, 160–161, 165–166
    baldness and, 547–548
    beauty products and, 545–546
    boomeritis syndrome and, 520–522
    eating disorders and, 159–161, 164–165, 546
    performance-enhancing substances and, 162–164
    plastic surgery and, 546–547
Body Mass Index (BMI), 332, 335, 394–395, 406–407
Bogues, Mugsy, 154
Boleyn, Ann, 22
bone development, 139, 156, 157, 245
Bonhomme, Jean, 9
boomeritis syndrome, 520–522
boot camp, 205–207
bowel movements, encopresis and, 126–127
boxer shorts, 482
boxing, 249
Boy Code
    components of, 68, 200–201
    denial and, 12–13
    emotional development of males and, 65–69, 75–88, 263–266
    fathers as role models and, 16–17, 68–69, 122–123, 217–218, 224–225
    male personality types and, 263–266
    risk taking and, 12–13, 68–69, 217–218, 224–225

Boykins, Earl, 154
Boys and Girls (Beal), 84, 228
brain
    development in adolescence, 181, 183, 191
    nicotine and, 191
    sexual orientation and, 229–230
    size, 23, 98–99
brain cancer, 273
Brannon, Robert, 68
Braun, Levine, Suzanne, 269
Braus, Patricia, 15
Brazelton, T. Berry, 121–123
breast cancer, 273–274, 460, 483–484
breast enlargement (gynecomastia), 175–177, 483
breast-feeding, 58, 60, 496
briefs, 482
Bris Milah, 45
Brody, Leslie, 67–68
Brown, Marc, 214
Brownell, Kelly D., 145–146, 401, 402, 403, 545
Bruss, Katherine, 469
Buchwald, Art, 508
bulimia, 160, 161
bullying, 104–107
Bully-Proofing Your Child (Garrity), 106
burnout, caregiver, 465–466
Bushman, Brad, 503–504
Buss, Arnold, 79

Caballero, Benjamin, 317
Cacioppo, John, 271
CAGE questionnaire, 445
calcium, 139, 320, 486
calcium channel blockers, 381, 423
Califano, Joseph, 193–194
calorie counting, 432
Cameron, James, 76–78
Caminiti, Ken, 162
cancer, 452–471
    alcohol use and, 314
    caregiver role in, 452–455, 458, 460–467
    childhood, 72
    diet, 306
    from environmental toxins, 73
    male response to diagnosis, 458–460
    oncologist selection for, 455–457
    second opinions and, 456–457
    sexuality and, 469
    smoking and, 347–348, 350
    support network in, 16, 457–458, 465, 467–469
    treatment for, 460
    see also specific types of cancer
Canseco, Jose, 162
Caprio, Sonia, 141–142

car accidents
  in adolescence, 186, 187–190
  alcohol use and, 180, 187, 189, 315
  pedestrians and, 112–113
  sleep deprivation and, 516, 518–519
  in young adulthood, 266–267
carbohydrates, 139, 296, 299–301, 430–432
cardiac rehabilitation, 383–384
cardiac resynchronization, 385
cardiac stress test, 333, 343–344
Carducci, Bernardo, 79
caregiver role, 259–263
  with cancer, 452–455, 458, 460–467
  gender gap in, 14–16, 18, 262–263, 268–270
  letting go of, 17, 18, 200–201
  nature of, 14–16, 262–263, 269–270, 324–326,
    369, 436–438
  stress of, 17–18, 269–270, 272, 391–392,
    448–451, 458, 465–466
  support for, 448–449, 465, 467
Carey, William, 77, 80, 100, 101
carotid dissection, 388–389
carpal tunnel syndrome, 397
Case for Marriage, The (Waite and Gallagher), 15,
    17, 271
Caucasians
  osteoporosis and, 485
  testicular cancer and, 173
Cavett, Dick, 511
centenarians, 9
cervical cancer, 44
Cesarean delivery (C-section), 32
Chalmers, Karen, 430
change, 274–284
  dietary, 306–307, 311–314, 406–407
  helping partners with, 275–276
  modeling, 282
  nagging and, 282–283
  stages of, 277–282
  in tactics, 283–284
Chase, Cheryl, 57–58
Chassin, Laurie, 190
Chess, Stella, 75–76
chest x-ray, 344–345
chewing tobacco, 193, 348–349
childbirth process, 32–34
child care, gender gap in, 14, 18
chlamydia, 171, 476
Chlamydia pneumonia, 415
cholesterol
  HDL, 293, 336–337, 407–408
  LDL, 293, 336–337, 407–412, 415
  total, 336, 407–408
  see also high cholesterol
cholesterol-lowering drugs, 381

cholesterol particle size, 416
chordee, 53
chores, 312–313
chorionic villus sampling (CVS), 28
Christensen, Andrew, 282–283
chromosomes
  abnormalities of, 36–37
  in fertilization process, 21–23
Cialis (taldenafil), 539
cigar-smoking, 347–348
circumcision, 39–48
  defined, 39
  emergency, 168
  history of, 39–40
  hypospadias and, 53
  pain and, 45
  procedure for, 45
  pros and cons of, 42–45
  rates in other countries, 41
  risks of, 45–47
Clarke, Peter, 457
claudication, 435
cleft lip and cleft palate, 38
clitorectomy, 57
clitoris, 55–56, 230
clubfoot, 37
clumsiness, 131–132
coaches, 240, 241–242, 248
cocaine, 137, 195, 388
Cochran, Sam, 506, 511
cognitive-behavioral therapy, 64–65
Cohn, Leigh, 546
Colapinto, John, 56–57
colonoscopy, 340, 341
color blindness, 34
colorectal cancer, 380, 397
  screening for, 11, 332, 334, 340–342, 471
  warning signs of, 366
Coltrane, Scott, 273, 295, 312–313
coming out, 231–233
Committed to Kids, 150
Commonwealth Fund, 10–11, 13, 201, 266
communication
  about alcohol and drug use, 195–198
  about alcoholism, 448–451
  bullying and, 106–107
  about cancer, 458–460, 467–469
  about health care, 255–256
  about sexuality, 210, 213–220, 535–536
  about smoking, 191–193
  stuttering and, 127–129
  about suicide, 203–205
Complete Blood Count (CBC), 333, 342
Complete Idiot's Guide to Managed Health Care,
    The (Korczyk and Witte), 325

computers, lack of exercise and, 152–154
conception process, 21–23, 214
concussion, 244, 247–249
condoms, 222–224
confidentiality laws, 135–136
congenital adrenal hyperplasia (CAH), 54–56, 230
congestive heart failure, 272, 385
constipation, avoiding, 480
constitutional delay, 156
Consumer Lab, 320
Consumer Product Safety Commission, 112
contemplation stage of change, 279–280
Cope, John R., 460
coronary artery bypass surgery, 17, 262, 382
corticosteroid (cortisone), 54
cortisol, 502
Couples Confronting Cancer (Fincannon and Bruss), 469
Courage to Raise Good Men, The (Silverstein), 31
Coyne, James, 272
CPR (cardiopulmonary resuscitation), 373–374
crack cocaine, 388
C-reactive protein, 372–373, 415
creatine, 162, 163–164, 165, 250
cremaster, 178
crime
    adolescence and, 186, 199
    boot camp/wilderness therapy, 205–207
    bullying and, 105
cryptosporidium, 73
cytomegalovirus (CMV), 415

Dabbs, James, 488–489
DASH diet, 316, 421
David, Deborah S., 68
Davidson, Karina, 504–505
Davis, Laura, 117–118
DDT (dichlorodiphenyltrichloroethane), 70
death
    from car accidents, 188
    from diabetes, 426
    from ephedra (ma huang) use, 164
    from falls, 114
    gender gap in mortality, 1–2, 8–9, 23, 268
    from heatstroke, 205, 206, 249–250
    leading causes of childhood, 109
    in lead poisoning, 72
    motorcycles and, 356–357
    risks in adolescence, 180
    from undetected heart abnormalities, 136–137, 142, 158–159, 261–262
    see also suicide

DeCherney, Alan H., 26
decongestants, 480
default sex, 22, 23
defibrillation, 373–374
DEHP (di-ethylexyl phthalate), 70–71
dehydration, 240–241
    avoiding, 139
    treatment of, 60, 250
    warning signs of, 60
demand-withdrawal response, 282–283
denial
    by African Americans, 9
    of alcoholism, 445–446
    Boy Code and, 12–13
    of cancer, 458–460
    causes of, 12–13
    of diabetes, 436–438
    in emergencies, 360, 361
    gender gap and, 10–13
    pathological stoicism and, 9
    prevalence of, 10–12
    price of, 261–262
    of vulnerability, 513–515
dental care, 333, 344, 372–373
depression, 105
    in adolescence, 199–202, 234
    family history of, 256
    in men, 505–515
    prevalence of, 200–201
    strokes and, 387
    treatment of, 507–508, 509–511
    warning signs of, 201–202, 508–509, 515
    see also suicide
DES (diethylstilbestrol), 71
desmopressin acetate (DDAVP), 126
Deutsch, Francine M., 312
DeVault, Marjorie, 294–295
developmental coordination disorder, 97, 131–132
developmental dyspraxia, 97, 131–132
DHEA, 165, 491–492, 543
diabetes, 125, 141–142, 267, 424–438
    diet and, 297, 300, 302
    gestational, 33, 141
    with obesity/overweight, 141–142, 397
    prevention and treatment of, 430–435, 438
    risk factors for, 427
    risks of, 426
    screening for, 332, 337–338, 428–429
    in specific ethnic groups, 142, 427, 435, 438
    types of, 141
    warning signs of, 364, 438
Diabetic Man, The (Lodewick et al.), 436
Diagnosis Cancer (Harpham), 454–455
Diagnostic and Statistical Manual of Mental Disorders (DSM-IV), 99–100

Diamond, Jed, 489–490
diastolic blood pressure, 417–418
Diclemente, Carlos, 277
dietary supplements, 162–164, 165, 315–321
diets and dieting
    for adults, 302, 310, 311, 406–407, 411–412,
        421, 430–432
    Atkins Diet, 302
    for children and adolescents, 147–149, 161,
        165
    DASH diet, 316, 421
    Mediterranean diet, 303–304
    Okinawa diet, 304–305
    see also food; nutrition; obesity/overweight
        condition
Dietz, William, 147
DiFranza, Joseph, 190–191
digital rectal exam (DRI), 334, 340
dihydrotestosterone (DHT), 487
Diller, Lawrence, 92
DiNubile, Nicholas A., 520–522
dioxin, 71, 74
discipline, 86, 91, 93
diuretics, 164, 423
diving accidents, 111
divorce
    job stress and, 498
    laws concerning, 15–16
DNA, in fertilization process, 21–23
doctors
    adolescents and, 134–137
    adults and, 321–331, 450
    attitudes toward patients, 13, 144, 325,
        330–331
    in discussions of alcoholism, 450
    preparation for visits, 327–329
    second opinions and, 456–457
    selecting, 14, 135–136, 325–327, 455–456
    sports physicals, 136–137, 159, 182, 262
dog bites, 114–115
Dollinger, Malin, 455
Don't Let Your HMO Kill You (Theodosakis and
        Feinberg), 325
double-contrast barium enema, 341
Down's syndrome, 481
"Dr. Mom" syndrome. see caregiver role
Dreaming for Two (Grill et al.), 30
dreams, of mothers during pregnancy, 30–31
dressing up, 215, 227, 228
drinking. see alcohol use
driving
    in adolescence, 186, 187–190
    alcohol and drug use and, 179, 180, 187, 189,
        190, 315, 357, 443, 444
    road rage and, 354–356

safety tips, 188–190
sleep deprivation and, 518–519
drowning, 110–111
drug use
    during adolescence, 186, 193–197,
        224
    driving and, 187, 189, 190
    prescription drugs. see medications
    sexual activity and, 224
    sports involvement and, 235
    in young adulthood, 266–267
Dryfoos, Joy G., 185, 195, 196–197
Duchenne's muscular dystrophy, 34–35
Dunkel-Schetter, Christine, 460
dyscalcula, 97
dysgraphia, 97
dyslexia, 94–97
dyspareunia, 533, 543
dyspraxia, 97, 131–132

Eat, Drink and Be Healthy (Willett), 296, 300, 303
eating disorders, 159–161, 164–165, 546
    types of, 160–161
    warning signs of, 161
Eat More, Weigh Less (Ornish), 405
echocardiograms, 158–159
Edison, Thomas, 96
eggs, 311
Eichner, Randy, 136–137
Einstein, Albert, 96
ejaculation, 220–221, 528–529, 531–532, 533
Elder, Sean, 445
electrocardiogram (ECG), 333, 343
electroconvulsive therapy (ECT), 511
Elkin, Allen, 495, 500, 504
embolism, warning signs of, 5
embryo, 22
embryonic/fetal stages, 28–31
emergencies, 358–363
    calling 911, 358–359, 361, 363
    emergency plan, 359–360
    genital, 168–173
    handling specific, 360–367
emergency room visits, 110, 114, 199, 208,
        243–244, 262, 358–359, 361, 363
EMLA, 45
emotional development
    gender gap in, 65–69, 75–88
    male personality types, 263–266
empathy, 107
employment
    during adolescence, 192, 208–209
    job stress and, 497–498
    on-the-job injuries, 2, 110, 208–209, 497
encopresis, 126–127

endocrine disrupters, 69–71
enemas, 127
enuresis, 123–126
environmental toxins, 69–74
enzyme deficiencies, 61
ephedra, 164, 165, 250, 316
epididymis, 138, 170–171, 174
epididymitis, 170–171
epididymo-orchitis, 170
epilepsy, 65
epiphysis, 251
epispadias, 53
Epstein, Leonard, 146, 147, 150
erectile dysfunction, 529–530, 534–537
    treatment of, 534–537, 538–539
    warning signs of, 529–530
Ericsson, Ronald J., 25
Eros-CTD, 543–544
esophageal cancer, 348, 367
estrogen, 59
    breast enlargement and, 175
    endocrine disrupters and, 69–71
Evans, Susan, 457
Everybody's Guide to Cancer Therapy (Dollinger et al.), 455
evidence-based medicine, 456
evolutionary conditioning, 12
Ewing, Marty, 239
exercise
    for adults, 285–294, 412, 422, 430, 433–434, 438
    for children and adolescents, 145–147, 150–154, 250
    couples working out together, 285–287
    encouraging, 150, 151–154, 250
    excessive, 165
    fitness tests, 287–293
    high blood pressure and, 422
    importance of, 13, 285, 379
    obesity and, 145, 146–147, 151–154, 399
    realistic approach to, 293–294
    see also sports
extreme sports, 238–239
Eyre, Harmon, 453

facial expressions, 67
Fallopian tubes, 22
falls, 114
family dinner, 313–314
Family Man (Coltrane), 273
Family Man personality, 264, 275
family medical history
    adolescent checkups and, 136
    alcoholism in, 442–443
    bedwetting and, 124, 125

birth defects and, 37
    communicating, 256
    obesity and, 143, 144–145
    in visits to doctor, 328, 329–330
family therapy, 64
Farkas, Arthur, 191–192
farm accidents, 110
fast food, 145, 147, 148–149, 308–309, 310, 398–399
fasting blood glucose test, 428
fathers
    gender orientation of sons and, 231–233
    as role models for sons, 16–17, 68–69, 122–123, 217–218, 224–225
    see also mothers; parents
fats in diet, 296, 297–299, 302, 306, 307, 311, 379, 411
fecal occult blood test (FOBT), 341
Feeding the Family (DeVault), 294–295
Feinberg, David T., 325
fertility clinics, 25–26
fertilization process, 21–23, 25–26
fetus, 21–31
    "boy anxiety" of mothers, 3, 29–31
    guessing sex of, 27–29
    influencing sex of, 24–27
    see also infancy; pregnancy
fiber, 300, 301, 412
fibric acids, 414
fight-or-flight mode, 12
finasteride, 479
Fincannon, Joy, 469
fires, 110
Fisch, Harry, 481–482
Fischer, Kurt, 84–85, 93
Fischhoff, Baruch, 198
fish, 63, 74, 308
Fisher, Helen, 488
Fisher, Martin, 134–135
fitness tests, 287–293
flavonoids, 310
Fleisig, Glenn, 246–247
Fleming, Megan, 527, 535
Flier, Jeffrey S., 371
flu shots, 345
folic acid/folate, 38, 319
food
    fast food, 145, 147, 148–149, 308–309, 310, 398–399
    mercury in, 63, 64
    organic, 74
    pesticides and, 73, 74
    as reward, 149
    sensitivities to, 63
    see also diets and dieting; nutrition; obesity/overweight condition

Food Fight (Brownell), 145–146
football, 242, 243–244, 249–250, 254
forceps delivery, 32
foreskin, 23
    circumcision and, 39–48
    restoring circumcised, 41
    in uncircumcised males, 46–48, 167–169
For Men Only (Imber), 547
For Women Only (Berman and Berman),
        540–541, 543
Foss, Robert, 189
fragile X syndrome, 35
Framingham Heart Study, 408
Freed, Rachael, 375–376, 383
free radicals, 318
Freud, Sigmund, 503, 515
Friedman, Jeff, 496

Gallagher, Maggie, 15–16, 271
Gallo, Betty, 16
Gallo, Dean, 16
Gametrics Ltd., 25
Garagiola, Joe, 349
Garrett, Floyd, 448
Garrity, Carla, 106–107
gastroenteritis, 59, 60
gatekeeping role, 18
Gatorade, 250
gay boys and men, 226–234
    coming out, 231–233
    health care and, 233–234
    homophobia and, 232–233
    nature versus nurture and, 229–230
    suicide and, 199, 234
gender-based medicine, 18
gender dysphoria, 228–229
gender gap
    in accidents and injuries, 108–110, 118–120
    in aggression, 84
    in body control, 121, 124
    in caregiving, 14–16, 18, 262–263, 268–270
    in cognitive development, 89–94
    in coping with stress, 495–497
    in emotional development, 65–69, 75–88,
        263–266
    in handling depression, 512–515
    in handling with sexuality problems, 526–527,
        539–540
    in health, 1–2, 7–18, 23, 32–39, 59–61, 69
    in health care, 3–5, 10–13, 133, 134, 278–279,
        322–323, 435–438
    in mortality rates, 1–2, 8–9, 23, 268
    in newborns, 32–34, 58–59
    in parental health care for children, 14, 18
    performance gap and, 93–94

    in personality, 65–69, 75–88
    in physical development, 23, 139
    in preferences for sex of baby, 24–27
    in schooling, 93–94
    in school readiness, 89–92
    in sexual double standard, 212–213
    in temperament, 77–88
gender orientation/identity
    of gay boys and men, 227–229
    of intersex children, 54–58
    see also sex of baby
gender roles
    in caregiving, 14–16, 18, 262–263, 268–270
    in nutrition, 294–295, 306–307, 311–312
    in play, 226–228
gender vertigo, 17
Gender Vertigo (Risman), 269–270
genes
    in fertilization process, 21–23
    see also family medical history
genetic disorders
    chromosomal abnormalities, 36–37
    sex-linked, 34–35
genitals
    ambiguous, 54–58, 230
    "buried," 49
    circumcision, 39–48
    development of, 22, 23
    of newborns and baby boys, 48–54
    normal variations in, 48–50
    protecting, 171, 252–253
    talking about, 214–215
    see also penis; prostate gland; sexuality;
        testicles
genital tubercle, 23
gestational diabetes, 33, 141
Giametti, Charlene, 219
Giedd, Jay, 183
GI Jim personality, 265, 274
Gilligan, Carol, 93–94
Glantz, Michael, 273
Glassberg, Alan, 455
Glaxo SmithKline, 81–82
glucose-6-phosphate-dehydrogenase (G6PD),
        61
glycemic index, 301, 431
glycemic load, 301
GnRH (gonadotropin-releasing hormone), 158
Goldberg, Kenneth, 264, 275, 322
Goldman, Ronald and Juliette, 216
Goldstein, Michael G., 325
gonorrhea, 171, 476
Goodman, Robin, 76, 80–81
Gottman, John, 272–273, 504
gout, 397

Graedon, Joe and Teresa, 320
Great Procrastinator personality, 265, 274
Green, Tom, 172, 173
Greer, Brian F., 124
Gremillion, David H., 265, 274–275
Grill, Hillary, 30–31
growth spurts, 139, 146, 154, 156, 181, 251, 472, 487
Guide for Cancer Supporters (Bloch and Bloch), 455, 461–462
gum disease, 372–373
guns, 86, 110, 115–118
    adolescence and, 179, 186
    safety tips, 116–117
    school shootings, 105
    toy gun play, 117–118
gymnastics, injuries, 242
gynecomastia (breast enlargement), 175–177, 483

Haffner, Debra, 215, 217–218, 226
Hailoo, Wajdy, 322
hair
    baldness and, 547–548
    facial, pubic, and armpit, 181
    wrapped around penis, 54
Hall, G. Stanley, 183
Halperin, Daniel, 43
Halving It All (Deutsch), 312
Hamilton, S. Sutton, 132
Hank Hardbody personality, 265–266, 274
Harpham, Wendy Schlessel, 454–455, 464, 468–469
Harrison, James, 69
Havas, Stephen, 422–423
Haynes, Tony, 205, 206
HDL (high-density lipoprotein) cholesterol, 293, 336–337, 407–408
heading, in soccer, 248
head injury
    in bike accidents, 111–112
    in precocious puberty, 157–158
health care
    communicating with boys about, 255–256
    gender gap in, 3–5, 10–13
health care information
    on alcoholism, 448–449
    on cancer, 453–455
    gender gap in use of, 15, 278–279
    on nutrition, 295–296, 311
    during puberty, 182–183
    sexuality and, 212–213
health insurance
    of African Americans, 8
    decisions concerning, 15

health screenings, 11, 324, 331–346
heart attack, 370–385
    CPR and, 373–374
    from diuretic use, 164
    emergency care for, 360–362
    follow-up care, 375–378
    impact on spouses, 17
    recovering from, 382–385
    risk factors for, 371–373, 378, 380, 426
    warning signs of, 2, 3, 10, 11, 360–362, 373
heart disease, 267, 369–385
    in African Americans, 8
    anger and, 502
    with diabetes, 142
    diagnostic procedures for, 382
    diet and, 297, 300, 302, 303, 317, 318, 319, 406–407, 411–412
    with obesity, 142, 405
    risk factors for, 13, 350, 408–412
    screening for, 333, 343–344
    treatment of, 378–382, 406–416
    warning signs of, 140
Heartmates (Freed), 375–376, 383
heat exhaustion, 244
heatstroke, 249–250
Heber, David, 308
height, 154–159
    short children, 154–157
    tall children, 157–159
helmets, 111–112, 246, 253, 254, 356–357, 522
hemoglobin A1C or HBA1C test, 429
hemophilia, 24, 34, 35
hemorrhagic strokes, 387
hemorrhoids, 334, 367
Henry VIII, 22
Henschke, Claudia, 470
Hensley, Scott, 5
hepatitis, 346, 398
herbal supplements, 320–321, 475, 476, 480
Herman-Giddens, Marcia, 181
hermaphrodites, 54–58
hernias, 51–52, 171, 173–175
Heroes, Rogues, and Lovers (Dabbs), 488–489
heroin, 195
Heyman, Richard, 255
HGH (human growth hormone), 156–157
Hickman, Clark, 473, 476
high blood pressure, 267, 416–424
    in African Americans, 8
    monitoring, 423–424
    primer on, 417–418
    risks of, 417
    screening for, 332, 335
    treatment for, 419–424
    warning signs of, 364

high cholesterol
  in adulthood, 267, 407–416
  risk factors for, 408–409, 415–416
  screening for, 332, 335–337
  treatment for, 407–416
Hippocrates, 27, 37, 128
Hirschprung's disease, 61
Hispanics
  circumcision and, 41
  diabetes and, 142, 427, 435
HIV infection, 42–43, 194, 211, 212, 213, 223, 224, 234
HMOs (health maintenance organizations), 325–326, 456
Hoban, Timothy, 130
Hochschild, Arlie, 295
hockey, 242, 249
Holbrook, Thomas, 546
Holland, Jimmie, 458–460, 468
Hollis, Zak, 104–106
Holmes, T. H., 500
Holzman, Ian R., 33
Home First Aid Kit, 359, 360
homicide, 266–267
homocysteine, 319, 415, 502
homophobia, 232–233
homosexuality. *see* gay boys and men
hooking up, 224
hormone replacement therapy (HRT), for men, 491–493
hostility, 501–505
How Healthy Is Your Family Tree? (Krause), 329
How to Change Your Spouse and Change Your Marriage (Kotin), 276, 283–284
How to Choose the Sex of Your Baby (Shettles), 25
H.pylori bacterium, 415
human genome, 66
human growth hormone (HGH), 156–157
human papilloma virus (HPV), 44
Human Side of Cancer, The (Holland), 458–460
Humatrope, 156–157
humor, 273, 504
hydroceles, 51–52
hydrogenation, 299
hygiene
  neglect of, in suicidal behavior, 204, 363
  for penis, 45, 46–48, 167, 168, 169
hypertension. *see* high blood pressure
hypnosis, 27–28
hypoglycemia, 433
hypogonadism, 490–493
hypospadias, 52–53, 69, 70, 71
hypothalamus, sexual orientation and, 229–230
hypoxia, 397

Iannini, Paul B., 14
I Don't Want to Talk About It (Real), 200, 506
Imber, Gerald, 547
imipramine, 126
impotence. *see* erectile dysfunction
impulsivity, 99–100
inattention, 99
Indestructo Man personality, 264, 274
infancy
  circumcision in, 39–48
  mortality rates in, 1
  sleep patterns in, 38–39
  see also fetus
infarction. *see* heart attack
Informed Decisions (American Cancer Society), 466
inguinal canal, 50–52
inguinal hernias, 51–52, 173–174
inhibited temperament, 78–81, 85
injuries. *see* accidents and injuries
in-line skating, 238, 246, 253
Inside the Teenage Brain (PBS program), 183
insulin resistance, 439–440
intercourse
  sex of baby and timing of, 25
  teenage sexuality and, 218–220, 222–224
  see also sexuality
Internet
  health information on, 221–222, 453–454
  pornography on, 221–222
intersex babies, 54–58
interventions, for alcoholism, 450–451
in vitro fertilization, 26
Ireland, Mary Lloyd, 245
iron, 317
ischemic stroke, 386

Jacobson, Neil S., 270–271, 282–283
James, Leon, 355–356
Jenkins, David, 301
Jennings, Kevin, 232
Jensen, Peter, 103–104
Jewish faith, circumcision in, 39–40, 45
jobs. *see* employment
job stress, 497–498
Johnson, Alex, 171–172
judgment, risk-taking behavior and, 120
junk food, 145, 147, 148–149, 308–309, 310, 398–399
juvenile detention facilities, 199

Kagan, Jerome, 79
Kaiser Permanente, 77
Kaminetsky, Jed, 543
Karlin, Elyse Zorn, 216

Kellner, Steven, 14
Kennedy, Christina M., 119
Keyser, Janis, 117–118
Kids & Sports (Small), 136
Kiecolt-Glaser, Janice, 272
kindergarten, 89–92, 106
Kindlon, Dan, 68, 83, 91, 200–202
Kirkendall, Donald, 248
Klein, Carol, 30, 31
Klein, Rachel G., 101
Kligfield, Paul, 380, 383
Klinefelter, Harry, 36
Klinefelter's syndrome, 36, 176, 177, 483
Klish, William, 140–141
Korczhk, Sophie M., 325
Kotin, Joel, 276, 277, 283–284
Kraemer, Sebastian, 7
Krasny, Laurie, 214
Krause, Carol, 329

labia, 54
LaCour, Judy, 306–307
Laken, Virginia and Keith, 469, 534
L-arginine, 543
La Rosa, John, 407
larynx cancer, 348
late bloomers, 156, 225
later adulthood stage, 268
Latinos. *see* Hispanics
Laumann, Edward O., 44
laxatives, 127
LDL (low-density lipoprotein) cholesterol, 293,
    336–337, 407–412, 415
lead poisoning, 72–73, 74
learning disabilities, 33–34, 93, 94–98, 131–132
learning styles, 90–91
LeFever, Gretchen, 100
Lerner, Jacqueline, 75–76
LeVay, Simon, 229–230
Leventhal, Bennett L., 185
Levine, Laurence A., 529
Levine, Mel, 95
Levinson, Daniel, 266
Levitra (vadenafil), 381, 539
lidocaine, 45
life expectancy
    of African Americans, 8
    gender gap in, 1–2, 8–9, 23, 268
life stages of men, 266–268
Lincoln, Abraham, 159
Lincoln, Gerald, 496
lipoproteins, 299, 416
Little League elbow, 245–246
Lodewick, Peter A., 436
loneliness, 271

Long, Charles E., III, 206
longevity gap, 1–2, 8–9, 23, 268
    closing, 16–17
    men's health crisis and, 9
    racial divide in, 8–9
low birth weight, 38–39
LSD, 195
Ludwig, David, 431
lung cancer, 347–348, 350
    screening for, 333, 344–345, 470
    warning signs of, 365–366
Lung Cancer (McCarthy and Wernick), 470
Lyden, Patrick, 388–389

Macken, Lynn, 378
ma huang, 164, 165
maintenance stage of change, 281
male menopause, 489–493
Male Menopause (Diamond), 489–490
managed care, 325–326, 331, 456
managed health care, 18
Manning, John, 372
Marfan syndrome, 158–159
marijuana, 176, 194–195
Maris, Roger, 162
Marketing Health Care to Women (Braus), 15
marriage
    divorce and, 15–16, 498
    impact on men's health, 15–16, 270–274,
        400–403
    impact on women's health, 17–18, 270–274
    see also sexuality
masturbation, 215, 218, 220–221, 222
mathematics, dyscalcula and, 97
Mayle, Peter, 214
McCarthy, Peggy, 470
McGorry, Mary, 110–111
McGwire, Mark, 162, 487
measles immunizations, 63
medical history. *see* family medical history
medications
    for AD/HD, 98, 100–102, 103–104
    for bedwetting, 126
    birth defects and, 38
    breast enlargement and, 483
    for cancer, 460
    for depression, 507–508, 509–511
    for diabetes, 430, 433–434
    in emergency plan, 360
    for enlarged prostate, 478–479
    for epilepsy, 65
    for erectile dysfunction, 385, 510, 529–530,
        534, 538–539, 542
    for female sexual response problems, 543–544
    gender gap in use of, 11

medications (*cont.*)
   for heart disease, 377, 379–381, 385, 412–416
   for high blood pressure, 423
   for high cholesterol, 412–414
   for obsessive-compulsive disorder, 64–65
   for osteoporosis, 485
   for prostatitis, 475
   psychiatric, 199
   shopping for, 15
   for social anxiety disorder (SAD), 81–82
   for stroke, 389
   for tics, 64
   in visits to doctor, 328–329
Mediterranean diet, 303–304
Mège-Mouriès, Hippolyte, 299
men's health clinics, at colleges and universities, 18
mental health counseling, 11, 64–65, 82, 102–103, 515
mercury, 63, 74, 308, 424
metabolic syndrome (Syndrome X), 439–440
micropenis, 49
MicroSort, 26
middle adulthood stage, 1, 267
Middle Ages, 24, 27
migraine headaches, 387–388
Milburn, Heather J., 28
Miller, Ann, 374
Miller, George, 206
Miller-Kovach, Karen, 15, 400–401
Mind at a Time, A (Levine), 95
minerals, 320
ministroke, 362, 387, 388
miscarriage, 23
Mismeasure of Desire, The (Stein), 229
mixed messages, on sexuality, 217–218
mohel, 45
Molzen, George, 390
Money, John, 56–57
monounsaturated fats, 298, 299
Morley, John, 491–493
Morrongiello, Barbara A., 119–120
Morse, Robert, 449, 450
mortality rates
   gender gap in, 1–2, 8–9, 23, 268
   health care and, 11
   on the job, 2
Mosca, Lori, 330–331, 376, 379
Mosher, Nancy, 213
mothers
   communicating about health care, 255–256
   communicating about sexuality, 210, 213–220
   as leaders in health care issues, 3–5, 14–16
   relationship with adolescent sons, 197–198, 203, 210, 213–220
   see also fathers; parents

Mothers and Sons (Klein), 31
motorcycles, 356–357
mouth cancer, 348–349
Multimodal Treatment Study (MTA study), 103–104
multivitamins, 302, 317
mumps, 63, 170
Murray, Karen, 158–159
muscle dysmorphia, 160
muscular dystrophy, 24, 34–35
myocardial infarction. *see* heart attack

nagging, 282–283, 349–350, 437
Nahl, Diane, 355–356
narcolepsy, 518–519
Nasrallah, Phillip, 46–47, 52, 166
National Center on Addition and Substance Abuse (CASA), 186, 193–194, 195
National Eating Disorders Screening Program, 161
National Health and Social Life Survey, 524, 542
National Intervention Network, 451
National Men's Health Week, 18, 275
National SAFE KIDS Campaign, 109, 110, 113
National Survey of Adolescent Males, 12
Native Americans
   cleft lip and cleft palate, 38
   diabetes and, 142, 427, 428
NeeDell, Elise, 455
Needleman, Robert, 121
negotiation, of change, 313
Nelson, Charles, 183
Nelson, Jennifer, 253–254
Nelson, Suzanne, 139
neonatal intensive care, 33
New Male Sexuality, The (Zilbergeld), 531–532, 536
New York Longitudinal Study, 75–76
nicotine, 190–191
nicotine gum, 352–353
nicotine skin patch, 353
nicotinic acid, 414
night terrors, 131
night training, 123–126
nitroglycerin, 385, 538
nocturnal enuresis (bedwetting), 123–126
Nolen-Hoeksema, Susan, 496–497
nonalcoholic steatohepatitis (NASH), 398
non-Hodgkin's lymphoma, 452
non-REM sleep, 131
Normann, Wilhelm, 299
Northouse, Laurel, 457, 458, 460, 463, 464, 465
nudity, 216
nutrition, 294–314
   change and, 306–307, 311–314, 406–407
   for diabetes, 430–432

diets and, 147–149, 161, 165, 302, 310, 311, 406–407, 411–412, 421, 430–432
food police, 295
guidelines for, 147–148, 150, 296, 297–306
junk food and, 145, 147, 148–149, 308–309, 310, 398–399
principles of, 307–311
salt and, 420, 421, 422–423
see also diets and dieting; food

obesity hypoventilization syndrome (OHS), 397
obesity/overweight condition, 138, 140–154, 393–407
in adults, 393–407, 432
breast enlargement in, 176
defining, 394–396
diabetes and, 141–142, 397
exercise and, 145, 146–147, 151–154, 399
high blood pressure and, 419–420
preventing, 146–154
problems of, 140–144, 397–398
reasons for, 144–146, 398–399
risks of, 371–372, 396–398, 412
support for spouse, 400–406
obsessive-compulsive disorder, 64–65
occupational therapy, 132
Offer, Daniel, 184
Office of Men's Health (proposed), U.S. Department of Health and Human Services, 18
Office of Women's Health, U.S. Department of Health and Human Services, 18
Okinawa diet, 304–305, 310
Olivardia, Roberto, 160–161, 163, 165–166, 240
Olweus, Dan, 105–106
omega-3 fatty acids, 308
oncologists, 455–457
on-the-job injuries, 2, 110, 208–209, 497
oral glucose tolerance test, 429
oral rehydration, 60, 250
oral sex, 219, 224
orchidometer, 177
orchiopexy, 50–51
orchitis, 170
organic food, 74
orgasm, 528–529
orgasmic disorder, 533, 542–543
Ornish, Dean, 278–279, 283, 305–306, 350, 402, 405, 413–414
Osgood-Schlatter disease, 251–252
osteoporosis, 320, 484–486
Out of Touch (Commonwealth Fund), 10–11, 266, 322–323
overuse injuries, 245–246, 397, 520–521

ovulation, 25
oxytocin, 32, 496

Pacific Islanders. see Asians and Pacific Islanders
Page, John, 467
paraphimosis, 168
parents
body image problems and, 164–165
bullying and, 106–107
communication about sexuality, 210, 213–220
involvement in sports, 239–242
obesity prevention and, 146–154
risk-taking behavior and, 119–120
as role models for children, 16–17, 68–69, 86, 122–123, 144–145, 146–154, 191–193, 217–218, 224–225, 255–256
smoking by adolescents and, 191–193
spending time with children, 196–198
temperament of child and, 76
toy gun play and, 117–118
in treatment of AD/HD, 102–103
see also fathers; mothers
partial AIS (androgen insensitivity syndrome), 55
pathological stoicism, 9
Paxil, 81–82
PCBs (polychlorinated biphenyls), 71, 74
pedestrian accidents, 112–113
pediatric endocrinologists, 157
pediatricians, 14, 135–136
peer pressure
alcohol and drug use and, 195
circumcision and, 44
obesity and, 144
resisting, 198
sexuality and, 225–226
penile cancer, 43
penile injections, 534, 537
penis
bending or curving, 53
circumcised, 39–40
hygiene for, 45, 46–48, 167, 168, 169
in normal sexual response, 528–529
problems with, 43–44, 52–54, 69, 70, 71, 167–169, 533
reconstruction of, 56–57
size of, 48–50, 49, 55, 177–178
uncircumcised, 46–48, 167–169
see also erectile dysfunction
performance-enhancing substances, 162–164, 165, 320–321, 487
peripheral vascular disease, 435
Perls, Fritz, 503
personality
gender gap and, 65–69, 75–88
male types, 263–266

pervasive developmental disorders (PDD), 61–63
Pescovitz, Ora, 155
pesticides, 73, 74
Peyronie's disease, 533
Peyrot, Mark, 435–436, 437
Phillips, Katherine A., 160–161, 165–166
phimosis, 43–44, 167
phthalates, 70–71, 74
physical abuse, 30, 201
physical exams
    annual checkups, 11, 134–136
    screening tests, 11, 324, 331–346
    sports physicals, 136–137, 159, 182, 262
    testicle self-exam, 137–138
Physical Fitness Specialist Manual, The, 288–292
physicians. *see* doctors
Pickwickian syndrome, 397
pipe-smoking, 348
Planned Parenthood, 213
plantar fasciitis, 520–521
Plante, Thomas, 286, 294
plaque, arterial, 142, 408
plastic surgery, 546–547
platelets, 319
play
    gender differences in, 66–67
    gender roles in, 226–228
    sex play, 215
    toy guns, 117–118
Pleck, Joe, 224
Plumert, Jodie, 120
pneumococcal vaccine, 333, 346
Pollack, William, 12, 68, 94, 200, 202, 511
pollution, 72–74
polysomnograph, 517–518
polyunsaturated fats, 298, 299
Ponton, Lynn E., 184, 186, 188, 197–198, 212,
    218, 225–226
Pope, Harrison, 159–161, 165–166
pornography, 221–222
portion control, 308–309
post-traumatic stress disorder (PTSD), 383
potassium, 422
potty training, 121–123, 126
Potty Training the Brazelton Way (Brazelton and
    Sprague), 122–123
poverty, adolescence and, 199
precocious puberty, 157–158
precontemplation stage of change, 278–279
prediabetes, 141, 428, 430
preeclampsia, 32–33
pregnancy
    birth defects and other problems, 34–39
    "boy anxiety" of mothers, 3, 29–31
    childbirth process, 32–34

    conception and, 21–23
    gestational diabetes, 33, 141
    guessing sex of baby, 27–29
    influencing sex of baby, 24–27
    premarital, 211, 212, 223
    protecting baby during, 38–39, 74
    smoking during, 27, 33, 38–39
preimplantation genetic diagnosis (PGD), 26
premature birth, 33
premature ejaculation, 531–532
preparation stage of change, 280
preschool years
    school preparation in, 89–92
    sports in, 236–237
    warning signs of violence in, 88
preteen years
    preparation for puberty, 182–183, 216–218
    sex education in, 216–218
    sports in, 237–239
    warning signs of violence in, 88
Preventive Ounce, The, 76–77
problem-solving skills, 86
Prochaska, James, 277–282
prostate cancer
    family history of, 13
    impact on spouses, 16, 262–263, 463–464, 534
    screening for, 11, 332, 338–340
    selenium and, 320
    support for, 16, 262–263
    treatment of, 306, 538
    warning signs of, 366
prostate gland, 472–482
    enlarged, 473, 476–480
    fertility and, 480–482
    prostatitis, 473–476
Prostate Specific Antigen (PSA), 338–340
prostatitis, 473–476
prostitution, 42
protein, 139, 163, 165, 296, 301–302
Psyching Out Diabetes (Rubin), 436
psychosis, 204
puberty
    breast enlargement during, 175, 176
    precocious, 157–158
    preparation for, 182–183, 216–218
    sexual orientation and, 230–231
    signs of, 180–182, 472, 487
    see also adolescence
pubic hair, 181
punishment, 85, 86
Pursch, Joseph A., 442, 446, 450
pyloric stenosis, 61

Rabinowitz, Rachel, 506–507
Rahe, R. H., 500

Raising Cain (Kindlon and Thompson), 68, 91
Raising Children to Resist Violence, 85–88
reading, 89
reading disabilities, 94–97
Real, Terrence, 200, 203, 506, 511, 512–515
Real Boys (Pollock), 12, 68
Reaven, Gerald, 439–440
Reconcilable Differences (Christensen), 282–283
red-green color blindness, 34
redshirting, 240
rehabilitation treatment, 383–384, 390
Reimer, David, 56–57
Reiter, Edward, 155
relational recovery therapy, 515
REM (rapid eye movement) sleep, 131
retractile testicles, 50, 174, 178
Reynolds, Cindy, 374
risk taking, 118–120
    in adolescence, 179–180, 184–197, 224–225
    in adulthood, 13, 265, 274, 356–357
    Boy Code and, 12–13, 68–69, 217–218,
        224–225
    health care and, 133
    healthy risks, 197–198
    sexuality and, 224–225
    sports and, 235
Risky Business Man personality, 265, 274
Risman, Barbara, 17, 269–270
Ritalin, 98, 103
Road Rage and Aggressive Driving (James and
    Nahl), 355–356
Robins, Arthur, 214
Robinson, Arthur, 36
Rock, Joyce and Calvin, 231–232
Rohrbaugh, Michael, 349–350, 351
role models
    parents as, 16–17, 68–69, 86, 122–123,
        144–145, 146–154, 191–193, 217–218,
        224–225, 255–256
    partners as, 282
Rollerblading, 238, 246, 253
Romance of Risk, The (Ponton), 184–185, 212,
    225–226
Rosemond, John, 122
Rosenbaum, Ernest H., 455
Rosenbaum, Isadora, 455
rough boys, 83–85
rubella immunizations, 63
Rubin, Richard, 435–437

Sabo, Don, 235, 239–242, 244
sadness, 68
Safe Passage (Dryfoos), 185
Salant, Robert, 473
salt in diet, 420, 421, 422–423

salt-wasting CAH, 54–55
Sargarese, Margaret, 219
Satcher, David, 140, 198–199, 211–212, 393–394,
    396–397
saturated fats, 298, 299, 302, 307, 407, 411
Savard, Marie, 329
Savard Health Record, The (Savard), 329
Savin-Williams, Richard, 233
saw palmetto, 475, 476, 480
Sawyer, Diane, 488
Sax, Leonard, 90–91
Schilling, Curt, 348–349
schizophrenia, 481
Schlussel, Richard, 170
Schmitt, Larry R., 114
schools, 89–107
    abstinence-only sex education, 211–213,
        223
    active boys in, 83
    aggression in, 84
    bullying and, 104–107
    discipline and, 91, 93
    fast food and, 145
    gay boys and, 233–234
    learning disabilities and, 94–98
    preparation for, 89–92, 106
    risky behavior and, 185–186
    rough boys and, 83–85
    single-sex education, 90–91
    smoking-cessation programs, 193
    sports in, 237
    violence in, 88, 105
Schover, Leslie R., 469
Schumacher, Heidi, 149–154
Schwartz, Pepper, 527, 531, 535–541
Schwebel, David, 112–113, 119–120
scooter injuries, 247
screening tests, 11, 324, 331–346
scrotum, 50–52
Seasons of a Man's Life, The (Levinson), 266
seat belt use, 187, 189
secondhand emotions, 498–499
secondhand smoke, 73, 350
second-impact syndrome, 249
second opinions, 456–457
selective mutism, 81–82
selenium, 320
Semans, James, 532
seminal vesicles, 22
sensate focus therapy, 536
sensory processing disorders, 97–98
Seven Principles for Making Marriage Work
    (Gottman), 272–273
Sex, Love and Health in America (Laumann), 44
Sex and the City (TV program), 527, 529

sex education
  abstinence-only programs, 211–213, 223
  by age, 214, 216–218
sex of baby
  "boy anxiety" of mothers, 3, 29–31
  factors determining, 21–23
  guessing, 27–29
  preferences for, 24–27
  selecting, 24–27
sexual abuse, 30, 125, 201
sexual arousal disorder, 542
sexual aversion disorder, 542
sexual desire disorder, 542
sexuality
  abstinence-education programs, 211–213, 223
  in adolescence, 210–234
  in adulthood, 523–544
  cancer and, 469
  condoms, 222–224
  of gay boys and men, 226–234
  hooking up, 224
  Internet health information and, 221–222
  masculinity and, 217–218, 224–225
  masturbation, 215, 218, 220–221, 222
  myths concerning, 523–526
  nudity around children, 216
  peer pressure and, 225–226
  physiology of male, 528–529
  post-heart attack, 384–385
  problems with female, 539–543
  problems with male, 526–539
  sex education by age, 214, 216–220
  sex play and, 215
  talking about, 210, 213–220
Sexuality and Fertility After Cancer (Schover), 469
sexually transmitted diseases (STDs), 211, 212, 223, 224, 234
  alcohol use and, 194
  balanitis and, 168
  circumcision and, 42–43
  epididymitis and, 171
  prostatitis and, 476
sexual orientation, 227–234
Shapiro, Pat, 232
Sheehy, Gail, 266
Shephard, Roy J., 288
Sher, Tamara, 18, 271
Shettles, Landrum B., 25
Shikany, James, 307, 311
short children, 154–157
shyness, 78–81, 85
sickle-cell anemia, 26
sigmoidoscopy, 341

Silverman, Doris, 67
Silverstein, Olga, 31
Singh, Narendra, 482
single mothers, 14
single-sex education, 90–91
Skakkabak, Niels, 69–70
skateboarding, 247
skin cancer, 334
Slap, Gail, 134
sleep apnea, 129–131, 365, 398, 516–518
sleep patterns, 516–519
  accidents and, 516, 518–519
  gender gap in, 11, 58–59
  infant, 38–39
  night terrors, 131
  sleep apnea and, 129–131, 365, 398, 516–518
  sleepwalking, 131
  snoring, 129–131, 365, 398, 516–518
sleep-wake cycle, 33
sleepwalking, 131
slipped capital femoral epiphysis, 251
Small, Eric, 136–137, 236, 238–242
Small, Gary, 10, 264
smegma, 47, 169
smiling, emotional development and, 67
Smith, Bernie, 273–274
smokeless tobacco, 193, 348–349
smoking
  during adolescence, 179, 186, 190–193
  in adulthood, 347–348
  during pregnancy, 27, 33, 38–39
  quitting, 193, 349–354
  risks of, 13, 74, 142, 318, 347–348
  secondhand smoke, 73, 350
  sports involvement and, 235
smoking-cessation programs, 193, 349–354
snow-shoveling, 369–370
Sobal, Jeffrey, 400, 402
soccer, 239, 240, 242–243, 247–248, 249, 253
social anxiety disorder (SAD), 81–82
social phobia, 81–82
social support
  cancer and, 16, 262–263, 457–458, 465, 467–469
  for caregiver role, 448–449, 465, 467
  importance of, 18
softball, 254
Sommers, Christina Hoff, 94
Sonenstein, Freya, 223, 225
Sonnett, Meredith, 199
sonograms, 27
Sothern, Melinda, 145, 146, 149–154
Sparrow, Joshua, 122–123
special education services, 93

Speck, Richard, 37
speech therapy, for stuttering, 129
sperm
    fertility problems and, 69, 319, 481–482
    in fertilization process, 21–23, 50
spermatic cord, 52
spermatocele, 174
sperm spinning, 25–26
spinal muscular atrophy, 26
Spock, Benjamin, 41
sports, 235–256
    by age, 236–239
    coaches and, 240, 241–242, 248
    equipment for, 243, 246, 253–254, 522
    exercise and, 150, 151–152
    injuries from, 242–253, 520–522
    nutrition for, 139
    parent role in, 241–242
    performance-enhancing substances and,
        162–164
    pressure in, 239–241
    sports physicals, 136–137, 159, 182, 252
sports drinks, 250
SRY (sex-determining region Y), 22–23
SSRIs (selective serotonin reuptake inhibitors),
    510
Stages of Change, 277–282
Stampfer, Meir, 317
standardized testing, 92
statins, 412–414
stature. see height
STDs. see sexually transmitted diseases (STDs)
Stein, Edward, 229
Stein, Ethel, 477
stents, 382
stereotypies, 62
steroids, anabolic, 137, 160, 162–163, 165, 176
Stock, Rich, 273
stoicism. see Boy Code
stomach ulcers, 415
stool toileting refusers, 126–127
Stop Handgun Violence, 115
street-crossing, 112–113
stress, 494–505
    of alcoholism in family, 441–442, 448–451
    anger and hostility in, 501–505
    of caregiver role, 17–18, 269–270, 272,
        391–392, 448–451, 458, 465–466
    gender gap in coping with, 495–497
    Generation Stress, 199–200
    of heart attack, 383
    job stress, 497–498
    measuring, 500–501
    secondhand emotions and, 498–499
    in sports participation, 239–241

testosterone levels and, 488
    warning signs of, 499
Stress Management for Dummies (Elkin), 504
stroke, 362–363, 380, 385–392
    in African Americans, 8
    alcohol use and, 314
    impact on family, 390–392
    risk factors for, 387–389, 426
    treatment of, 389–390
    warning signs of, 362, 385–387
stuttering, 127–129
Styron, William, 508
sudden infant death syndrome (SIDS), 1, 33,
        38–39, 73
suicide, 199, 363
    adolescence and, 179, 180, 203–205, 234
    body dysmorphic disorder (BDD) and,
        160–161
    bullying and, 105
    depression and, 509, 511
    sports involvement and, 235
    warning signs of, 204, 363
    young adulthood and, 266–267
    see also depression
sulfa drugs, 61
Supporter Cancer Care (Rosenbaum et al.), 455
surgery
    for breast enlargement, 175
    bypass, 17, 262, 382
    circumcision, 39–48, 53, 168
    for cleft palate, 38
    for clubfoot, 37
    for hernias, 173
    prostate, 306, 479–480, 534, 538
    reconstructive, 56–57
    sex-reassignment, 228
    for sleep apnea, 518
    for testicular cancer, 172
    for testicular torsion, 170
    for undescended testicles, 50–51
Svec, Carol, 455, 457
swimming accidents, 110–111
Syndrome X (metabolic syndrome), 439–440
systolic blood pressure, 417–418

tackling, in football, 244
tall children, 157–159
Tanner, James, 181
Tanner stages, 181
Taubman, Bruce, 127
Taylor, Shelley, 495
TB skin test, 333, 343
tea, 310
team sports. see sports
teenagers. see adolescence

television
    impact on children, 67
    lack of exercise and, 152–154
    media literacy, 153
    sexuality and, 210, 527, 529
    smoking and, 192
    violence and, 87
temperament, 75–88, 255
    active boys, 82–83
    gender gap, 77–88
    rough boys, 83–85
    shyness, 78–81
    social anxiety disorder (SAD), 81–82
Tempero, Margaret, 455
tennis, 240
termination stage of change, 282
testicles, 23
    cancer of, 50, 69, 70, 71, 137–138, 171–173,
        174–175, 182, 483
    emergencies of, 169–173
    of intersex babies, 54
    measurement of, 177
    problems with, 50–52, 69–71, 169–175, 178
    removal of, 57
    retractile, 50, 174, 178
    self-exam, 137–138
    undescended, 23, 50–51, 55, 69, 70, 172–175
testicular dysgenesis syndrome (TDS), 69
testicular torsion, 52, 170, 171
testes, 23, 55, 483, 487
testosterone
    anabolic steroids, 137, 160, 162–163, 165, 176
    in baldness, 547–548
    breast enlargement and, 175, 176–177, 483
    endocrine disrupters and, 69–71
    in male fetus and infant, 12, 23, 28, 32–33, 53,
        59, 230, 487
    male menopause and, 489–493, 528
    for micropenis, 49
    obesity/overweight and, 397
    osteoporosis and, 485
    shifts in levels of, 486–493
    for short stature, 156
tetanus booster, 333, 345
Theodosakis, Jason, 325
Therapeutic Lifestyle Changes (TLC), 409–412,
    413
Things the Family Should Avoid (Brownell), 403
Thomas, Alexander, 75–76
Thompson, Michael, 68, 83, 91, 200–202, 221, 222
Thompson, Tommy, 194
throat cancer, 348
thyroid function, 176–177
tic disorders, 63–64
Tiefer, Leonore, 541

tissue plasminogen activators (tPAs), 386
toilet training, 121–123, 126
Toohey, Barbara, 436
tooth and gum care, 333, 344, 372–373
Torre, Ali, 16, 262–263
Torre, Joe, 16, 262–263
total cholesterol, 336, 407–408
Tourette's syndrome, 33–34, 63–64, 104–106
toys
    guns, 117–118
    phthalates in, 71
    see also play
traffic accidents, 112–113
Trager, Jonathan, 134–136
trans fats, 299, 307, 411
transgender, 228
transient ischemic attack (TIA), 362, 387, 388
transillumination, 51
transsexuals, 228–229
Tremblay, Richard, 83, 85
triglycerides, 299, 336, 439–440
Trim Kids (Sothern et al.), 149–154
Tronick, Edward Z., 65
Tseng, David, 232, 233–234
Tunnel Visionary personality, 264–265
Turner, Samuel, 82
type A personality, 502
type 1 diabetes, 141, 337, 426. see also diabetes
type 2 diabetes, 141, 277, 337, 425, 426, 427. see
    also diabetes

Udesky, Laurie, 506–507
Ultimate Sports Nation (Steen), 139
ultrasound, 28
umbilical hernias, 52
Understanding Men's Passages (Sheehy), 266
Understanding Your Child's Temperament (Carey),
    77, 80
undescended testicles (cryptorchidism), 23, 50–51,
    55, 69, 70, 172–175
U.S. Department of Agriculture, 73, 74, 300, 302,
    309
U.S. Department of Education, 90, 92, 93, 94
U.S. Department of Health and Human Services
    Office of Men's Health (proposed), 18
    Office of Women's Health, 18
U.S. Department of Labor, 15, 208
U.S. Food and Drug Administration (FDA), 26,
    70, 74, 81–82, 156–157, 163, 316, 319
unsaturated fats, 298
Uprima (apomorphine), 539
urethra, 23, 53, 472
urethral stricture, 475
urinalysis, 333, 343
urinary retention, 477

urinary tract infections (UTIs), 42, 125, 170–171
Us Too!, 467
uterus, 22

vaccines and vaccination, 63, 333, 345–346
Vargas, Deborah, 206–207
varicocele, 174, 481
vas deferens, 22
vasodilators, 381
vasopressin, 124, 126
venting anger, 386, 503–504
ventricular fibrillation, 373
Vermillion, Jack, 105–106
Viagra, 385, 510, 529–530, 534, 537, 538–539,
542
victims
    of bullying, 104–106
    of violence, 87
violence
    adolescence and, 180, 186, 199
    bullying, 104–107
    guns and, 86, 105, 110, 115–118, 179, 186
    healthy risks and, 197–198
    preventing, 85–87, 105
    rough boys, 83–85
    school shootings, 105
    warning signs of, 88
    young adulthood and, 266–267
vision tests, 333, 344
vitamins and minerals, 38, 302, 315–320, 486
voice changes, 181
volleyball, 242
Von Alman, Kristian, 149–154
Von Roenn, Jamie, 458
vulva, 56

Waite, Linda J., 15–16, 271
Wakefield, Andrew, 63
walking, 293
Wallace, Janet, 285–286
Wallace, Mike, 507–508
Walter, Paul, 214
War Against Boys, The (Sommers), 94
warfarin, 389
warm baths, 480
water accidents, 110–111
water pollution, 72–74
Waters, Maury, 328
Waters, Rob, 5–6, 21, 66–67, 104, 156, 239, 294,
328
weapons. see guns

Weight Watchers, 15
Weinberg, Clarice, 25
Weinberg, M. Katherine, 65, 67
Well Spouse, 467
Wernick, Sarah, 470
Wessex Growth Study, 155
Westheimer, Ruth, 214
Westmoreland, William, 507, 508
wet dreams, 219, 220–221
What's the Big Secret? (Krasny and Brown), 214
When a Parent Has Cancer (Harpham), 468–469
When Life Becomes Precious (NeeDell), 455
Where Did I Come From? (Mayle et al.), 214
white-coat hypertension, 419
Whites. see Caucasians
Who Am I? Where Did I Come From?
    (Westheimer), 214
wilderness therapy, 205–207
Willett, Walter, 296, 300, 302, 303, 305–306, 317,
320
Williams, Janice, 502
Williams, Redford, 505
Wing, Rena, 403
Wiswell, Tom, 42
Witte, Hazel A., 325–326
Women's Health Initiative (WHI), 306–307
work. see employment

X chromosomes
    disorders linked to, 24, 34–39
    in fetal development, 21–23, 26
    in selecting sex of baby, 24–27
XXY males, 36
XYY males, 36–37

Y chromosomes
    in fetal development, 21–23, 26
    in selecting sex of baby, 24–27
York, Merle James, 175
young adulthood stage
    drug and alcohol use during, 266–267
    mortality rates in, 1
    nature of, 266–267
    suicide and, 266–267
    violence in, 266–267
Your Adolescent, 231
Youth Risk Behavior Survey (YRBS), 179–180,
    185, 190

Zilbergeld, Bernie, 531–532, 536
Zyban (bupropion), 353–354

Symptoms Index

abusive behavior
    in depression, 509, 513
academic performance problems
    in depression, 202
    in suicidal behavior, 204
accident proneness
    with stress, 499
    see also clumsiness
acne
    with male hormone therapy, 492
    with steroid use, 163, 165
    in XYY males, 36–37
adenoid enlargement
    in sleep apnea, 130–131
adrenal gland enlargement
    in congenital adrenal hyperplasia (CAH), 54–55
aggression
    with depression, 202, 509, 513
    with male hormone therapy, 492
    in rough boys, 85
    with steroid use, 163
alcohol use
    with depression, 202, 506, 509
    in eating disorders, 161
    with stress, 499
    in suicidal behavior, 204, 363
allergies
    in autism, 63
amnesia. *see* memory problems/amnesia
anger, 501–505
    in depression, 509
anxiety
    in depression, 509
    in eating disorders, 161
    in encopresis, 126
    in heart attack, 360
    in hypoglycemia, 433
    in sleep apnea, 517
    with stress, 499
appetite loss
    in colorectal cancer, 366
    in depression, 509
    with stress, 499
    in suicidal behavior, 204, 363
    see also weight loss
arthritis
    with obesity/overweight, 397

attention problems, 88, 92
    in AD/HD, 64, 98–102
    in concussion, 248
    in depression, 202, 509
    in fragile X syndrome, 35
    in male menopause, 490
    in reading disabilities, 97
    in sleep apnea, 129–130, 517
    with stress, 499

back pain
    in heart attack, 2, 3, 360
    in lung cancer, 365
    with obesity/overweight, 397
    in osteoporosis, 485
    in prostate cancer, 366
    in prostatitis, 474
    with stress, 499
balance problems
    in strokes, 362
    see also clumsiness
bedwetting, 59
    in diabetes, 125
    from early toilet training, 122
    from emotional trauma, 125
    in sexual abuse, 125
    in sleep apnea, 130
    in urinary tract infections, 125
behavioral problems, 92
    in autism, 62
    in fragile X syndrome, 35
    in lead poisoning, 72
    in suicidal behavior, 363
    in very short children, 154–155
binge eating
    in eating disorders, 161
bizarre thoughts
    in psychosis, 204
blackouts
    in alcoholism, 442, 443
bleeding, 359
    in hemophilia, 35
blood clots
    circumcision and, 48
    in embolisms, 5
blurred vision
    in diabetes, 426

blurred vision (*cont.*)
    in heart attack, 11
    in high blood pressure, 364
    in testicular cancer, 172
body image problems
    in Adonis Complex, 160–161, 165–166
    in eating disorders, 159–161
    see also self-esteem problems
bowel problems, 59
    in colorectal cancer, 366
    in encopresis, 126–127
    with stress, 499
brain damage
    in concussion, 248
brain swelling
    in concussion, 249
breast enlargement, 175–177
    in Klinefelter's syndrome, 176, 483
    in obesity/overweight, 176
    with steroid use, 163, 175–176, 483
    in XXY males, 36
breathing problems, 358
    in congestive heart failure, 385
    in glucose-6-phosphate-dehydrogenase
      (G6PD), 61
    in heart attack, 2, 11, 360, 374
    in lung cancer, 365
    in obesity/overweight, 130, 140, 397
    in sleep apnea, 129–131, 365
broken bones
    in osteoporosis, 485
bronchitis
    in lung cancer, 365

carpal tunnel syndrome
    with obesity/overweight, 397
cataracts
    with obesity/overweight, 397
change resistance
    in autism, 62
    in shyness, 79
chest indentation/protrusion
    in Marfan syndrome, 159
chest pain, 358
    with ephedra use, 164
    in heart abnormality, 136–137
    in heart attack, 2, 11, 360
    in lung cancer, 365
chills
    in prostatitis, 474
clingy behavior
    in shyness, 80
clumsiness
    in dyspraxia, 97, 131–132
    in heatstroke, 250

    in reading disabilities, 97
    with stress, 499
    in strokes, 362
cold sweat
    in heart attack, 360
coma
    in diabetes, 426
    in heart attack, 374
    in lead poisoning, 72
    in strokes, 362
confusion, 358
    in diabetes, 427
    in heatstroke, 250
    in hypoglycemia, 433
    with stress, 499
    in strokes, 362
connective tissue problems
    in Marfan syndrome, 158–159
consciousness, loss of
    in concussion, 248
    in heart attack, 374
    in stroke, 386
constipation
    in colorectal cancer, 366
    from early toilet training, 122
    from encopresis, 127
    with stress, 499
contact avoidance
    in autism, 62
convulsions
    in strokes, 362
coordination problems
    in strokes, 362
coughing up blood, 359
    in lung cancer, 365
    in testicular cancer, 172
cramping
    in colorectal cancer, 366
    with creatine use, 163–164
    in heatstroke, 250
cysts
    epididymal, 71
    in scrotum, 174

dehydration
    with creatine use, 163–164
    in gastroenteritis, 60
    in heatstroke, 206, 249–250
depression, 367
    in alcoholism, 442
    from bullying, 105
    of caregivers, 17, 376
    in eating disorders, 161
    in male menopause, 489, 490
    from physical abuse, 200, 201

post-heart attack, 377–378, 383–384
    from sexual abuse, 201
    in sleep apnea, 517
    with stress, 499
diarrhea
    in colorectal cancer, 366
    in gastroenteritis, 60
    with stress, 499
disorientation
    in stroke, 386
distractibility
    in AD/HD, 99–100
dizziness, 358
    in concussion, 248
    in dehydration, 60
    in heart attack, 360
    in hypoglycemia, 433
    with stress, 499
    in strokes, 362
drawing problems
    in dyspraxia, 131–132
drooping eyes
    in stroke, 386
drug use
    with depression, 202, 509
    in eating disorders, 161
    with stress, 499
    in suicidal behavior, 204, 363
dry lips and mouth
    in dehydration, 60
    in stress, 499
dry skin
    in diabetes, 364, 426

ear enlargement
    in fragile X syndrome, 35
ear infections, 33–34
    in cleft lip and cleft palate, 38
    from environmental toxins, 73
eating habits. see appetite loss; hunger
emotional trauma
    from dog bites, 114–115
    of heart attack, 383
empty feelings
    in depression, 509
erectile dysfunction
    in cancer, 469, 530, 534
    with depression, 510
    in diabetes, 435, 530
    in male menopause, 490
    prostate surgery and, 339, 534
    in prostatitis, 476
    in sleep apnea, 517
    smoking and, 350, 530
eye-contact problems

in autism, 62
    in overarousal and overstimulation,
        67
    in shyness, 78
eye problems. see vision problems

facial-hair sparseness
    in XXY males, 36
fainting, 358
    in heart abnormality, 136–137
    in strokes, 362
fatigue
    in cancer, 469
    in colorectal cancer, 366
    in congestive heart failure, 385
    in depression, 509
    in diabetes, 364, 426
    with diuretic use, 164
    in glucose-6-phosphate-dehydrogenase
        (G6PD), 61
    in heart attack, 10, 360
    in male menopause, 490
    in prostatitis, 474
    in sleep apnea, 365
    with stress, 499
fear, lack of
    in autism, 62
fertility problems
    in androgen insensitivity syndrome (AIS),
        55
    from environmental toxins, 69–74
    with male hormone therapy, 492
    from testicular injury, 171
    with varicocele, 174, 481
    in XXY males, 36
    see also erectile dysfunction
fever
    in cancer, 365, 452
    circumcision and, 48
    in gastroenteritis, 60
    in prostatitis, 474
flat feet
    in Marfan syndrome, 159
flulike symptoms
    in prostatitis, 474
food sensitivities
    in autism, 63
foot problems
    in club foot, 37
    in gout, 397
    in Marfan syndrome, 159
foreskin ballooning, 169
foreskin infections, 40, 43–44
foreskin swelling and pain
    in paraphimosis, 168

fussiness
    in hernias, 51–52
    in hydroceles, 51–52
    in testicular torsion, 52

gallstones
    with obesity/overweight, 397
gas pains
    in colorectal cancer, 366
genital sores
    in sexually transmitted diseases (STDs), 42–43
giggling inappropriately
    in autism, 62
growth delays
    from hormone deficiencies, 156–157
    in sleep apnea, 130
gum disease
    with diabetes, 426
    with obesity/overweight, 397
    from smokeless tobacco, 193

hair growth
    with male hormone therapy, 492
hair sparseness/loss
    with steroid use, 163
    in XXY males, 36
hallucinations
    in heatstroke, 206
    in psychosis, 204
handedness problems
    in reading disabilities, 97
handwriting problems
    in dyspraxia, 131–132
headache, 367
    in concussion, 248
    in depression, 509
    in heart attack, 10
    in high blood pressure, 364
    in sleep apnea, 129–131, 365, 517
    with stress, 499
    in strokes, 362, 386, 387–388
    in testicular cancer, 172
head trauma
    in precocious puberty, 157–158
hearing loss
    in cleft lip and cleft palate, 38
heartburn
    in esophageal cancer, 367
heart disease
    with diabetes, 142
    with obesity/overweight, 142
hernias
    with obesity/overweight, 397
high blood pressure
    with alcohol use, 314, 442

with ephedra use, 164
    with obesity/overweight, 143
    in sleep apnea, 130, 517
    with steroid use, 163
    in Syndrome X, 439–440
    from urinary tract infections (UTIs), 42
high cholesterol
    with obesity/overweight, 143, 397
    with steroid use, 163
    in Syndrome X, 439–440
hip pain
    from osteoporosis, 484–485
    in slipped capital femoral epiphysis, 251
hoarseness
    in lung cancer, 365
hopelessness
    in depression, 509
hunger
    in diabetes, 364, 426
    in hypoglycemia, 433
    with stress, 499
    in suicidal behavior, 204, 363
    see also weight gain

immune system problems
    from diabetes, 426
    from environmental toxins, 73
    marriage problems and, 272–273
impotence. see erectile dysfunction
impulsivity, 93
    in AD/HD, 99–100
    with stress, 499
incontinence
    prostate surgery and, 339
indigestion
    with stress, 499
infections, increase in
    in diabetes, 364, 426
insulin resistance
    in Syndrome X, 439–440
IQ reduction
    in lead poisoning, 72
    see also learning problems
irritability
    in depression, 509, 513
    in male menopause, 489, 490
    in sleep apnea, 517
    with stress, 499

joint and ligament looseness
    in Marfan syndrome, 159

kidney disease
    with diabetes, 142, 338, 426
    in urinary tract infections (UTIs), 42

knee swelling/tenderness
  in Osgood-Schlatter disease, 251–252

language problems
  see also speech delay
laughing inappropriately
  in autism, 62
  in stress, 499
learning problems
  in dyspraxia, 131–132
  in lead poisoning, 72
  in sleep apnea, 517
leg pain
  in diabetes, 435
  in embolisms, 5
leg swelling
  in congestive heart failure, 385
lesions
  in sexually transmitted diseases (STDs),
    42–43
lightheadedness
  in heart attack, 360
  in hypoglycemia, 433
limb pain
  in stroke, 386
lip bleeding
  from smokeless tobacco, 193
lip malformation
  in cleft lip and cleft palate, 38
listlessness
  in active boys, 83
  in pyloric stenosis, 61
liver damage
  with alcohol use, 314, 442
  with nonalcoholic steatohepatitis (NASH),
    398
long limbs
  in Marfan syndrome, 159
loss of limbs
  with diabetes, 142

memory problems/amnesia
  in AD/HD, 99
  in alcoholism, 442
  in concussion, 248
  in depression, 509
  in heart attack, 374
  in male menopause, 490
  in sleep apnea, 129–130, 517
mental retardation
  in fragile X syndrome, 35
mood swings, 367
  in depression, 202
  with male hormone therapy, 492
  in male menopause, 490

with steroid use, 163, 165
  with stress, 499
  in suicidal behavior, 363
motor skills problems
  in autism, 62
  in dyspraxia, 131–132
  see also clumsiness
motor tics
  in Tourette's syndrome, 63–64,
    104–105
mouth malformation
  in cleft lip and cleft palate, 38
mouth sores
  from smokeless tobacco, 193
muscle aches
  in prostatitis, 474
muscle loss
  in male menopause, 490
muscle spasms
  in heatstroke, 250
muscle strains
  with creatine use, 163–164

nausea
  in cancer, 469
  in gastroenteritis, 60
  in heart attack, 360
  of mother during pregnancy, 28
  in prostatitis, 474
  with stress, 499
  in strokes, 362
nearsightedness
  in Marfan syndrome, 159
neck pain
  in heart attack, 262, 360
  with stress, 499
numbness of body part
  from bike riding, 482
  in diabetes, 364
  in strokes, 362

orgasm pain
  in prostatitis, 474
orthopedic problems
  in clubfoot, 37
  from sports injuries, 243–246, 251–252,
    520–522
overactivity, 33–34, 82–83, 92
  in active boys, 83
  in AD/HD, 98–100
  in autism, 62
  in sleep apnea, 129–130
  with stress, 499
overworking
  with depression, 202

pain sensitivity
in autism, 62
pale skin/eyes
in glucose-6-phosphate-dehydrogenase
(G6PD), 61
pancreatitis
with alcohol use, 314
passivity
in autism, 62
pelvic pain
in prostate cancer, 366
penile bleeding
circumcision and, 46, 48
penile discharge
circumcision and, 48
penile infections
in balanitis, 167, 168
circumcision and, 40, 43–44, 47
penile numbness
from bike riding, 482
penile pain
circumcision and, 45
penile shrinkage
in male menopause, 490
personal neglect
in suicidal behavior, 204, 363
playing problems
in AD/HD, 100
in autism, 62
pneumonia
in lung cancer, 365
psychosis
with male hormone therapy, 492
in suicidal behavior, 204

rapid heart rate
with ephedra use, 164
in glucose-6-phosphate-dehydrogenase
(G6PD), 61
in high reactors, 59, 66, 79
rectal pain
in hemorrhoids, 367
in prostatitis, 474
repetitive speech
in autism, 62
respiratory infections
from environmental toxins, 73
respiratory problems, 59
ritualistic behaviors
in autism, 62
run-down feeling
in heart attack, 10

scrotum discoloration, 169
in blue balls, 178

scrotum fluid
in testicular cancer, 138
scrotum pain
in epididymitis, 170–171
with mumps, 170
in prostatitis, 473
seizures
in epilepsy, 65
in lead poisoning, 72
self-esteem problems
in Adonis Complex, 160–161, 165–166
in depression, 202
in eating disorders, 159–161
in male menopause, 490
of nonathletes, 236
sex drive/response problems
blue balls and, 178
circumcision and, 44
in male menopause, 490
see also erectile dysfunction
shame
from bedwetting, 124, 125
from breast enlargement, 176
with depression, 513–514
in obesity/overweight, 144
shortness of breath, 358
in congestive heart failure, 385
in glucose-6-phosphate-dehydrogenase
(G6PD), 61
in heart attack, 2, 11, 360
in lung cancer, 365
short stature
from hormone deficiencies, 156–157
in late bloomers, 156
shoulder pain
in heart attack, 262, 360
sleepiness, 358
in hypoglycemia, 433
in sleep apnea, 517
sleep problems
in depression, 202, 509
infant, 33
in male menopause, 490
in obesity/overweight, 130, 398, 516–517,
518
with stress, 499
in suicidal behavior, 204, 363
smoking increase
with stress, 499
snoring
in sleep apnea, 129–131, 365, 516–518
social skills problems
in autism, 62, 63
social withdrawal
in alcoholism, 442, 444

in autism, 62, 63
in depression, 202, 513
in shyness, 80
in suicidal behavior, 204, 363
sores not healing
in diabetes, 364, 426, 427
speech delay, 93
in autism, 62
in reading disabilities, 96
in XXY males, 36
speech disturbances
in fragile X syndrome, 35
in hypoglycemia, 433
in social anxiety disorder, 81
stuttering, 127–129
spinal curvature
in Marfan syndrome, 159
in osteoporosis, 485
stomach pain, 358
in colorectal cancer, 366
in gastroenteritis, 60
in heart attack, 10, 360
in Hirschsprung's disease, 61
with stress, 499
in testicular torsion, 52, 170
stuttering, 33–34, 127–129
sunken eyes
in dehydration, 60
swearing
in Tourette's syndrome, 63–64
sweating
in hypoglycemia, 433
in social anxiety disorder (SAD), 81

tall stature
in Marfan syndrome, 158–159
in precocious puberty, 157–158
in XYY males, 36–37
tarry stools
in colorectal cancer, 366
teeth grinding
with stress, 499
testicle enlargement
in fragile X syndrome, 35
testicle shrinkage
with male hormone therapy, 492
in male menopause, 490
with steroid use, 163
in XXY males, 36
testicle swelling/tenderness, 169
at birth, 48–49
in epididymitis, 171
in hernias, 51–52
in hydroceles, 51–52
in testicular cancer, 138, 172

in testicular torsion, 52, 170, 171
with varicocele, 174
thigh pain
in prostate cancer, 366
thirst
in diabetes, 364
tics
with stress, 499
in Tourette's syndrome, 63–64, 104–105
tingling of body part
from bike riding, 482
in diabetes, 364
tonsil enlargement
in sleep apnea, 130–131
tremors
in social anxiety disorder (SAD), 81

urination frequency
in diabetes, 364, 426
with diuretic use, 164
with enlarged prostate, 477, 478
in prostate cancer, 366
in prostatitis, 474
with stress, 499
urination problems
circumcision and, 46, 47, 48
with enlarged prostate, 477, 478
in hypospadias, 52–53
lack of circumcision and, 169
in prostate cancer, 366
in prostatitis, 473, 474
urine darkness
in dehydration, 60
in glucose-6-phosphate-dehydrogenase
(G6PD), 61

violent behavior
in depression, 202, 509, 513
in rough boys, 85
with steroid use, 163
in suicidal behavior, 204
in XXY males, 37
vision problems, 358
with diabetes, 142, 338, 426
in heart attack, 11
in high blood pressure, 364
in Marfan syndrome, 159
in strokes, 362
in testicular cancer, 172
see also blurred vision
vocal tics
in Tourette's syndrome, 63–64, 104–105
vomiting
with creatine use, 163–164
in eating disorders, 161

vomiting (*cont.*)
  in gastroenteritis, 60
  in Hirschsprung's disease, 61
  in hydroceles, 51–52
  of mother during pregnancy, 28
  in prostatitis, 474
  in pyloric stenosis, 61
  in social anxiety disorder (SAD), 81
  in strokes, 362
  in testicular torsion, 52, 170
vomiting blood, 359

weakness, muscle
  in colorectal cancer, 366
  in heart attack, 360
  in hypoglycemia, 433
  in male menopause, 490
  in muscular dystrophy, 34–35
  with stress, 499
weight gain
  in Adonis Complex, 165

in depression, 202, 509
in male menopause, 489
see also hunger
weight loss
  in Adonis Complex, 165
  in colorectal cancer, 366
  in depression, 202, 509
  in diabetes, 364, 426
  with diuretic use, 164
  in lung cancer, 365
  in pyloric stenosis, 61
  see also appetite loss
wheezing
  in congestive heart failure, 385
  in lung cancer, 365
worrying
  in obsessive-compulsive disorder, 64

yellow skin/eyes
  in glucose-6-phosphate-dehydrogenase
    (G6PD), 61

ABOUT THE AUTHORS

EMILY SENAY, M.D., is a medical correspondent for CBS News *The Early Show* and *CBS News Sunday Morning*. She graduated from the University of Chicago with a degree in biology and from Mt. Sinai School of Medicine in New York City. She worked as a physician at clinics in the New York City area, making house calls to homebound patients on the Lower East Side; on the Floating Hospital, caring for homeless and battered women and children; and on Rikers Island, one of the largest municipal jails in the world. She also cared for hospitalized patients at Beth Israel Medical Center and at Doctors Hospital in Manhattan.

She began her career in journalism as a writer and producer of physician education programs at Lifetime Medical Television and later anchored Medical News Network. She shifted her focus to lay journalism, beginning at CBS News in 1995. In 2002, she received the Society for Women's Health Research Excellence in Women's Health Research Journalism Award. Dr. Senay is also currently a resident in the Mount Sinai General Preventive Medicine Residency Program in New York City. She lives in New York City with her husband, son, and twin daughters.

ROB WATERS is a former staff writer for *Health* magazine and a former senior editor for *Web*MD, where he edited the men's health section. He is a contributing editor to the *Psychotherapy Networker* magazine and has written for many other publications, including *Reader's Digest, Parenting, FamilyCircle*, and the *Los Angeles Times*. In 2001, he was a fellow with the University of Maryland's Journalism Fellowships in Child and Family Policy. He lives and works as a health and mental health writer and editor in Berkeley, California.